Donald School ***Textbook of***

PowerPoint Presentation on

Advanced Ultrasound in

OBSTETRICS & GYNECOLOGY

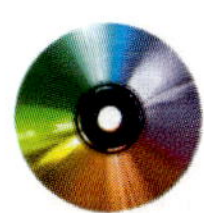

System requirement:

- Operating System - Windows Vista or above
- Web Browser – Internet Explorer 8 or above, Google Chrome & Mozilla Firefox
- Essential plugins – Java & PDF Reader
  - Facing problems in viewing content – it may be your system does not have java enabled.
  - You can test java and download PDF reader by using the links from the help section of the CD/DVD.

Accompanying CD/DVD Rom is playable only in Computer and not in DVD player.

CD/DVD has Autorun function – it may take few seconds to load on your computer. If it does not works for you then follow the steps below to access the contents manually:

- Click on my computer
- Select the CD/DVD drive and click open/explore – this will show list of files in the CD/DVD
- Find and double click file – "launch.html"

For more information about troubleshoot of Autorun click on:

http://support.microsoft.com/kb/330135

Donald School ***Textbook of PowerPoint Presentation on Advanced Ultrasound in*** OBSTETRICS & GYNECOLOGY

Tuangsit Wataganara MD
Associate Professor
Division of Maternal Fetal Medicine
Department of Obstetrics and Gynecology
Faculty of Medicine, Siriraj Hospital, Thailand

Ritsuko Kimata Pooh MD PhD
President
CRIFM Clinical Research Institute of
Fetal Medicine PMC, Osaka, Japan

Asim Kurjak MD PhD
Professor of Obstetrics and Gynecology
Medical School Universities of Zagreb and Sarajevo
Croatia

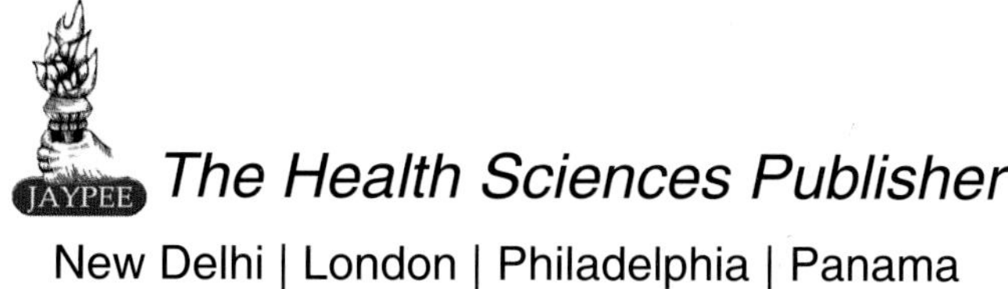

New Delhi | London | Philadelphia | Panama

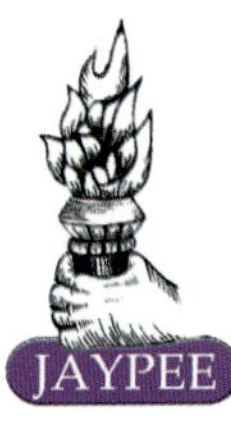

Jaypee Brothers Medical Publishers (P) Ltd

Headquarters

Jaypee Brothers Medical Publishers (P) Ltd
4838/24, Ansari Road, Daryaganj
New Delhi 110 002, India
Phone: +91-11-43574357
Fax: +91-11-43574314
Email: jaypee@jaypeebrothers.com

Overseas Offices

J.P. Medical Ltd
83 Victoria Street, London
SW1H 0HW (UK)
Phone: +44 20 3170 8910
Fax: +44 (0)20 3008 6180
Email: info@jpmedpub.com

Jaypee-Highlights Medical Publishers Inc.
City of Knowledge, Bld. 237, Clayton
Panama City, Panama
Phone: +1 507-301-0496
Fax: +1 507-301-0499
Email: cservice@jphmedical.com

Jaypee Medical Inc.
The Bourse
111 South Independence Mall East
Suite 835, Philadelphia, PA 19106, USA
Phone: +1 267-519-9789
Email: jpmed.us@gmail.com

Jaypee Brothers Medical Publishers (P) Ltd
17/1-B Babar Road, Block-B, Shaymali
Mohammadpur, Dhaka-1207
Bangladesh
Mobile: +08801912003485
Email: jaypeedhaka@gmail.com

Jaypee Brothers Medical Publishers (P) Ltd
Bhotahity, Kathmandu, Nepal
Phone: +977-9741283608
Email: kathmandu@jaypeebrothers.com

Website: www.jaypeebrothers.com
Website: www.jaypeedigital.com

Inquiries for bulk sales may be solicited at: jaypee@jaypeebrothers.com

Donald School Textbook of PowerPoint Presentation on Advanced Ultrasound in Obstetrics & Gynecology

First Edition: **2016**

ISBN: 978-93-5152-920-0

Printed at: Ajanta Offset & Packagings Ltd., New Delhi

Contributors

Aliyu Labaran Dayyabu MBBS MSc FWACS
Senior Lecturer
Head of Perinatal Medicine Unit, Obstetrics and Gynecology Department, Abubakar Tafawa Balewa University Teaching Hospital, Bauchi, Nigeria

Aris Antsaklis MD PhD FRCOG (Hon)
Professor, Department of Obstetrics and Gynecology
University of Athens, Greece

Ashok Khurana MBBS MD (Radiodiagnosis)
Chairman, The Ultrasound Lab, C 584,
Defence Colony, New Delhi, India

Asim Kurjak MD PhD
Professor of Obstetrics and Gynecology
Medical School Universities of Zagreb and Sarajevo
Croatia

Azen Salim MD MSc
Consultant Gulardi Center
Indonesian Society of Maternal Fetal Medicine
Jakarta, Indonesia

Badreldeen Ahmed MBCHB MD MFFP FRCOG CCST
Professor, Hamad Medical Corporation
Department of Obstetrics and Gynecology
Doha, Qatar

CB Nagori MD DGO
Director, Dr. Nagori's Institute for Infertility and IVF
Ahmedabad, India

Carmina Comas MD PhD
Director, Research and Development, Fetal Medicine Unit
Department of Obstetrics and Gynecology
Hospital Universitari Quirón Dexeus
Barcelona, Spain

Cihat Sen MD
Professor and Chairman
Department of Perinatal Medicine
Cerrahpasa Medical School
Istanbul University, Turkey

Corazon Yabes-Almirante MD MSc PhD
Center Chief, Perinatal-Neonatology-Pediatric Gynecology Center, Philippine Children's Medical Center, Philippines

Dominic Iliescu MD
Assistant Professor, Prenatal Diagnostic Unit
Department of Obstetrics and Gynecology
University of Medicine and Pharmacy
Craiova, Romania

Eleni Anastasiou
Consultant, Department of Endocrinology, "Alexandra" Maternity Hospital
University of Athens, Athens, Greece

Frank A Chervenak MD
Professor and Chairman
Department of Obstetrics and Gynecology
Weill Medical College of Cornell University
Obstetrician and Gynecologist-in-Chief
New York Presbyterian Hospital
New York, USA

Giovanni Monni MD
Head, Department of Obstetrics and Gynecology
Microcitemico Hospital, Cagliari, Italy

Giuseppe Cali MD MSc
Head, Maternal-Fetal Medicine Unit
AORNAS Civico, Palermo, Italy

Guillermo Azumendi MD PhD
Head, Clinica Gutenberg, Malaga, Spain

Gwang Jun Kim MD PhD
Professor and Chairman, Department of Obstetrics and Gynecology, Chung-Ang University Hospital
Seoul, South Korea

Ivica Zalud MD PhD
Professor and Chairman
Department of Obstetrics and Gynecology, and Women's Health, John A Burns School of Medicine, University of Hawaii, Honolulu, USA

Jaideep Malholtra MD FICOG
Director, Rainbow-IVF-ART Ltd.
Malholtra Nursing & Maternity Home, India

Kazuo Maeda MD PhD
Honorary Professor, Department of Obstetrics and Gynecology, Tottori University Medical School, Japan

Lara Spalldi Barišic MD
Assistant Professor
Dubrovnik International University, Croatia

Mandy Abushama FRCOG DFFP Dobs MSc
Consultant
The Feto Maternal Medical Center
Doha, Qatar

Milan Stanojevic MD PhD
Professor, Department of Obstetrics and Gynecology
Neonatal Unit
Medical School University of Zagreb, Croatia

Mónica Echevarria MD
Consultant, Fetal Medicine Unit
Department of Obstetrics and Gynecology
Hospital Universitari Quirón Dexeus, Barcelona, Spain

Narendra Malhotra MD FICOG FRCOG
Director, Global Rainbow Healthcare
Malholtra Nursing and Maternity Home Ltd., India
New York Weill Cornell Medical Center, USA

Panos Antsaklis
Consultant
First Department of Obstetrics and Gynecology
Alexandra Maternity Hospital
University of Athens, Athens, Greece

Radu Vladareanu MD PhD
Professor and Chairman
Department of Obstetrics and Gynecology
Carol Davila University of Medicine
Elias University Hospital
Bucharest, Romania

Ritsuko Kimata Pooh MD PhD
President
CRIFM Clinical Research Institute of
Fetal Medicine PMC, Osaka, Japan

Simona Vladareanu MD PhD
Associate Professor
Carol Davila University of Medicine
Elias University Hospital, Bucharest, Romania

Sonal Panchal MD
Consultant
Dr Nagori's Institute for Infertility and IVF
Ahmedabad, India

Tamara Illescas MD
Consultant
Delta Ultrasound Diagnostic Center in Obstetrics and Gynecology
Madrid, Spain

Tuangsit Wataganara MD
Associate Professor
Division of Maternal Fetal Medicine
Department of Obstetrics and Gynecology
Faculty of Medicine, Siriraj Hospital, Thailand

Vincenzo D'Addario MD
Associate Professor
Department of Obstetrics and Gynecology
Medical School, University of Bari, Italy

Vlad Zamfirescu MD
Assistant Professor
Carol Davila University of Medicine
Elias University Hospital, Bucharest, Romania

Preface

Donald School Textbook of PowerPoint Presentation on Advanced Ultrasound in Obstetrics and Gynecology is essentially a combination between an Atlas and a Textbook. Currently, there are a number of Atlases and Textbooks on Ultrasound in Obstetrics and Gynecology in the market. In order to facilitate the learning process of the readers, we chose PowerPoint Presentation platform to present the latest advancement of ultrasound application in Obstetrics and Gynecology. This project is a novel textbook concept that applies PowerPoint Presentation to demonstrate key learning points that are essential to the readers. Each chapter was assigned to one of our 34 corresponding authors according to their specialty. The learning objectives for each chapter were set, and the authors are responsible to crystalize the content into only a few sentences on each PowerPoint slide. The corresponding authors are responsible for the originality of their materials. Intellectual proprietary is being protected by obtaining permission from the responsible parties whenever the material that does not belong to the authors is used.

In order to comply with an obligation of standard textbook, all the data shown in each chapter are properly quoted. The list of literature reference is provided at the end of each chapter. Our 42 chapters cover all the essential basic knowledge, as well as the recent developments in the field of Ultrasound in Obstetrics and Gynecology. PowerPoint Presentation is an important teaching tool, and teaching is the core of Ian Donald Inter-University School of Ultrasound in Medicine. The primary objective of this project is to enhance the learning experience of our readers through the strength of PowerPoint Presentation, yet the skill for preparing a teaching slide set can also be appreciated from this textbook.

This textbook project is one of a kind. The editorial work itself took us one and a half years. We enjoyed witnessing the transformation of PowerPoint Presentation into the real textbook. We hope that the readers will equally enjoy this learning experience, and be inspired by not only the learning, but the teaching as well.

Tuangsit Wataganara
Ritsuko Kimata Pooh
Asim Kurjak

Contents

Chapter

1

Sonoembryology

Ritsuko Kimata Pooh

3D ULTRASOUND IN EARLY PREGNANCY

Transvaginal Approach Yields Better Image Quality

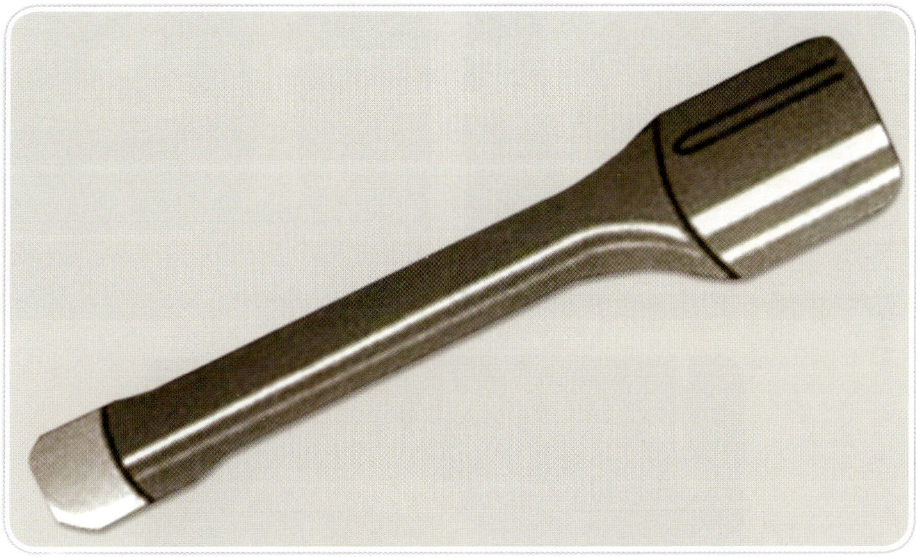

Sonoembryology: Embryology in vivo

3D Surface-Render of a 6 Weeks' Embryo

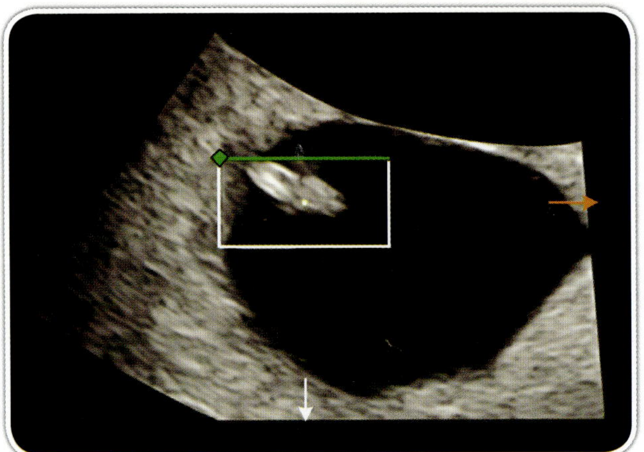

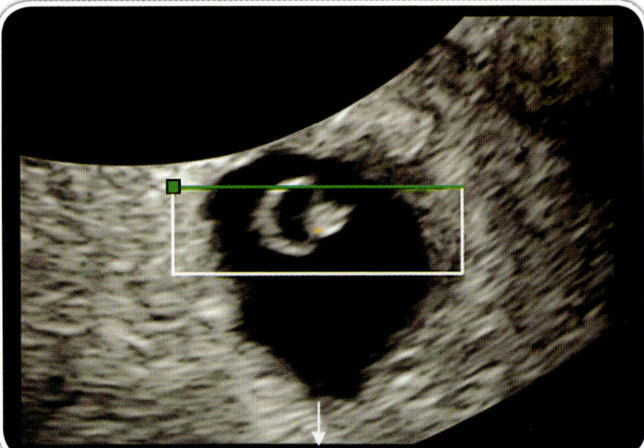

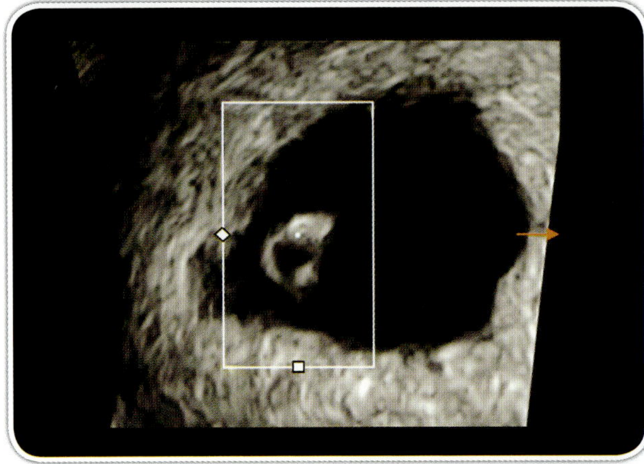

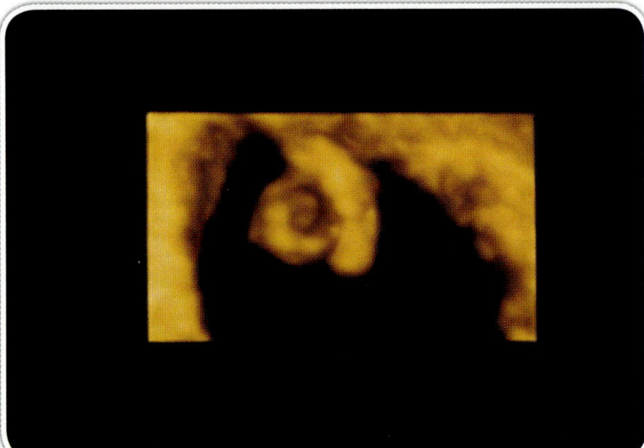

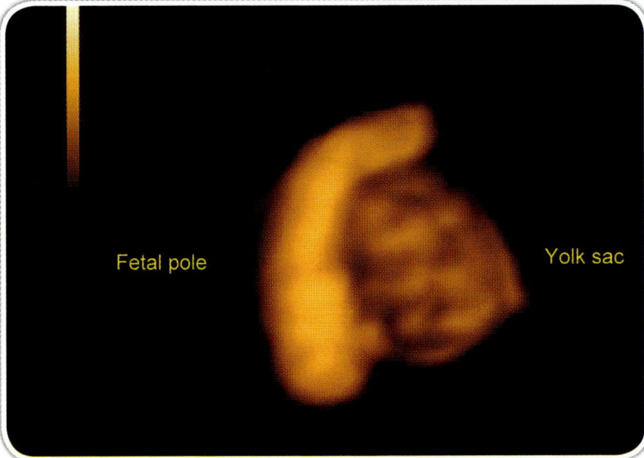

For complete presentation, please refer the accompanying CD-ROM...

SUGGESTED READING

1. Benoit B, Chaoui R. Three-dimensional ultrasound with maximal mode rendering: a novel technique for the diagnosis of bilateral or unilateral absence or hypoplasia of nasal bones in second-trimester screening for Down syndrome. Ultrasound Obstet Gynecol. 2005;25:19-24.
2. Benoit B, Hafner T, Kurjak A, Kupesic S, Bekavac I, Bozek T. Three-dimensional sonoembryology. J Perinat Med. 2002;30:63-73.
3. Blaas HG, Eik-Nes SH, Isaksen CV. The detection of spina bifida before 10 gestational weeks using two- and three-dimensional ultrasound. Ultrasound Obstet Gynecol. 2000;16:25-9.
4. Bolitho DG. Hand, Congenital hand deformities. emedicine 2006. http://www.emedicine.com/plastic/TOPIC298.HTM.
5. Carbillon L, Seince N, Largillière C, Bucourt M, Uzan M. First-trimester diagnosis of sirenomelia. A case report. Fetal Diagn Ther. 2001;16(5):284-8.
6. Chaoui R, Benoit B, Mitkowska-Wozniak H, Heling KS, Nicolaides KH. Assessment of intracranial translucency (IT) in the detection of spina bifida at the 11–13-week scan. Ultrasound Obstet Gynecol. 2009;34:249-52.
7. Chaoui R, Levaillant JM, Benoit B, Faro C, Wegrzyn P, Nicolaides KH. Three-dimensional sonographic description of abnormal metopic suture in second- and third-trimester fetuses. Ultrasound Obstet Gynecol. 2005;26:761-4.
8. Cicero S, Avgidou K, Rembouskos G, Kagan KO, Nicolaides KH. Nasal bone in first-trimester screening for trisomy 21. Am J Obstet Gynecol. 2006;195:109-14.
9. Cicero S, Curcio P, Rembouskos G, Sonek J, Nicolaides KH. Maxillary length at 11-14 weeks of gestation in fetuses with trisomy 21. Ultrasound Obstet Gynecol. 2004;24:19-22.
10. Cicero S, Rembouskos G, Vandecruys H, Hogg M, Nicolaides KH. Likelihood ratio for trisomy 21 in fetuses with absent nasal bone at the 11-14-week scan. Ultrasound Obstet Gynecol. 2004;23:218-23.
11. Daskalakis G, Anastasakis E, Lyberopoulos E, Antsaklis A. Prenatal detection of congenital cataract in a fetus with Lowe syndrome. J Obstet Gynaecol. 2010;30(4):409-10.
12. Dugoff L, Thieme G, Hobbins JC. First trimester prenatal diagnosis of chondroectodermal dysplasia (Ellis-van Creveld syndrome) with ultrasound. Ultrasound Obstet Gynecol. 2001;17:86-8.
13. Francis PJ, Berry V, Bhattacharya SS, Moore AT. The genetics of childhood cataract. J Med Genet. 2000;37:481-488.
14. Hata T, Dai SY, Kanenishi K, Tanaka H. Three-dimensional volume-rendered imaging of embryonic brain vesicles using inversion mode. J Obstet Gynaecol Res. 2009;35:2:258-61.
15. Karkinen-Jääskeläinen M, Saxen L, Vaheri A, Leinikki P. Rubella cataract in vitro: sensitive period of the developing human lens. J Exp Med. 1975;141:1238-48.
16. Kim MS, Jeanty P, Turner C, Benoit B. Three-dimensional sonographic evaluations of embryonic brain development. J Ultrasound Med. 2008;27:119-124.
17. Kurjak A, Pooh RK, Merce LT, Carrera JM, Salihagic-Kadic A, Andonotopo W. Structural and functional early human development assessed by three-dimensional and four-dimensional sonography. Fertil Steril. 2005;84:1285-99.
18. Kurjak A, Schulman H, Predanic A, Predanic M, Kupesic S, Zalud I. Fetal choroid plexus vascularization assessed by color flow ultrasonography. J Ultrasound Med. 1994;13:841-4.
19. Kurjak A, Zudenigo D, Predanic M, Kupesic S. Recent advances in the Doppler study of early fetomaternal circulation. J Perinat Med. 1993;21:419-39.
20. Léonard A, Bernard P, Hiel AL, Hubinont C. Prenatal diagnosis of fetal cataract: case report and review of the literature. Fetal Diagn Ther. 2009;26(2):61-7. Epub 2009 Sep 11.
21. Monteagudo A, Mayberry P, Rebarber A, Paidas M, Timor-Tritsch IE. Sirenomelia sequence: first-trimester diagnosis with both two- and three-dimensional sonography. J Ultrasound Med. 2002;21:915-20.
22. Pedreira DA, Diniz EM, Schultz R, Faro LB, Zugaib M. Fetal cataract in congenital toxoplasmosis. Ultrasound Obstet Gynecol. 1999;13(4):266-7.
23. Pooh RK, Kurjak A. Novel application of three-dimensional HDlive imaging in prenatal diagnosis from the first trimester. Perinat Med. 2014 Jul 11. pii: /j/jpme.ahead-of-print/jpm-2014-0157/jpm-2014-0157.xml. doi: 10.1515/jpm-2014-0157.
24. Pooh RK, Kurjak A. Three-dimensional/Four-dimensional sonography moved prenatal diagnosis of fetal anomalies from the second to the first trimester of pregnancy. Donald School Journal of Ultrasound in Obstetrics and Gynecology, October-December 2012;6(4):376-90.
25. Pooh RK, Shiota K, Kurjak A. Imaging of the human embryo with magnetic resonance imaging microscopy and high-resolution transvaginal three-dimensional sonography: human embryology in the 21st century. Am J Obstet Gynecol. 2011;204:77-9.
26. Reches A, Yaron Y, Burdon K, Crystal-Shalit O, Kidron D, Malcov M, Tepper R. Prenatal detection of congenital bilateral cataract leading to the diagnosis of Nance-Horan syndrome in the extended family. Prenat Diagn. 2007;27(7):662-4.
27. Rembouskos G, Cicero S, Longo D, Vandecruys H, Nicolaides KH. Assessment of the fetal nasal bone at 11-14 weeks of gestation by three-dimensional ultrasound. Ultrasound Obstet Gynecol. 2004 ;23:232-6.
28. Romain M, Awoust J, Dugauquier C, Van Maldergem L. Prenatal ultrasound detection of congenital cataract in trisomy 21. Prenat Diagn. 1999;19(8):780-2.

29. Schiesser M, Holzgreve W, Lapaire O, Willi N, Lüthi H, Lopez R, Tercanli S. Sirenomelia, the mermaid syndrome--detection in the first trimester. Prenat Diagn. 2003;23:493-5.
30. Teoh M, Meagher S. First-trimester diagnosis of micrognathia as a presentation of Pierre Robin syndrome. Ultrasound Obstet Gynecol. 2003;21:616-8.
31. Thut CJ, Rountree RB, Hwa M, Kingsley DM. A large-scale in situ screen provides molecular evidence for the induction of eye anterior segment structures by the developing lens. Dev Biol. 2001;231:63-76.
32. Timor-Tritsch IE, Peisner DB, Raju S. Sonoembryology: an organ-oriented approach using a high-frequency vaginal probe. J Clin Ultrasound. 1990;18:286-98.
33. Tsai MY, Lan KC, Ou CY, Chen JH, Chang SY, Hsu TY. Assessment of the facial features and chin development of fetuses with use of serial three-dimensional sonography and the mandibular size monogram in a Chinese population. AmJ Obstet Gynecol. 2004;190: 541-6.
34. Zoppi MA, Ibba RM, Axiana C, Floris M, Manca F, Monni G. Absence of fetal nasal bone and aneuploidies at first-trimester nuchal translucency screening in unselected pregnancies. Prenat Diagn. 2003;23:496-500.

Chapter 2

Bleeding in the First Trimester of Pregnancy

Azen Salim

CLASSIFICATION

Bleeding during first trimester pregnancy can be classified into:

A. Normal pregnancy

B. Abnormal pregnancy
   1. Intrauterine pregnancy
   2. Extrauterine pregnancy.

Etiology During Normal Pregnancy

- Subchorionic bleeding
- Abnormal shape of the uterus
- Cervical polyp
- Cervical malignancy
- Low site placentation/placenta previa
- Fibroid
- Cervical surface erosion.

SUBCHORIONIC BLEEDING

- Can cause miscarriage or premature delivery
- Appears as an anechoic area
- The echogenicity of this anechoic area can increase greatly over time.

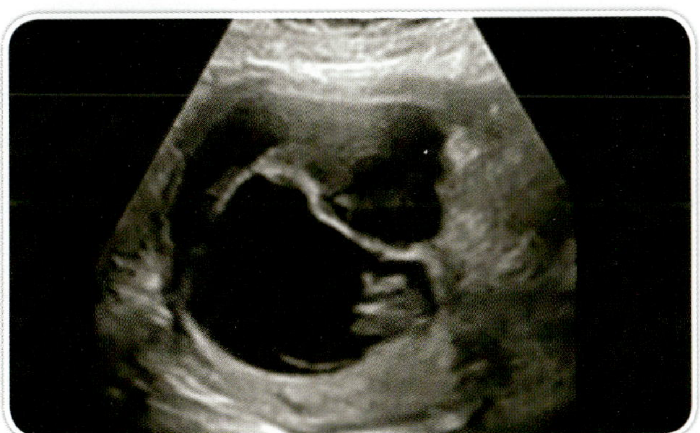
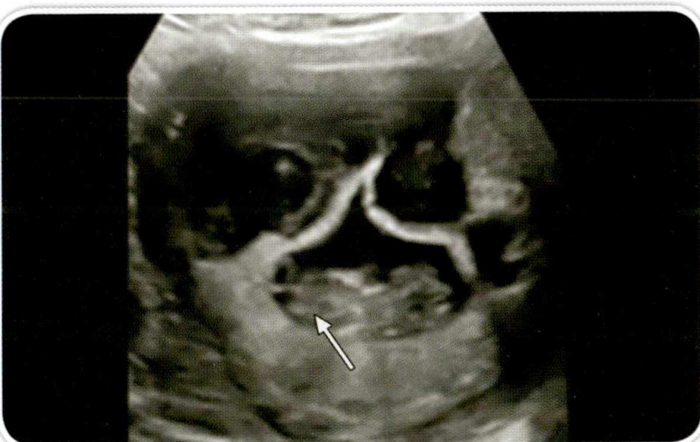

Severe subchorionic bleeding in 9 weeks of gestation

CHORIONIC BUMP

- Appear as a convex, polypoid bulge into the chorionic cavity that is sometimes seen at first-trimester ultrasound examination
- Echolucent lesion arising within the chorion (i.e. trophoblast) immediately beneath the chorionic membrane, bulging into the gestational sac.

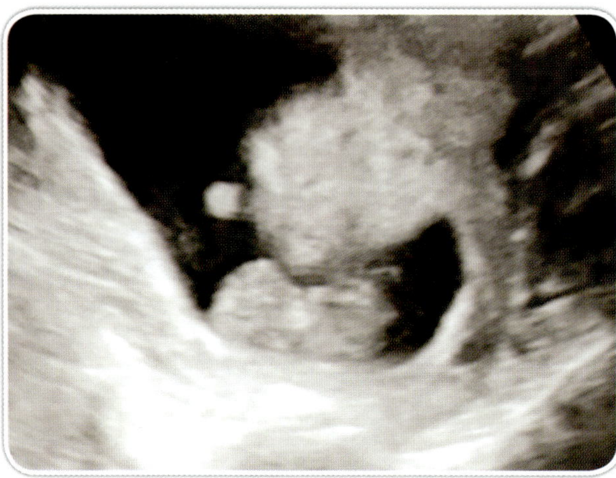

Chorionic bump

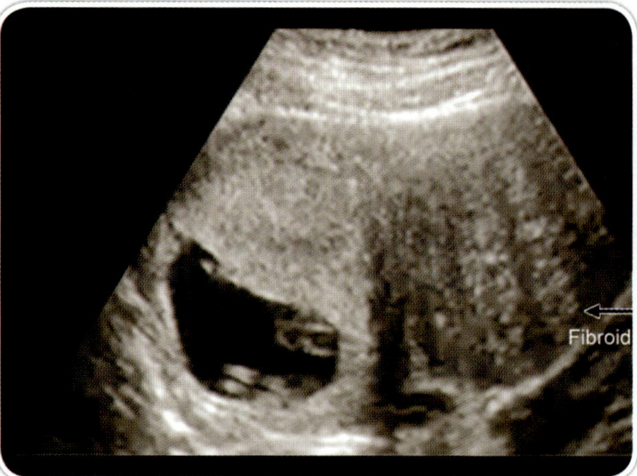

8 weeks pregnancy with large intramural fibroid

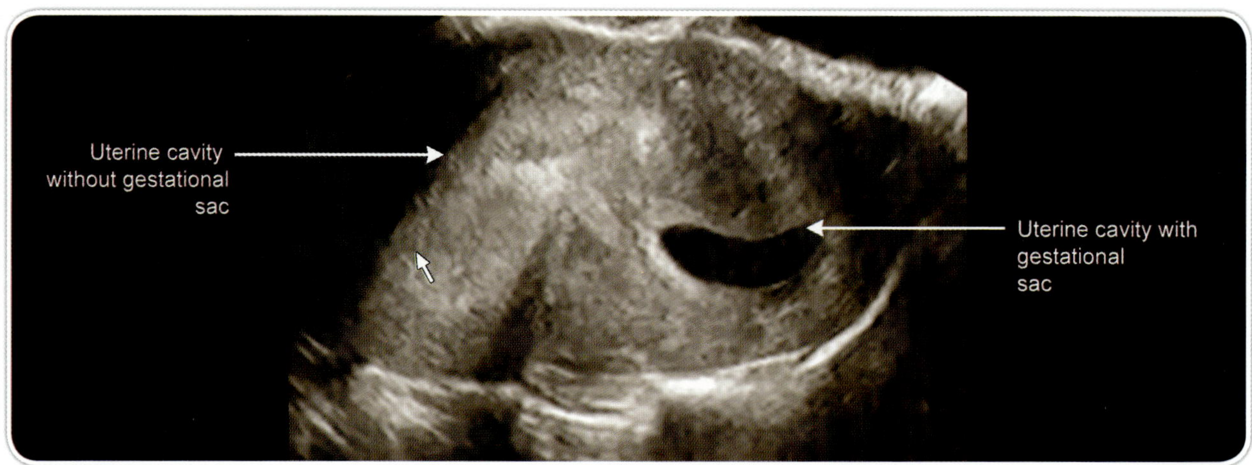

5 weeks gestational age with severe arcuate uterus

For complete presentation, please refer the accompanying CD-ROM...

SUGGESTED READING

1. Acharya et al. JCU. 2002.
2. Campbell J et al. BJOG. 1992.
3. Espinosa J, et al. The prevalence and clinical significance of amniotic fluid "sludge" in patients with preterm labor and intact membranes. Ultrasound Obstet Gynecol 2005;25:346-52
4. Filly, et al. JUM. 2010.
5. Goldstein SR, Subramanyam BR, et al. Subchorionic bleeding in threatened abortion : sonographic findings and significance. Am J Roentgenol. 1983;141:975-8.
6. Harris RD, Couto C, Karpovsky C, et al. The chorionic bump: a first trimester pregnancy sonographic finding associated with a guarded prognosis. J Ultrasound Med. 2006:25;757-63.
7. Hately W, Case J, Campbell S. Establishing the death of an embryo by ultrasound: report of a public enquiry with recommendation. Ultrasound Obstet Gynecol. 1995;5:353-7
8. Jurkovic D, et al. Cesarean scar pregnancy. Ultrasound Obstet Gynecol. 2003;21:310.
9. Jurkovic D, et al. First trimester diagnosis and management of pregnancies implanted into the lower uterine segment cesarean section scar. Ultrasound Obstet Gynecol. 2003;21:220-7.
10. Lindsay et al. Radiology 1992
11. Makikallio, et al. Ultrasound Obstet Gynecol 1999
12. Mantoni M, Pedersen JF. Intrauterine hematoma : an ultrasound study of threatened abortion. Br J Obstet Gynecoll. 1981;88:47-51.
13. Odeh et al. JUM. 2008
14. Romero R, et al. Detection of microbial biofilm in intraamniotic infection. 2008;198:135,e1-5.
15. Romero R, et al. What is amniotic fluid. "Sludge" Ultrasound Obstet Gynecol. 2007;30:793-8.
16. Tan, et al. JUM. 2011.
17. Tan, et al. JUM. 2012.
18. Yegul, et al. JUM. 2009.

Chapter

3

11 to 14 Weeks' Scan

Tamara Illescas

OBJECTIVES

- Basics:
  - Viability
  - Number of fetuses
  - Chorionicity
  - Estimation of gestational age
  - Placenta, uterus and adnexa
- Screening for aneuploidies
- Anatomy anomalies.

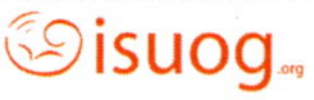
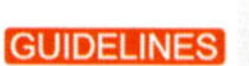

ISUOG Practice Guidelines: performance of first-trimester fetal ultrasound scan

BASICS

- Patient's background.
- Probe:

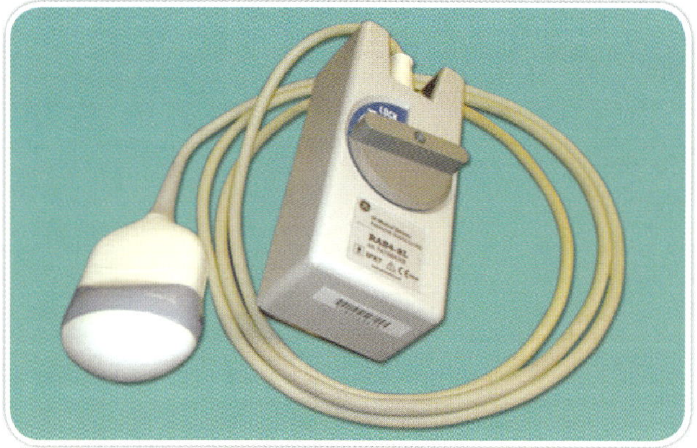

TA: Curvilinear transducer (4–7 MHz probe) to obtain a global view of the pelvis and exclude any pelvic pathology

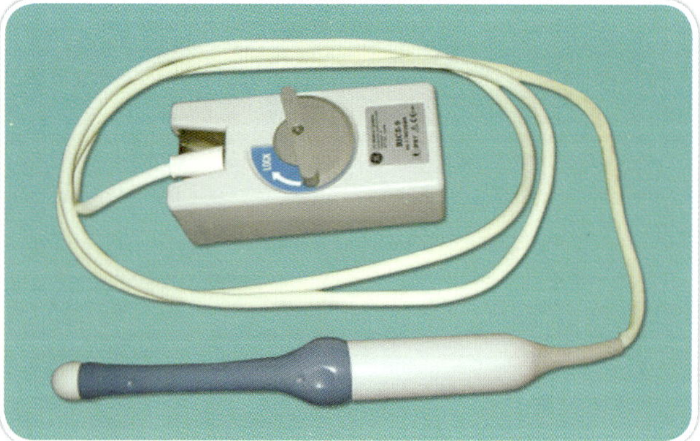

TV: Curvilinear high-frequency transducer (9–12 MHz probe). Closer proximity of the transducer to the fetus results in a better display of the anatomy

---

1. The origin of the images is cited when not belonging to the author.
2. When not indicated, the images are the author's own original pictures, the vast majority of which were obtained at **Delta Ultrasound Diagnostic Center** in Obstetrics and Gynecology, Madrid, Spain.

- **Survey scan:** Global view → transverse and longitudinal planes. At 11–14 weeks of gestation, an intrauterine pregnancy should be obvious with a sonographic window created by the amniotic sac filled with echonegative amniotic fluid and the fetus inside.

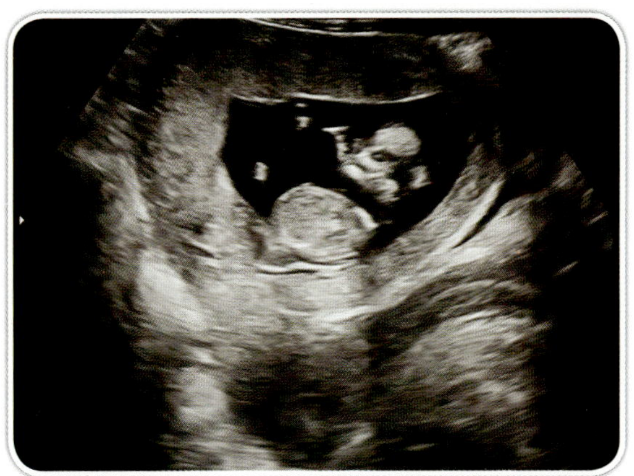

  - Look for any obvious myometrial or cervical pathology
  - Describe any uterine malformations
  - Both adnexa should be scanned entirely, excluding any obvious ovarian pathology or adnexal masses.

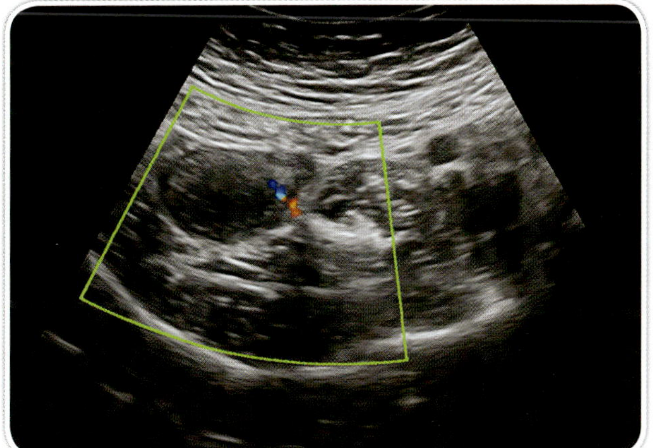

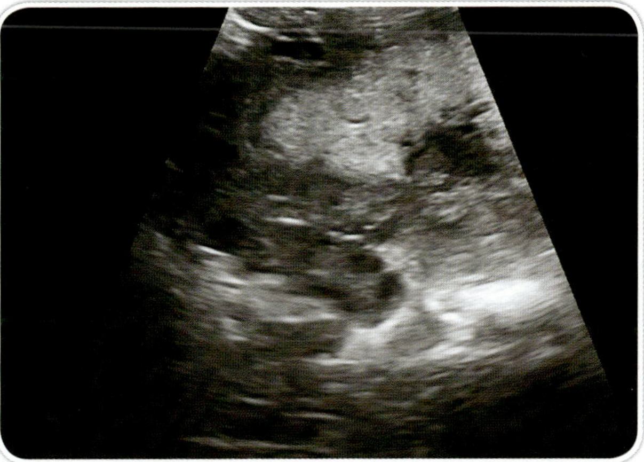

Normal ovaries

(ISUOG Guidelines, 2013)

- **Viability**
  - The visualization of the fetal heart rate in the fetal chest confirms fetal viability
  - The fetal heart rate can be measured by implementing the pulsed Doppler.

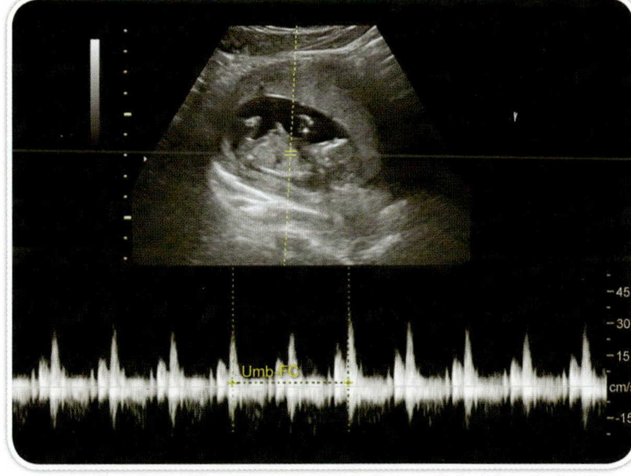

For complete presentation, please refer the accompanying CD-ROM...

SUGGESTED READING

1. Adiego B, Martinez-Ten P, Perez-Pedregosa J, Crespo A, Santacruz B, Illescas T, Barron E. Determinación del sexo fetal en el primer trimestre de la gestación: estudio prospectivo. Rev Chil Obstet Ginecol. 2010;75:117-23.
2. Borenstein M, Persico N, Kagan KO, Gazzoni A, Nicolaides KH. Frontomaxillary facial angle in screening for trisomy 21 at 11 + 0 to 13 + 6 weeks. Ultrasound Obstet Gynecol. 2008;32:5-11.
3. Borrell A. Promises and pitfalls of first trimester sonographic markers in the detection of fetal aneuploidy. Prenatl Diagn. 2009; 29: 62-8.
4. Chaoui R, Benoit B, Mitkowska-Wozniak H, Heling KS, Nicolaides KH. Assessment of intracranial translucency (IT) in the detection of spina bífida at the 11-13-week scan. Ultrsound Obstet Gynecol. 2009;34:249-52.
5. Comas C, Prats P. Echocardiography in Early Pregnancy. Donald School J Ultrasound Obstet Gynecol. 2013;7:168-81.
6. Dagklis T, Plasencia W, Maiz N, Duarte L, Nicolaides KH. Choroid plexus cyst, intracardiac echogenic focus, hyperecogenic bowel and hydronephrosis in screening for trisomy 21 at 11 + 0 to 13 + 6 weeks. Ultrasound Obstet Gynecol. 2008;31:132-5.
7. Kagan KO, Cicero S, Staboulidou I, Wright D, Nicolaides KH. Fetal nasal bone in screening for trisomies 21, 18 and 13 and Turner síndrome at 11-13 weeks of gestation. Ultrasound Obstet Gynecol. 2009;33:259-64.
8. Kagan KO, Valencia C, Livanos P, Wright D, Nicolaides KH. Tricuspid regurgitation in screening for trisomies 21, 18 and 13 and Turner síndrome at 11 + 0 to 13 + 6 weeks of gestation. Ultrasound Obstet Gynecol. 2009;33:18-22.
9. Lachmann R, Picciarelli G, Moratalla J, Greene N, Nicolaides KH. Frontomaxillary facial angle in fetuses with spina bífida at 11-13 weeks' gestation. Ultrasound Obstet Gynecol. 2010;36:268-71.
10. Maiz N, Valencia C, Kagan KO, Wright D, Nicolaides KH. Ductus venosus Doppler in screening for trisomies 21, 18 and 13 and Turner síndrome at 11-13 weeks of gestation. Ultrasound Obstet Gynecol. 2009;33:512-7.
11. Martinez-Ten P, Adiego B, Illescas T, Bermejo C, Wong AE, Sepulveda W. First-trimester diagnosis of cleft lip and palate using three-dimensional ultrasound. Ultrasound Obstet Gynecol. 2012;40(1):40-6.
12. Martinez-Ten P, Adiego B, Perez-Pedregosa J, Illescas T, Wong AE, Sepulveda W. First-trimester assessment of the nasal bones using the retronasal triangle view. J Ultrasound Med. 2010;29:1555-61.
13. Nicolaides KH, Azar G, Byrne D, Mansur C, Marks K. Fetal nuchal translucency: ultrasound screening for chromosomal defects in first trimester of pregnancy. BMJ. 1992;304:867-9.
14. Nicolaides KH. A model for a new pyramid of prenatal care based on the 11 to 13 weeks' assessment. Prenat Diagn. 2011;31:3-6.
15. Nicolaides KH. Screening for fetal aneuploidies at 11 to 13 weeks. Prenat Diagn. 2011;31:7-15.
16. Nicolaides KH. The 11-13+6 weeks scan. The Fetal Medicine Foundation. http://www.fetalmedicine.com.
17. Salomon LJ, Alfirevic Z, Bilardo CM, Chalouhi GE, Ghi T, Kagan KO, et al. ISUOG practice guidelines: performance of first-trimester fetal ultrasound scan. Ultrasound Obstet Gynecol. 2013; 41: 102-13.
18. Sepulveda W, Illescas T, Adiego B, Martinez-Ten P. Prenatal Detection of Fetal Anomalies at the 11-to-13-week Scan – Part I: Brain, Face and Neck. Donald School J Ultrasound Obstet Gynecol. 2013;7(4):359-68.
19. Sepulveda W, Wong AE, Martinez-Ten P, Perez-Pedregosa J. Retronasal triangle: a sonographic landmark for the screening of cleft palate in the first trimester. Ultrasound Obstet Gynecol. 2010;35:7-13.
20. Sepulveda W, Wong AE, Viñals F, Andreeva E, Adzehova N, Martinez-Ten P. Absent mandibular gap in the retronasal triangle view: a clue to the diagnosis of micrognathia in the first trimester. Ultrasound Obstet Gynecol. 2012;39:152-6.
21. Sonek J, Borenstein M, Dagklis T, Persico N, Nicolaides KH. Frontomaxillary facial angle in fetuses with trisomy 21 at 11-13+6 weeks. Am J Obstet Gynecol. 2007;196:271.e1-271.e4.
22. Zvanca M, Gielchinksky Y, Abdeljawad F, Bilardo CM, Nicolaides KH. Hepatic artery Doppler in trisomy 21 and euploid fetuses at 11-13 weeks. Prenat Diagn. 2011;31:22-7.

Chapter 4

Gestational Trophoblastic Diseases

Kazuo Maeda

CLASSIFICATIONS

Abnormal Trophoblasts of Placental Origin

- Gestational trophoblastic diseases and tumors
- Non-gestational choriocarcinoma

Gestational trophoblastic diseases and tumors	Non-gestational choriocarcinoma
• Hydatidiform mole – Complete hydatidiform mole – Partial hydatidiform mole – Invasive mole • Persistent trophoblastic disease • Choriocarcinoma • Placental site trophoblastic tumor (PSTT) • Epithelioid trophoblastic tumor (ETT)	• Primary gonadal choriocarcinoma in ovary or testis • Metamorphosis of other cancer, e.g. stomach cancer • Serum or urine hCG is positive, systemic metastases Non-gestational choriocarcinoma tends to resist methotrexate (MTX) therapy.

COMPLETE HYDATIDIFORM MOLE

- No fetus or fetal component
- Uterus is filled with cysts covered by trophoblasts
- Chromosomes are 46 XX, of which XX are both male origin (androgenesis)
- Maternal blood circulates in the uterine intercystic space.

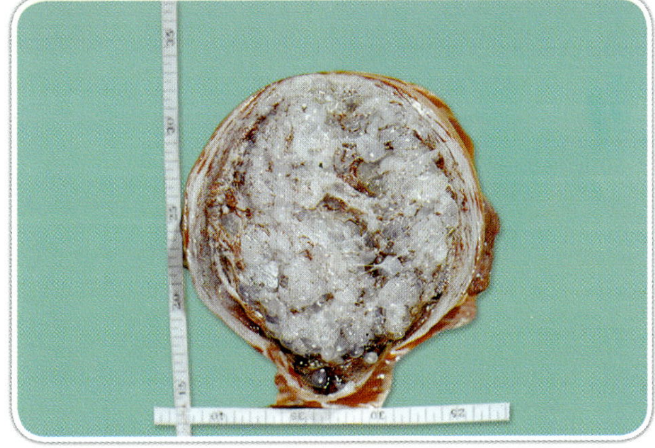

- Symptoms:
  - Enlarged uterus without the fetus
  - Vaginal hemorrhage, molar cyst expulsion
  - High human chorionic gonadotropin (hCG), e.g. urine hCG ≥ 100,000 IU/L
  - Hyperemesis, preeclamptic change (hypertension and proteinuria).

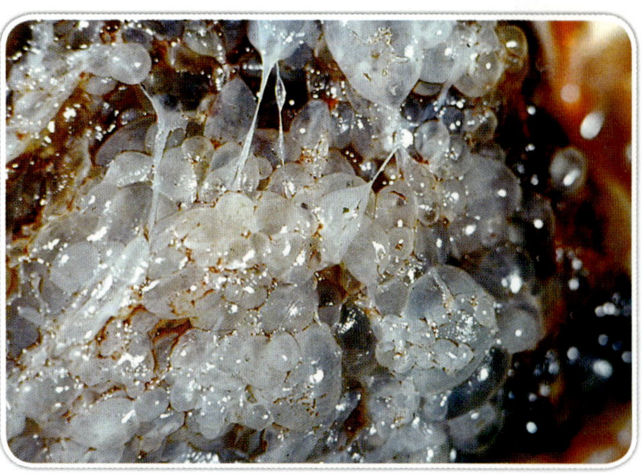

Pathologic classifications:

- Choriocarcinoma
- Invasive mole
- Placental site trophoblastic tumor (PSTT)
- Epithelioid trophoblastic tumor (ETT)
- Persistent trophoblastic disease.

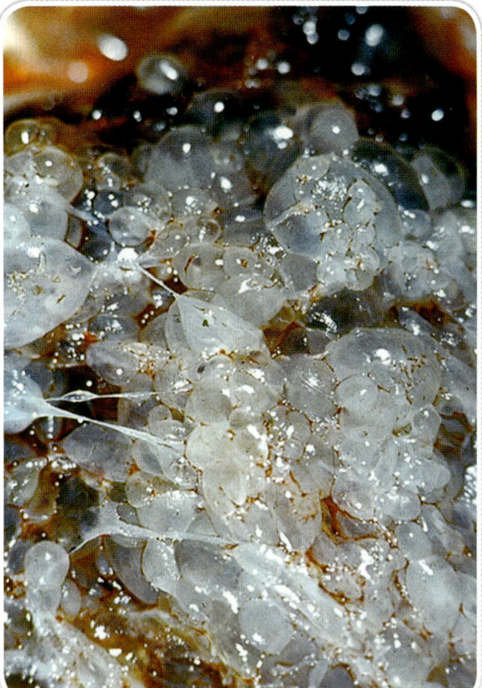

Real-time B-mode

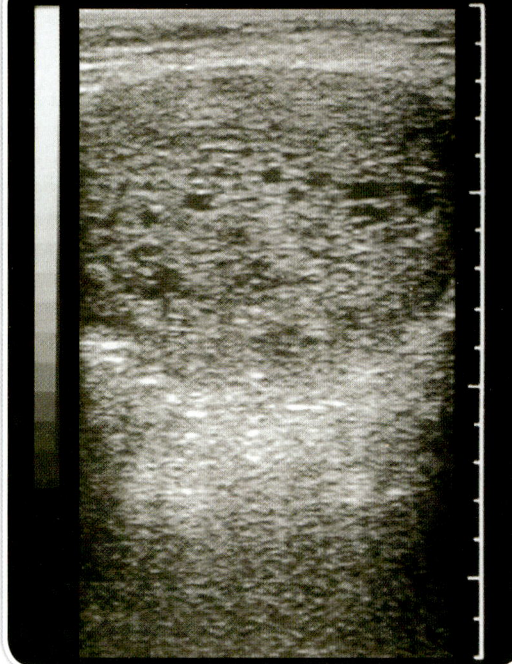

Molar cysts

12 weeks

No fetus

Multiple intrauterine cysts from ultrasound.

For complete presentation, please refer the accompanying CD-ROM...

SUGGESTED READING

1. Koga K, Maeda K, et al. Treatment of chorioepithelioma (chorio- carcinoma) of uterine cervix with hypogastric arterial infusion of MTX. J Jap Obstet Gynecol Soc. 1966;1:245-9.
2. Koga K, Maeda K. Prophylactic chemotherapy with amethopterin for prevention of choriocarcinoma following removal of hydatidiform mole. Am J Obstet Gynecol. 1968;100:270-5.

Chapter

5

Noninvasive Prenatal Testing (NIPT) for Aneuploidies

Carmina Comas, Mónica Echevarria

LEARNING OBJECTIVES

- Basics of molecular techniques for NIPT: Counting and non-counting methods
- Current commercial tests available
- Current performance, advantages and limitations
- Published studies
- Recommendations from scientific societies
- Future directions of NIPS.

DEVELOPMENT OF PRENATAL MOLECULAR GENETICS

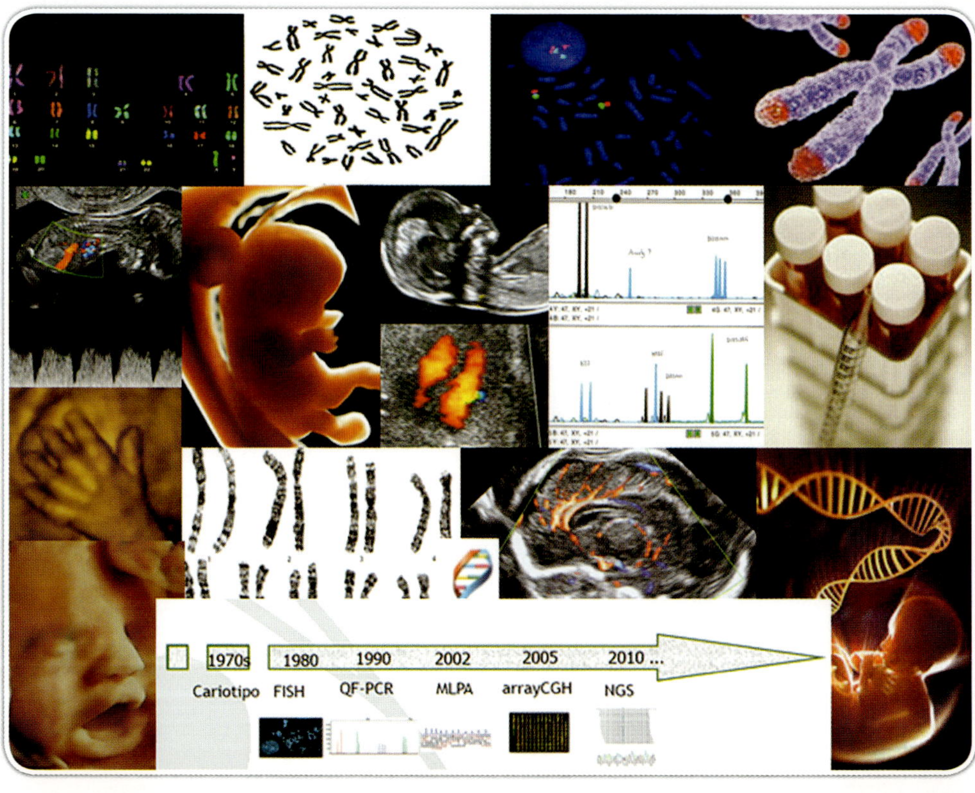

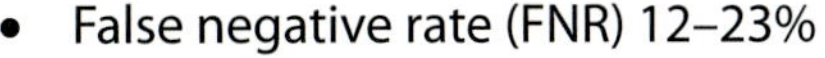

BACKGROUND: COMBINED US AND BIOCHEMICAL SERUM MARKERS

- False positive rate (FPR) 1.9–5.2%
- False negative rate (FNR) 12–23%

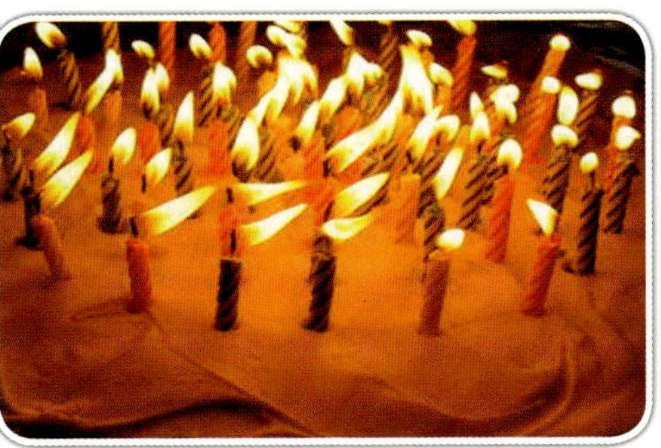

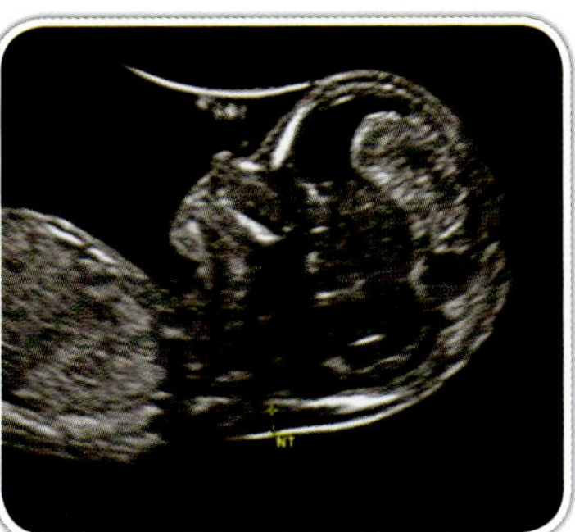

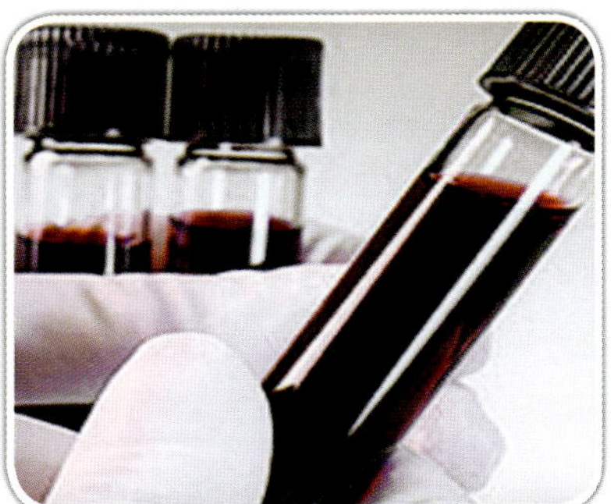

BACKGROUND: INVASIVE PRENATAL DIAGNOSTIC PROCEDURES

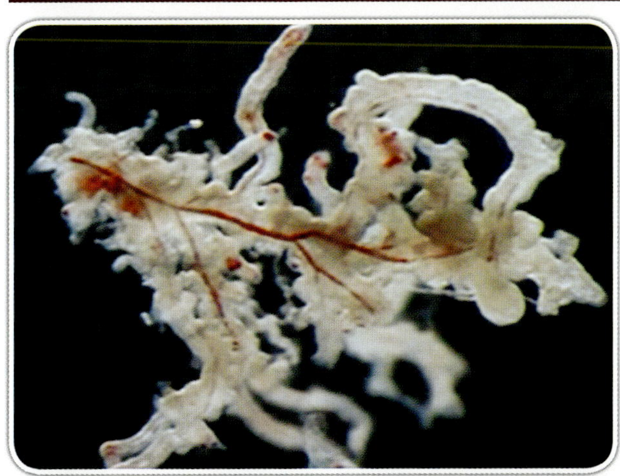

- Accuracy
  - 97.5–99.6% CVS
  - 99.4–99.8% AF
- Miscarriage rate
  - 0.6–2%

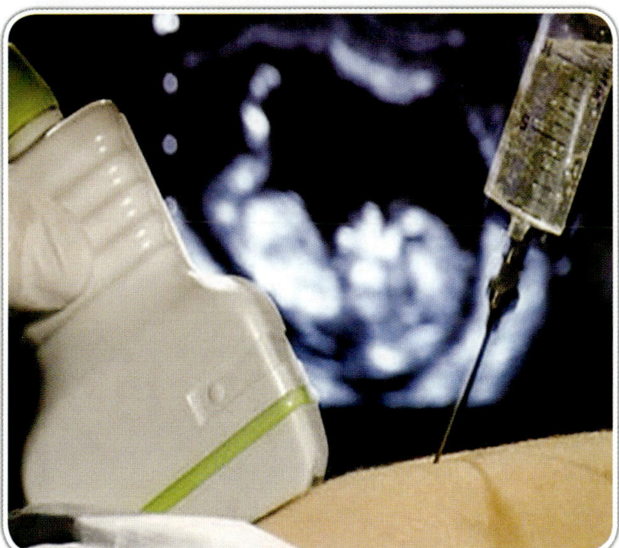

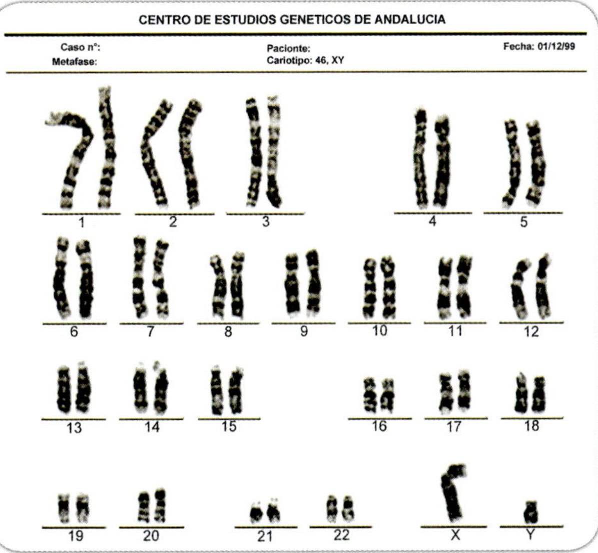

For complete presentation, please refer the accompanying CD-ROM...

SUGGESTED READING

1. Ashoor G, Poon L, Syngelaki A, Mosimann B, Nicolaides KH. Fetal fraction in maternal plasma cell-free DNA at 11–13weeks' gestation: effect of maternal and fetal factors. Fetal Diagn Ther. 2012;31:237-43.
2. Ashoor G, Syngelaki A, Wagner M, Birdir C, Nicolaides KH. Chromosome-selective sequencing of maternal plasma cell-free DNA for first-trimester detection of trisomy 21 and trisomy 18. Am J Obstet Gynecol. 2012;206:322.e1-5.
3. Bianchi DW, Parker RL, Wentworth J, Madankumar R, Saffer C, Das AF, et al. CARE Study Group. DAN Sequencing versus Standard Prenatal Aneuploidy Screening. N Engl J Med. 2014;370:799-808.
4. Bianchi DW, Platt LD, Goldberg JD, Abuhamad AZ, Sehnert AJ, Rava RP. On behalf of the Maternal BLood IS Source to Accurately diagnose fetal aneuploidy (MELISSA). Study Group. Genome-wide fetal aneuploidy detection by maternal plasma DNA sequencing. Obstet Gynecol. 2012;119:890-901.
5. Canick JA, Palomaki GE, Kloza EM, Lambert-Messerlian GM, Haddow JE. The impact of maternal plasma DNA fetal fraction on next generation sequencing tests for common fetal aneuploidies. Prenat Diagn. 2013;33:667-74.
6. Chiu RW, Akolekar R, Zheng YW, Leung TY, Sun H, Chan KC,et al. Non-invasive prenatal assessment of trisomy 21 by multiplexed maternal plasma DNA sequencing: large scale validation study. BMJ. 2011;342:c7401.
7. Dan S, Wang W, Ren J, Li Y, Hu H, Xu Z, et al. Clinical application of massively parallel sequencing-based prenatal noninvasive fetal trisomy test for trisomies 21 and 18 in 11,105 pregnancies with mixed risk factors. Prenat Diagn. 2012;32:1225-32.
8. Ehrich M, Deciu C, Zweifellhofer T, Tynan JA, Cagasan L, Tim R, et al. Noninvasive detection of fetal trisomy 21 by sequencing of DNA in maternal blood: a study in a clinical setting. Am J Obstet Gynecol. 2011;204;205.e201-211.
9. Fairbrother G, Johnson S, Musci TJ, Song K. Clinical experience of noninvasive prenatal testing with cell-free DNA for fetal trisomies 21, 18, and 13, in a general screening population. Prenat Diagn. 2013;33:580-3.
10. Futch T, Spinosa J, Bhatt S, de Feo E, Rava RP, Sehnert AJ. Initial clinical laboratory experience in noninvasive prenatal testing for fetal aneuploidy from maternal plasma DNA samples. Prenat Diagn. 2013;33:569-74.
11. Garfield SS, Amstrong SO. Clinical and cost consequences of incorporating a novel non-invasive prenatal test into the diagnostic pathway for fetal trisomies. J Managed Care Medicine. 2012;15:34-41.
12. Gil MM, Quezada MS, Bregant B, Ferraro M, Nicolaides KH. Implementation of maternal blood cell-free DNA testing in early screening for aneuploidies. Ultrasound Obstet Gynecol. 2013;42:34-40.
13. Gratacós E, Nicolaides K. Clinical perspective of cell-free DNA testing for fetal aneuploidies. Fetal Diagn Ther. 2014;35:151-5.
14. Kagan KO, Etchegaray A, Zhou Y, Wright D, Nicolaides KH. Prospective validation of first trimester combined screening for trisomy 21. Ultrasound Obstet Gynecol. 2009;34:14-8.
15. Lau TK, Chan MK, Lo PS, et al. Clinical utility of noninvasive fetal trisomy (NIFTY) test-early experience. J Matern Fetal Neonatal Med. 2012;25:1856-9.
16. Malone FD, Canick JA, Ball RH, Nyberg DA, Comstock CH, Bukowski R, et al. First-trimester or second-trimester screening, or both, for Down's syndrome. N Engl J Med. 2005;353:2001-11.
17. Manegold-Brauer G, Kang Bellin A, Hahn S, De Geyter C, Buechel J, Hoesli I, Lapaire O. A new era in prenatal care: non-invasive prenatal testing in Switzerland. Swiss Med Wkly. 2014;144:w13915.
18. Nicolaides KH, Syngelaki A, Ashoor G, Birdir C, Touzet G. Noninvasive prenatal testing for fetal trisomies in a routinely screened first-trimester population. Am J Obstet Gynecol. 2012;207:374.
19. Nicolaides KH, Syngelaki A, Gil M, Atanasova V, Markova D. Validation of targeted sequencing of single-nucleotide polymorphisms for non-invasive prenatal detection of aneuploidy of chromosomes 13, 18, 21, X, and Y. Prenat Diagn. 2013;33:575-9.
20. Nicolaides KH. Screening for fetal aneuploidies at 11 to 13 weeks. Prenat Diagn. 2011;31:7-15.
21. Noninvasive prenatal testing for fetal aneuploidy. Committee Opinion No. 545. American College of Obstetricians and Gynecologists. Obstet Gynecol. 2012;120: 1532-4.
22. Norton ME, Brar H, Weiss J, Karimi A, Laurent LC, Caughey AB, et al. Non-Invasive Chromosomal Evaluation (NICE) Study: results of a multicenter prospective cohort study for detection of fetal trisomy 21 and trisomy 18. Am J Obstet Gynecol. 2012;207:137.e1-8.
23. Palomaki GE, Deciu C, Kloza EM, Lambert-Messerlian GM, Haddow JE, Neveux LM, et al DNA sequencing of maternal plasma reliably identifies trisomy 18 and trisomy 13 as well as Down syndrome: an international collaborative study. Genet Med 2012;14: 296-305.
24. Palomaki GE, Kloza EM, Lambert-Messerlian GM, Haddow JE, Neveux LM, Ehrich M, et al. DNA sequencing of maternal plasma to detect Down syndrome: an international clinical validation study. Genet Med. 2011;13:913-20.
25. Salomon LJ, Alfirevic Z, Audibert F, Kagan KO, Yeo G, Raine-Fenning N. On behalf of the ISUOG Clinical Standards Committee. US STATEMENT ISUOG consensus statement on the impact of non-invasive prenatal testing (NIPT) on prenatal ultrasound practice. Ultrasound Obstet Gynecol. 2014;44:122-3.
26. Song K, Musci TJ, Caughey AB. Clinical utility and cost of non-invasive prenatal testing with cfDNA analysis in high-risk women based on a US population. J Matern Fetal Neonatal Med. 2013;26:1180-5.

27. Song Y, Liu C, Qi H, Zhang Y, Bian X, Liu J. Noninvasive prenatal testing of fetal aneuploidies by massively parallel sequencing in a prospective Chinese population. Prenat Diagn. 2013;33:700-6.
28. Sparks AB, Struble CA, Wang ET, Song K, Oliphant A. Noninvasive prenatal detection and selective analysis of cell-free DNA obtained from maternal blood: evaluation for trisomy 21 and trisomy 18. Am J Obstet Gynecol. 2012;206:319.e1-9.
29. Stumm M, Entezami M, Haug K, Blank C, Wüstemann M, Schulze B, Diagnostic accuracy of random massively parallel sequencing for non-invasive prenatal detection of common autosomal aneuploidies: a collaborative study in Europe. Prenat Diagn. 2014;34:185-91.
30. Verweij EJ, Jacobsson B, van Scheltema PA, de Boer MA, Hoffer MJ, Hollemon D, et al European non-invasive trisomy evaluation (EU-NITE) study: a multicenter prospective cohort study for non-invasive fetal trisomy 21 testing. Prenat Diagn. 2013;33:996-1001.
31. Wang E, Batey A, Struble C, Musci T, Song K, Oliphant A. Gestational age and maternal weight effects on fetal cellfree DNA in maternal plasma. Prenat Diagn. 2013;33:662-6.
32. Zimmermann B, Hill M, Gemelos G, Demko Z, Banjevic M, Baner J,et al. Noninvasive prenatal aneuploidy testing of chromosomes 13, 18, 21, X, and Y, using targeted sequencing of polymorphic loci. Prenat Diagn. 2012;32:1233-41.

Chapter 6

Multifetal Pregnancies

Tuangsit Wataganara

SONOGRAPHIC EVALUATION OF MULTIFETAL PREGNANCY

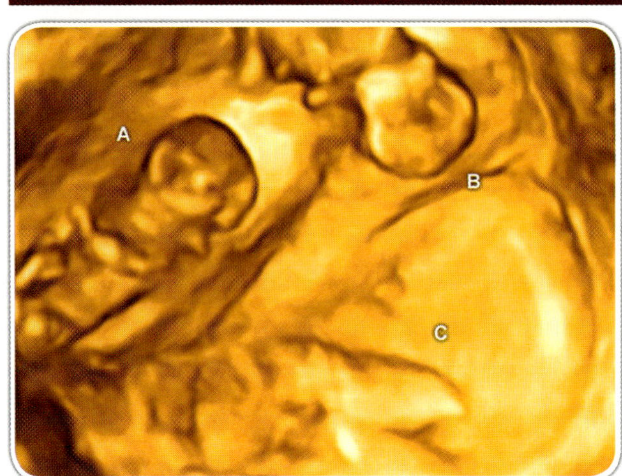

Scopes

- Number and viability of fetuses
- Chorionicity
- Growth and amniotic fluid.

Concordant Twins

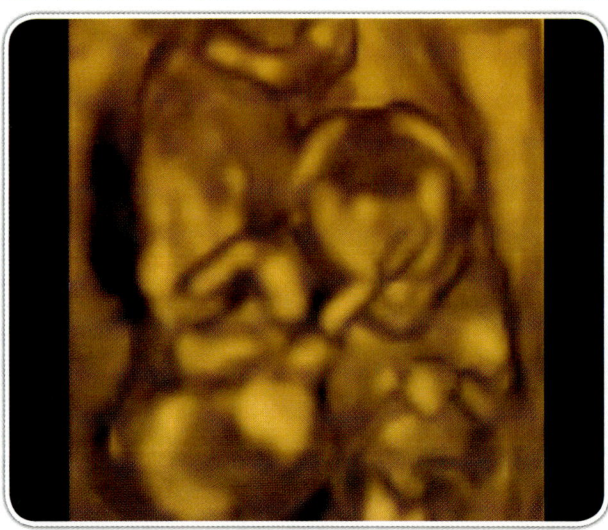

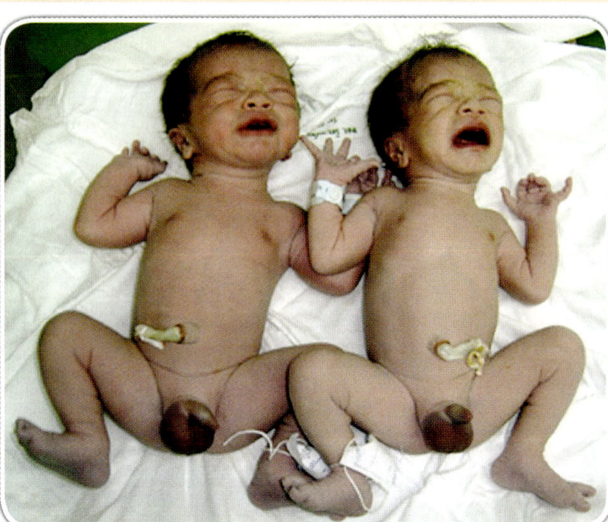

Determination of Chorionicity

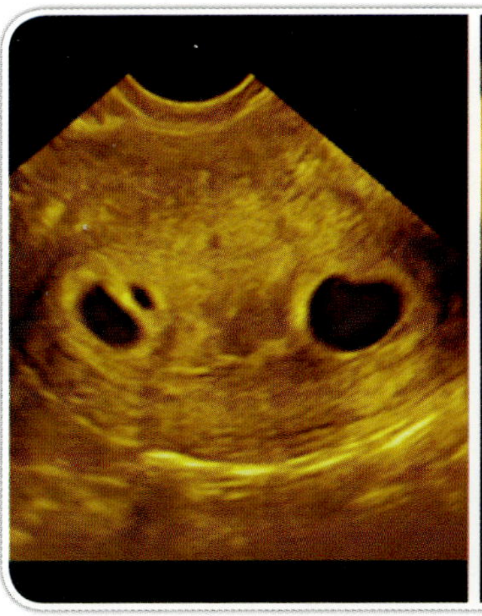
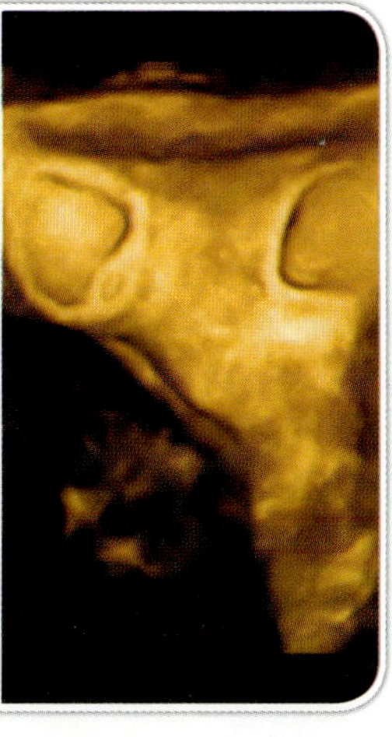

Location of gestational sacs: Dichorionic

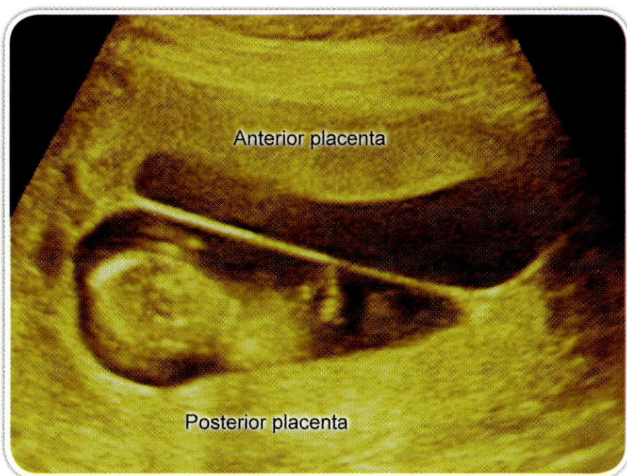

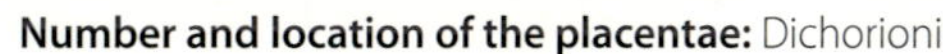

Number and location of the placentae: Dichorionic

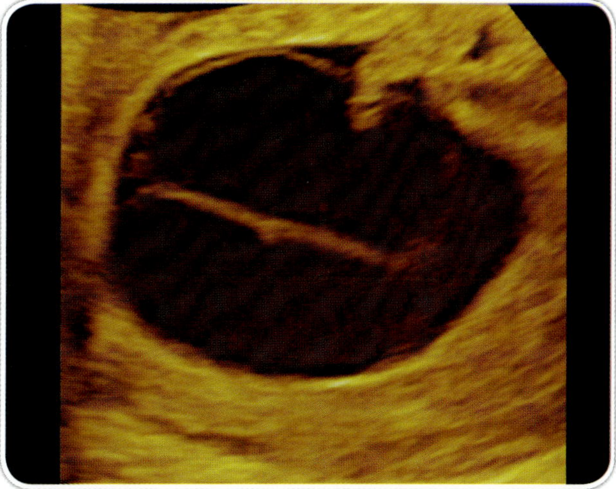

Monochorionic: "T" sign

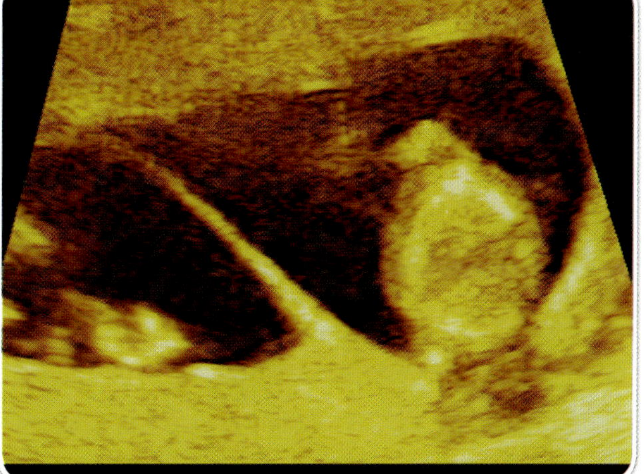

Dichorionic: "λ" sign

Monochorionic Diamniotic

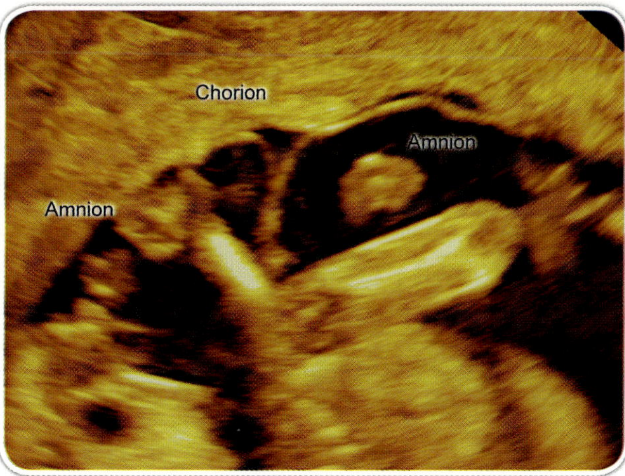

"λ" Sign in 3D

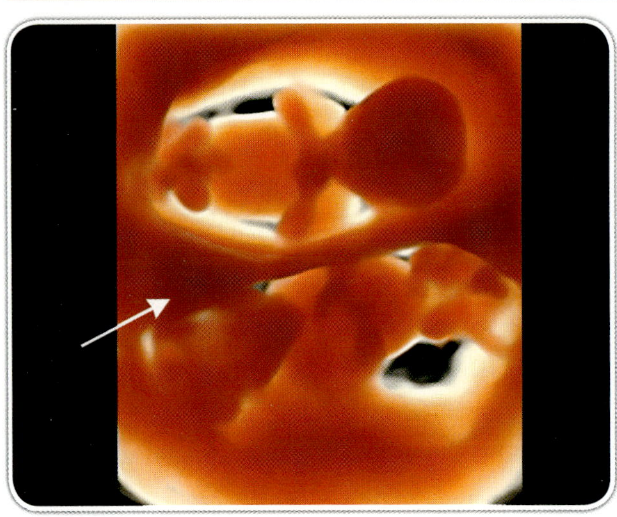

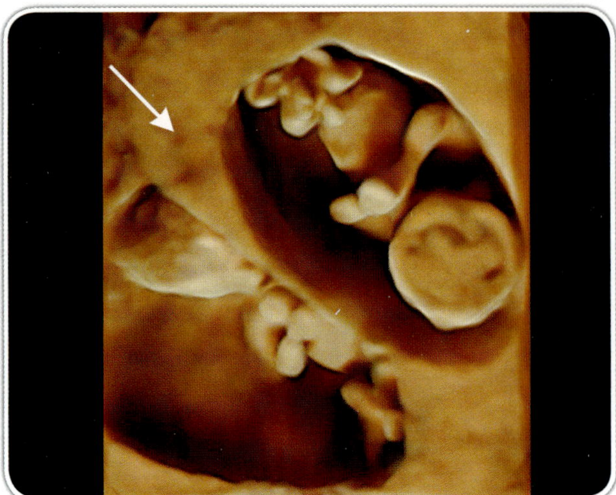

Fetal Viability

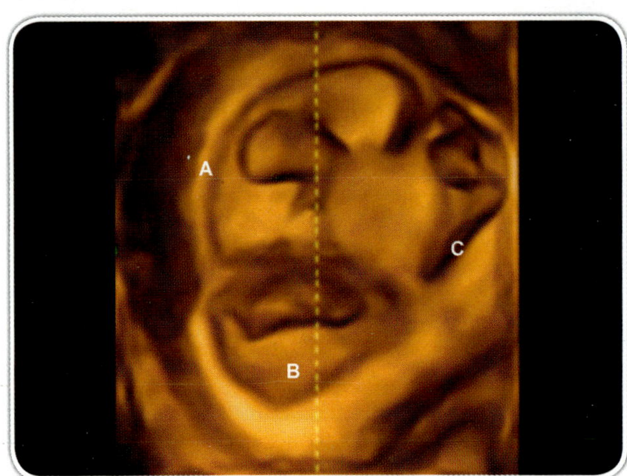

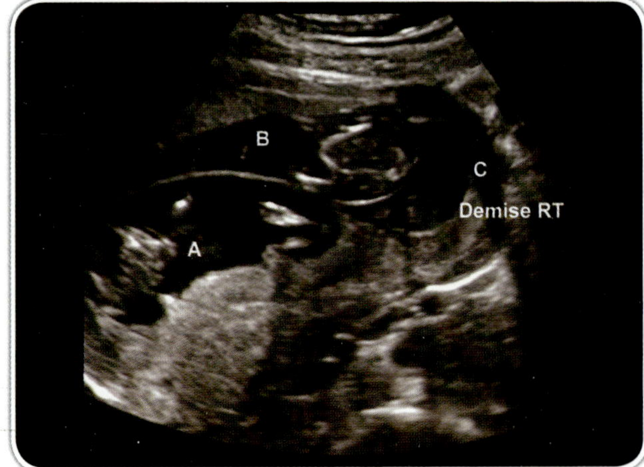

Trichorionic triamniotic triplets with 1 fetal demise

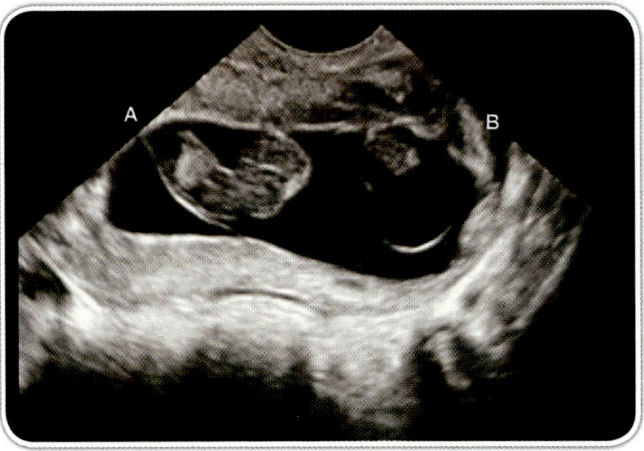

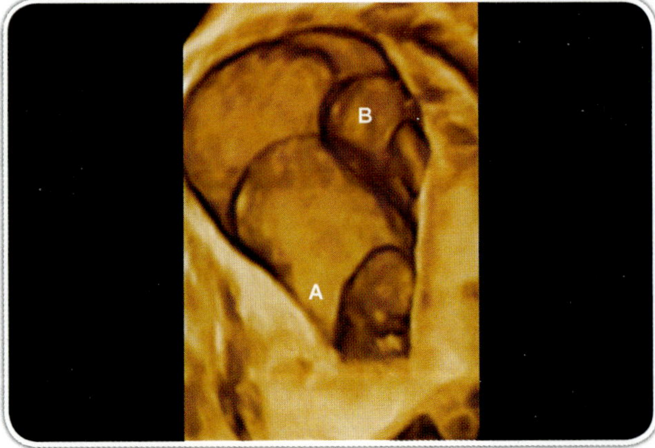

Early double demises of monochorionic twins

Monochorionic Twins

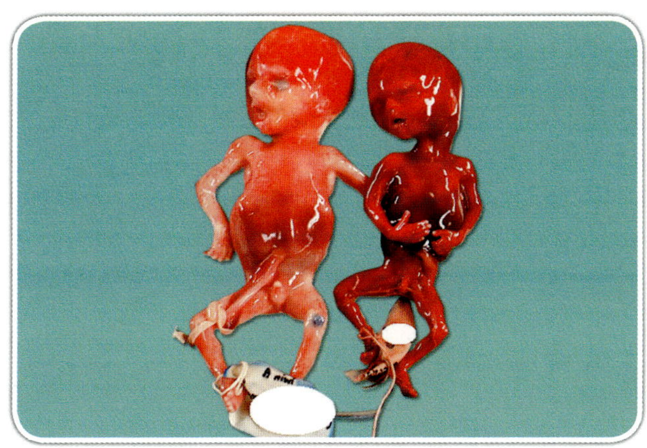

- Ever present vascular connection
- One fetal demise → Agonal hypotension → 25% demise of the co-twin → 25% of survivors suffer from cerebral palsy

(Dube et al. 2002)

Agonal Hypotension

Neurodevelopmental consequences

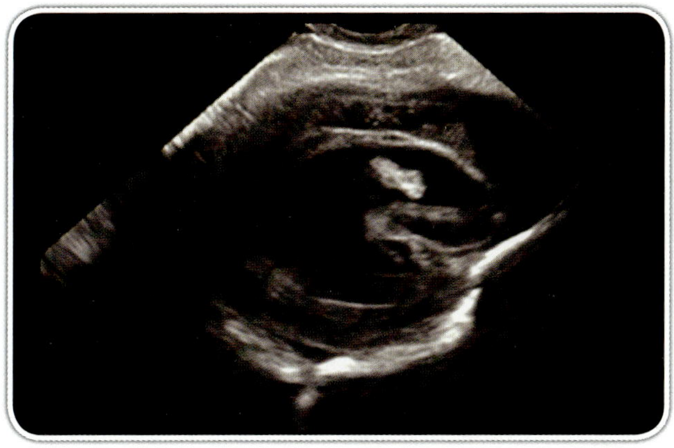

Cerebral damage

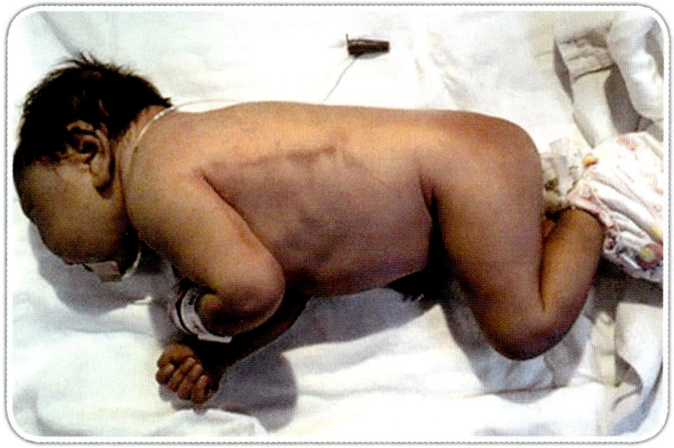

Microcephaly: Cerebral palsy

Porencephaly

as a result of agonal hypotension

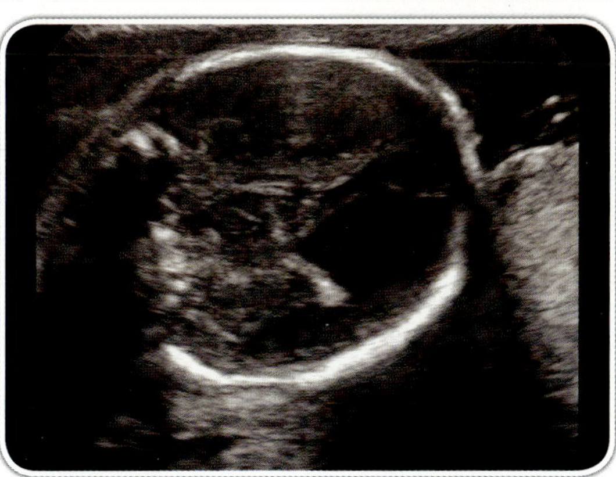

Complicated Monochorionic Twins

Intertwin transfusion related	Non-transfusion related
• Twin-twin transfusion syndrome	• Severe selective fetal growth restriction
• Reversed twin-twin transfusion syndrome	• Monoamniotic twins
• Twins anemic polycythemic sequence (TAPS)	• Conjoined twins
• Twins reversed arterial perfusion sequence (TRAPS) : Acardiac twins	

TWIN-TWIN TRANSFUSION SYNDROME (TTTS)

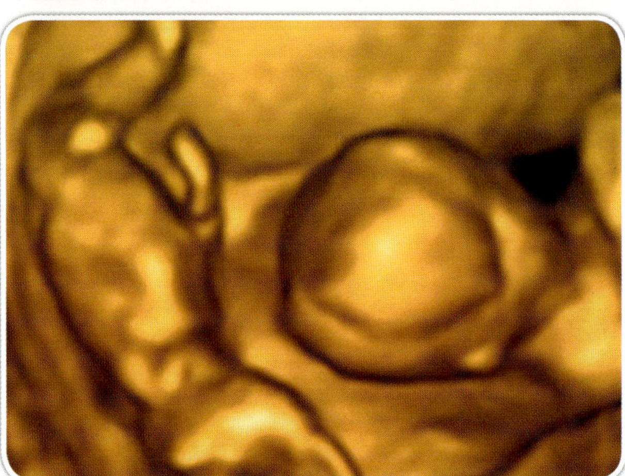

Scopes

- Clinical course
- Sonographic diagnosis
- Treatments

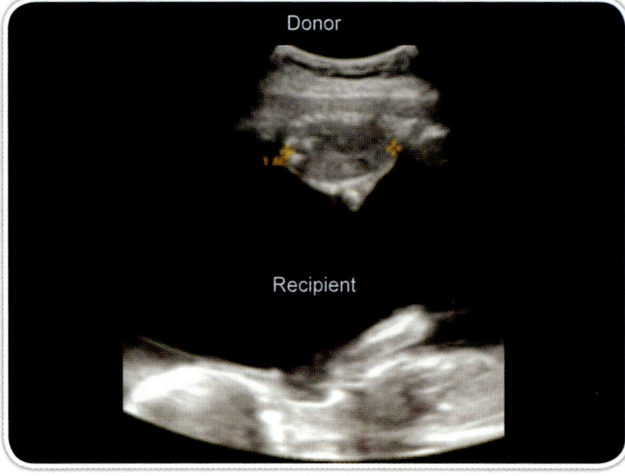

- Incidence: 5.5 – 17.5% of monochorionic twins *(Sebire et al. 1997)*
- High perinatal mortality
- Long-term neurological sequele of the surviving fetus
- Quintero's and Cincinnati's staging.

Quintero/Cincinnati TTTS

Stage 1

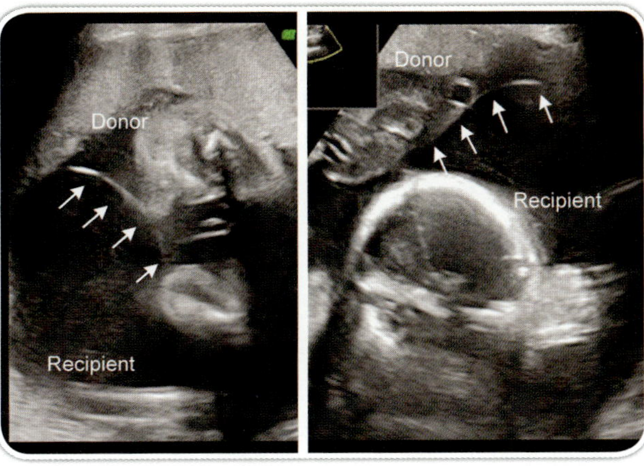

Oligo (DVP < 2 cm) Polyhydramniotic (DVP > 8 cm) sequence

Stage 2

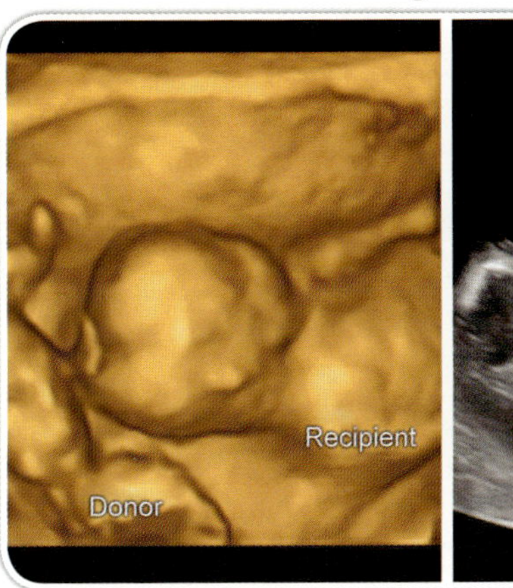

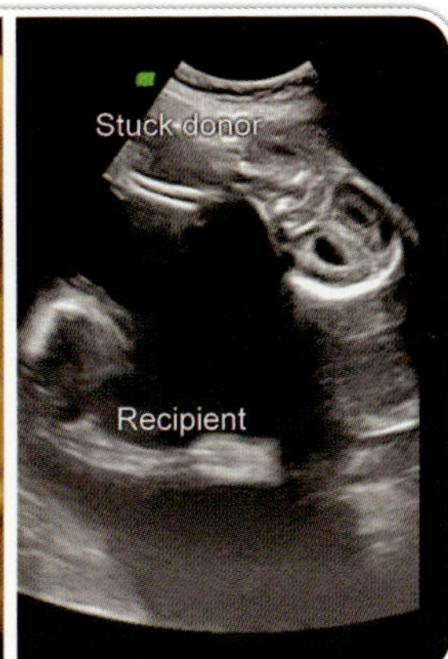

Absent urinary bladder of donor/ "stuck twin"

Stage 3A

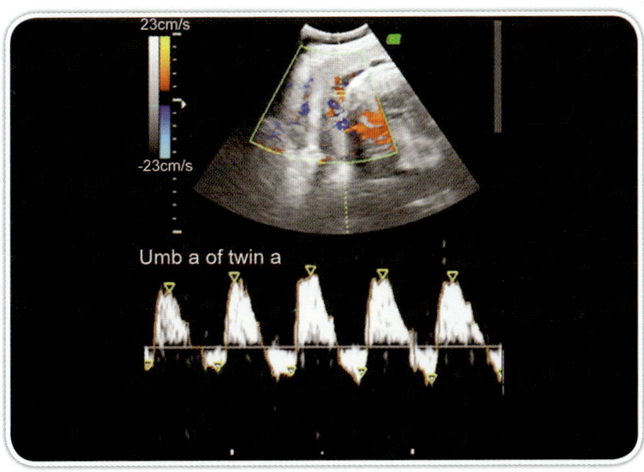

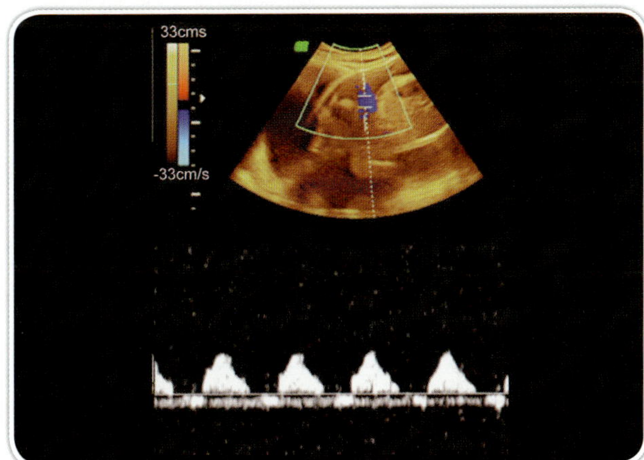

Doppler changes with intact cardiovascular profile

Stage 3B

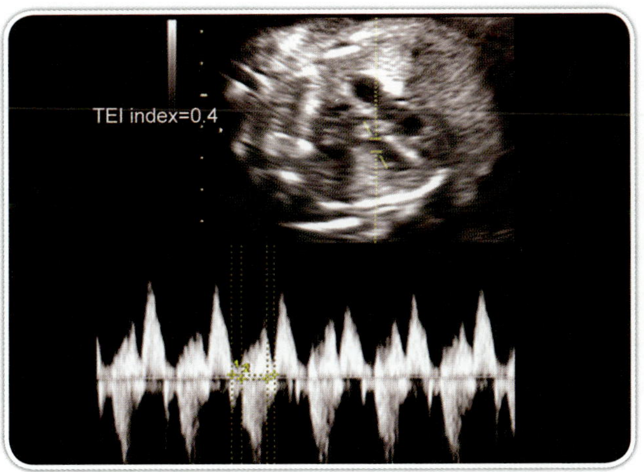

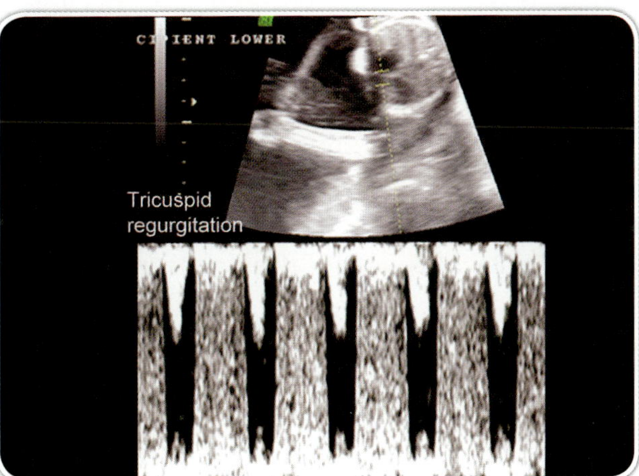

Doppler changes with impaired cardiovascular profile

Stage 4: Fetal hydrops

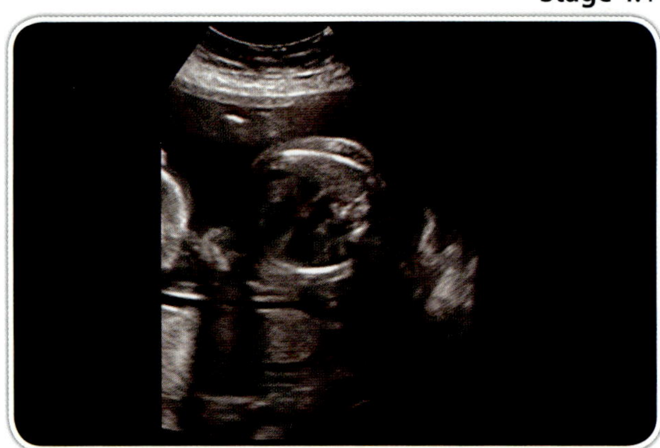

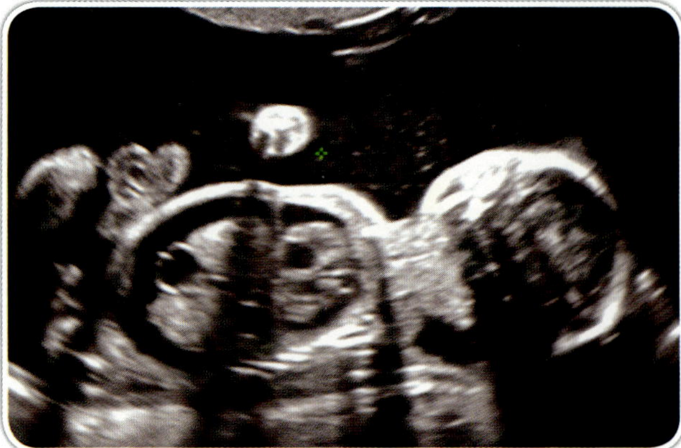

Quintero TTTS stage 5: Single/double fetal demises

Treatments of TTTS

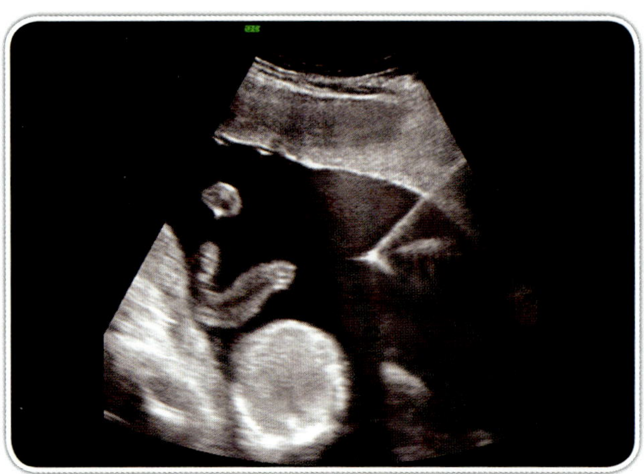

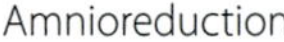

Amnioreduction

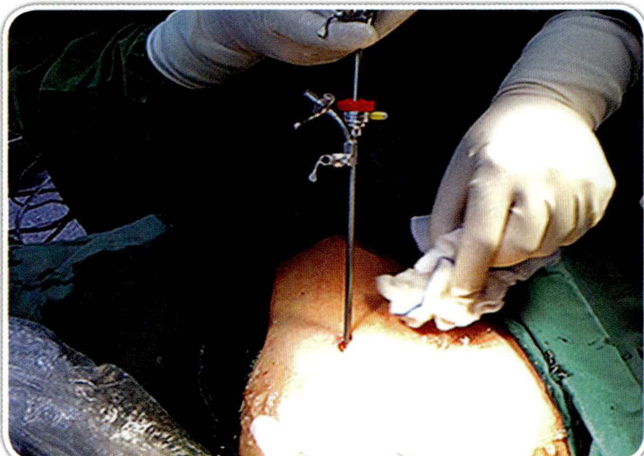

Laser photocoagulation

Chorionic Anastomoses

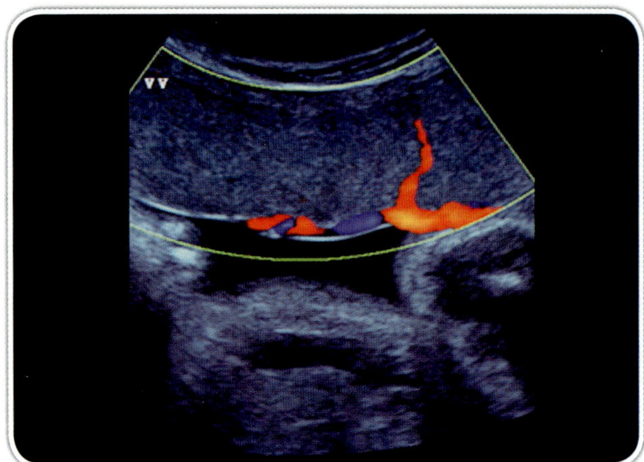

Sonographic identification

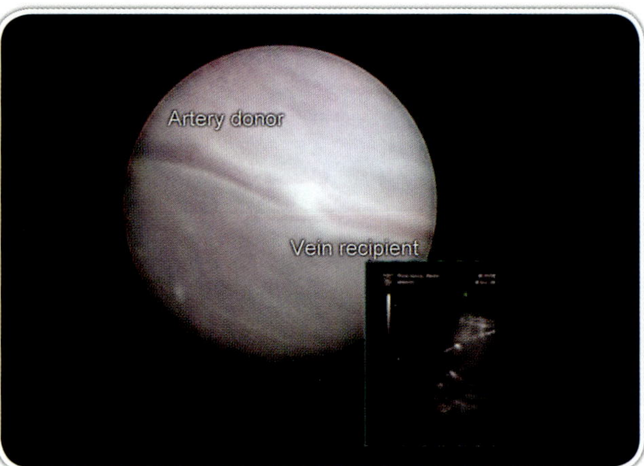

Fetoscopic identification

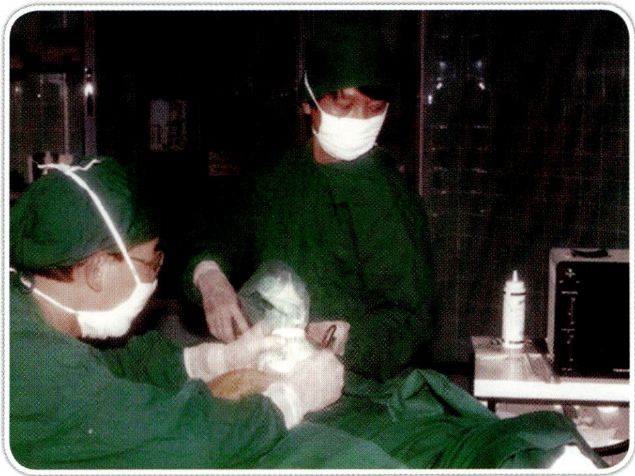

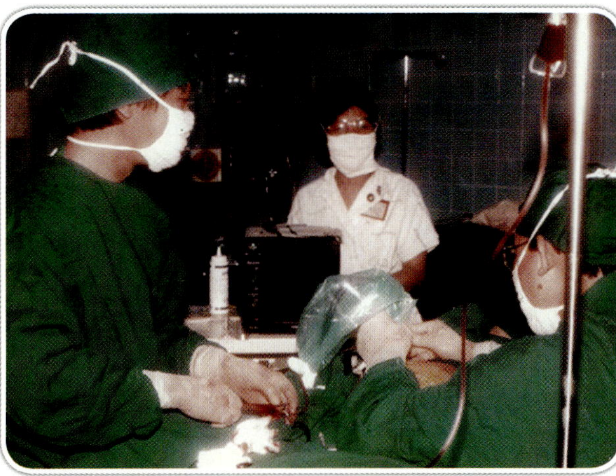

History of fetal therapy at Siriraj Hospital, Bangkok, THAILAND

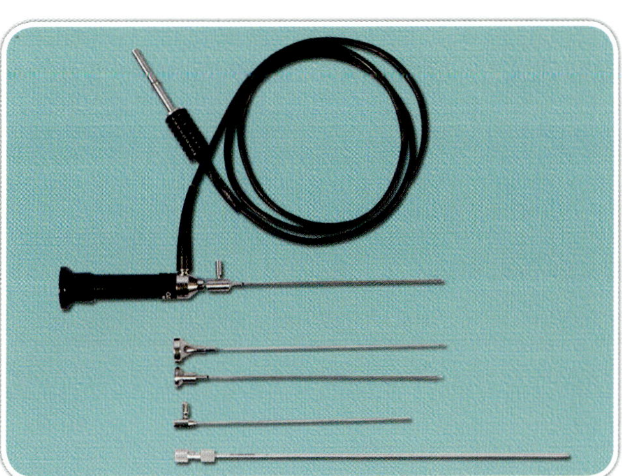

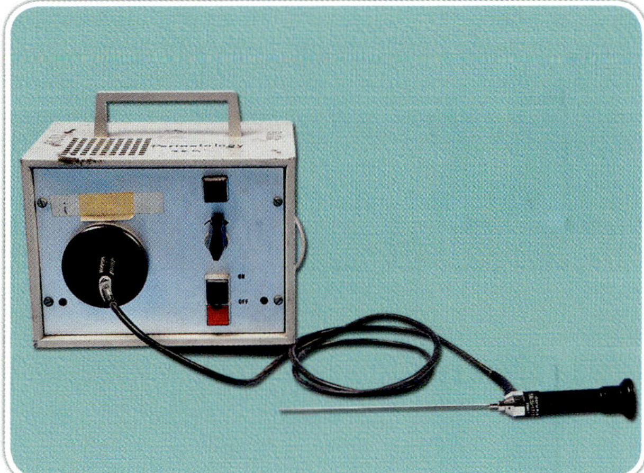

First fetoscopic set at Siriraj Hospital, Bangkok, THAILAND

Techniques of Fetoscopic Laser Photocoagulation

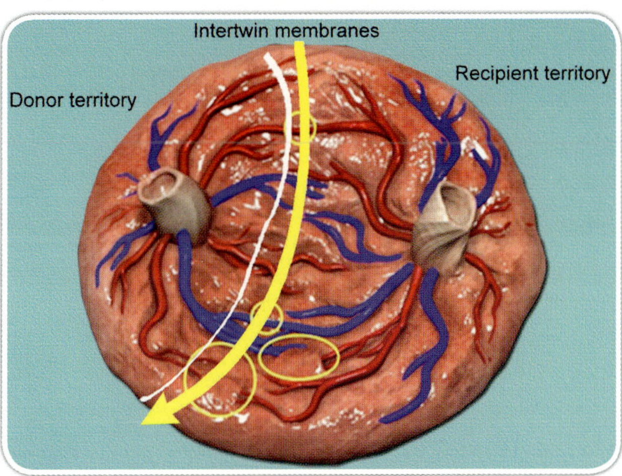

Non-selective: Along membrane equator

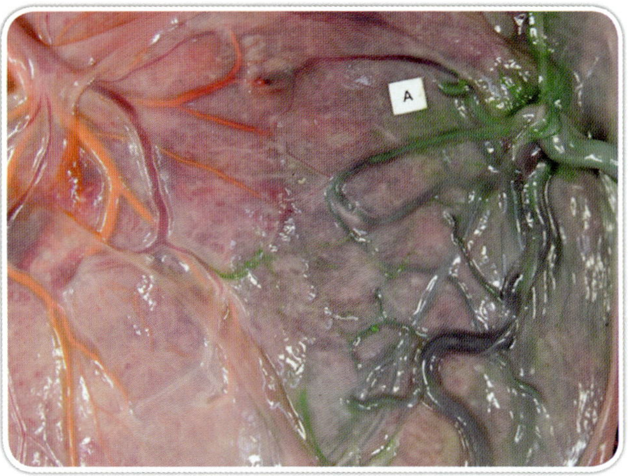

Dye injection study

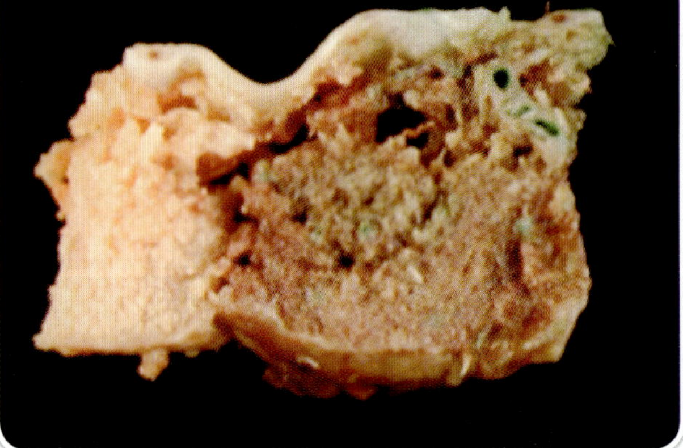

Cotyledon infarction following non-selective coagulation

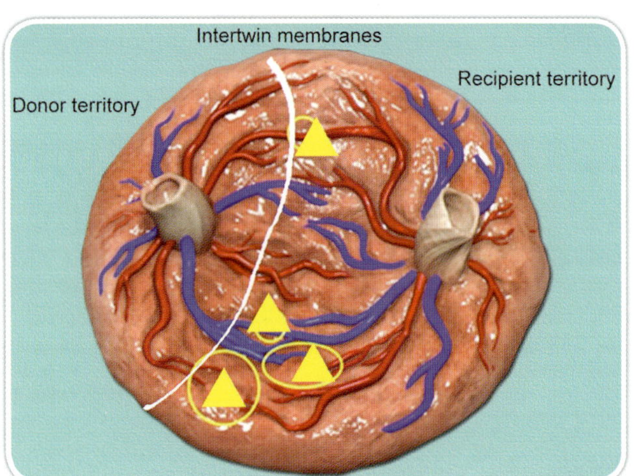

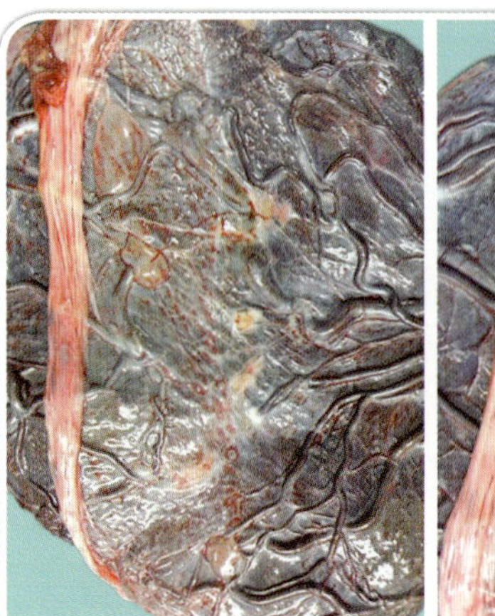

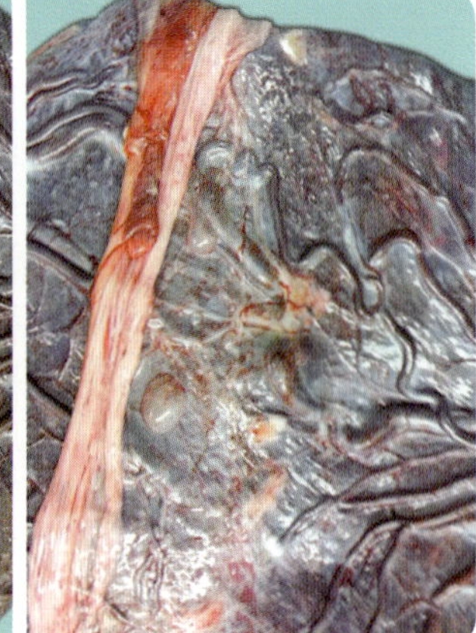

Selective: Only anastomoses

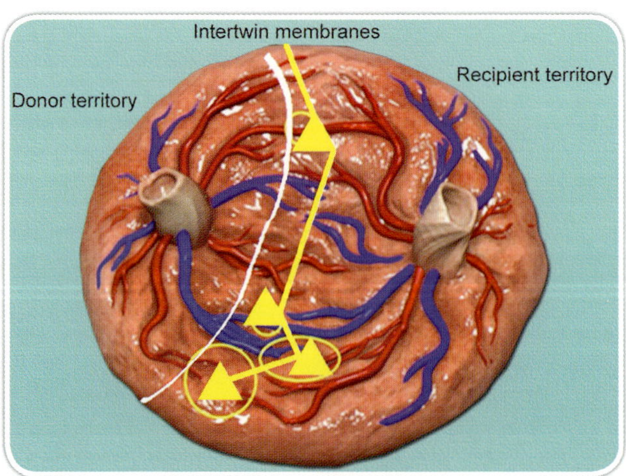

Equatorial: Selective, followed by non-selective along vascular equator

(Slaghekke et al. 2014)

Tricuspid Regurgitation and Pericardial Effusion (Transient Hydrops) in Ex-Donor

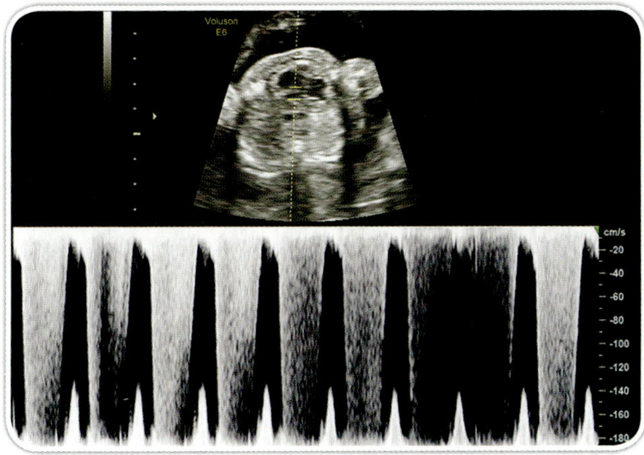

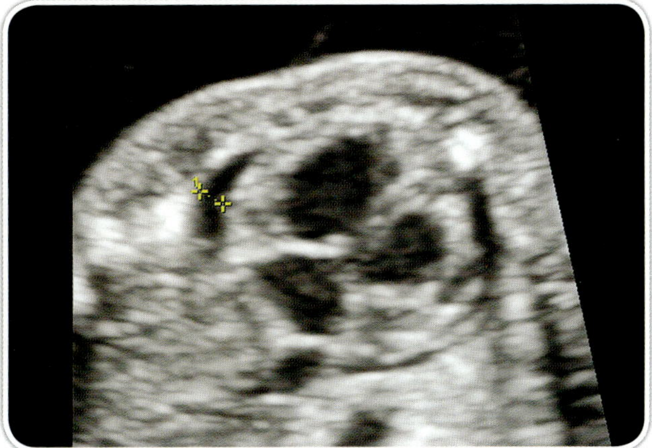

Day 1 after laser: Evidence of volume return to the ex-donor

Complications After Laser Surgery

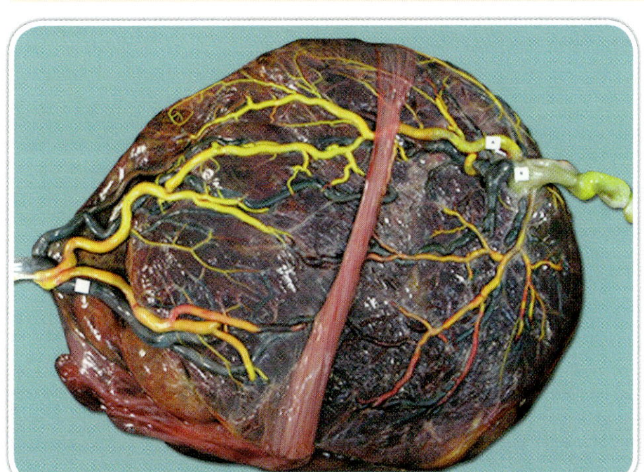

- Residual anastomoses 4–22%
- Persistent or recurrent TTTS
- TAPS
- Septostomy
- Rupture of the membranes.

(Wataganara and Kanokpongsakdi, 2008)

TTTS Stage 3 in MC Triplets

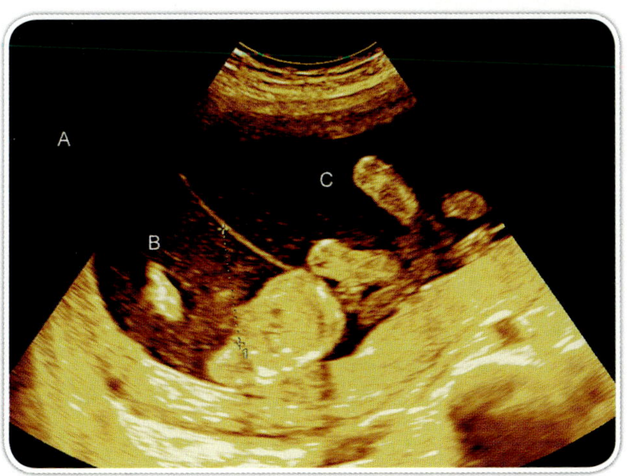

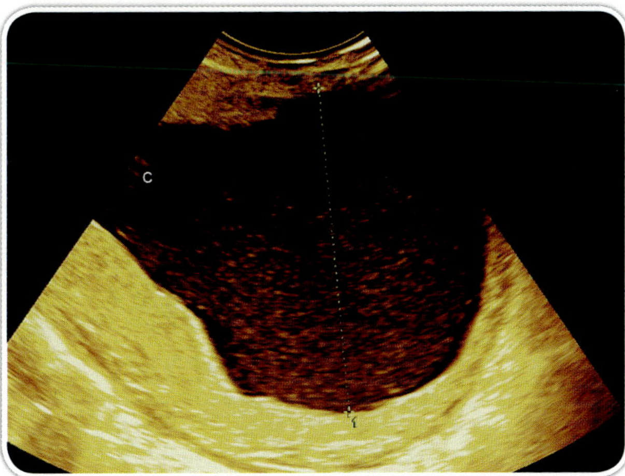

Reverse Twin-Twin Transfusion Syndrome after Fetoscopic Laser Photocoagulation of Chorionic Anastomoses: A Case Report

Tuangsit Wataganara[a] Pharuhas Chanprapaph[a] Tuenjai Chuangsuwanich[b]
Sujin Kanokpongsakdi[a] Prakong Chuenwattana[a] Vitaya Titapant[a]

[a]Division of Maternal-Fetal Medicine, Department of Obstetrics and Gynecology, and [b]Division of Pathology, Department of Medicine, Faculty of Medicine Siriraj Hospital, Bangkok, Thailand

Reverse TTTS: A unique complication from laser surgery in TTTS.

(Wataganara et al. 2009)

TWINS REVERSED ARTERIAL PERFUSION SEQUENCE (TRAPS)

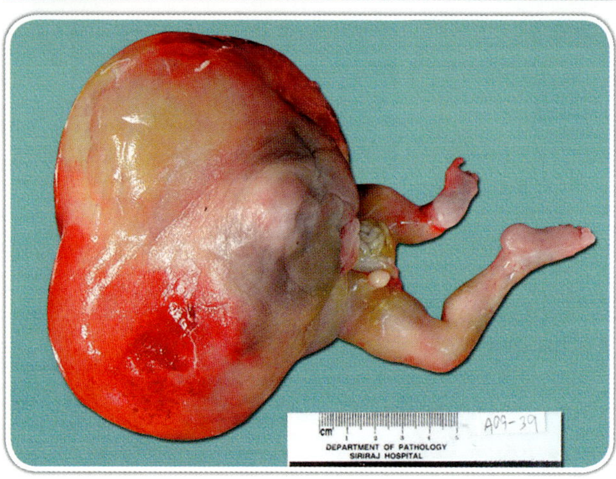

Scopes

- Sonographic diagnosis
- Clinical course
- Treatment options.

Clinical Course

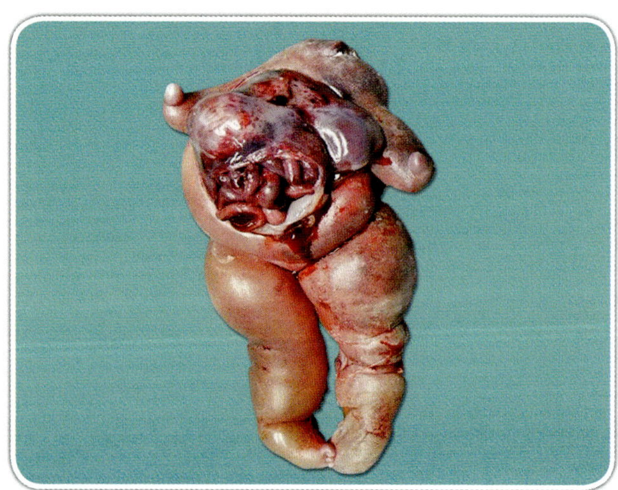

- 0.3/10,000 pregnancies

(Benirschke et al. 1977)

- The "pump twin" is smaller, but could suffer cardiac failure and hydrops
- The "acardiac twin" has atrophy of heart (acardia) and brain (acephalus).

Sonographic Diagnosis

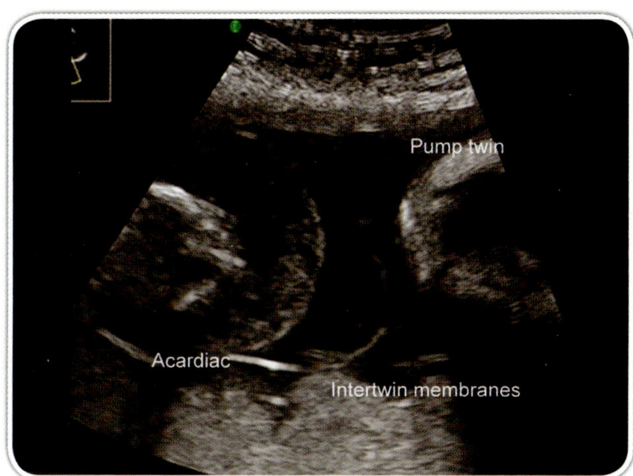

- 0.3/10,000 pregnancies

(Benirschke et al. 1977)

- Normal appearance of the 'pump twin'.

Amorphous Appearance of the Acardiac Twin

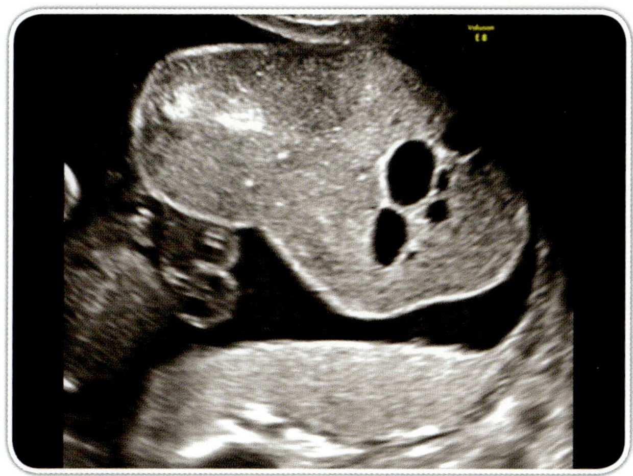

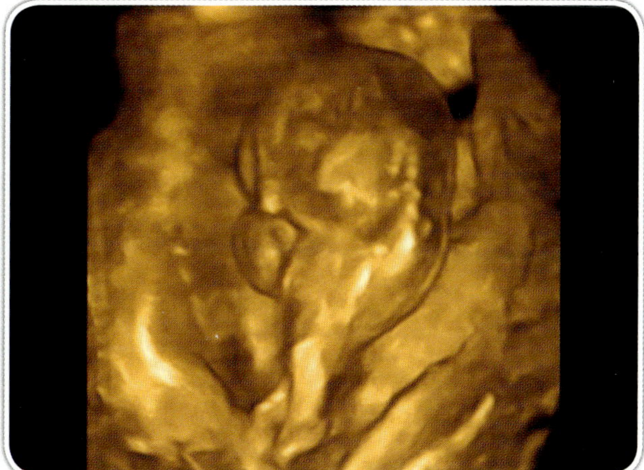

Polyhydramnios Associated with Acardiac Twin

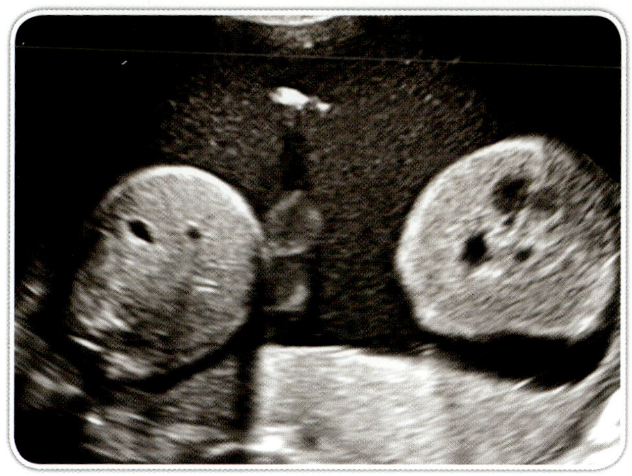

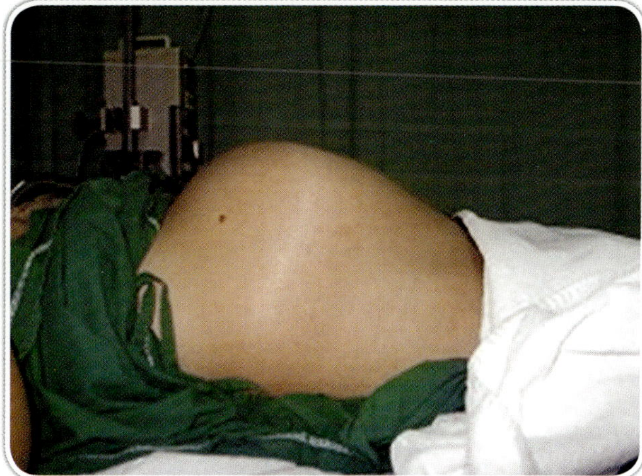

Diagnostic Appearance of the Umbilical Artery in the Acardiac Twin

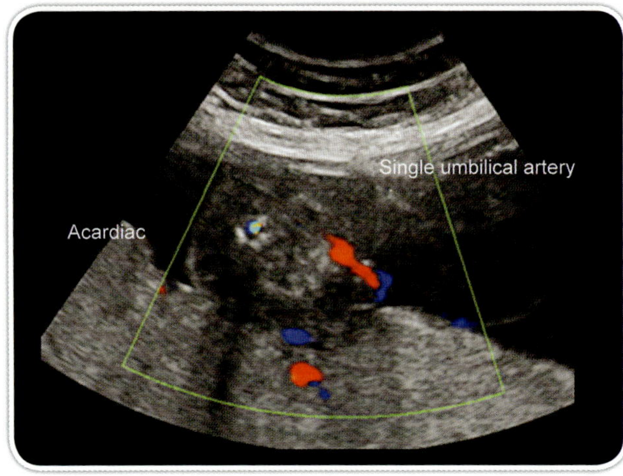

Single umbilical artery

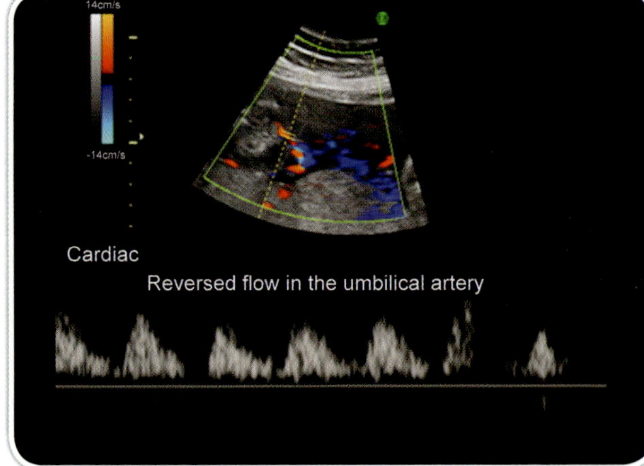

Reversed blood flow into the acardiac fetus

Volume Measurement of Acardiac Mass

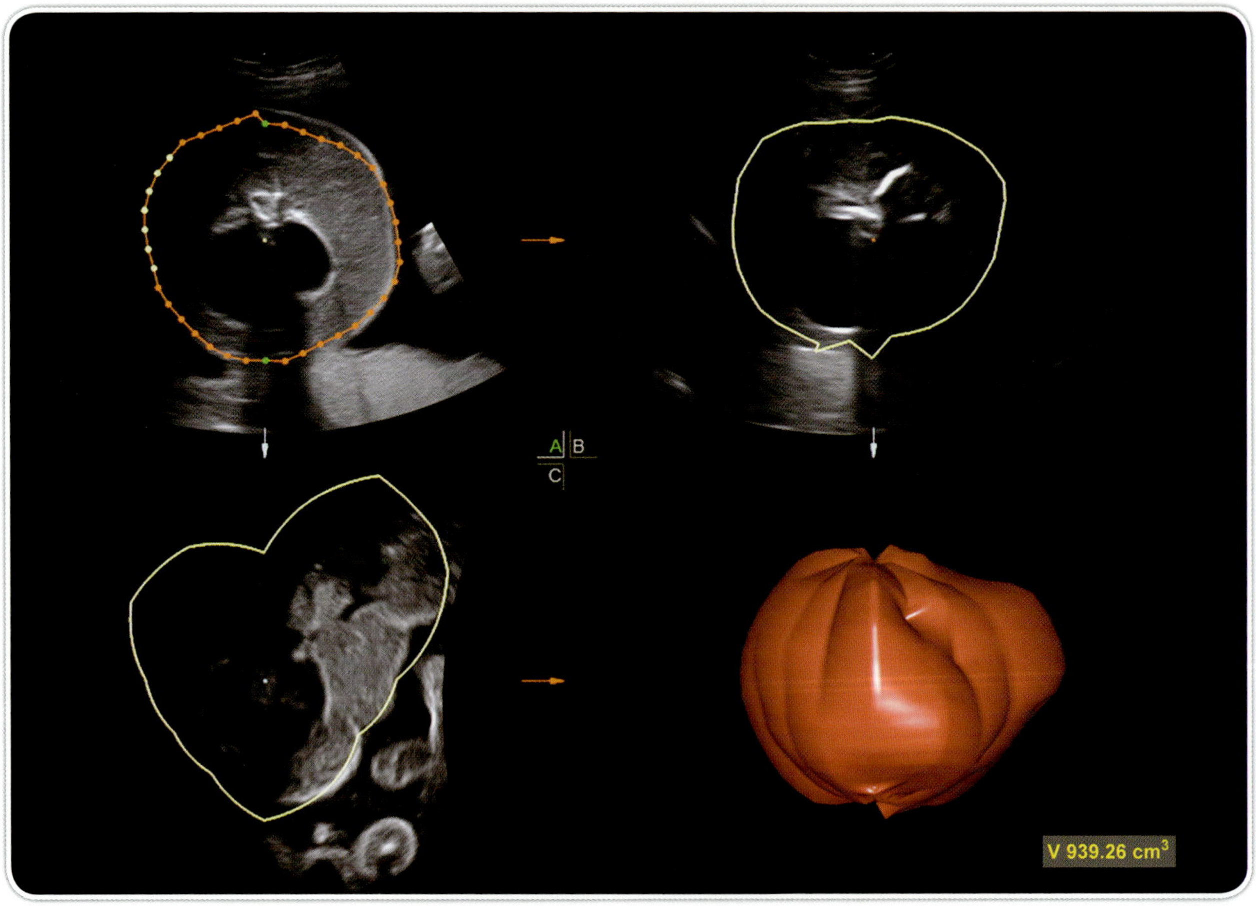

Post-termination X-ray and Angiogram

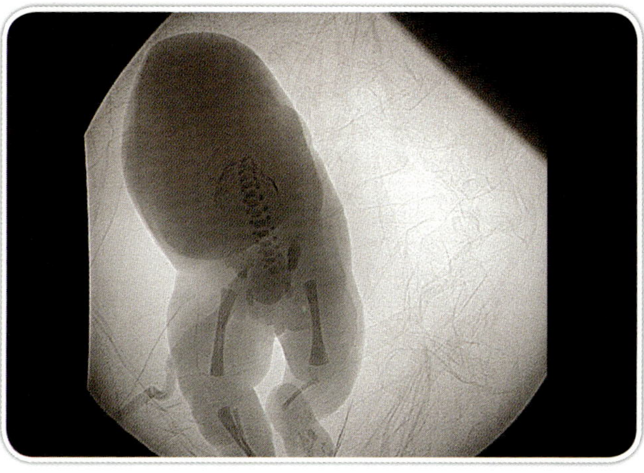

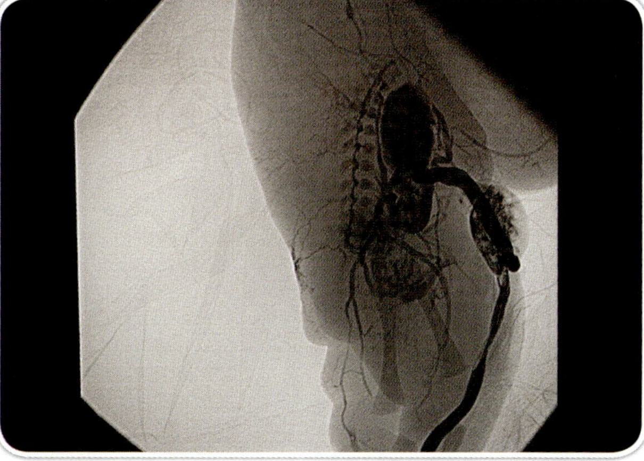

Acardiac twin has poorly developed upper torso and heart

Bipolar Coagulation of the Umbilical Cord

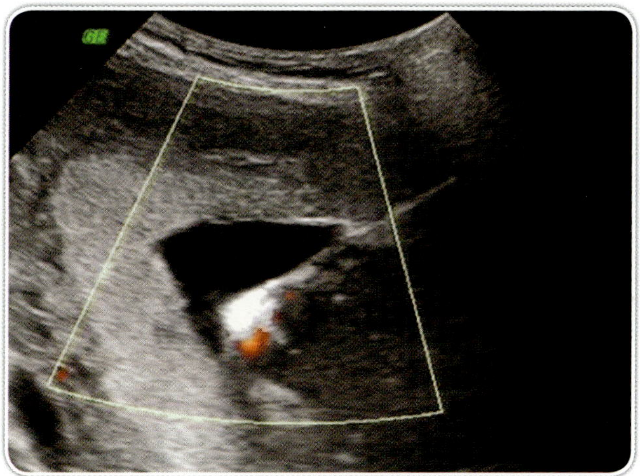

Outcomes of Bipolar Cord Occlusion

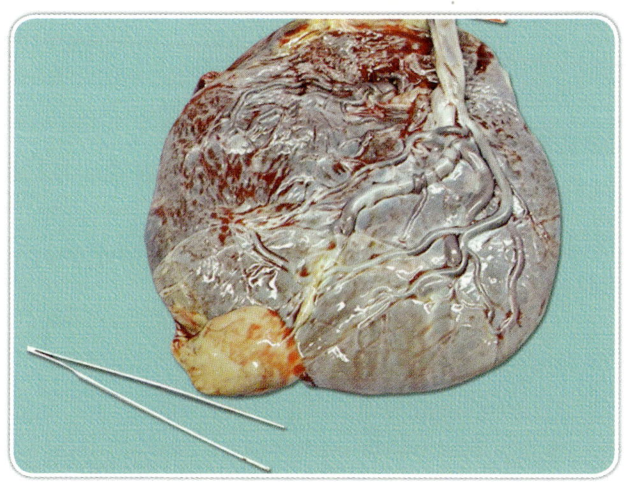

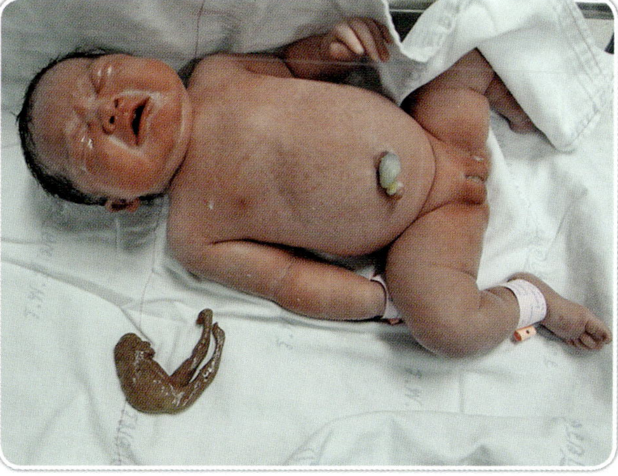

Radiofrequency Ablation (RFA)

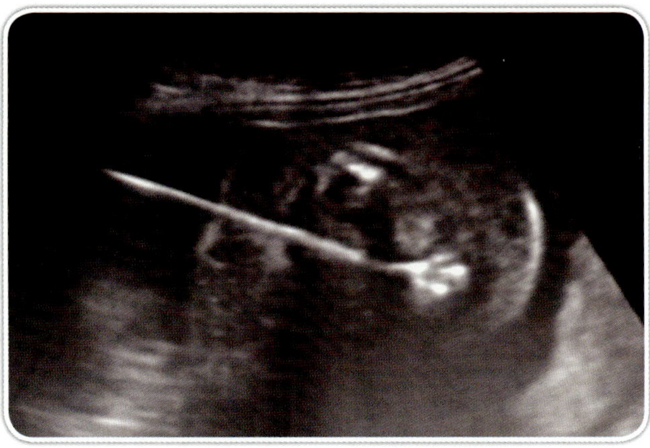

Coagulated Area Following RFA

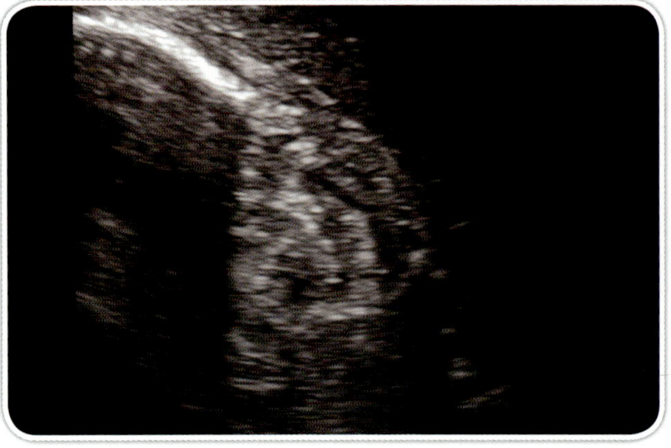

Note the golf ball hyperechoic area in the intrafetal part of umbilical vessels

(Wataganara et al. 2011)

Absence of Flow Following RFA

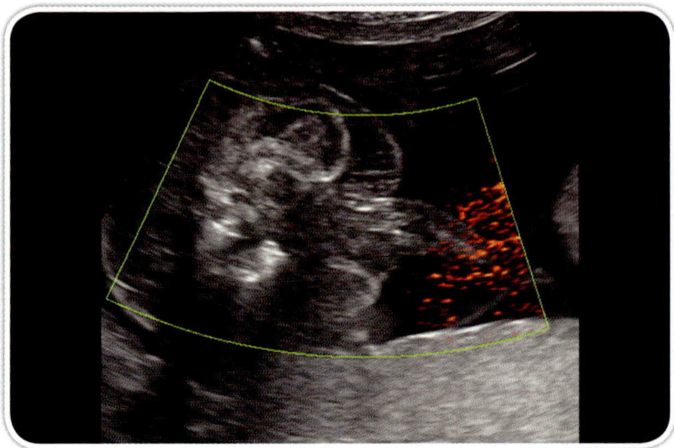

Power Doppler shows an absence of flow toward the acardiac mass

Outcomes of RFA

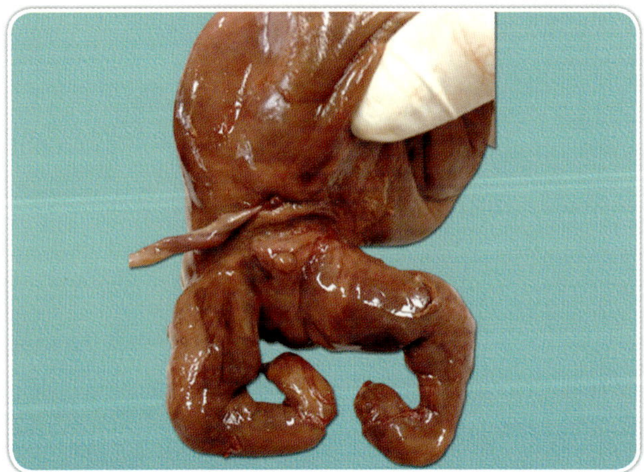

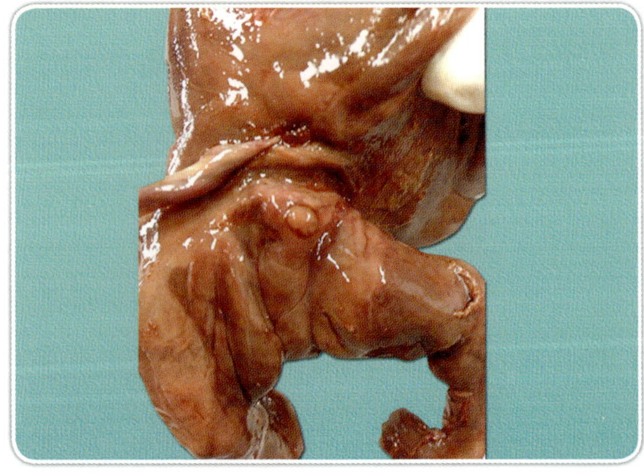

TWINS ANEMIC POLYCYTHEMIC SEQUENCE (TAPS)

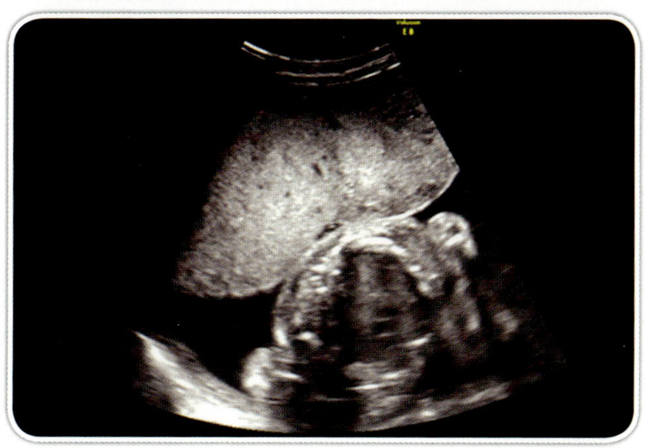

Scopes

- Sonographic diagnosis
- Clinical course
- Treatment options.

Sonographic Diagnosis

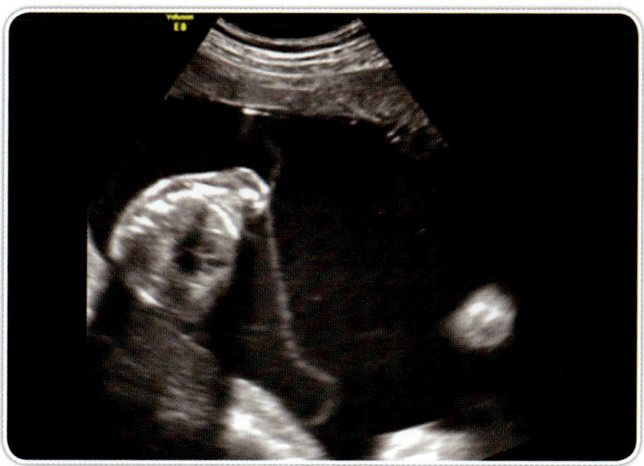

Growth and amniotic fluid discordance

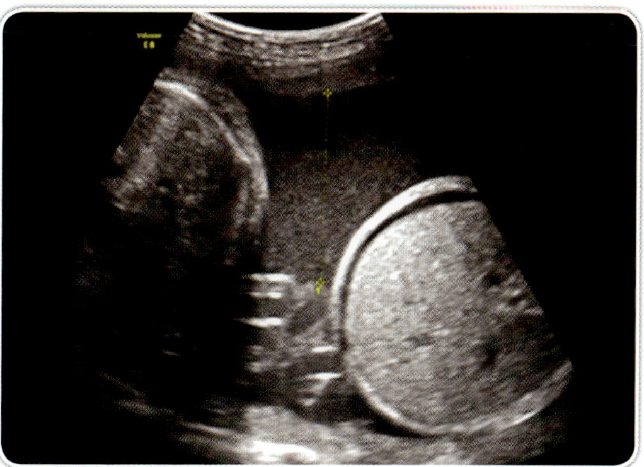

Hydrops could occur in either anemic or polycythemic twin

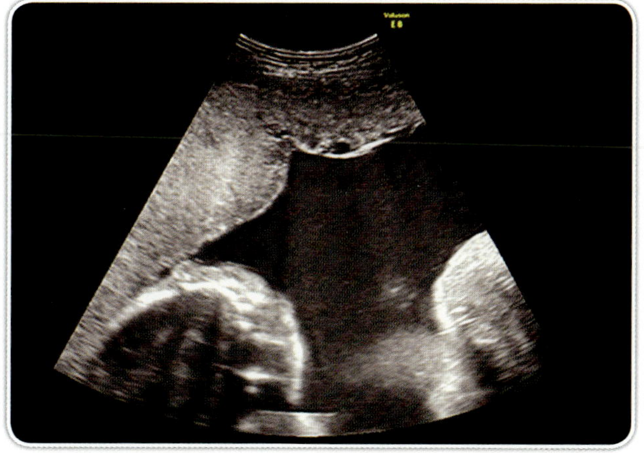

Placentomegaly reflects extramedullary hematopoiesis

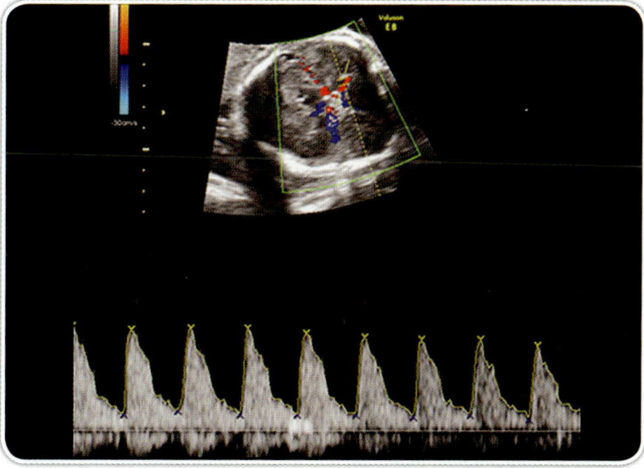

Fetal anemia can be detected by peak systolic velocity of the middle cerebral artery

SELECTIVE FETAL GROWTH RESTRICTION (sFGR)

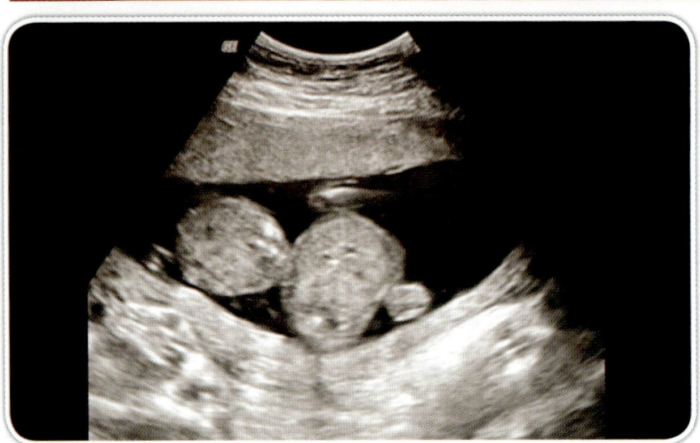

Scopes

- Sonographic diagnosis
- Clinical course
- Treatment options.

Sonographic Diagnosis

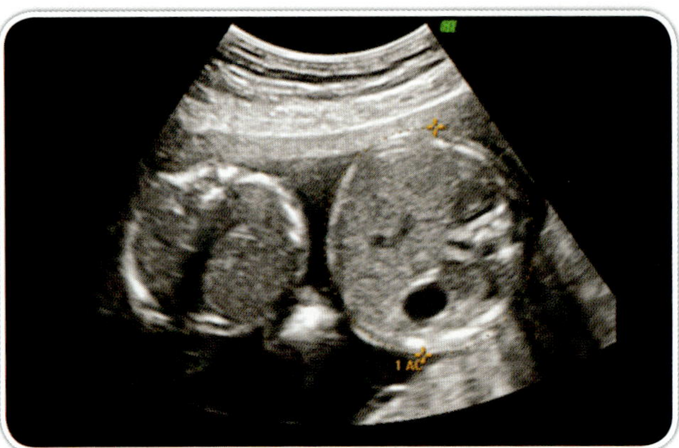

Discordant fetal weight > 25%

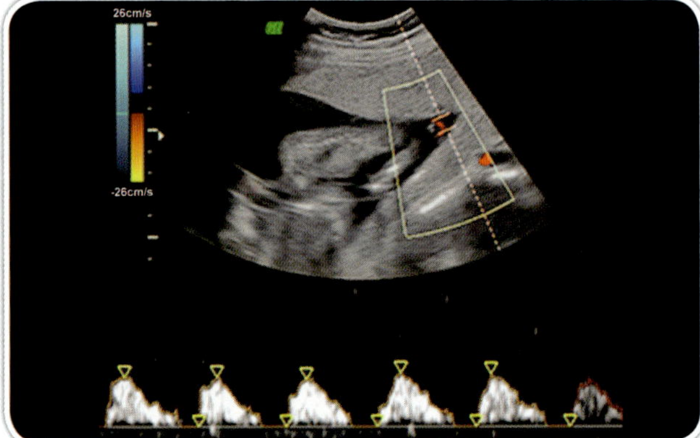

Critical Doppler changes (absent or reversed end-diastolic flow in the umbilical artery)

Marginal Umbilical Cord Insertion
Unequal Placental Territories

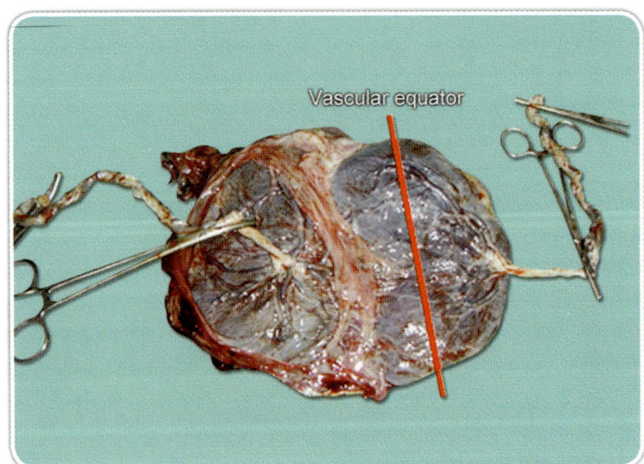

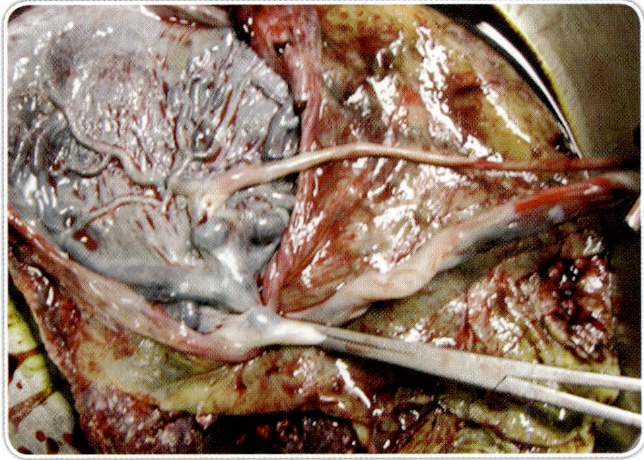

Note the difference in sizes of the umbilical cords

Prenatal Management

Expectant and timed delivery	Invasive approaches
• Close surveillance with non-stress test (NST) and Doppler	• Laser dichorionization
• Deliver when the tests are non-reassuring or at 34 to 36 weeks'	• Cord occlusion of the growth restricted fetus
• REFERENCES	

Cord Occlusion of the Growth Restricted Fetus

- **Rationale**
  - To prevent agonal hypotension that could lead to double fetal demises or brain damage if one twin dies.
- **Techniques**
  - Amnioinfusion
  - Bipolar, RFA, interstitial laser
  - Monitor for complete occlusion.

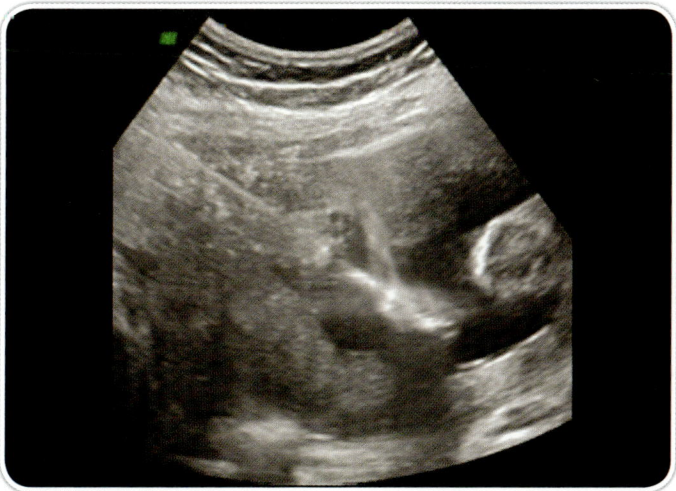

Outcome of Cord Occlusion in sFGR

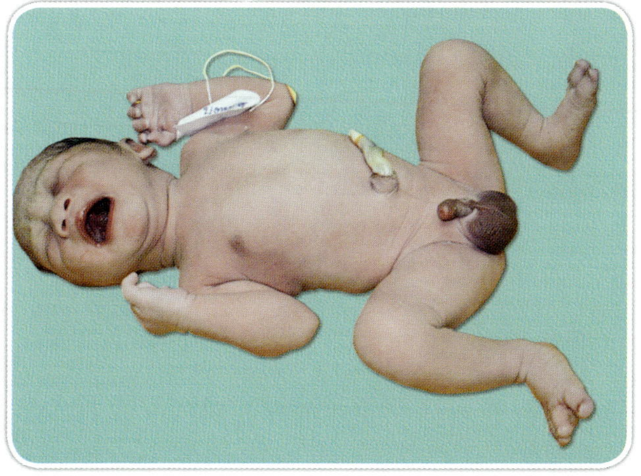

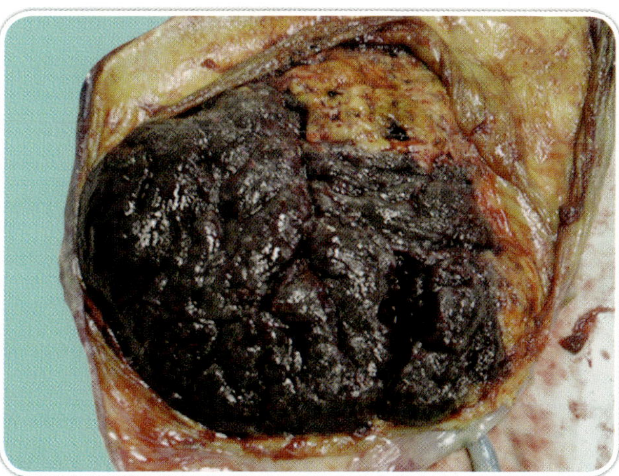

Note the infarct placental territory of the FGR fetus

DISCORDANT FETAL MALFORMATIONS IN MONOCHORIONIC TWINS

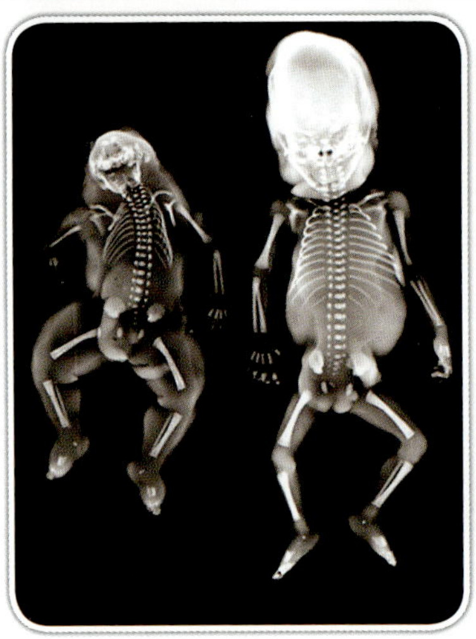

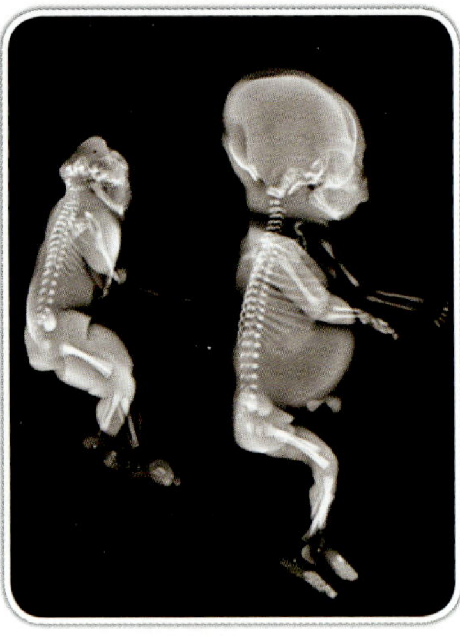

Scopes

- Sonographic diagnosis
- Clinical course
- Treatment options.

Discordant Fetal Acrania Detected During 1st Trimester Screening

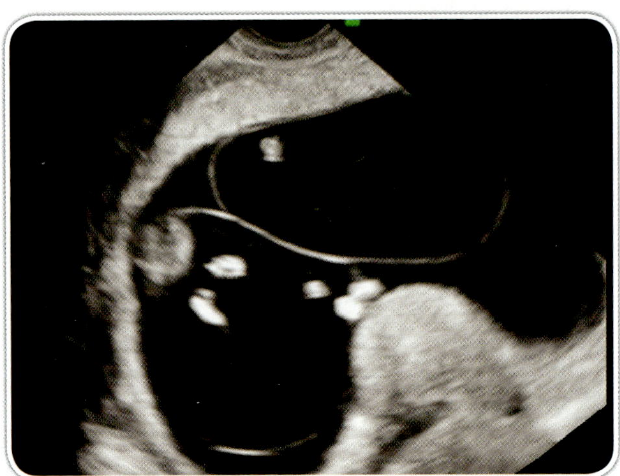

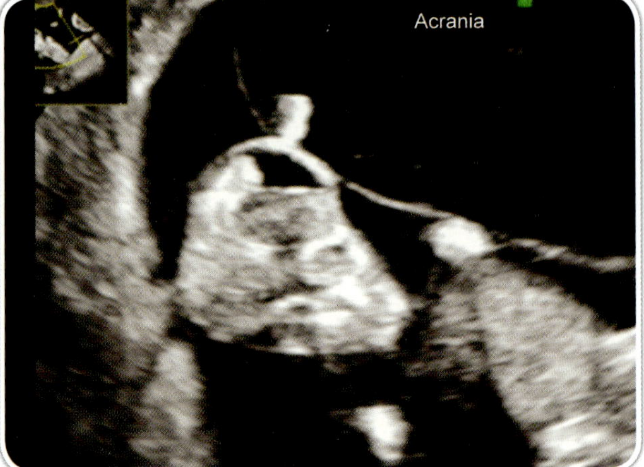

Note the ultrasound appearance of monochorionic diamniotic twins

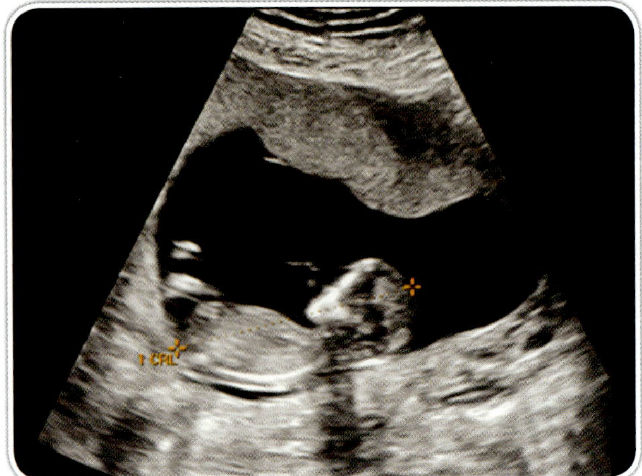

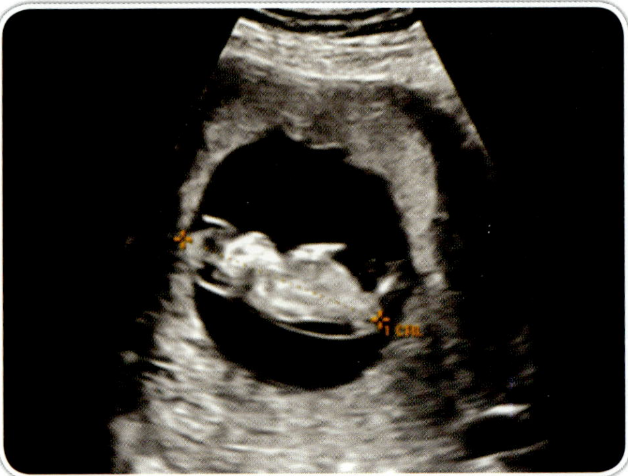

CLINICAL COURSE

- Anomalous twin could die, resulting in agonal hypotension in the other normal twin.
- Anomalous twin could have complications, such as polyhydramnios, which threaten loss of the whole pregnancy.

TREATMENT OPTIONS

- Expectant management with timed delivery
- Cord occlusion of the anomalous twin.
- Termination of the whole pregnancy

Termination of the Whole Pregnancy

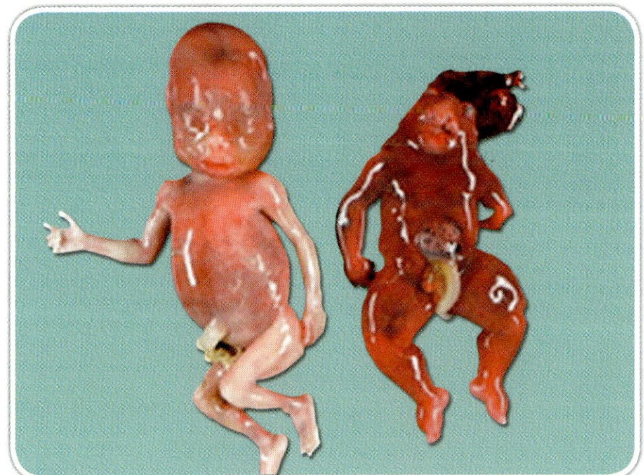

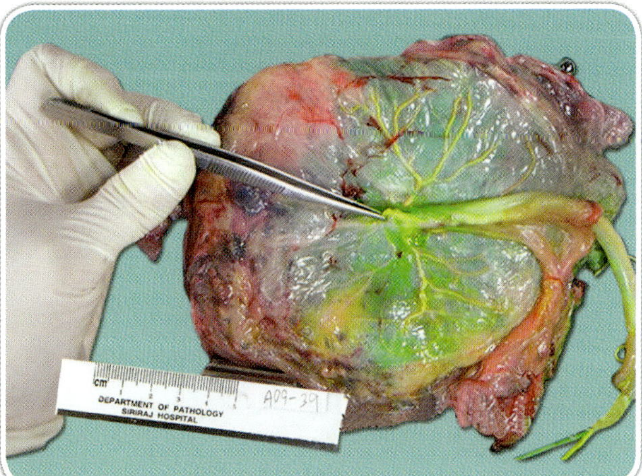

Note the communicating chorionic vessels

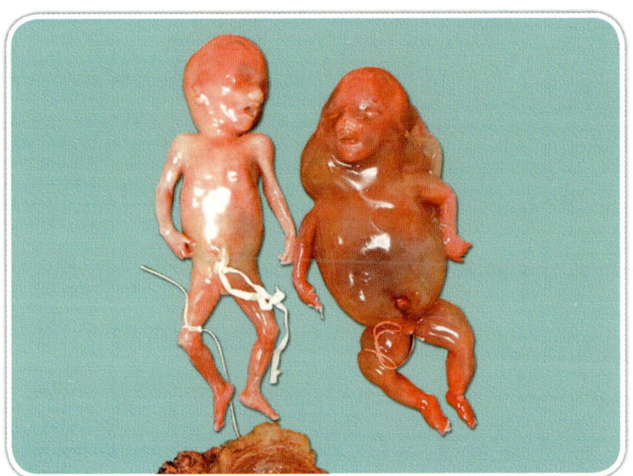

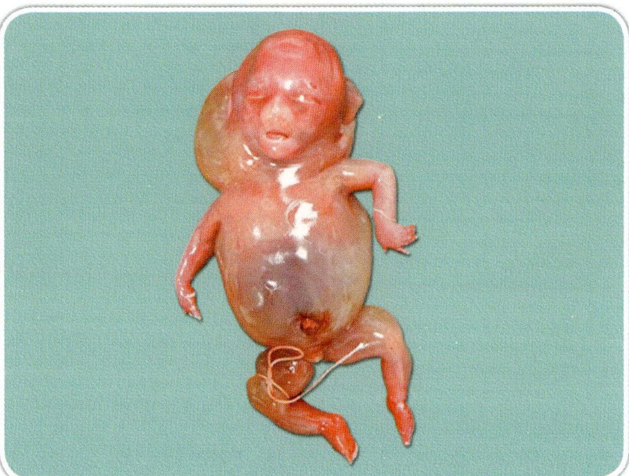

Discordant fetal cystic hygroma with hydrops

Cord Occlusion

Heterokaryotypic monochorionic twins

- Monochorionic twins with one male 46, XY and one female 45, XO
- Hydropic change in the female 45, XO fetus threatened loss of the whole pregnancy or agonal hypotension of the male 46, XY co-twin.

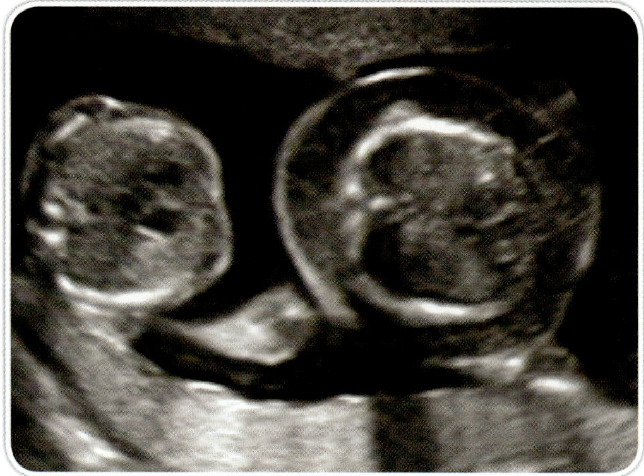

(Wataganara et al. 2012)

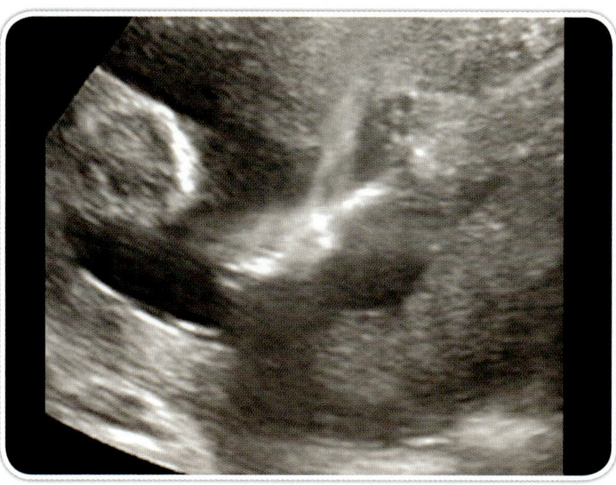

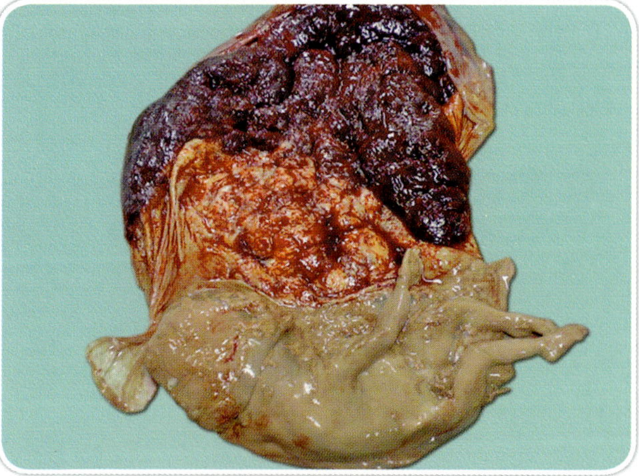

- Apparently healthy baby boy was delivered at 36 weeks'
- Note the cord-occluded 45, XO fetus with its infarct placental territory

Follow Up at 2 Years of Age

6% 45, XO mosaicism was diagnosed from fluorescent in situ hybridization (FISH) of the lymphocytes

(Wataganara et al. 2012)

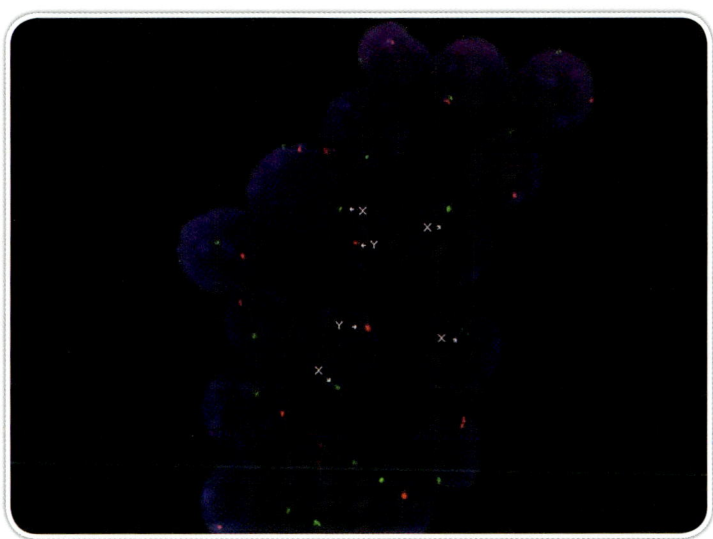

COMPLICATED MONOAMNIOTIC TWINS

Scopes

- Sonographic diagnosis
- Clinical course
- Treatment options.

Monoamniotic Twins

- Incidence: 1: 8,000 pregnancies or 5% of monochorionic twins.

(Sebire et al. 2000)

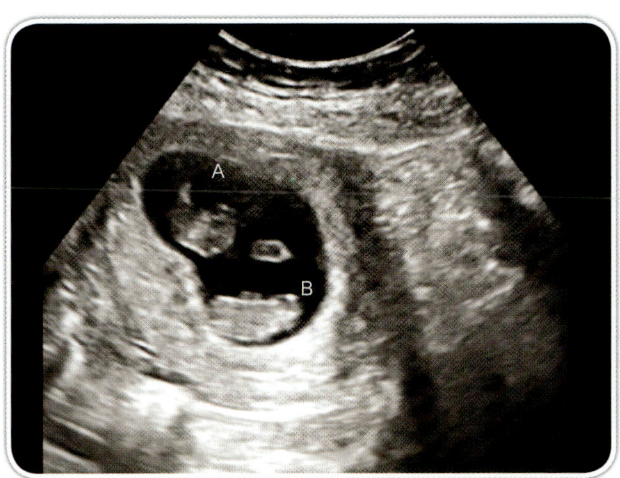

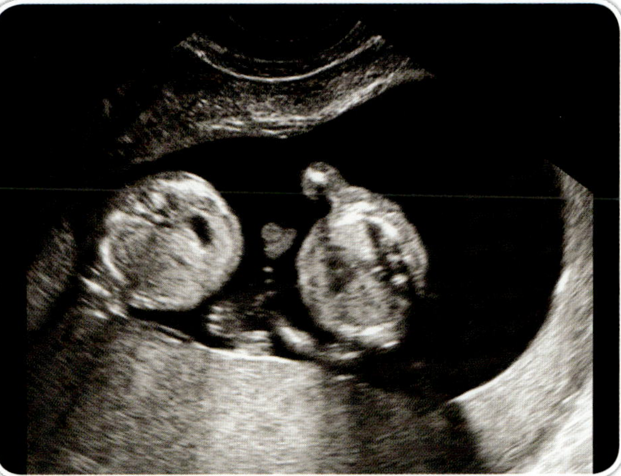

Umbilical Cord Entanglement

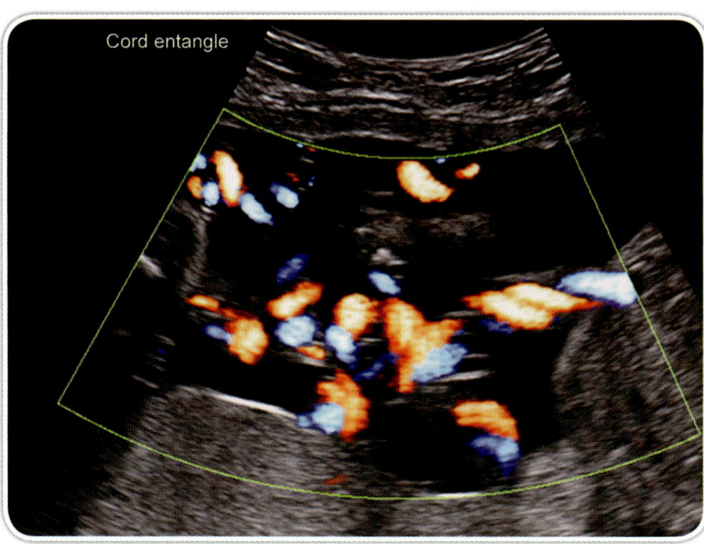

Umbilical Cord Entanglement 3D Sonoangiography

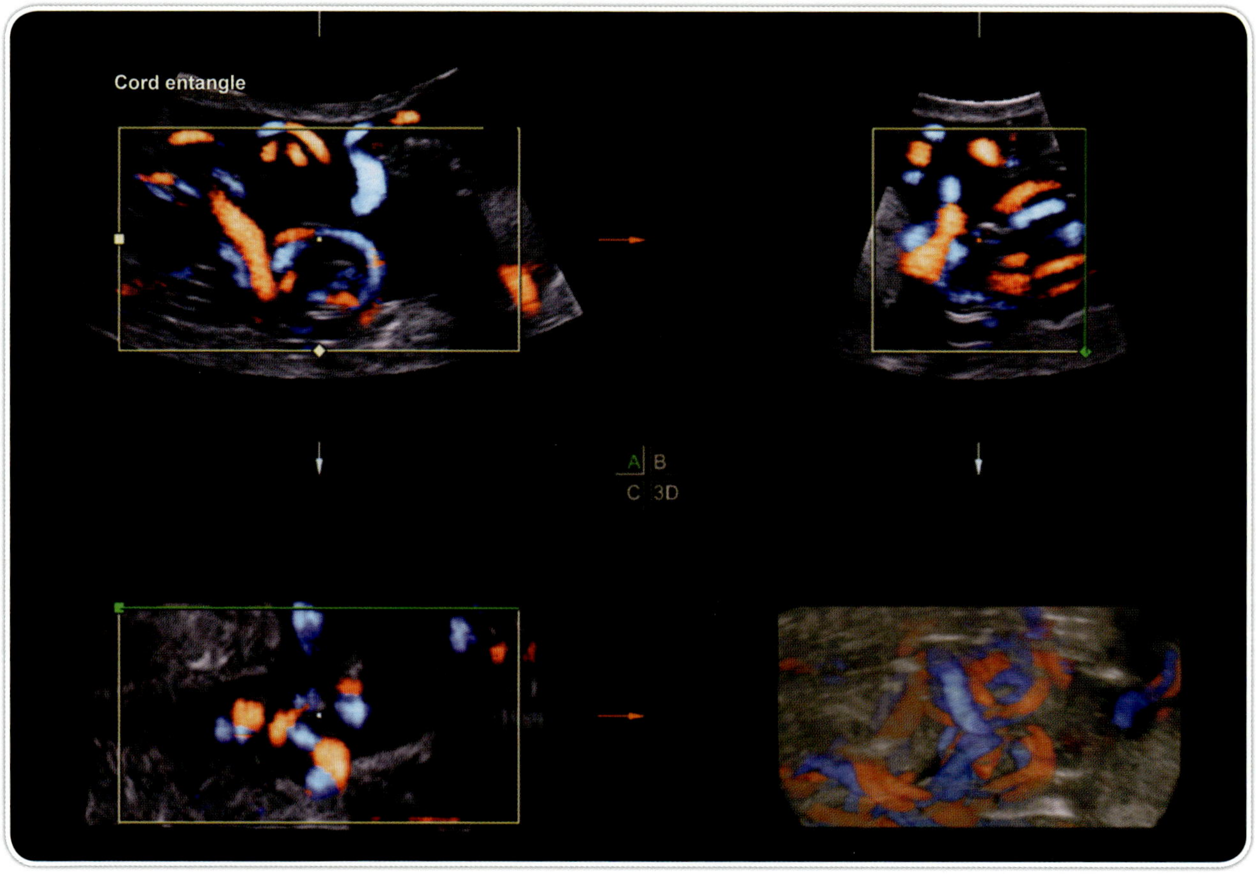

Umbilical Cord Entanglement Pulsed-Wave Ultrasound Examination

- Simultaneous recording of two different heart rates within the same pulsed-wave sampling gate

(Arabin et al. 1999)

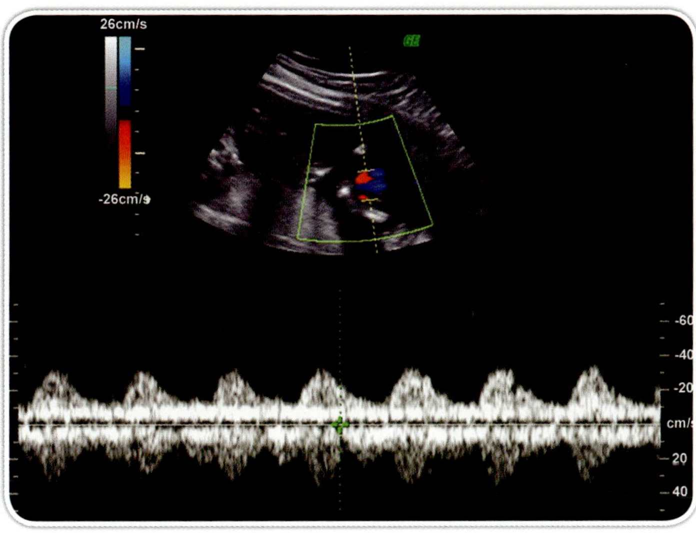

Clinical Impact of Umbilical Cord Entanglement

- Perinatal mortality in MA twins is mainly from conjoined twins, TRAP, discordant anomaly and spontaneous miscarriage
- Expectant management in cord entanglement has a very good prognosis
- The practice of early delivery should be reviewed.

(Dias et al. 2010)

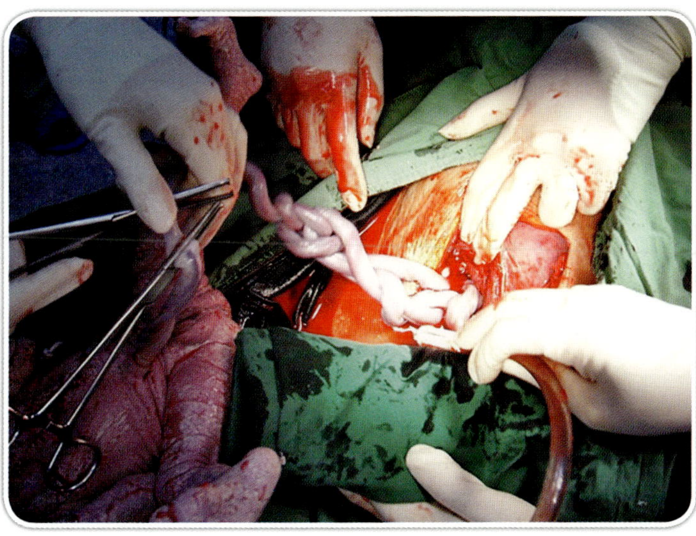

Cord Entanglement with Discordant Fetal Anomalies

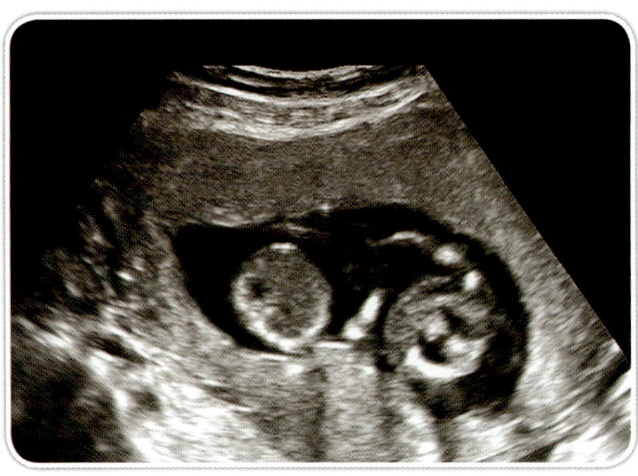

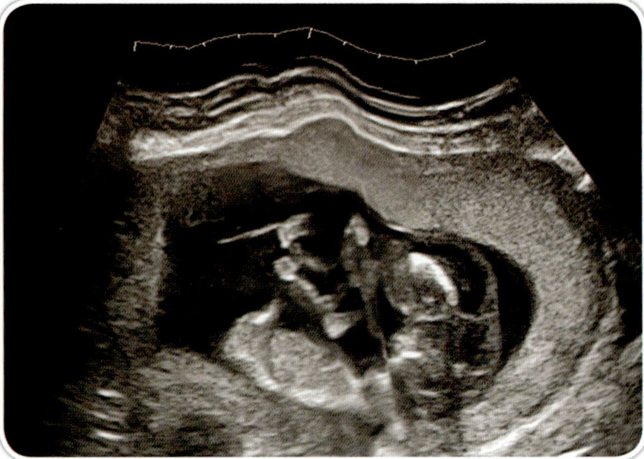

Note that one fetus has cystic hygroma with bilateral pleural effusion

Cord Entanglement with Discordant Fetal Anomalies: 3D US

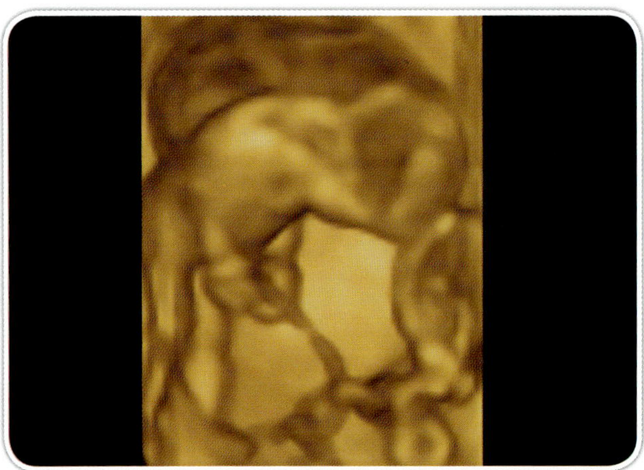

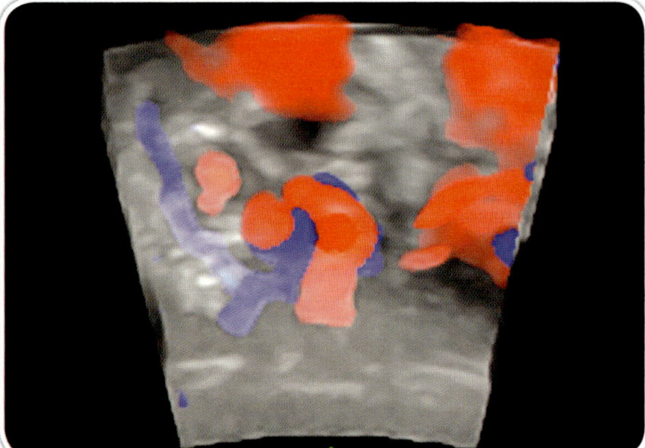

Cord Entanglement with Discordant Fetal Anomalies

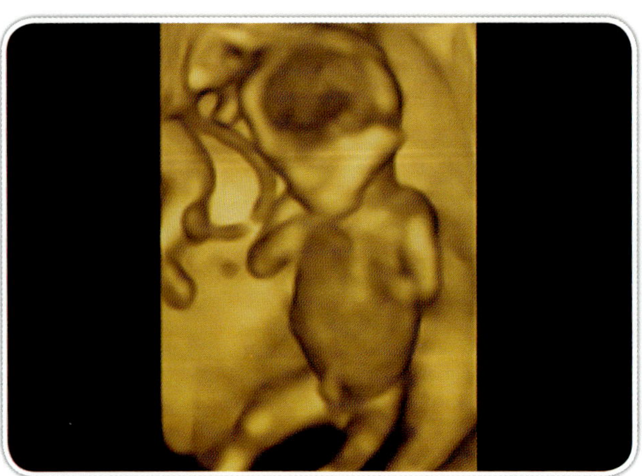

- If the fetus with cystic hygroma dies, the normal fetus can suffer from agonal hypotension.

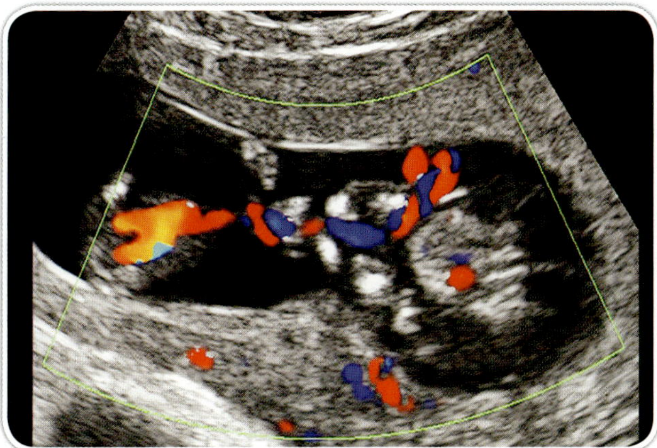

- Bipolar cord occlusion cannot be performed safely due to the cord entanglement.
- Interstitial laser or RFA, therefore, are more suitable.

Technique of Interstitial Laser

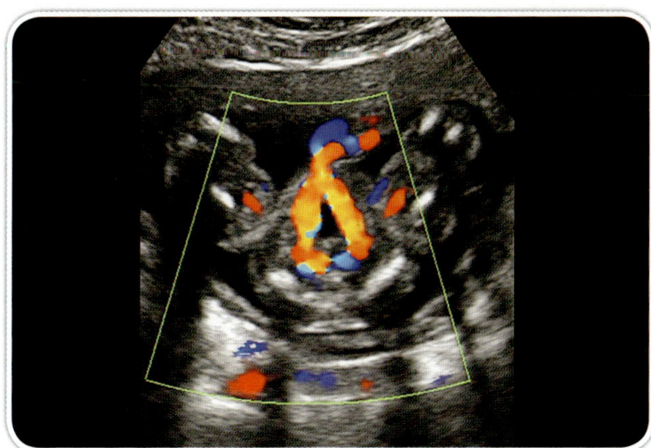

- Nd:YAG laser fiber is inserted through the chorionic villus sampling needle (16G)
- It is targeting at intrafetal part of the umbilical arteries.

Outcome of Interstitial Laser

Discordant fetal anomalies with cord entanglement

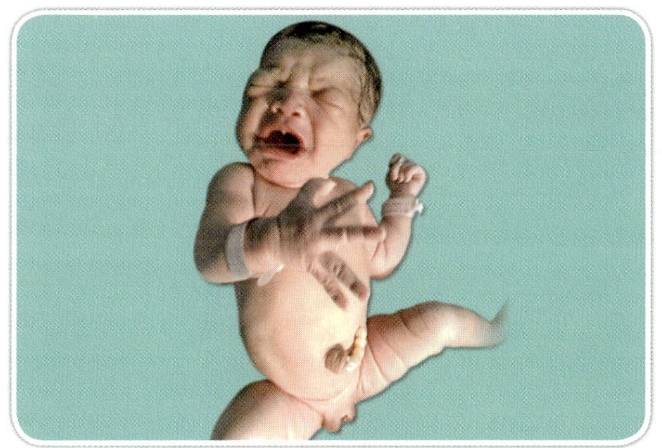

Normal fetus

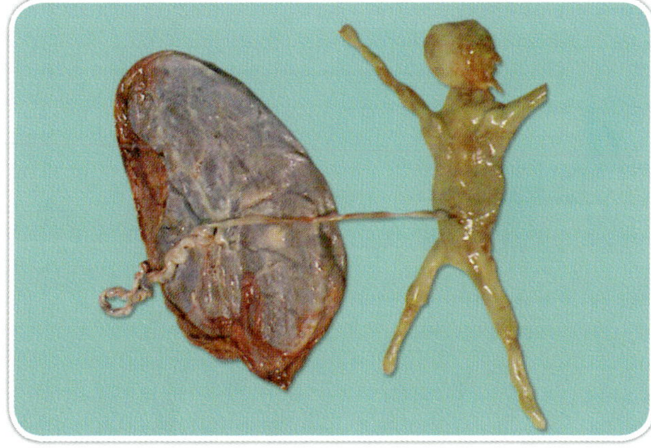

Fetus with cystic hygroma

Note the cord entanglement

Techniques for Cord Occlusion

Techniques	Success rate (technical/clinical)	
Sclerosing substances (i.e. ethanol) and embolization (i.e. coil)	33%	Recanalization or migration of coils
US or fetoscopic guided cord ligation	62%	PPROM 30%, technical difficulties, multiple ports
Monopolar thermocoagulation	?	
Laser cord transection		Higher failure with more advanced gestational age (> 20 wks')
Bipolar diathermy	80%	Higher failure with more advanced gestational age (> 20 wks')
Radiofrequency ablation	90%	Low chance of terminating the wrong fetus
Harmonic scalpel	?	Require laparotomy

Complications of Cord Occlusion Fetal

- Incomplete occlusion, leading to cerebral damages
- Ruptured cord, leading to exanguination
- Amniotic band sequence
- Preterm labor, preterm PROM
- Accidental septostomy, leading to cord accident or amniotic band sequence.

Complications of Cord Occlusion Maternal

- Myometrial bleeding
- Placental abruption
- Amniotic fluid leakage
- Infection
- Burn at the grounding plate

Screening Recommendation for the Surviving Fetus

- US on the following day, then weekly starting from 24 weeks'
- Specifically look for signs of exanguination (Vmax MCA) and cerebral damages (ventriculomegaly or porencephaly)
- MRI when there is a suspicion from the US, or at 30 weeks'.

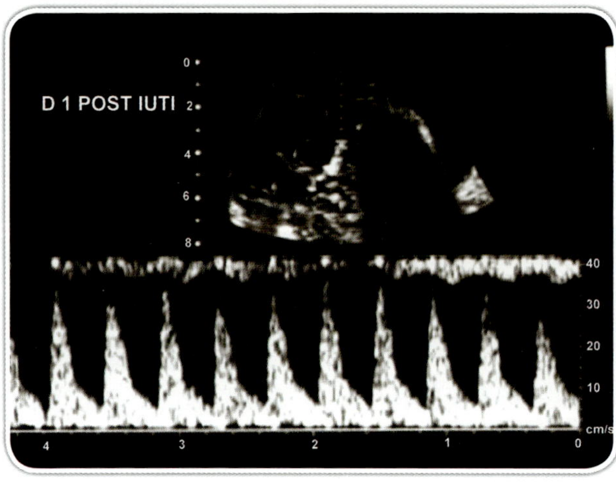

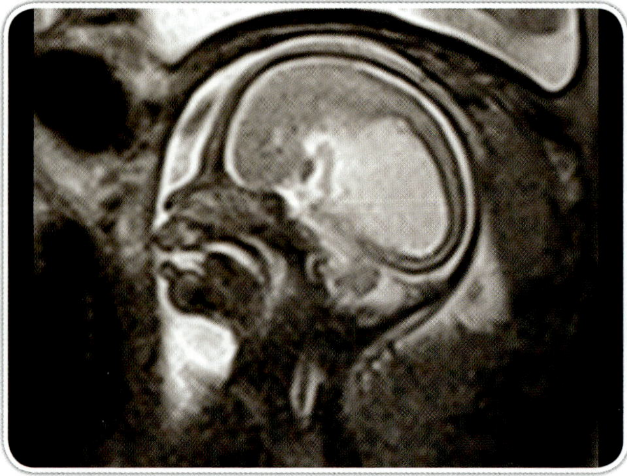

CONJOINED TWINS

Scopes

- Sonographic diagnosis
- Clinical course
- Treatment options

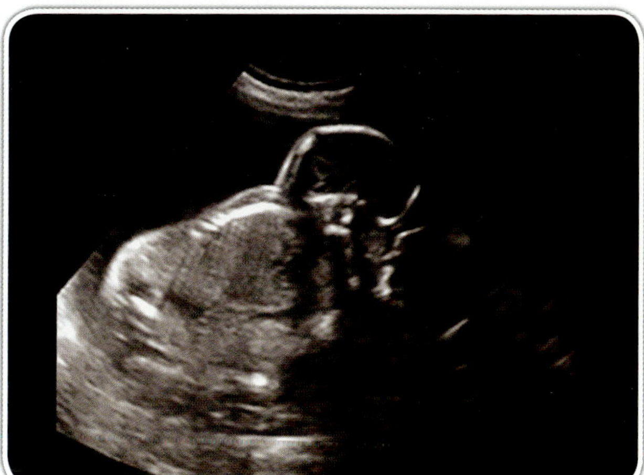

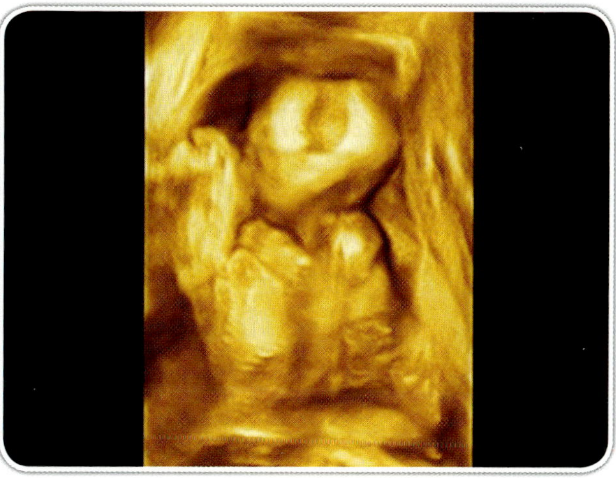

Conjoined Twins: Ultrasound Diagnosis

- Apparent fusion
- No separating membranes
- Anomalies in a twin pair
- More than three vessels in the umbilical cord

(Koontz et al. 1983)

- Both fetal heads persistently at the same level
- Backward flexion of the cervical and upper thoracic spine
- No change in the relative positions of the fetuses.

(Koontz et al. 1983)

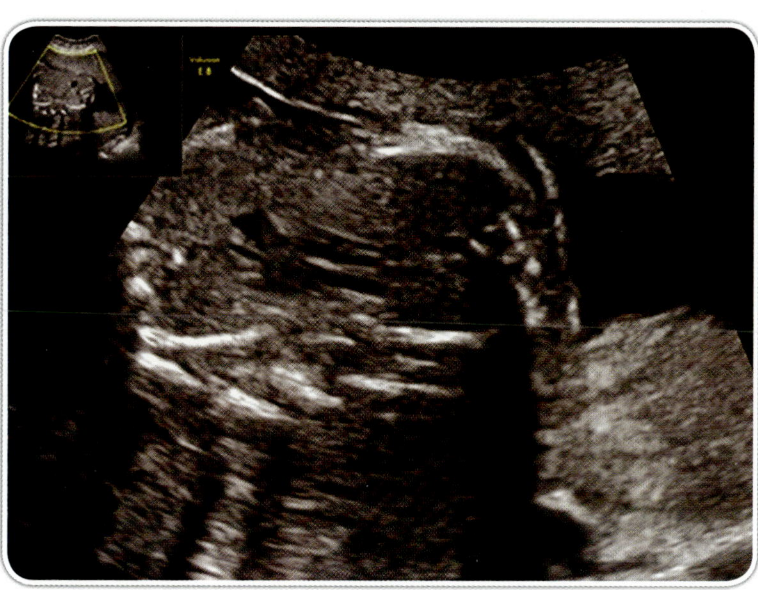

Conjoined Twins 5-Vessel Cord

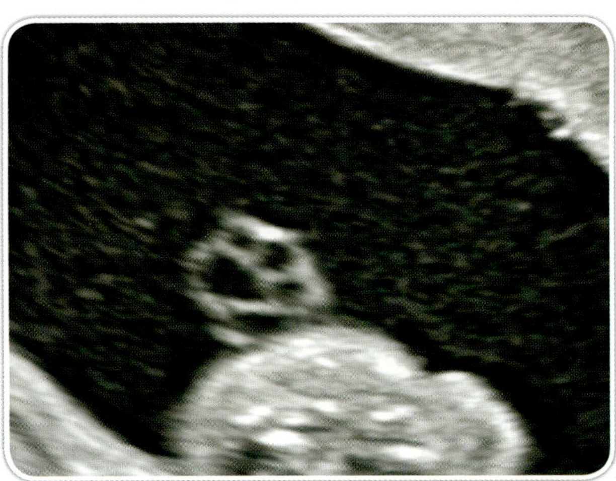

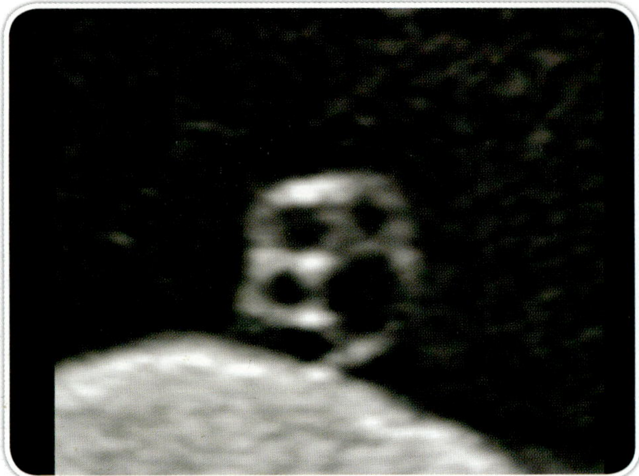

3D US Surface Thoraco-omphalopagous

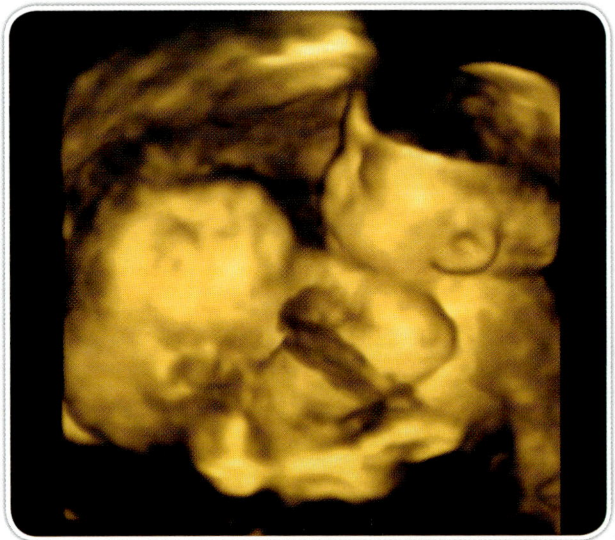

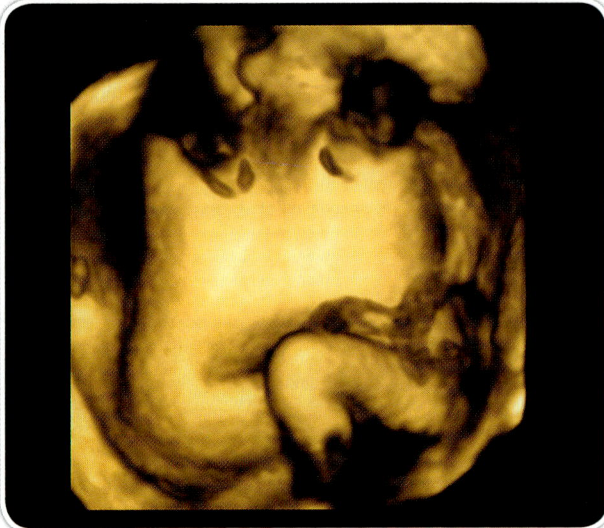

3DUS TUI Thoraco-omphalopagous

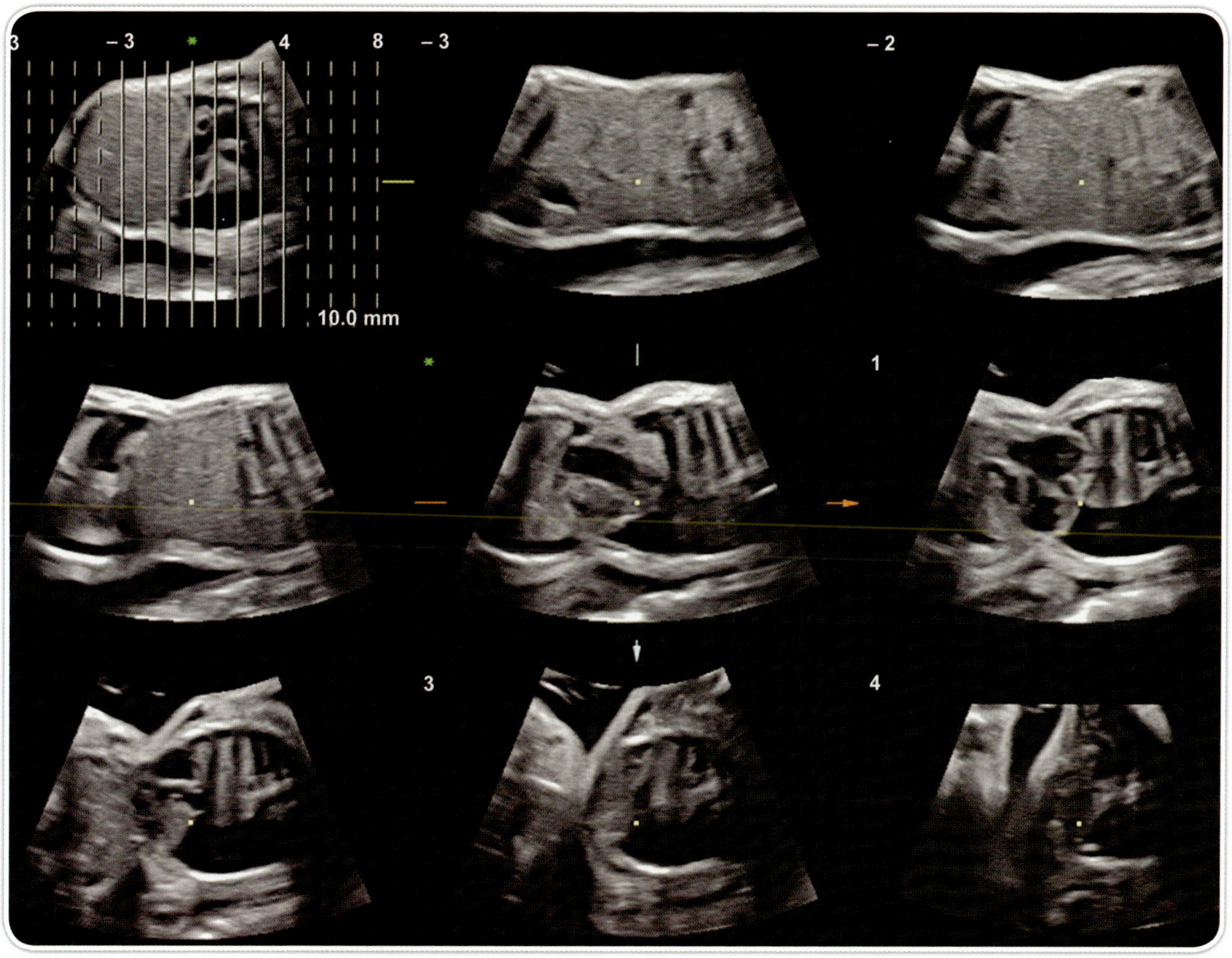

Thoraco-omphalopagous Conjoined

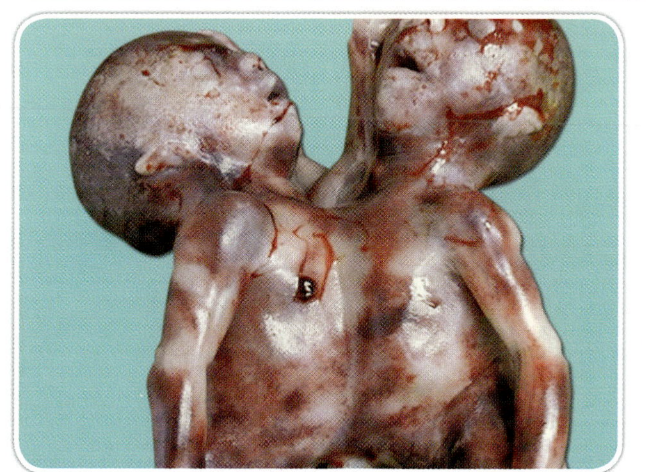

Type	Incidence	Organs shared
Thoracopagus	40%	Heart, liver, GI
Omphalopagus	34%	Liver, GI
Pygopagus	18%	Spine, GU, lower GI
Ischiopagus	6%	Pelvis, GU, GI, liver
Craniopagus	2%	Brain

Pygopagous Conjoined Twins

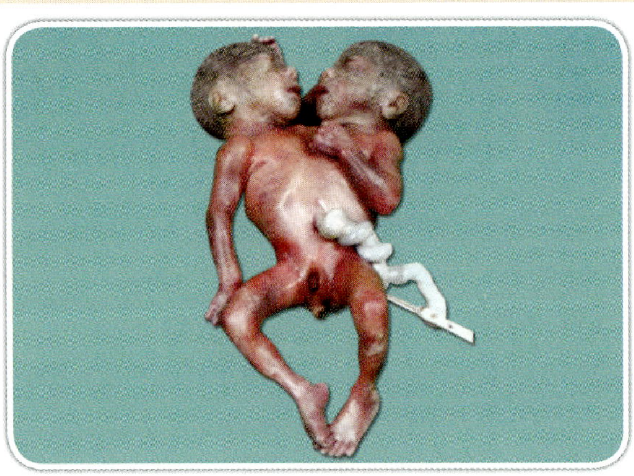

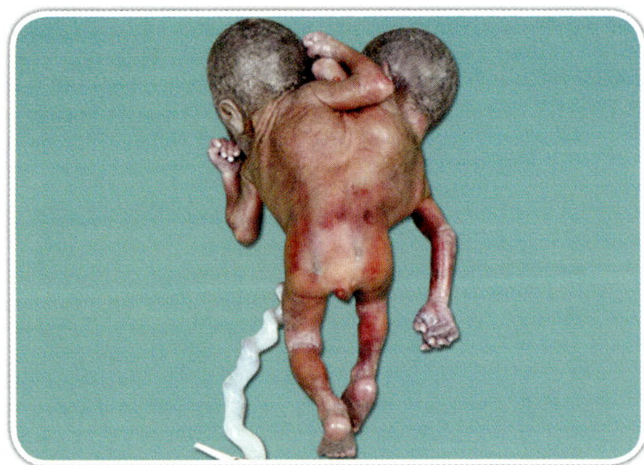

Janiceps Rarest form of Conjoined

- Janiceps conjoined twinning: 2 faces are attached but oriented in opposite directions
- Partial duplication of craniofacial, upper oropharyngeal, and cardiac organs.

(Kastenbaum et al. 2009)

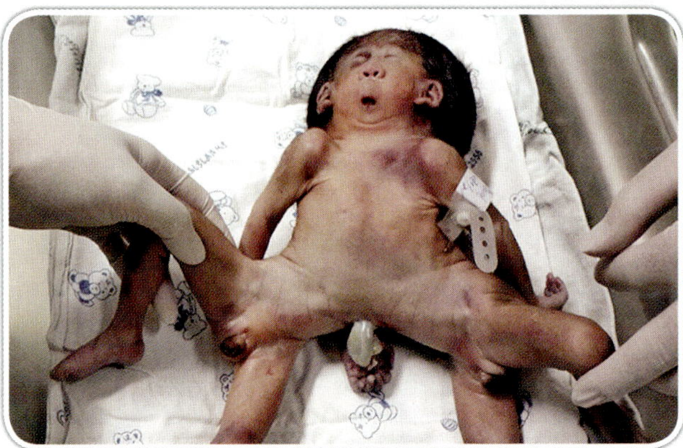

Janiceps Conjoined Twins 3DHD Demonstration

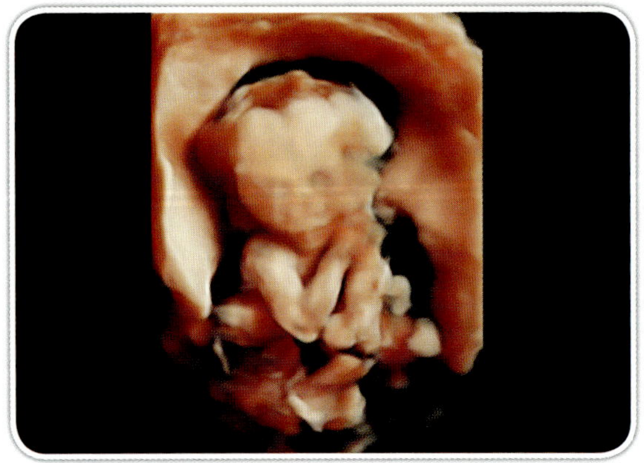

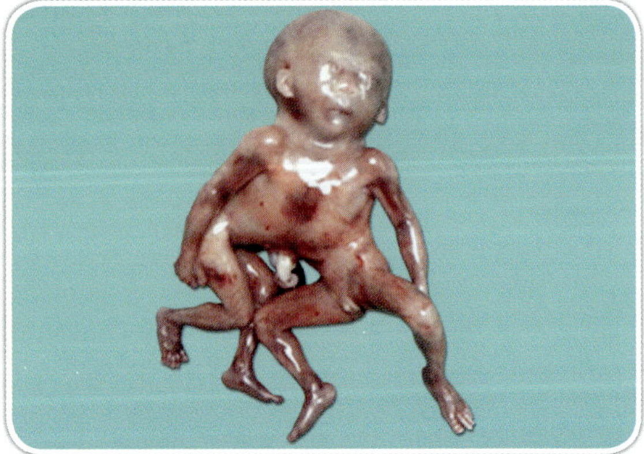

Thoraco-omphalopagous Conjoined

Possibility of separation?

- Sharing of cardiac structures
- Sharing of hepatic vasculature.

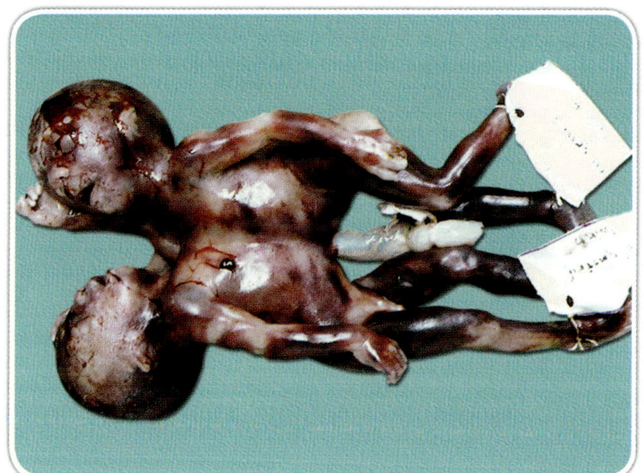

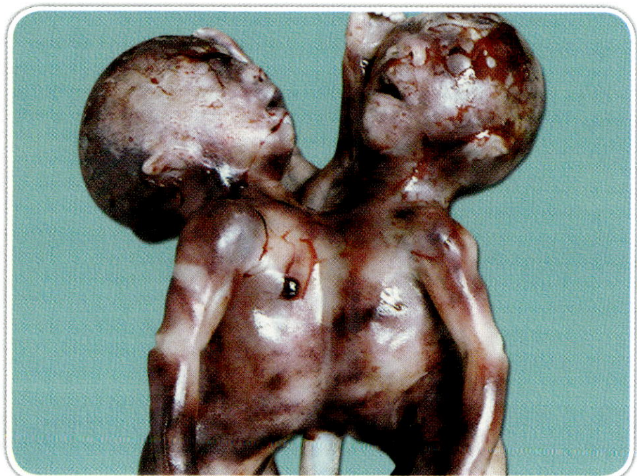

Postnatal Surgical Separation

- Cardiovascular sharing
- 3D US to determine the possibility of separation.

(Wataganara et al. 2008)

(Wen et al. 2013)

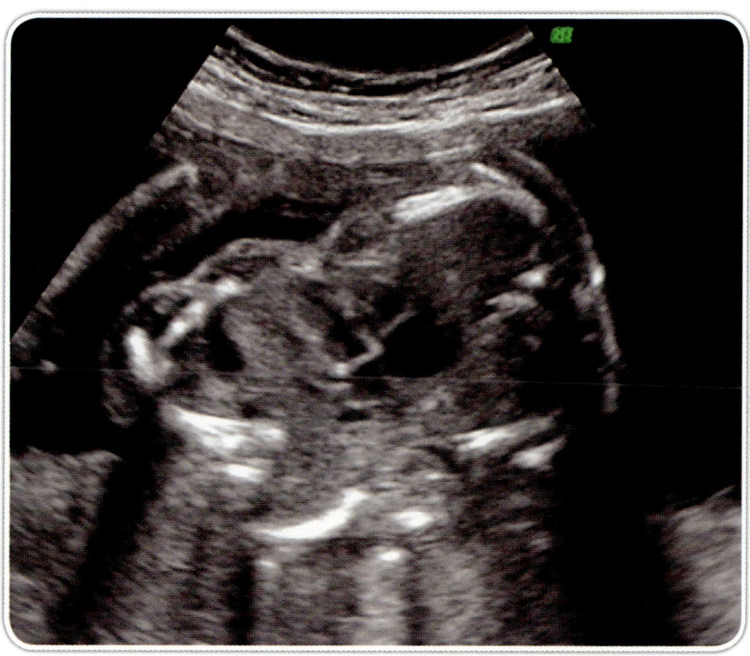

Thoraco-omphalopagous Conjoined Twins Topographic Ultrasound Imaging (TUI)

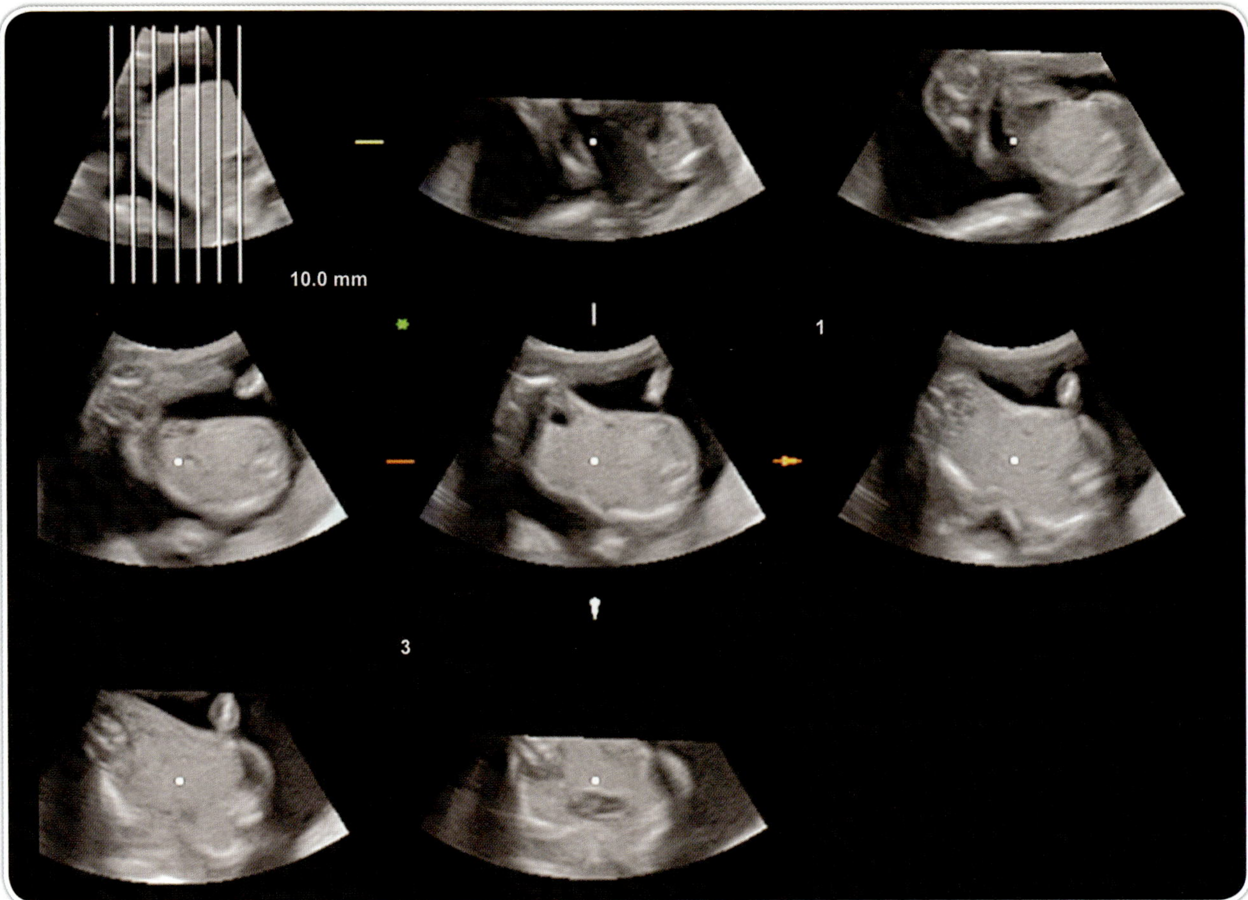

Ultrasound Obstet Gynecol 2008; 32: 236–238
Published online in Wiley InterScience (www.interscience.wiley.com).

Letters to the Editor

Three-dimensional power Doppler in the diagnosis and surgical management of thoraco-omphalopagus conjoined twins.

T. Wataganara *†, A. Sutanthaviboon†, S. Ngerndham‡ and C. Vantanasiri†
†Division of Maternal-Fetal Medicine, Department of Obstetrics and Gynecology, Faculty of Medicine Siriraj Hospital and ‡Division of Neonatology, Department of Pediatrics, Faculty of Medicine Siriraj Hospital, Mahidol University, 2 Prannok Road, Bangkoknoi, Bangkok, Thailand 10700
**Correspondence.*
(e-mail: sitwg@mahidol.ac.th)
DOI: 10.1002/uog.5326
Published online 11. June 2008

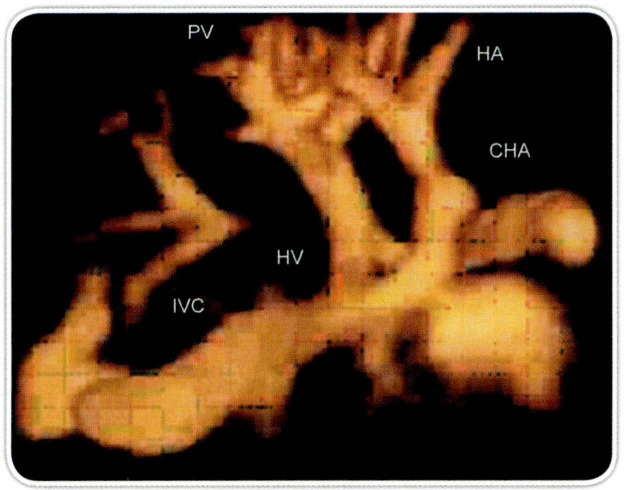

Three-dimensional power Doppler image (color mode i.e. with soft tissue subtraction) showing major intra-abdominal and intrahepatic vessels. CHA, common hepatic artery; HA, hepatic artery; HV, hepatic vein; IVC, inferior vena cava; PV, portal vein

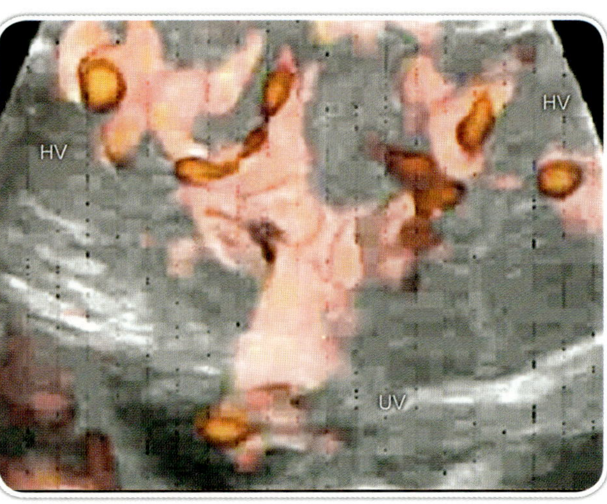

Three-dimensional power Doppler image (glass body mode) showing a single umbilical cord with an absence of intrahepatic shared vasculature. HV, hepatic vein; UV, umbilical vein

(Wataganara et al. 2008)

CONCLUSION

- Monochorionic twins are associated with higher complications
- Laser dichorionization and cord occlusion can help improving neonatal survival in complicated monochorionic twins
- Detailed ultrasound examination can help determine the possibility of separation in thoraco-omphalopagous conjoined twins.

SUGGESTED READING

1. Arabin B, Laurini RN, van Eyck J. Early prenatal diagnosis of cord entanglement in monoamniotic multiple pregnancies. Ultrasound in obstetrics & gynecology : the official journal of the International Society of Ultrasound in Obstetrics and Gynecology. 1999;13:181-6.
2. Benirschke K, des Roches Harper V. The acardiac anomaly. Teratology. 1977;15:311-6.
3. Dias T, Mahsud-Dornan S, Bhide A, Papageorghiou AT, Thilaganathan B. Cord entanglement and perinatal outcome in monoamniotic twin pregnancies. Ultrasound in obstetrics & gynecology : the official journal of the International Society of Ultrasound in Obstetrics and Gynecology. 2010;35:201-4.
4. Kastenbaum HA, McPherson EW, Murdoch GH, Ozolek JA. Janiceps conjoined twins with extreme asymmetry: case report with complete autopsy and histopathologic findings. Pediatric and developmental pathology : the official journal of the Society for Pediatric Pathology and the Paediatric Pathology Society. 2009;12:374-82.
5. Sebire NJ, Souka A, Skentou H, Geerts L, Nicolaides KH. First trimester diagnosis of monoamniotic twin pregnancies. Ultrasound in obstetrics & gynecology : the official journal of the International Society of Ultrasound in Obstetrics and Gynecology. 2000;16:223-5.
6. Wataganara T, Chanprapaph P, Chuangsuwanich T, Kanokpongsakdi S, Chuenwattana P, Titapant V. Reverse twin-twin transfusion syndrome after fetoscopic laser photocoagulation of chorionic anastomoses: a case report. Fetal diagnosis and therapy. 2009;26:111-4.
7. Wataganara T, Sutanthaviboon A, Ngerncham S, Vantanasiri C. Three-dimensional power Doppler in the diagnosis and surgical management of thoraco-omphalopagus conjoined twins. Ultrasound in obstetrics & gynecology : the official journal of the International Society of Ultrasound in Obstetrics and Gynecology. 2008;32:236-7.

Chapter

7

Fetal Neuroanatomy by Ultrasound

Ritsuko Kimata Pooh

FETAL BRAIN SCAN (CNS SCAN)

Why Brain Scan is Difficult??

Essential Knowledge of

- CNS anatomy
- How to cut the fetal brain by US
- CNS development during pregnancy
- CNS pathology.

Embryo CS 13–23

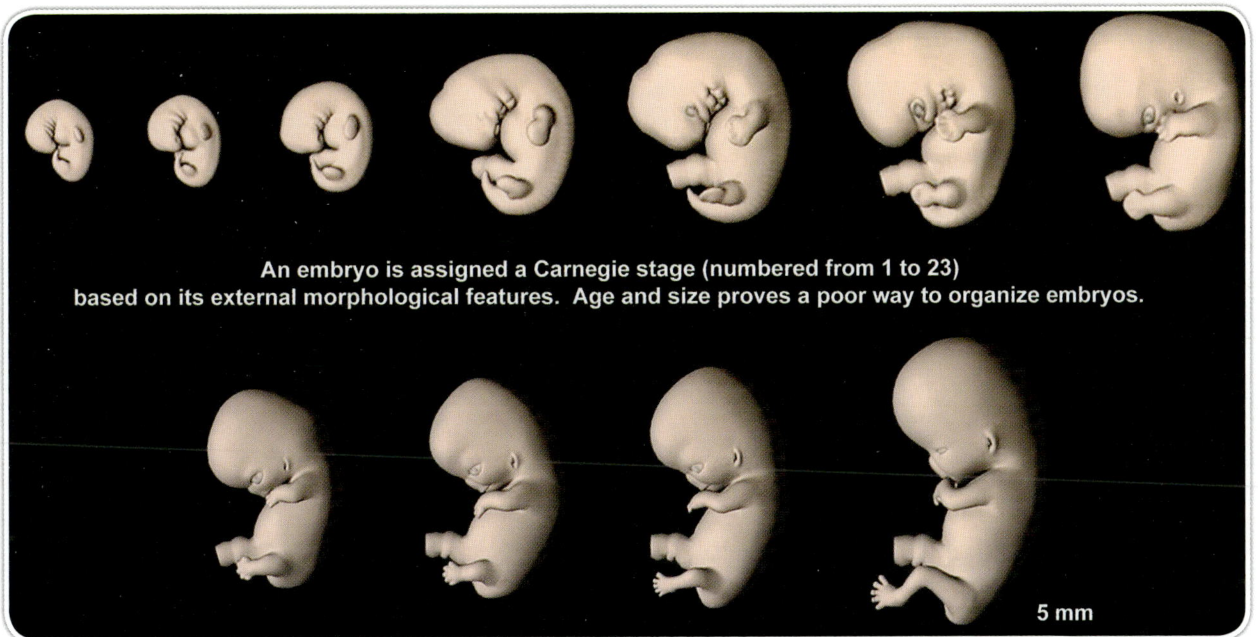

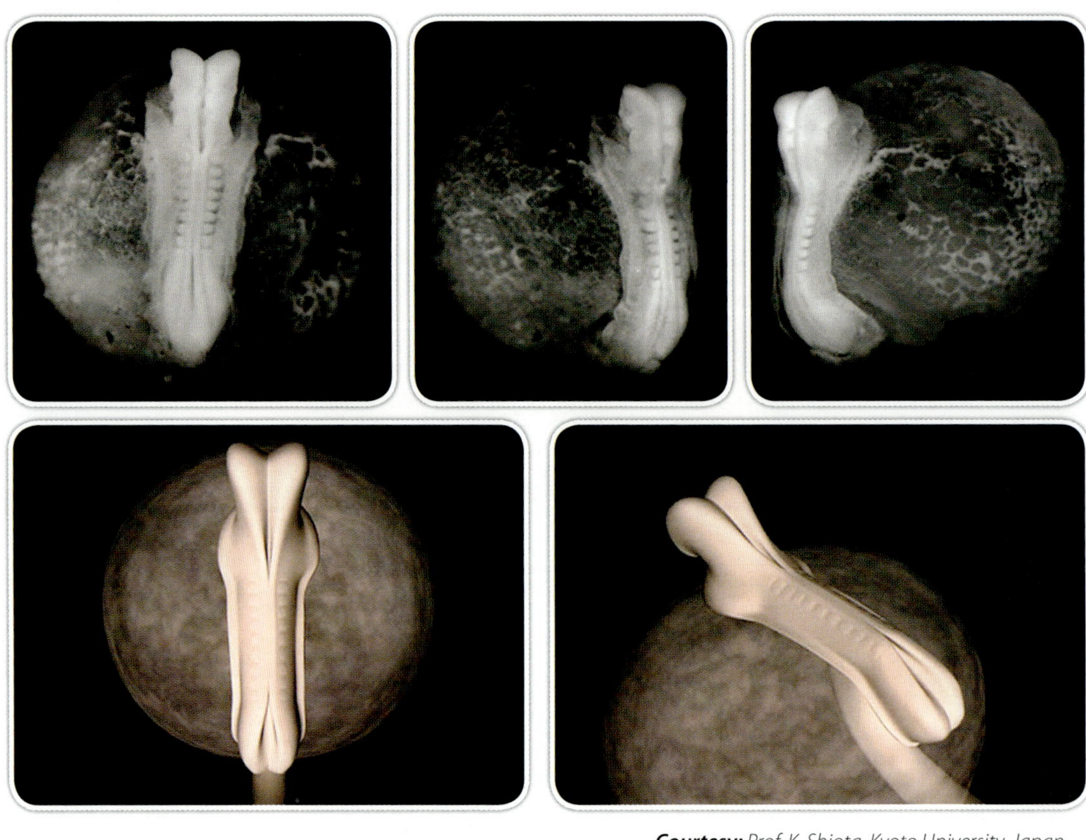

Courtesy: *Prof. K. Shiota, Kyoto University, Japan*

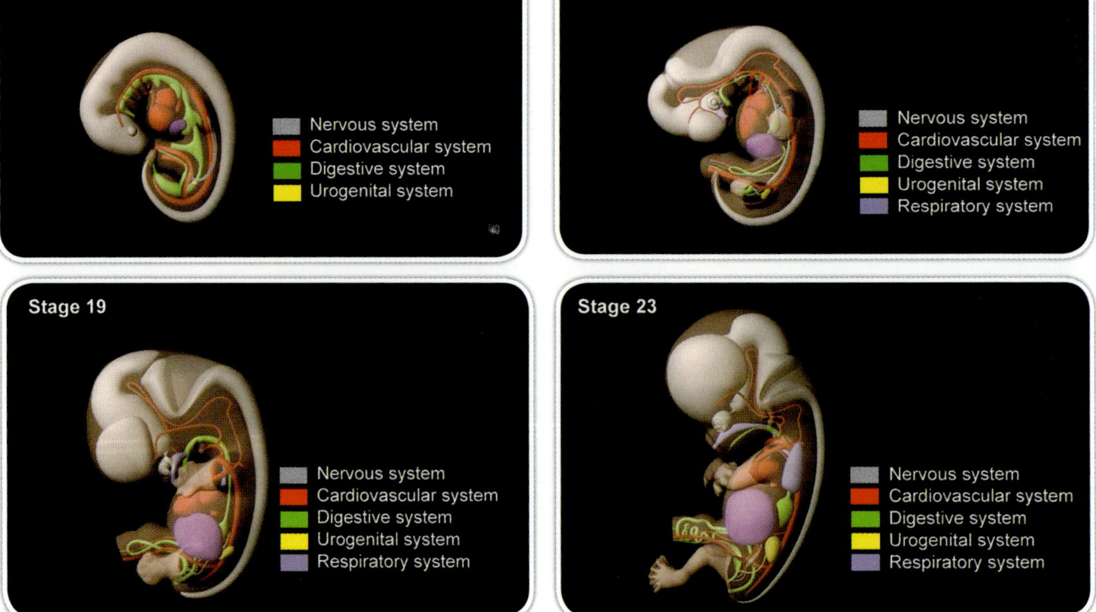

Courtesy: *Prof. K. Shiota, Kyoto University, Japan*

For complete presentation, please refer the accompanying CD-ROM...

SUGGESTED READING

1. Benacerraf BR. Inversion mode display of 3D sonography: applications in obstetric and gynecologic imaging. Am J Roentgenol. 2006 Oct;187(4):965-71.
2. Fetal Neurology, Pooh RK, Kurjak A. Jaypee Brothers Medical Publishers, New Delhi, 2009
3. Hata T, Dai SY, Kanenishi K, Tanaka H. Three-dimensional volume-rendered imaging of embryonic brain vesicles using inversion mode. J Obstet Gynaecol Res. 2009;35(2):258-61.
4. Kusanovic JP, Nien JK, Gonçalves LF, Espinoza J, Lee W, Balasubramaniam M, Soto E, Erez O, Romero R. The use of inversion mode and 3D manual segmentation in volume measurement of fetal fluid-filled structures: comparison with Virtual Organ Computer-aided AnaLysis (VOCAL). Ultrasound Obstet Gynecol. 2008;31(2):177-86.
5. Monteagudo A, Reuss ML, Timor-Tritsch IE. Imaging the fetal brain in the second and third trimesters using transvaginal sonography. Obstet Gynecol.1991:77:27-32.
6. Monteagudo A, Timor-Tritsch IE, Mayberry P. Three-dimensional transvaginal neurosonography of the fetal brain: 'navigating' in the volume scan. Ultrasound Obstet Gynecol. 2000;16:307-13.
7. Monteagudo A, Timor-Tritsch IE, Moomjy M. In utero detection of ventriculomegaly during the second and third trimesters by transvaginal sonography. Ultrasound Obstet Gynecol. 1994:4:193-8.
8. Pooh RK, Aono T. Transvaginal power Doppler angiography of the fetal brain. Ultrasound Obstet Gynecol. 1996:8:417-21.
9. Pooh RK, Kurjak A, Tikvica A. Normal and abnormal brain Vascularity, In Pooh RK, Kurjak A eds, Fetal Neurology,Jaypee Brothers Medical Publishers, New Delhi, 2009: pp 39-58.
10. Pooh RK, Kurjak A. 3D and 4D sonography and magnetic resonance in the assessment of normal and abnormal CNS development:alternative or complementary. L Perinat Med. 2011:39(1):3-13.
11. Pooh RK, Maeda K, Pooh KH, Kurjak A. Sonographic assessment of the fetal brain morphology. Prenat Neonat Med. 1999:4:18-38.
12. Pooh RK, Maeda K, Pooh KH. An Atlas of Fetal Central Nervous System Disease. Diagnosis and Management. Parthenon CRC Press, London, New York, 2003.
13. Pooh RK, Nagao Y, Pooh KH. Fetal neuroimaging by transvaginal 3D ultrasound and MRI. Ultrasound Rev Obstet Gynecol. 2006; 6: 123–34.
14. Pooh RK, Nakagawa Y, Nagamachi N, Pooh KH, Nakagawa Y, Maeda K, et al. Transvaginal sonography of the fetal brain: detection of abnormal morphology and circulation. Croat Med J. 1998:39:147-57.
15. Pooh RK, Neuroanatomy Visualized by 2D and 3D, In Pooh RK, Kurjak A eds Fetal Neurology, Jaypee Brothers Medical Publishers, New Delhi, 2009; pp 15-38.
16. Pooh RK, Pooh KH, Nakagawa Y, Nishida S, Ohno Y. Clinical application of three-dimensional ultrasound in fetal brain assessment. Croat Med J. 2000;41:245-51.
17. Pooh RK, Pooh KH. Fetal neuroimaging with new technology. Ultrasound Review Obstet Gynecol. 2002;2:178-181.
18. Pooh RK, Pooh KH. The assessment of fetal brain morphology and circulation by transvaginal 3D sonography and power Doppler. J Perinat Med. 2002:30:48-56.
19. Pooh RK, Pooh KH. Transvaginal 3D and Doppler ultrasonography of the fetal brain. Semin Perinatol. 2001;25:38-43.
20. Pooh RK, Shiota K, Kurjak A. Imaging of the human embryo with magnetic resonance imaging microscopy and high-resolution transvaginal 3-dimensional sonography: human embryology in the 21st century. Am J Obstet Gynecol. 2011;204(1):77.el-16.
21. Pooh RK. B-mode and Doppler studies of the abnormal fetus in the first trimester. In: Chervenak FA, Kurjak A editors. Fetal medicine. Parthenon Publishing, Carnforth 46-51,1999
22. Pooh RK. Fetal Brain Assessment by Three-Dimensional Ultrasound. In Kurjak A, Kupesic S eds. Clinical Application Of 3D Sonography. Carnforth, UK, Parthenon Publishing, 2000:171-9.
23. Pooh RK. Three-dimensional ultrasound of the fetal brain. In Kurjak A ed. Clinical application of 3D ultrasonography. Parthenon Publishing, Carnforth 2000;176-80.
24. Pooh RK. Two-dimensional and three-dimensional Doppler angiography in fetal brain circulation. In Kurjak A ed. 3D Power Doppler in Obstetrics and Gynecology. Parthenon Publishing, Carnforth, 1999:105-11.
25. Robinson AJ, Goldstein R. J Ultrasound Med 2007; 26:83-95
26. Sonographic examination of the fetal central nervous system: guidelines for performing the 'basic examination' and the 'fetal neurosonogram'. Ultrasound Obstet Gynecol. 2007;29:109-16
27. Timor-Tritsch IE, Monteagudo A, Mayberry P. Three-dimensional ultrasound evaluation of the fetal brain: the three horn view. Ultrasound Obstet Gynecol. 2000;16:302-6.
28. Timor-Tritsch IE, Monteagudo A. Transvaginal fetal neurosonography: standardization of the planes and sections by anatomic landmarks. Ultrasound Obstet Gynecol 1996:8:42-7.
29. Timor-Tritsch IE, Peisner DB, Raju S. Sonoembryology: an organ-oriented approach using a high-frequency vaginal probe. J Clin Ultrasound. 1990:18:286-98.

Chapter

8

Fetal Neuropathology

Ritsuko Kimata Pooh

CEREBRAL DEVELOPMENTAL STAGES

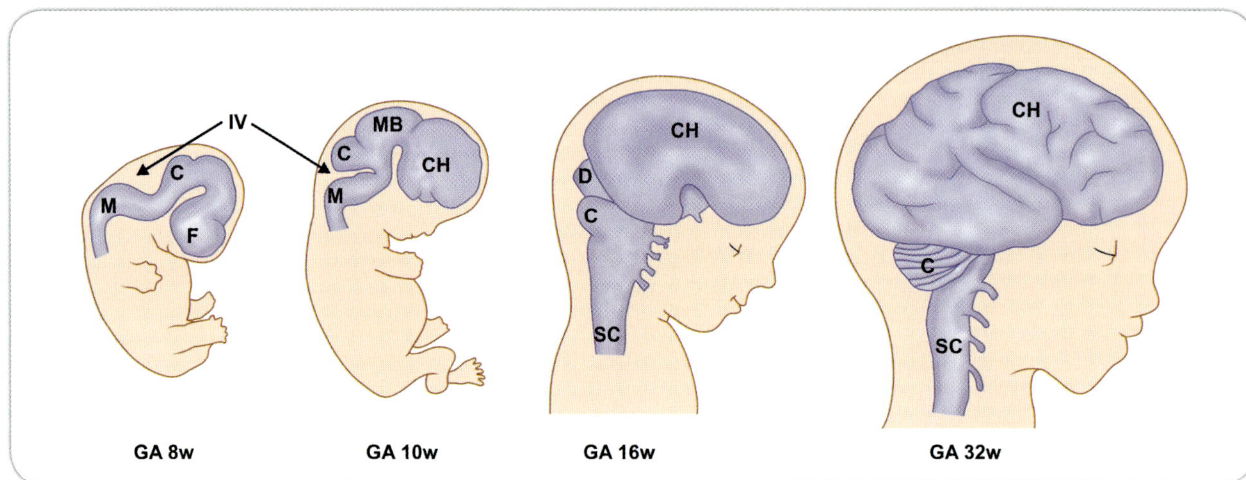

• Primary neurulation	(3–4 weeks' gestation)
• Secondary neurulation	(4 weeks' gestation)
• Procencephalic development	(2–3 months' gestation)
• Neuronal proliferation	(3–4 months' gestation)
• Neuronal migration	(3–5 months' gestation)
• Organization	(5 months' gestation –postnatal)
• Myelination	(5 months' gestation –postnatal)

CRANIUM/SPINA BIFIDA

Encephalocele

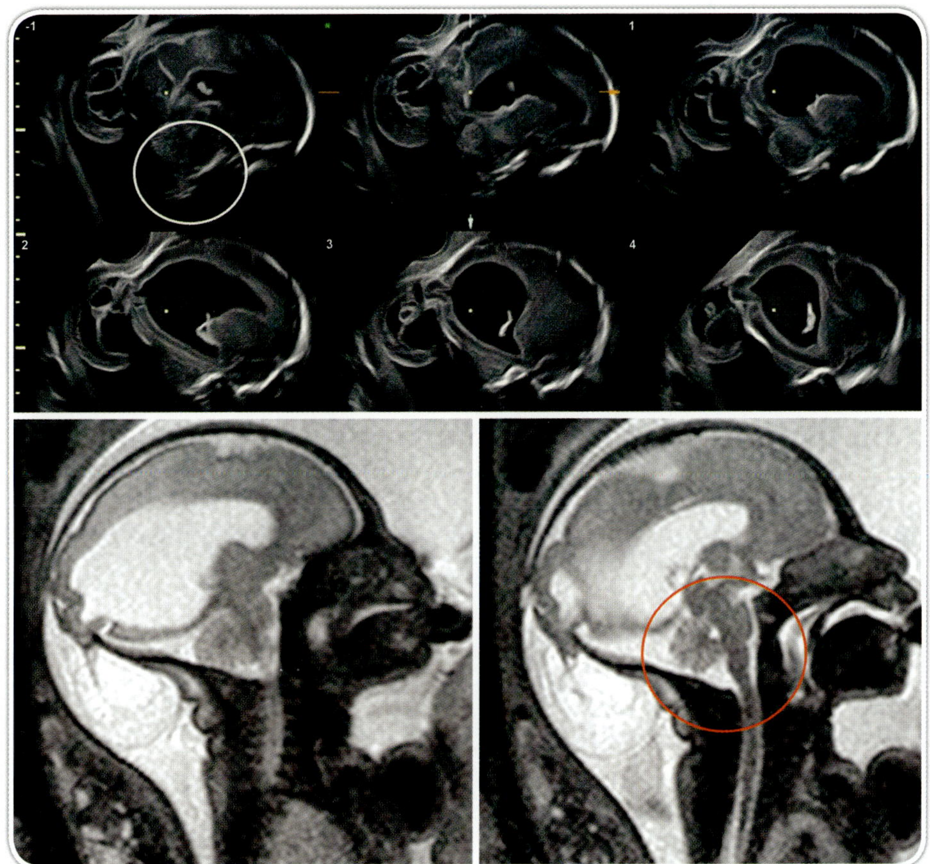

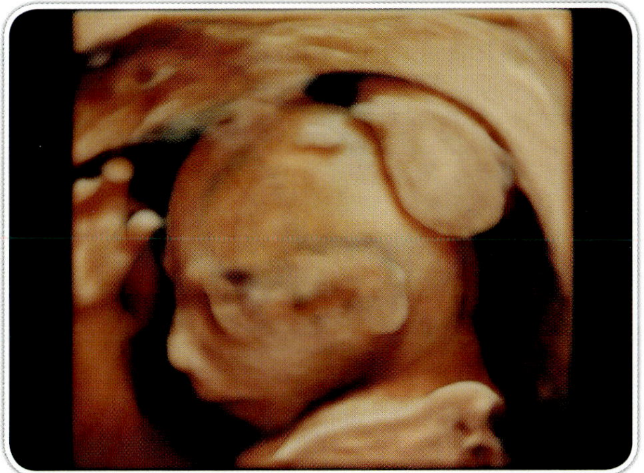

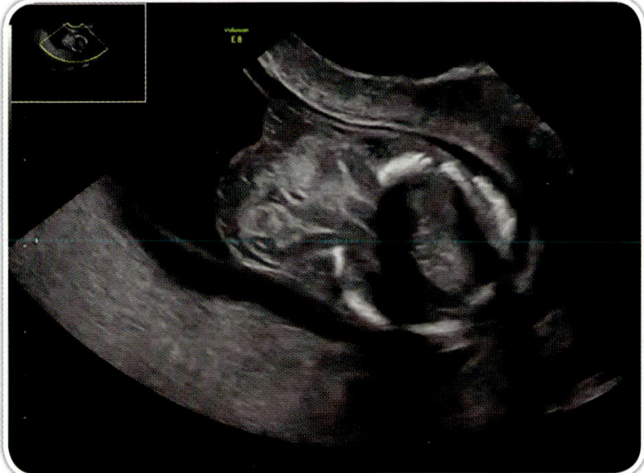

Encephalocele at 14 weeks of gestation: Ectopic cerebri, brainstem and posterior fossa

For complete presentation, please refer the accompanying CD-ROM...

SUGGESTED READING

1. Alagappan R, Browning PD, Laorr A, McGahan JP. Distal lateral ventricular atrium: reevaluation of normal range. Radiology. 1994;193:405-8
2. Almog B, Gamzu R, Achiron R et al. Fetal lateral ventricular width: what should be its upper limit? A prospective cohort study and reanalysis of the current and previous data. J Ultrasound Med. 2003;22:39-43.
3. Barkovich AJ, Kjos BO, Normal D, et al: Revised classification of the posterior fossa cysts and cyst-like malformations based on the results of multiplanar MR imaging. AJNR.1989;10:977-88.
4. Barkovich AJ, Simon EM, Walsh CA. Callosal agenesis with cyst: a better understanding and new classification. Neurology. 2001;23:56(2):220-7.
5. Benacerraf BR, Spiro R, Mitchell AG. Using three-dimensional ultrasound to detect craniosynostosis in a fetus with Pfeiffer syndrome. Ultrasound Obstet Gynecol. 2000;16:391-4.
6. Biggio JR Jr, Wenstrom KD, Owen J. Fetal open spina bifida: a natural history of disease progression in utero. Prenat Diagn. 2004;24(4):287-9.
7. Bretelle F, Senat MV, Bernard JP, Hillion Y, Ville Y. First-trimester diagnosis of fetal arachnoid cyst: prenatal implication. Ultrasound Obstet Gynecol. 2002;20:400-2.
8. de Laveaucoupet J, Audibert F, Guis F, Rambaud C, Suarez B, Boithias-Guerot C, et al. Fetal magnetic resonance imaging (MRI) of ischemic brain injury.Prenat Diagn. 2001 ;21:729-36
9. Demaerel P, Van de Gaer P, Wilms G, Baert AL. Interhemispheric lipoma with variable callosal dysgenesis: relationship between embryology, morphology, and symptomatology. Eur Radiol. 1996;6(6):904-9.
10. D'Addario V, Pinto V, Del Bianco A, Di Naro E, Tartagni M, Miniello G, et al. The clivus-supraocciput angle: a useful measurement to evaluate the shape and size of the fetal posterior fossa and to diagnose Chiari II malformation. Ultrasound Obstet Gynecol. 2001;18:146-9
11. Elchalal U, Yagel S, Gomori JM, Porat S, Beni-Adani L, Yanai N, et al. Fetal intracranial hemorrhage (fetal stroke): does grade matter? Ultrasound Obstet Gynecol 2005; 26: 233–43.
12. Endres LK, Cohen L. Reliability and validity of three-dimensional fetal brain volumes. J Ultrasound Med. 2001;20:1265-9.
13. Faro C, Chaoui R, Wegrzyn P, Levaillant JM, Benoit B, Nicolaides KH. Metopic suture in fetuses with Apert syndrome at 22-27 weeks of gestation. Ultrasound Obstet Gynecol. 2006 ;27:28-33.
14. Greco P, Resta M, Vimercati A, Dicuonzo F, Loverro G, Vicino M, et al. Antenatal diagnosis of isolated lissencephaly by ultrasound and magnetic resonance imaging. Ultrasound Obstet Gynecol. 1998;12:276-9.
15. Ickowitz V, Eurin D, Rypens F, Sonigo P, Simon I, David P, Brunelle F, Avni FE. Prenatal diagnosis and postnatal follow-up of pericallosal lipoma: report of seven new cases.AJNR 2001;22:767-72.
16. Isaacs H. Fetal brain tumors: a review of 154 cases. Am J Perinatol. 2009;26(6):453-66.
17. Jeanty P, Zaleski W, Fleischer AC. Prenatal sonographic diagnosis of lipoma of the corpus callosum in a fetus with GoldenharS syndrome. 1991;8(2):89-90.
18. Kobayashi K, Nakahori Y, Miyake M, Matsumura K, Kondo-Iida E, Nomura Y, et al. An ancient retrotransposal insertion causes Fukuyama-type congenital muscular dystrophy. Nature. 1998;23;394(6691):388-92.
19. Kojima K, Suzuki Y, Seki K, Yamamoto T, Sato T, Tanaka T, Suzumori K. Prenatal diagnosis of lissencephaly (type II) by ultrasound and fast magnetic resonance imaging. Fetal Diagn Ther. 2002;17:34-6.
20. Lasjaunias PL, Chng SM, Sachet M, Alvarez H, Rodesch G, Garcia-Monaco R. The management of vein of Galen aneurysmal malformations. Neurosurgery. 2006;59:S184-94.
21. Malinger G, Ben-Sira L, Lev D, Ben-Aroya Z, Kidron D., Lerman-Sagie T. Fetal brain imaging: a comparison between magnetic resonance imaging and dedicated neurosonography. Ultrasound Obstet Gynecol. 2004;23:33-40.
22. McGahan JP, Grix A, Gerscovich EO. Prenatal diagnosis of lissencephaly: Miller-Dieker syndrome. J Clin Ultrasound. 1994;22:560-3.
23. Meizner I, Elchalal U. Prenatal sonographic diagnosis of anterior fossa porencephaly. J Clin Ultrasound. 1996 ;24:96-9
24. Moinuddin A, McKinstry RC, Martin KA, Neil JJ. Intracranial hemorrhage progressing to porencephaly as a result of congenitally acquired cytomegalovirus infection--an illustrative report. Prenat Diagn. 2003:23:797-800.
25. Monteagudo A, Timor-Tritsch IE. Fetal Neurosonography of congenital brain anomalies. In Timor-Tritsch IE, Monteagudo A, Cohen HL. Ultrasonography of the Prenatal and Neonatal Brain, 2nd edn. McGraw-Hill, New York, 2001; pp 151-258
26. Nicolaides KH, Campbell S, Gabbe SG, Guidetti R Ultrasound screening for spina bifida: cranial and cerebellar signs. Lancet. 1986;12;2(8498):72-4.
27. Pilu G, Porelo A, Falco P, Visentin A. Median anomalies of the brain. in Timor-Tritsch IE, Monteagudo A, Cohen HL eds, Ultrasonography of the Prenatal and Neonatal Brain. 2nd edn. McGraw-Hill, New York, 2001; pp 259-76.
28. Pooh RK, Kurjak A. 3D and 4D sonography and magnetic resonance in the assessment of normal and abnormal CNS development: alternative or complementary. J Perinat Med. 2011;39:3-13.
29. Pooh RK, Kurjak A. Fetal Neurology. Jaypee Brothers Medical Publishers, New Delhi, 2009
30. Pooh RK, Kurjak A. Neuroscan of Normal and Abnormal Vertebrae and Spinal Cord. Fetal Neurology, Pooh RK, Kurjak A, Jaypee Brothers Medical Publishers, New Delhi, 2009 pp141-159

31. Pooh RK, Maeda K, Pooh KH, Kurjak A. Sonographic assessment of the fetal brain morphology. Prenat Neonat Med. 4:18-38,1999.
32. Pooh RK, Nagao Y, Pooh KH. Fetal neuroimaging by transvaginal 3D ultrasound and MRI. Ultrasound Rev Obstet Gynecol. 2006; 6: 123-34.
33. Pooh RK, Nakagawa Y, Pooh KH, Nakagawa Y, Nagamachi N. Fetal craniofacial structure and intracranial morphology in a case of Apert syndrome. Ultrasound Obstet Gynecol. 1999;13:274-80
34. Pooh RK, Pooh KH, Nakagawa Y, Maeda K, Fukui R, Aono T. Transvaginal Doppler assessment of fetal intracranial venous flow. Obstet Gynecol. 1999;93:697-701.
35. Pooh RK, Pooh KH, Nakagawa Y, Nishida S, Ohno Y. Clinical application of three-dimensional ultrasound in fetal brain assessment. Croat Med J. 2000;41:245-251.
36. Pooh RK, Pooh KH. Antenatal assessment of CNS anomalies, including neural tube defects. Fetal and Neonatal Neurology and Neurosurgery, 4th edition, Levene MI, Chervenak FA, Elsevier 2008; pp291-338.
37. Pooh RK, Pooh KH. Fetal neuroimaging. Fetal and Maternal Medicine Review, Cambridge University Press, 2008;19:1-31.
38. Pooh RK, Pooh KH. Fetal neuroimaging with new technology. Ultrasound Review Obstet Gynecol. 2002;2:178-81
39. Pooh RK, Pooh KH. Fetal Ventriculomegaly. Donald School J Ultrasound Obstet Gynecol. 2007; 2(2):40-46.
40. Pooh RK, Pooh KH. The assessment of fetal brain morphology and circulation by transvaginal 3D sonography and power Doppler. J Perinat Med. 2002;30:48-56.
41. Pooh RK, Pooh KH. Transvaginal 3D and Doppler ultrasonography of the fetal brain. Semin Perinatol. 2001;25:38-43.
42. Pooh RK. Contribution of transvaginal high-resolution ultrasound in fetal neurology. Donald School J Ultrasound Obstet Gynecol. 2011;5:93-99.
43. Pooh RK. Fetal brain assessment by three-dimensional ultrasound. In Kurjak A, Kupesic S eds. Clinical Application of 3D Sonography. Carnforth,UK:Parthenon Publishing 2000:171-9.
44. Pooh RK. Fetal central nervous system. Donald School Basic Textbook of Ultrasound in Obstetrics and Gynecology, Ahmed B, Adra A, Kavak ZN, Eds., Jaypee Brothers Medical Publishers, New Delhi, 2008; pp 326-49
45. Pooh RK. Fetal neuroimaging of neural migration disorder. Ultrasound Clinics, Lazebnik N, Lazebnik RS, Elsevier 2008;3(4):541-52.
46. Pooh RK. Neuroanatomy visualized by 2D and 3D. Fetal Neurology, Pooh RK, Kurjak A, Jaypee Brothers Medical Publishers, New Delhi, 2009; pp 15-38.
47. Pooh RK. Neuroscan of Congenital Brain Abnormality. Fetal Neurology, Pooh RK, Kurjak A, Jaypee Brothers Medical Publishers, New Delhi, 2009; pp 59-139
48. Pooh RK. Neuroscan of congenital brain abnormality. Fetal Neurology, Pooh RK, Kurjak A, Jaypee Brothers Medical Publishers, New Delhi, 2009; pp59-139.
49. Prayer D, Brugger PC, Kasprian G, Witzani L, Helmer H, Dietrich W, et al. MRI of fetal acquired brain lesions. Eur J Radiol. 2006;57(2):233-49.
50. Roelfsema NM, Hop WC, Boito SM, Wladimiroff JW. Three-dimensional sonographic measurement of normal fetal brain volume during the second half of pregnancy. Am J Obstet Gynecol. 2004;190(1):275-80
51. Schwarzler P, Homfray T, Bernard JP, Bland JM, Ville Y. Late onset microcephaly: failure of prenatal diagnosis. Ultrasound Obstet Gynecol. 2003;22(6):640-2
52. Sherer DM, Abramowicz JS, Eggers PC, Metlay LA, Sinkin RA, Woods JR. Jr. Prenatal ultrasonographic diagnosis of intracranial teratoma and massive craniomegaly with associated high-output cardiac failure. Am J Obstet Gynecol. 1993;168:97-9.
53. Sherer DM, Anyaegbunam A, Onyeije C. Antepartum fetal intracranial hemorrhage, predisposing factors and prenatal sonography: a review. Am J Perinatol. 1998;15:431-41
54. Tart RP, Quisling RG. Curvilinear and tubulonodular varieties of lipoma of the corpus callosum: an MR and CT study. J Comput Assist Tomogr. 1991;15:805-10.
55. Tonni G, Panteghini M, Rossi A, Baldi M, Magnani C, Ferrari B, Lituania M. Craniosynostosis: prenatal diagnosis by means of ultrasound and SSSE-MRI. Family series with report of neurodevelopmental outcome and review of the literature. Archives Gynecol Obstet. 2011;283:909-16.
56. Volpe JJ. Brain tumors and vein of Galen malformation. Neurology of the Newborn (4th edn). Philadelphia; WB Saunders.2001; pp 841-56.
57. Volpe JJ. Neural tube formation and prosencephalic development. Neurology of the Newborn (4th ed). Philadelphia; WB Saunders, 2001; pp 3-44
58. Volpe JJ. Neuronal proliferation, migration, organization and myelination. Neurology of the newborn. 4th ed. W.B. Saunders, USA, 2001; pp 45-99.

Chapter 9

Fetal Neurobehavior

Asim Kurjak, Lara Spalldi Barišić, Guillermo Azumendi

IS FETAL NEUROLOGICAL ASSESSMENT POSSIBLE?

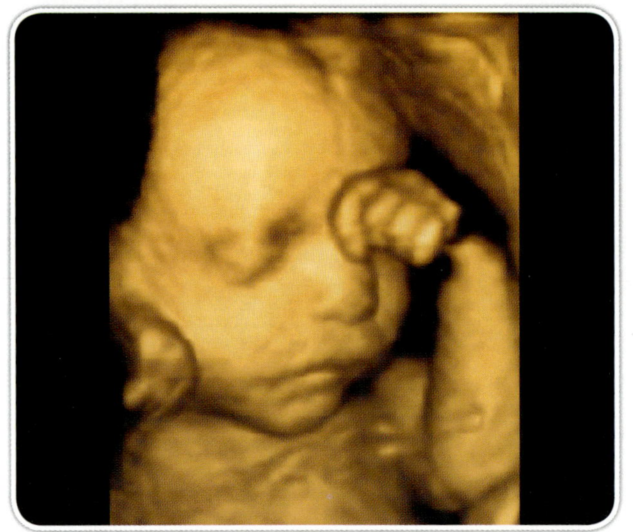

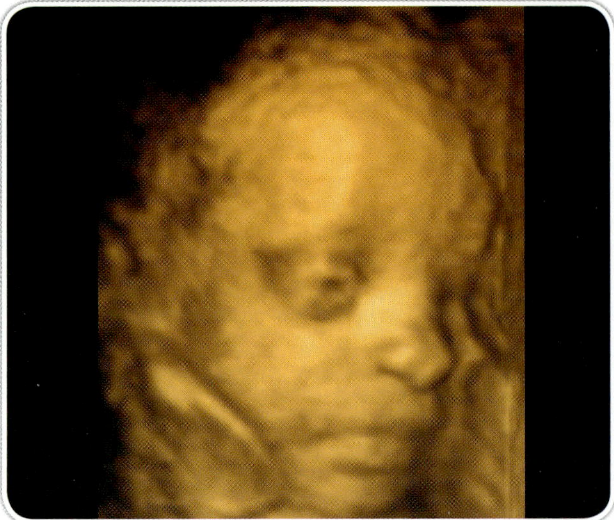

Courtesy: *Controversies in Obstetrics and Gynecology, Paris, Nov. 27-30:2008.*

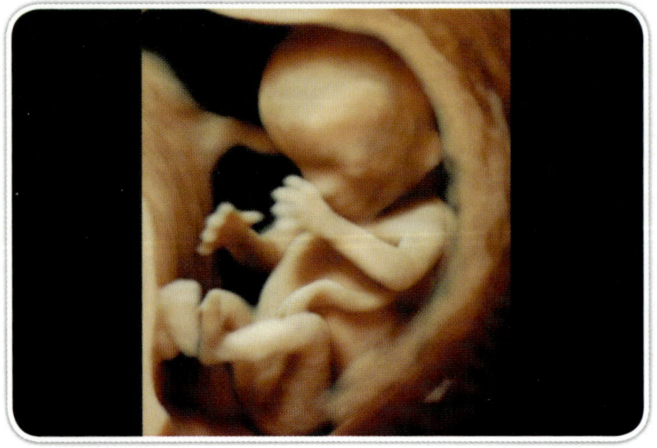

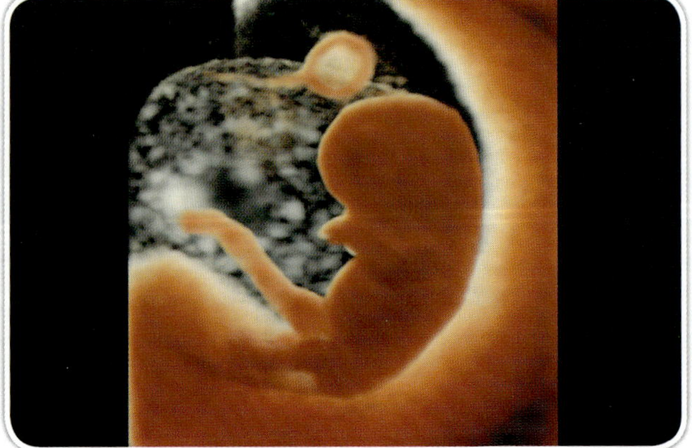

3DHD

Courtesy: *R. Pooh*

Quality of Images

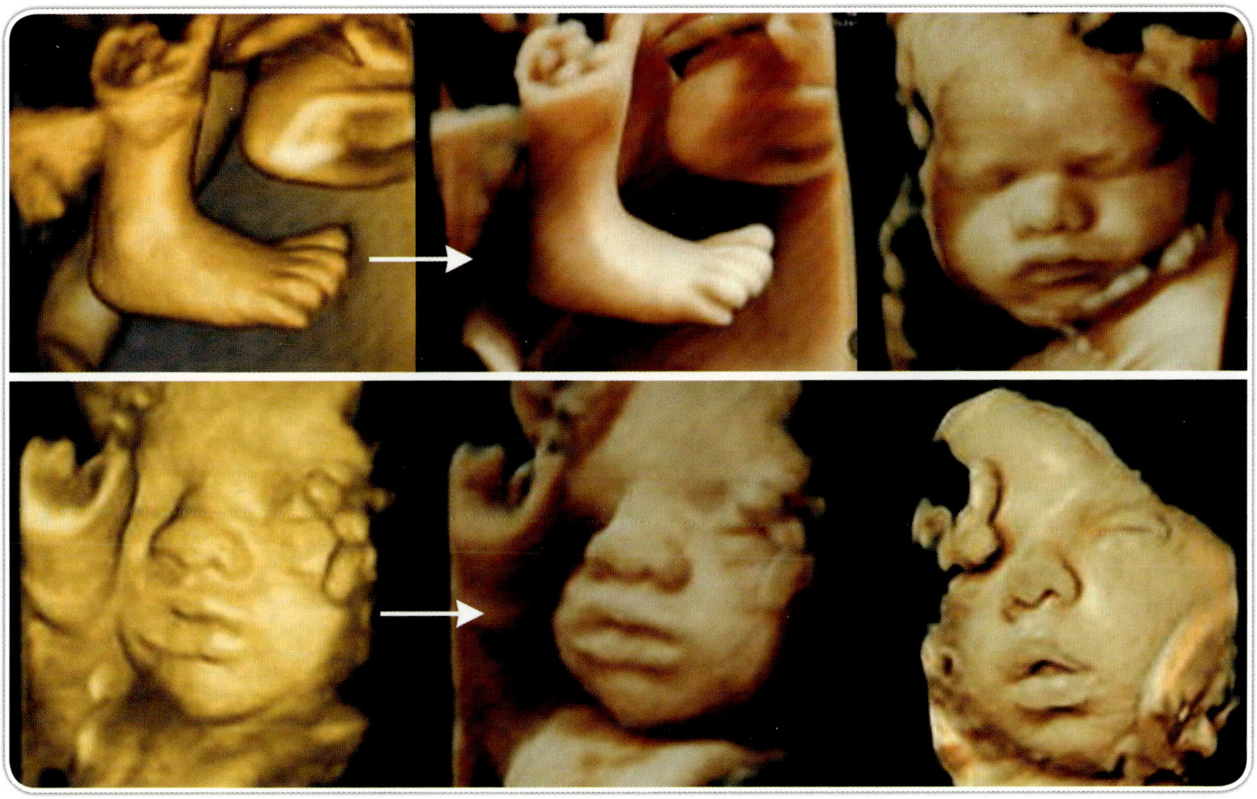

FETAL NEUROLOGY—INTRODUCTION

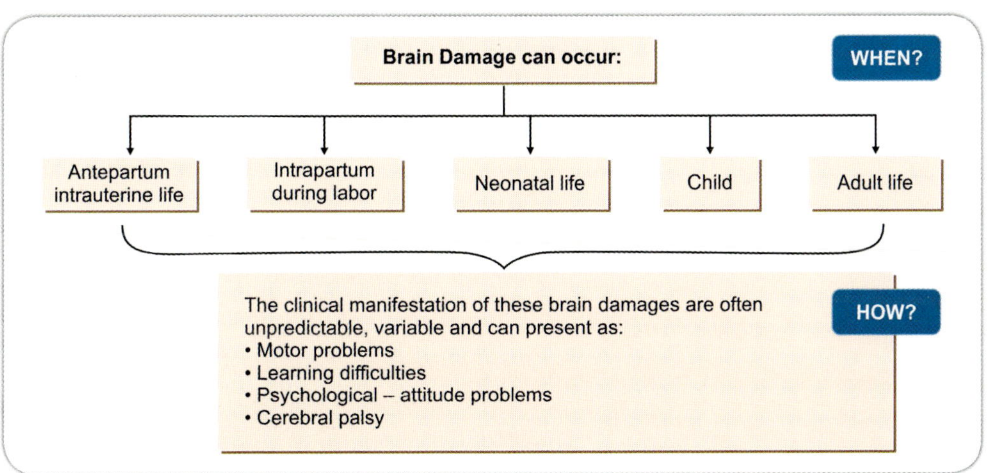

Kurjak et al. 2004

For complete presentation, please refer the accompanying CD-ROM…

SUGGESTED READING

1. Abo-Yaqoub S,Kurjak A, Mohammed AB,Shadad A, Abdel-Maaboud M. The role of 4-D ultrasonography in prenatal assessment of fetal neurobehaviour and prediction of neurological outcome.J Matern Fetal Neonatal Med. 2012;25(3):231-6
2. Adinolfi M. Dev Med Child Neurol. 1993:35:549-53.
3. Amiel-Tison C. Update of the Amiel-Tison neurologic assessment for the term neonate or at 40 weeks corrected age. 2002;27(3):196-212
4. Asim Kurjak, Salwa Abo-Yaqoub, Milan Stanojevic, Alin Basgul Yigiter, Oliver Vasilj, Daniela Lebit, et al. The potential of 4D sonography in the assessment of fetal neurobehavior – multicentric study in high-risk pregnancies. Jan. 2010. Journal of Perinatal Medicine. 2010; 38(1).
5. Dammann O, Leviton A. Maternal intrauterine infection, cytokines, and brain damage in the preterm newborn. Pediatr Res.1997:42(1):1-8.
6. Kurjak, et al. Intrauterine growth restriction and cerebral palsy. Acta Inform Med. 2010;18(2): 64-82.
7. Kurjak A, Ana Tikvica, Milan Stanojevic, Berivoj Miskovic, Baldreldeen Ahmed, Guillermo Azumendi, et al. The Assessment of Fetal Neurobehavior by Three-dimensional and Four-dimensional Ultrasound. 2008;21(10):675-84.
8. Kurjak A, Andonotopo W, Hafner T, Kadic AS, Stanojevic M, Azumendi G, et al. Normal standards for fetal neurobehavioral developments – longitudinal quantification by four-dimensional sonography. Journal of Perinatal Medicine. 2006:34(1).
9. Kurjak A, et al. New scoring system for fetal neurobehavior assessed by three- and fourdimensional sonography. B J Perinat Med. 2008;36:73-81.
10. Kurjak A. et al. Three- and four-dimensional ultrasonography for the structural and functional evaluation of the fetal face. Am J Obstet Gynecol. 2007:196:16-28.
11. Pooh RK, Shiota K, Kurjak A. Imaging of the human embryo with magnetic resonance imaging microscopy and high-resolution transvaginal 3-dimensional sonography: human embryology in the 21st century. Am J Obstet Gynecol. 2011:204:77.e1-16.
12. Stanojevic M, et al. Continuity between fetal and neonatal neurobehavior. Seminars in Fetal and Neonatal Medicine.2012:17(6):324-329. Fetal Neurology:Volume-II.
13. Stanojevic M, Talic A, Miskovic B,Vasilj O, Shaddad AN, Ahmed B,et al. An Attempt to Standardize Kurjak's Antenatal Neurodevelopmental Test: Osaka Consensus Statement.DSJUOG.2011;5:317-29.

Chapter 10

Fetal Neurobehavioral Development in Twin Pregnancies

Lara Spalldi Barišić, Asim Kurjak

The Beliefs of Great Philosopher Socrates....

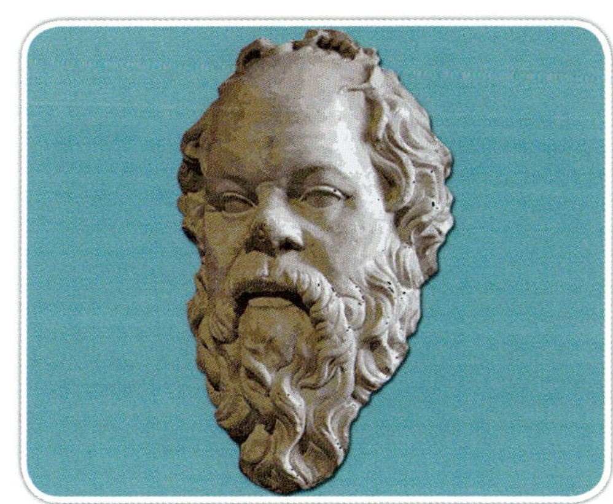

"THE SECRET OF CHANGE IS TO FOCUS ALL OF YOUR ENERGY, NOT ON FIGHTING THE OLD, BUT ON BUILDING THE NEW."

~ **SOCRATES**

Keep on Educating Ourselves ...

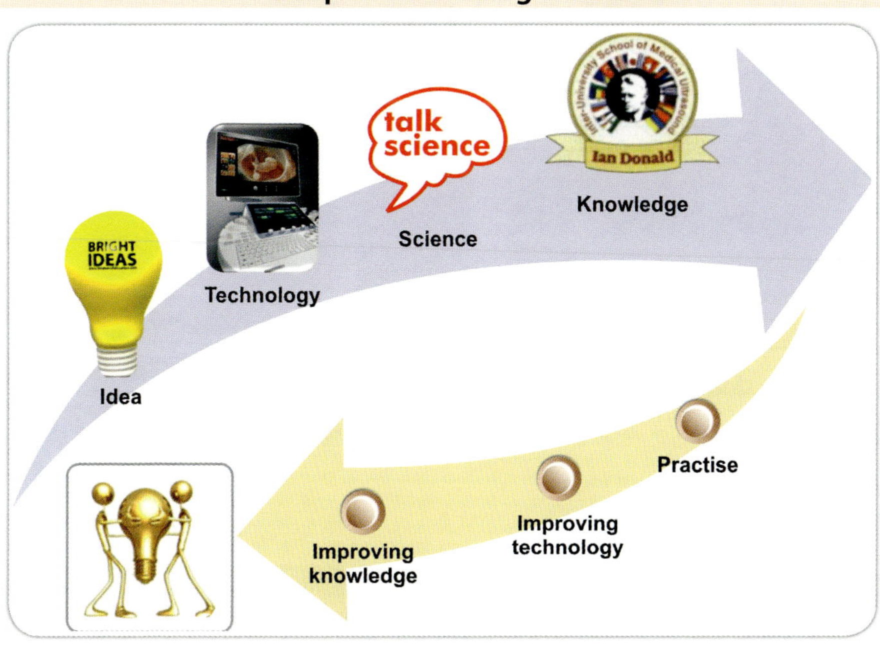

- With the rapid advances in technology **and improvement of image resolution, especially in 3D/4D ultrasound...**
  ...Over the years, ultrasonographic studies have showed **a fascinating details of fetal anatomy and diversity of fetal intrauterine activities.**

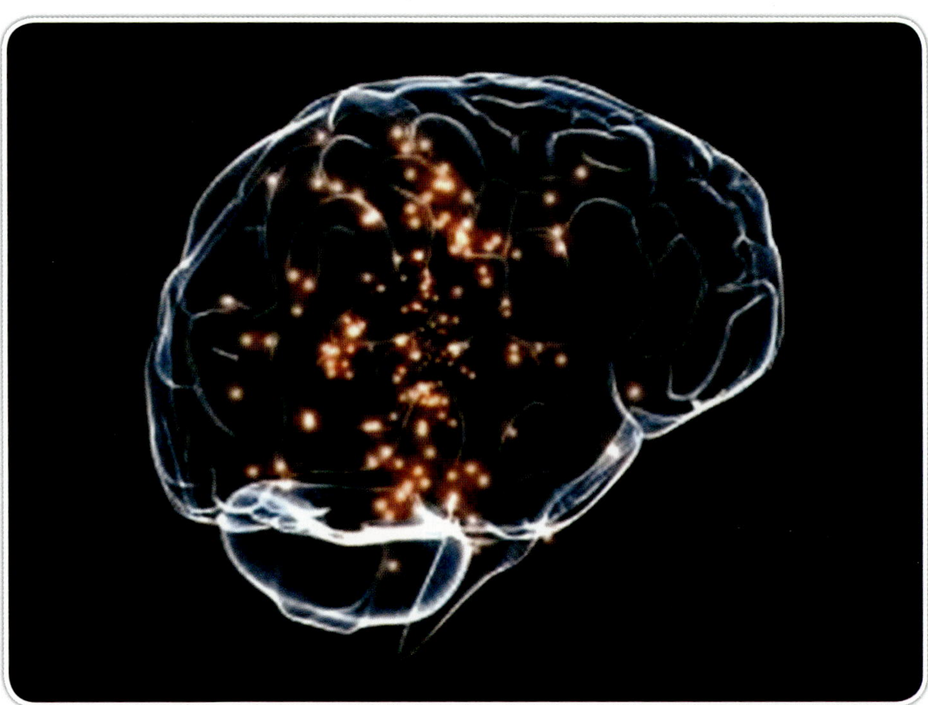

Dichorionic Diamniotic (DCDA) Twins 11 wks'

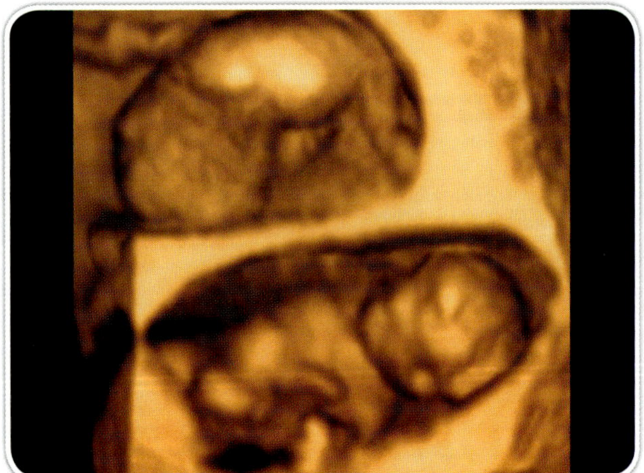

Spontaneous and independent movement of the twins

Courtesy: G. Azumendi

DCDA Twins 8 wks'

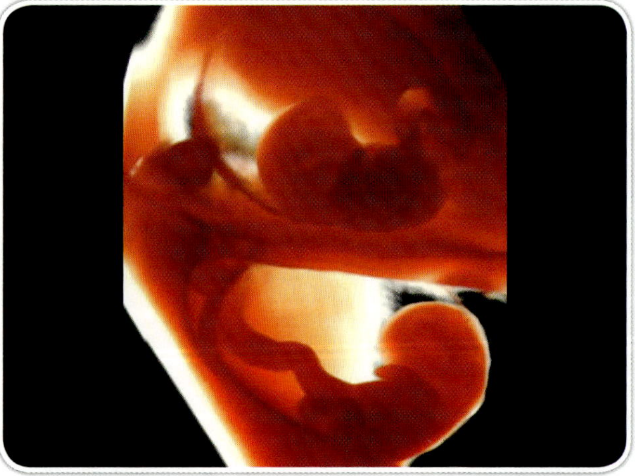

Dr. Bernard Benoit—Courtesy of GE Healthcare

For complete presentation, please refer the accompanying CD-ROM...

SUGGESTED READING

1. Amiel-Tison C, et al. From neonatal to fetal neurology: some clues for interpreting fetal findings. Pooh RK, Kurjak A. (Eds). Fetal Neurology. 2009;12:374-401.
2. Antsaklis P, Antsaklis A. The Assessment of Fetal Neurobehavior with Four-dimensional Ultrasound: The Kurjak Antenatal Neurodevelopmental Test. Donald School Journal of Ultrasound in Obstet and Gyne. 2012;6(4):362-375363.
3. Antsaklis P, et al. The assessment of fetal neurobehavior with 4D ultrasound: the KANET test. Current Health Sciences Journal 2013;39(1).
4. Arabin B, Bos R, Rijlaarsdam R, Mohnhaupt A, von Eyck J. The onset of inter-human contacts. Longitudinal ultrasound observations in early twin pregnancies. Ultrasound Obstet Gynecol 1996;8:199-173.
5. Arabin B, et al. Ultrasound Obstet Gynecol . 1996.
6. Callen DF, Fernandez H, Hull YJ, Svigos JM, Chambers HM, Sutherland GR. A normal 46,XX infant with a 46,XX/69,XXY placenta: a major contribution to the placenta is from a resorbed twin. Prenat Diagn. 1991;11(7):437-42.
7. De Vries JIP, Visser GHA, Prechtl HFR. The emergence of fetal behaviour. Qualitative Aspects- Early Human Development, 1982.
8. Dimitriou G,Pharoah PO,Nicolaides KH,Greenough A. Cerebral palsy in triplet pregnancies with and without iatrogenic reduction. Eur J Pediatr.2004;163(8):449-51. Epub.
9. Hata T, Sasaki M, Yanagihara T. Difference in the frequency of types of inter-twin contact at 10–13 weeks' gestation: preliminary four-dimensional sonographic study. Matern Fetal Neonatal Med. 2012;25:226-30.
10. Hepper,P. Fetal behavior: Why so sceptical? 1996. In : Ultrasound in Obstetrics and Gynecology. 1996:8:145-8.
11. Honemeyer U, Kurjak A. Prenatal beginnings of temperament formation – myth or reality? Case study of a twin pregnancy, Issued on Donald School Journal of Ultrasound in Obstetrics and Gynecology 2012;6(2):148-53.
12. Kandel, et al. The brain and behaviour. Principles of Neural Science NY: Mc Graw-Hill, 2000.
13. Kurjak A, Azumendi G, Andonotopo W, Salihagic-Kadic A. Three- and four-dimensional ultrasonography for the structural and functional evaluation of the fetal face. Am J Obstet Gynecol. 2007;196(1):16-28
14. Kurjak A, et al. Assessment of fetal behaviour by 3D and 4D sonography. In Hata T, Kurjak A, Kozuma S (Eds): Current Topics on Fetal 3D/4D Ultrasound. Bentham Science Publishers, pp. 234-65.
15. Kurjak A, et al. New scoring system for fetal neurobehavior assessed by three- and four-dimensional sonography. J Perinat Med. 2008;36(1):73-81
16. Kurjak A, Talic A, Stanojevic M, Honemeyer U, Serra B, Prats P, et al. The study of neurobehavior in twins in all three trimesters of pregnancy, 2013.
17. Landy HJ, Weiner S, Corson SL, et al. The "vanishing twin": ultrasonographic assessment of fetal disappearance in the first trimester. Am J Obstet Gynecol. 1986;155(1):14-9.
18. Lloveras E, Lecumberri JM, Pérez C, Melero C, Zamora L, Sánchez MA, et al. A female infant with a 46,XX/48,XY, +8, +10 karyotype in prenatal diagnosis: a 'vanishing twin' phenomenon? Prenat Diagn. 2001;21(10):896-7.
19. Mulder EJ, Visser GH, Bekedam DJ, Prechtl HF. Emergence of behavioural states in fetuses of type-1-diabetic women. Early Human Development. 1987;15(4):231-51.
20. Mulder EJH, Derks JB, de Laat MWM,Visser GHA. Fetal behavior in normal dichorionic twin pregnancy. Early Hman Development. 2011; 88(3):129-34
21. Nijhuis JG (Ed). 1992. Fetal Behaviour: Developmental and Perinatal Aspects. Oxford: Oxford University Press, 1992.
22. Nijhuis JG. Fetal behavior. Neurobiol Aging. 2003:24 (1):S41-6; discussion S47-9, S51-2.
23. Pharoah PO, Cooke RW. A hypothesis for the aetiology of spastic cerebral palsy--the vanishing twin. Dev Med Child Neurol. 1997;39(5):292-6.
24. Pharoah PO. Prevalence and pathogenesis of congenital anomalies in cerebral palsy. Arch Dis Child Fetal Neonatal Ed. 2007;92(6): F489-93.
25. Pharoah POD,.et al. Twins and locomotor disorder in children. J. Bone Joint Surg. 2006;88(B no. 3):295-7.
26. Pharoah POD, Cooke T. Cerebral palsy and multiple births. Arch Dis Child . Fetal Neonatal Ed. 1996;75:174-7.
27. Prats P, Vecek N, Andonotopo W, Carrera JM, Kurjak A. Assessment of multifetal pregnancies. In Carrera JM, Kurjak A (Eds): Donald School Atlas of Clinical Application of Ultrasound in Obstetrics and Gynecology. Jaypee Brothers: New Delhi. 2006; 133-64.
28. Prechtl H. 1997. State of the art of a new functional assessment of the young nervous system. An early predictor of cerebral palsy. Early Human Development 1997:50(1):1–11.
29. Reddy KS, Petersen MB, Antonarakis SE, Blakemore KJ . The vanishing twin: an explanation for discordance between chorionic villus karyotype and fetal phenotype. Prenat Diagn. 1991;11(9):679-84.
30. Reinold E. 1973. Clinical value of fetal spontaneous movements in early pregnancy. J Perinat Med. 1973;1:65-72.
31. Salihagic Kadic A, Predojević M, Kurjak A. Advances in Fetal Neurophysiology. In: Pooh RK, Kurjak A. Fetal Neurology. Jaypee Brothers: New Delhi, 2009.
32. Sampson A, de Crespigny LC. Vanishing twins: the frequency of spontaneous fetal reduction of a twin pregnancy. Ultrasound Obstet Gynecol. 1992;2(2):107-9

33. Stanojevic M,. et al. Continuity between fetal and neonatal neurobehavior. Semin Fetal Neonatal Med. 2012;17(6):324-9.
34. Stanojević M, et al. An attempt to standardize. Kurjak's Antenatal Neurodevelopmental Test: Osaka Consensus Statement. DSJUOG. 2011;5:317-29.
35. Tendais I, Visser GHA, Figueiredo B, Montenegro N, Mulder EJH. Fetal Behavior and Heart Rate in Twin Pregnancy: A Review. 2013;16(02).
36. Vecek N, Kurjak A, Azumendi G. Fetal behaviour in multiple pregnancies studied by four-dimensional sonography. Ultrasound Rev Obstet Gynecol. 2004;4:52-8.
37. Watson L, Stanley F. Report of the Western Australian Cerebral Palsy Register. Perth, Western Australia: TVW Telethon Institute for Child Health Research, 1999.

Chapter 11

Fetal Therapy

Tuangsit Wataganara

Types of Intrauterine Interventions

- Medical treatment
  - Transplacental
  - Intra-amniotic
  - Intraumbilical
  - Intramuscular
- Gene therapy and stem cell transplant
- Minimally invasive procedure
  - Needling procedures
  - Shunting procedures
  - Fetoscopic procedures
- Open fetal surgery
  - Repair of myelomeningoceles
  - Microcystic congenital pulmonary airway malformation (CPAM)
  - Resection of fetal tumors.

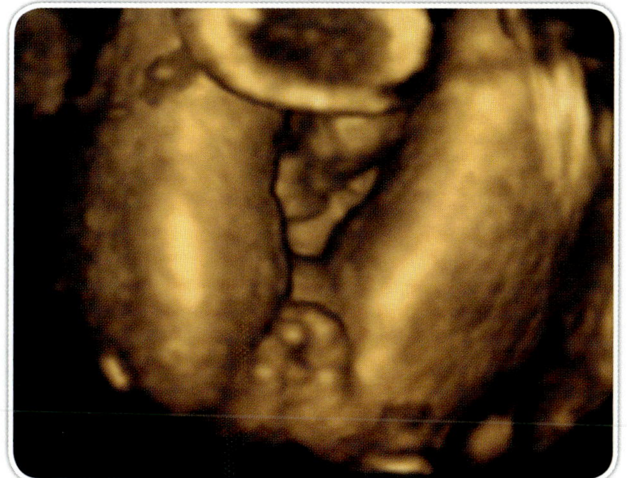

Congenital adrenal hyperplasia

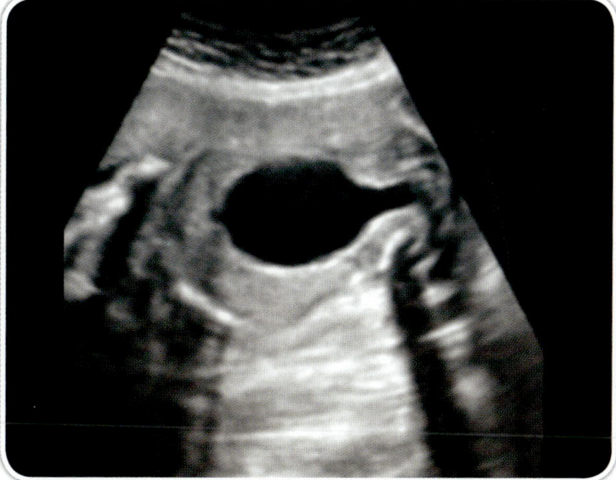

Posterior urethral valve

(Ville 2011)

Medical Treatment

- Administration of therapeutic substances through
  - The mother (transplacental)
  - Intra-amniotic fluid
  - Intraumbilical vein
  - Intramuscular.

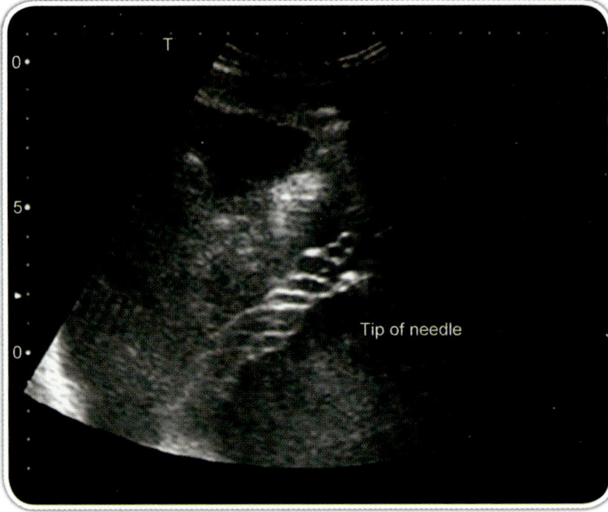

Intraumbilical vein fetal blood transfusion

Transplacental Administration

- Steroids administration to accelerate fetal lung maturity
- Anti-retroviral administration to prevent vertical HIV transmission

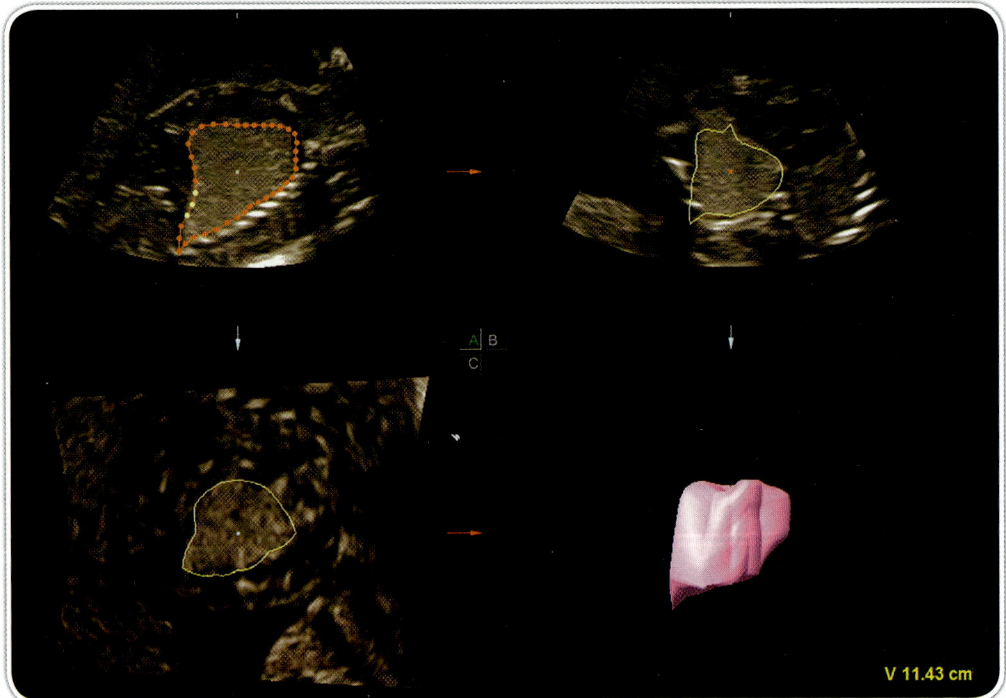

- Administration of antiarrhythmic agents (e.g. digoxin, sotalol, flecanide, amiodarone) to treat fetal tachyarrhythmia
- Administration of dexamethasone to treat fetal bradyarrhythmia (immunogenic atrioventricular blockade).

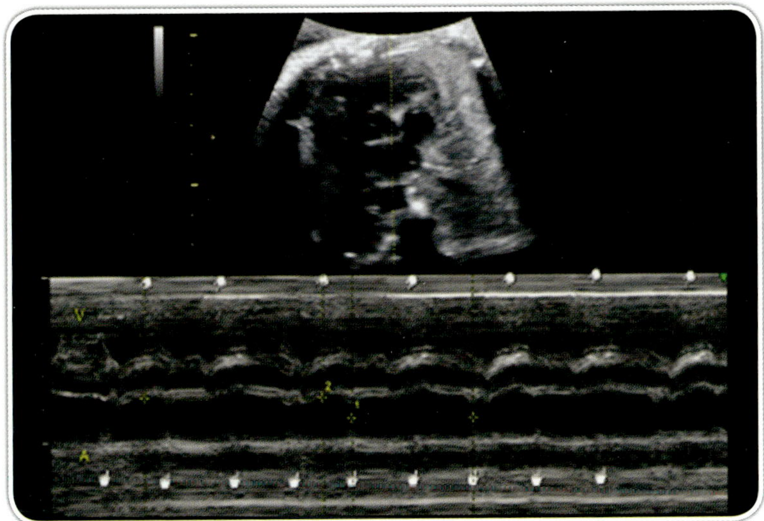

(Anuwutnavin et al. 2013)

Transamniotic Fluid

- Levothyroxine administration in the treatment of fetal goiter (as a result of fetal hypothyroidism)
- Dexamethasone (0.5–2 mg/D) administration to prevent virilization from congenital adrenal hyperplasia from 21-hydroxylase deficiency

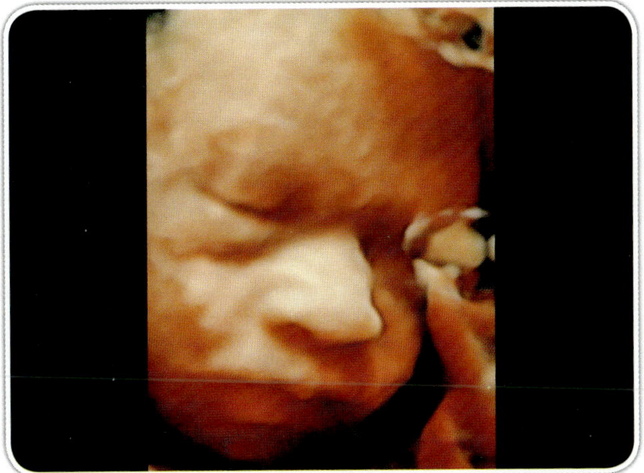

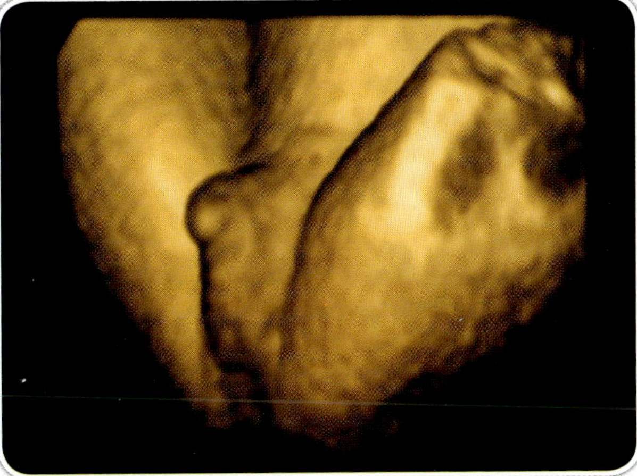

CONGENITAL ADRENAL HYPERPLASIA

Treatment Options: Prenatal Dexamethasone

- Autosomal recessive inherited. Fetal hyperandrogenemia
- Carrier couple has a chance of 1 in 4 of having an affected fetus
- Virilization (ambiguous genitalia) can occur in female fetus
- Early prenatal administration of dexamethasone can prevent virilization.

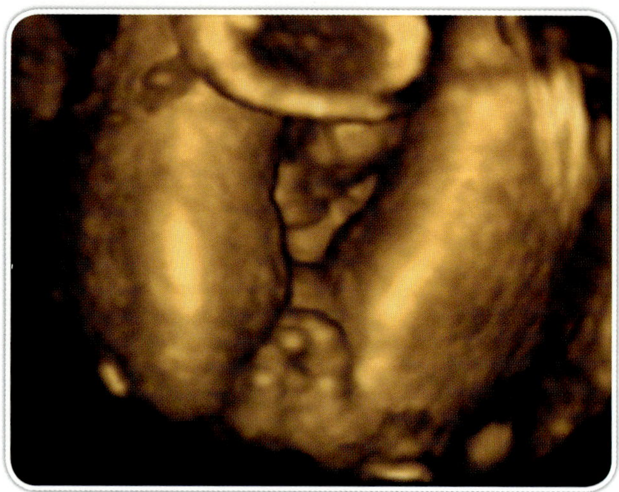

Congenital Adrenal Hyperplasia Fetal Gender Determination

Invasive: CVS

- Risks of pregnancy loss
- Too late to prevent virilization in female fetus.

Noninvasive: cff-DNA

- No risks of pregnancy loss
- Detected as early as 7 menstrual weeks' with nearly 100% accuracy for fetal gender determination.

GENE THERAPY AND STEM CELL TRANSPLANT

To alleviate the severity of certain genetic diseases, i.e. thalassemia

Fetal Gene Therapy

- Gene therapy = delivering of genetic material into the cells to treat diseases (e.g. Duchenne muscular dystrophy, cystic fibrosis)
- In utero stem cell transplant = targets at stem cells, which are rapidly expanding

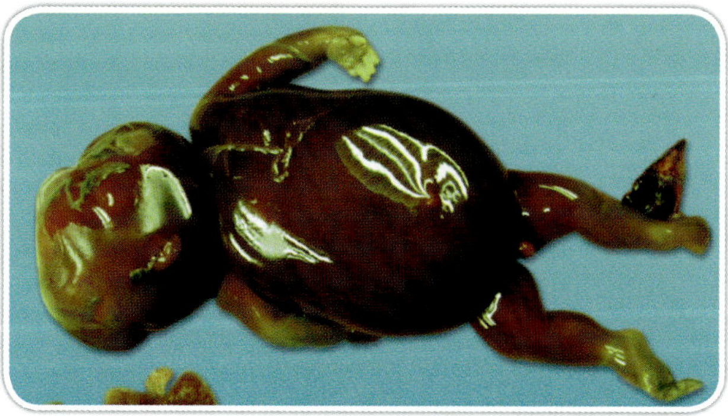

Fetal Bart's hydrops

- Long-term immune tolerance can be induced by either gene therapy or fetal stem cell transplant
- The treatment can be repeated after birth.

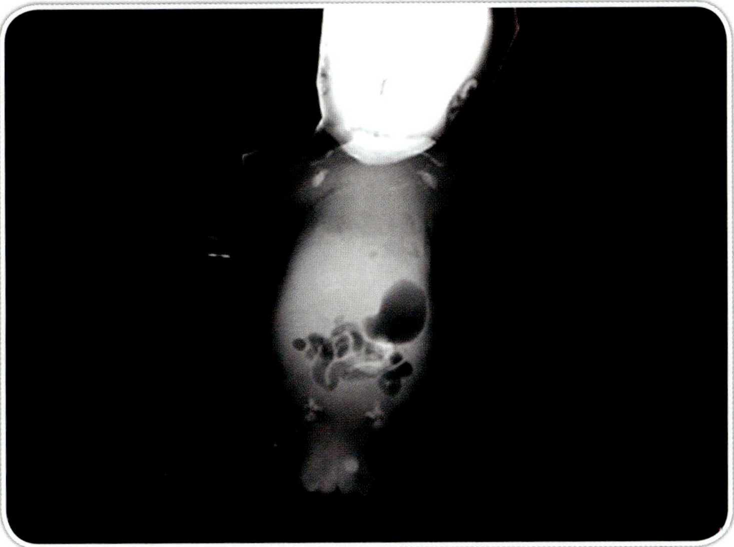

(Fetal achondrogenesis; Wataganara et al. 2006)

Fetal Stem Cell Transplant

- A large number of cells can be transferred in an early stage of life
- There is also an advantage of physiologic fetal stem cell migration and development
- During fetal life, the capacity to mount an immune response to allogeneic cells is impaired compared with adult life
- This provides an opportunity to induce tolerance to alloantigens without a prior myeloablation
- This approach can be particularly applicable in severe thalassemia diseases.

(Touraine et al. 1989)

MINIMALLY INVASIVE PROCEDURES

- Needle intervention
- Shunting procedures
- Fetoscopic interventions

Fetal Conditions Amendable for Minimally Invasive Procedures

Complicated monochorionic twins
- Twin-twin transfusion syndrome (TTTS)
- Twins reversed arterial perfusion sequence (TRAPS or Acardiac twin)
- Twin anemic-polycythemic sequence (TAPS)
- Discordant lethal fetal malformations
- Fetal anemia
- Shunting procedures
- Congenital diaphragmatic hernia
- Cardiac malformations
- Amniotic band
- Chorioangioma.

Serial Amniodrainage

Serial amniodrainage can be useful in polyhydramnios that threatened loss of the pregnancy, such as twin-twin transfusion syndrome, placental chorioangioma, etc.

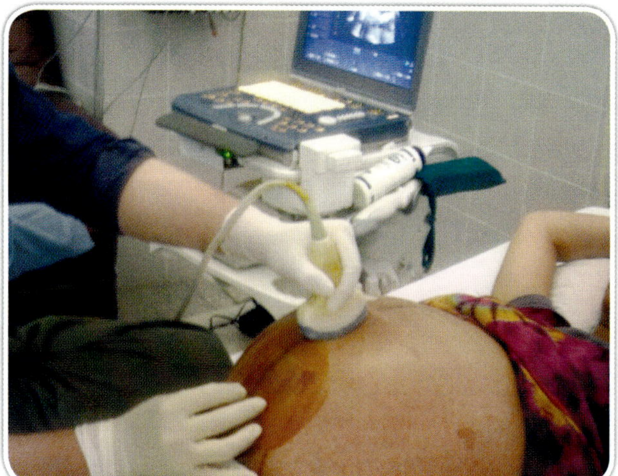

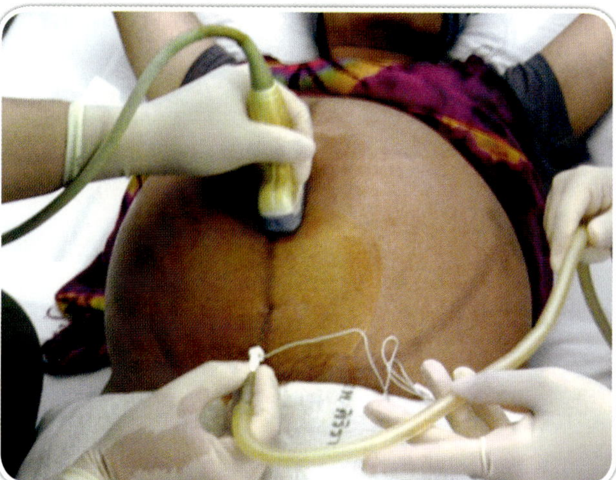

(Moise et al. 2005)

FETAL ANEMIA

Treatment options: Intrauterine blood transfusion

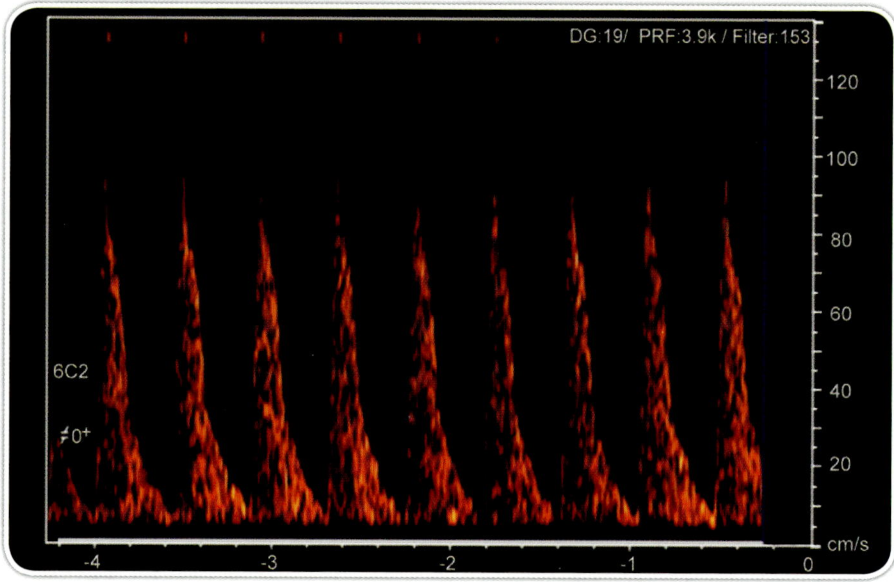

- Severe anemia in the fetus can cause hydrops and fetal death.
- Increased peak systolic velocity of the middle cerebral artery can be used to noninvasive diagnosed fetal anemia, and guide the intrauterine blood transfusion.

(Wataganara et al. 2006)

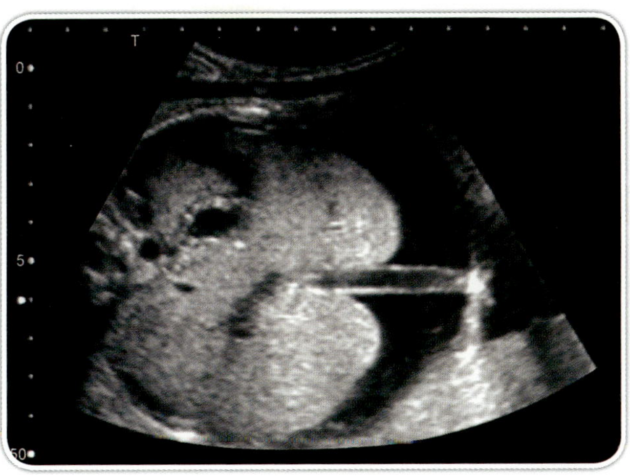

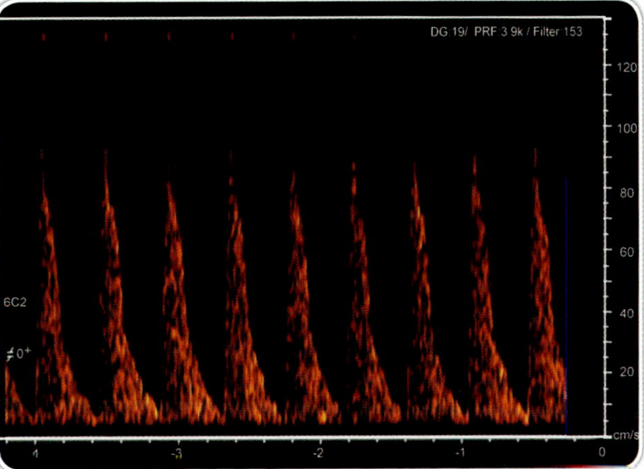

Intrauterine Fetal Blood Transfusion

- Fetal blood transfusion is life-saving
- It can be repeated if the cause of fetal anemia is persistent.

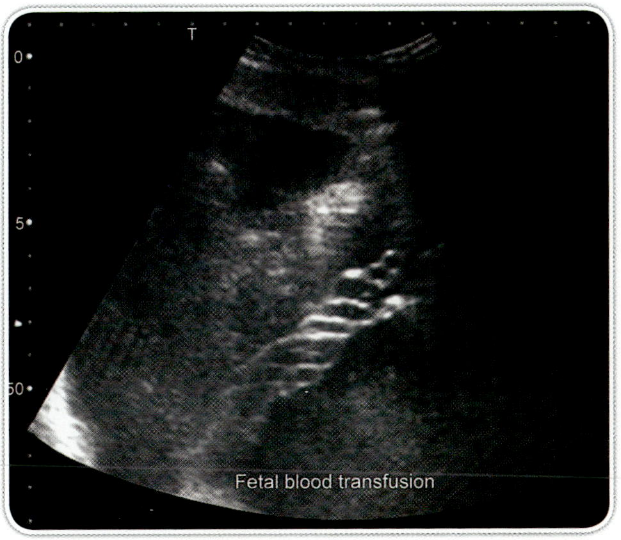

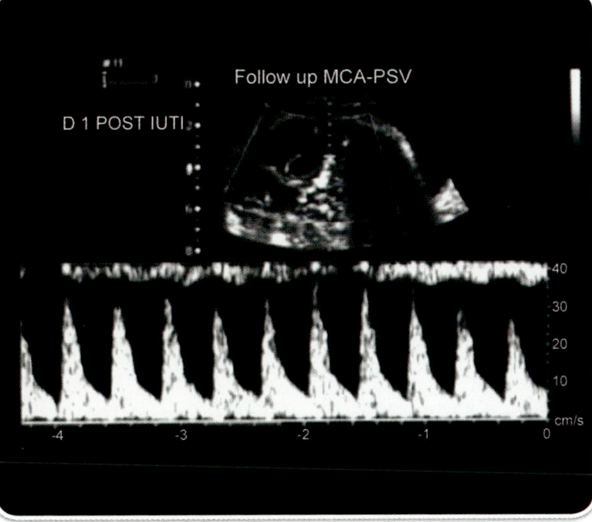

- This child received in utero transfusion due to anemic hydrops
- The hydrops was converted
- Diagnosis was hemoglobin Constant Spring Homozygote, with in-utero hemolytic crisis.

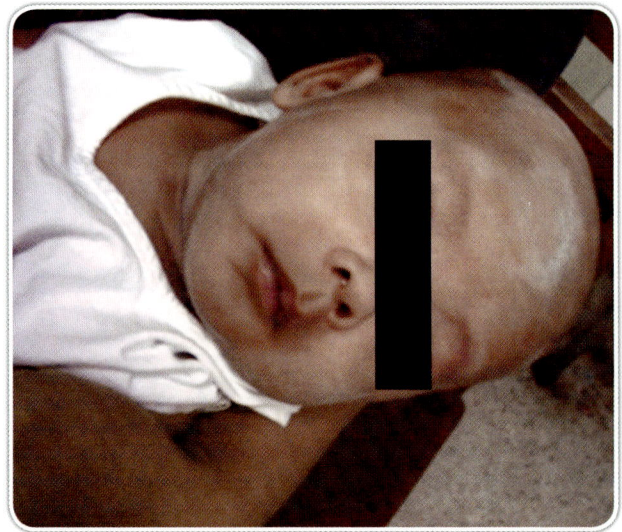

(Wataganara et al. 2006)

Fetal Intrathoracic Lesions

- Treatment options: Thoracocentesis
  Pleuro-amniotic shunting

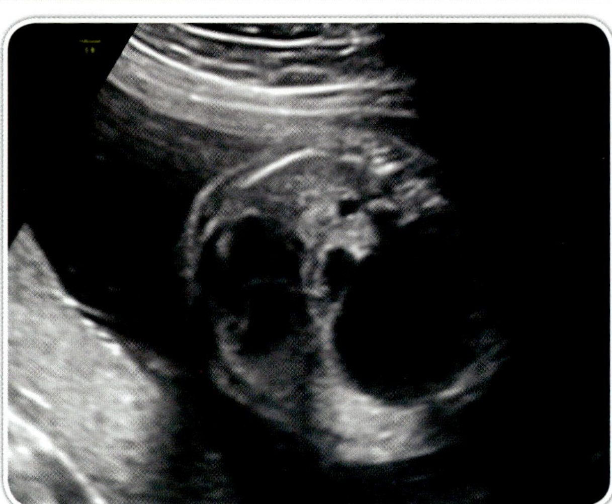

In Utero Management of Fetal Intrathoracic Lesions

Interventions	Diseases
Thoracocentesis (tapping)	Primary pleural effusion Macrocystic CPAM
Pleuro-amniotic shunting	Primary pleural effusion Macrocystic CPAM
Pleurodesis	Primary pleural effusion
Open fetal surgery (removal)	Microcystic CPAM Solid lesion

CPAM = congenital pulmonary airway malformation

Thoracocentesis

- Out patient setting
- Strict aseptic technique
- Fetal analgesia
- Tocolysis
- Technical considerations
- Fetal immobilization
- Anatomical consideration
- Fluid characteristics
- Possible adverse events
- Follow up.

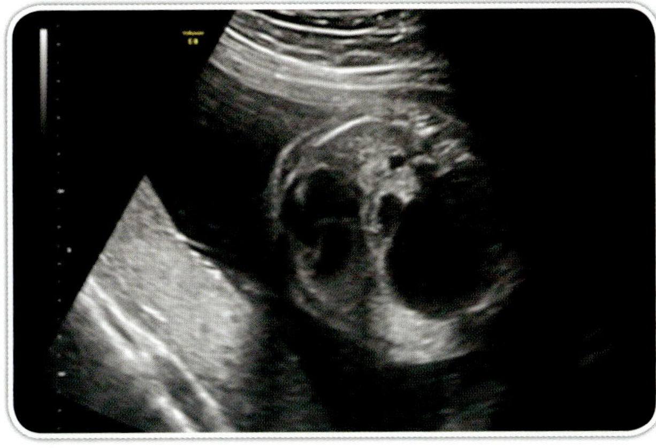

Pleuro-amniotic Shunting

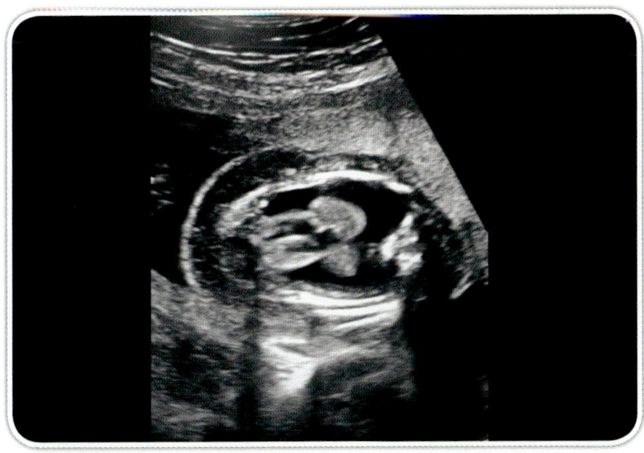

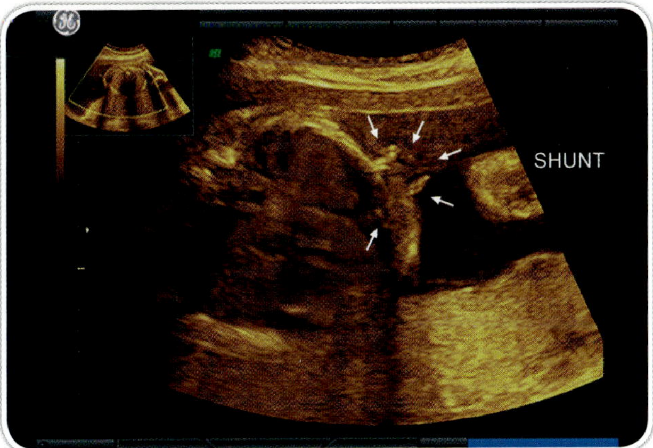

- **Rapid enlargement** of pleural effusion, especially with **mediastinal shift** and/or **hydrops**, is an indication for urgent decompression
- This will also allow for normal alveolar development
- Pleuro-amniotic shunting provides effective ongoing drainage

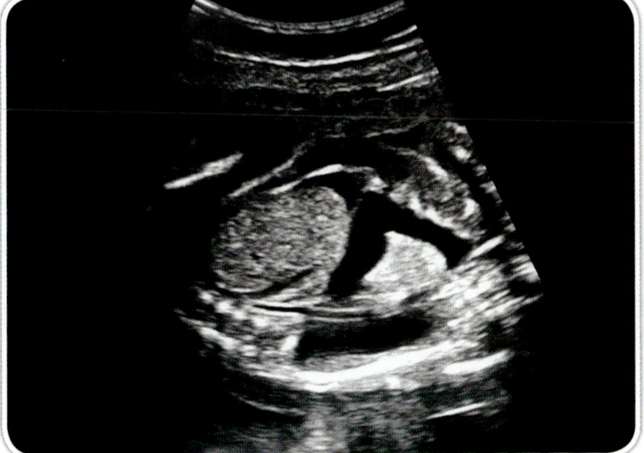

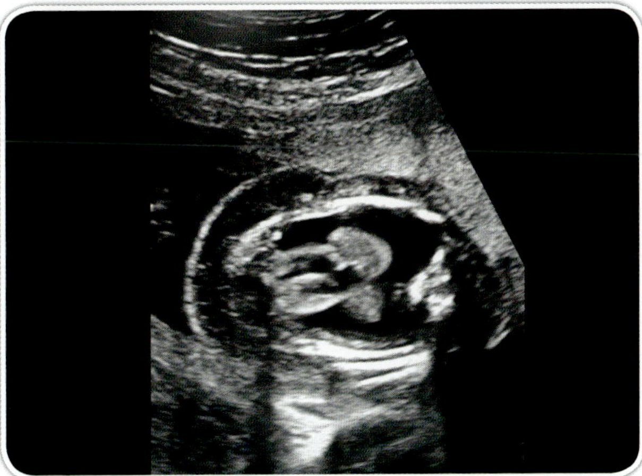

- Types of shunt
  - Basket shunt
  - Rocket shunt
  - Harrison bladder shunt

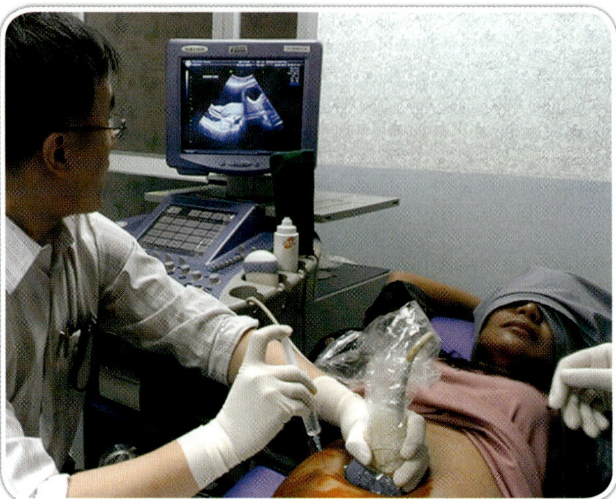

- Seldinger technique
- Equalization of the pressures in the pleural and amniotic cavity

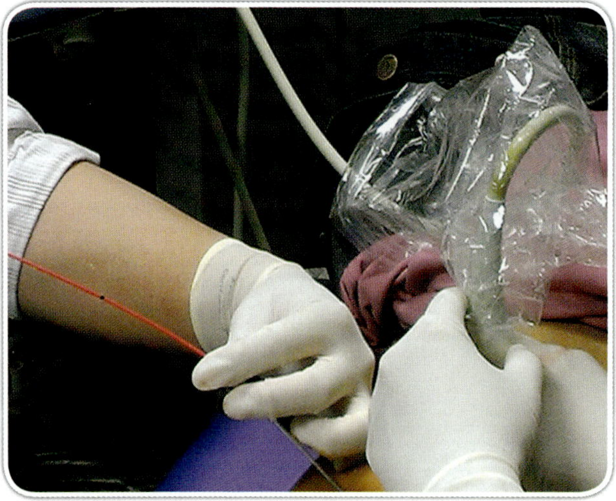

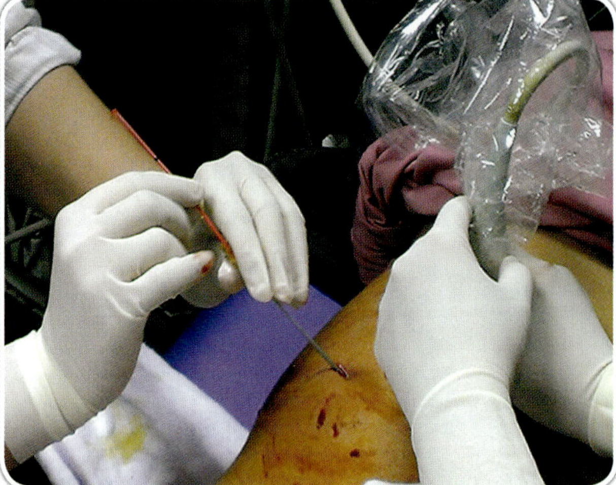

- Complications of shunting
  - Catheter migration
  - Shunt obstruction
  - Shunt reversal
  - Preterm premature rupture of membranes (PPROM)
  - Chorioamnionitis
- 10–20% of fetal shunts need to be repeated.

Shunt Migration

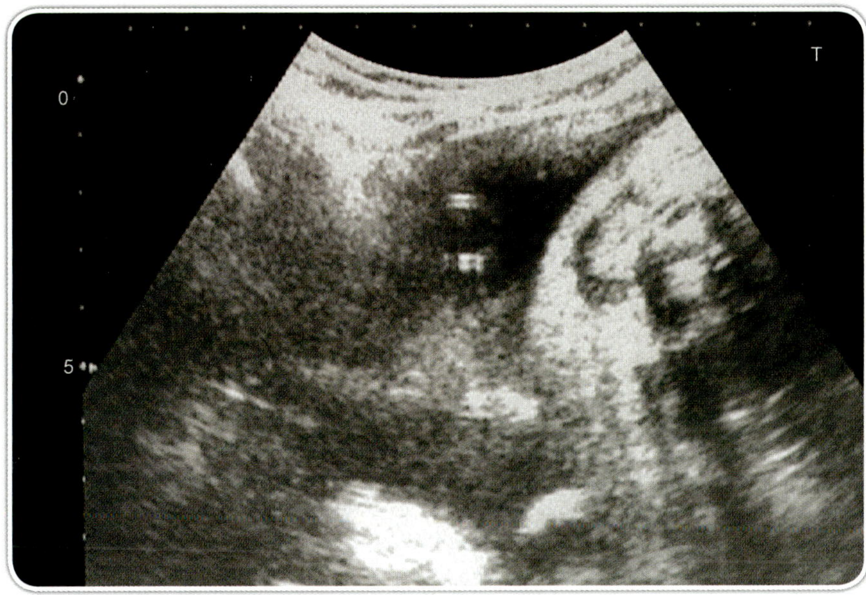

Pleuro-amniotic Shunting

- Follow up
    - Weekly ultrasound surveillance
        - progression/regression of the disease
        - shunt complications
    - Repeat shunting
    - Timing of delivery

(Nicolaides and Azar 1990)

In Utero Treatment of Fetal Lung Lesions

Pleurodesis	Open surgery
• Failed or repeated thoracocentesis	• Microcystic CPAM
• Failed or repeated shunting	• Solid lesions

FETAL POSTERIOR URETHRAL VALVE

- Treatment options
  - Vesicocentesis
  - Fetoscopic cystoscopy with valve ablation
  - Vesico-amniotic shunting
  - Open fetal surgery (no longer an option)

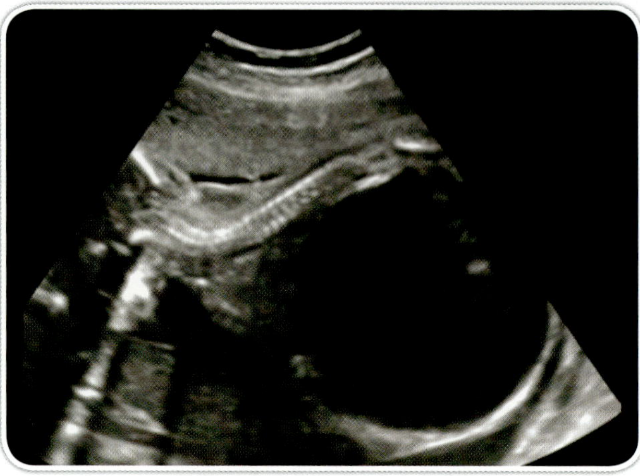

Posterior Urethral Valve

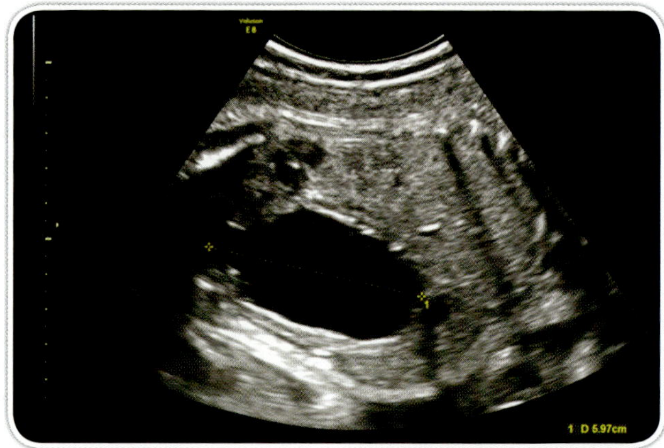

Congenital membranes obstructing the posterior urethra

Sonographic findings:

- Distended urinary bladder and proximal urethra ('keyhole sign')
- Oligohydramnios
- Hydronephrosis
- Renal cortical damages.

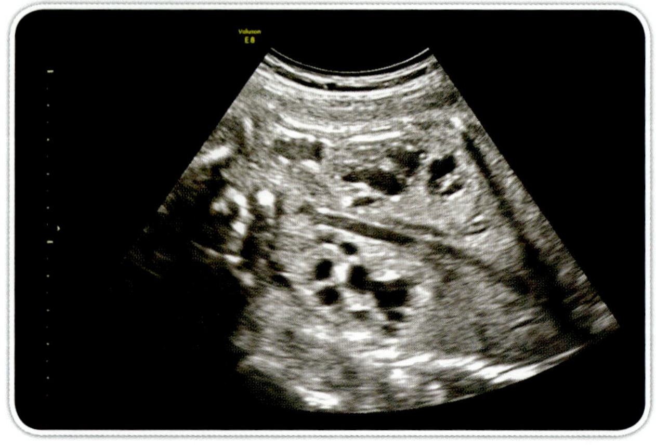

- The baby may die in utero, or suffers long-term consequences
  - Lung hypoplasia
  - Renal damages
  - Potter's syndrome
  - Prune belly syndrome.
- Approximately 1/3 of fetus with posterior urethral valve have abnormal karyotype.

(Haeri et al. 2013)

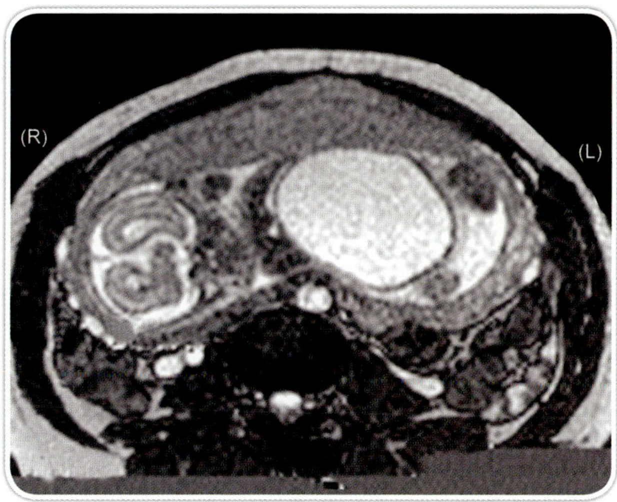

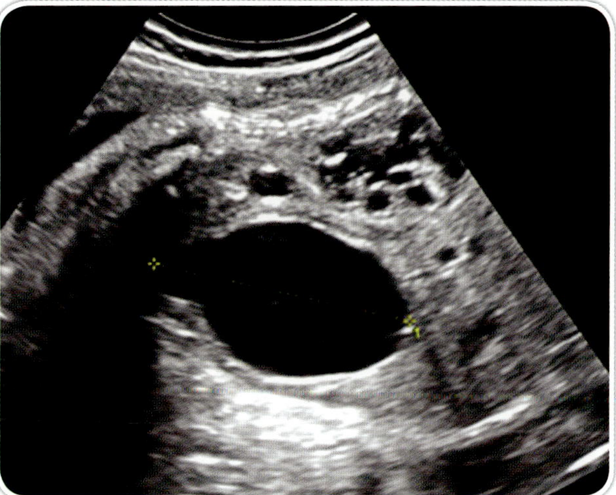

Renal Cystic Changes Resulting from Posterior Urethral Valve

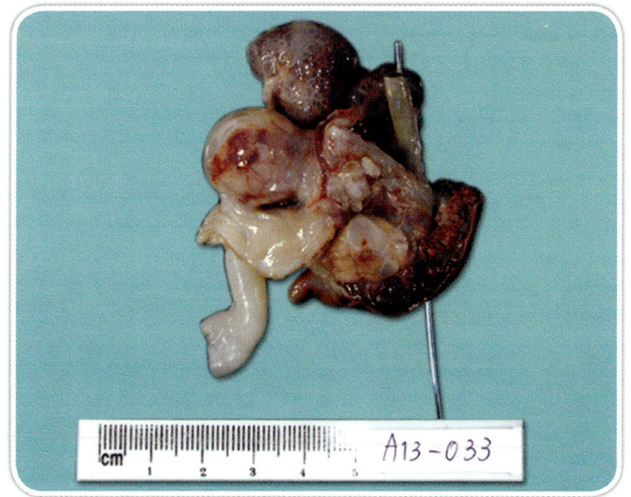

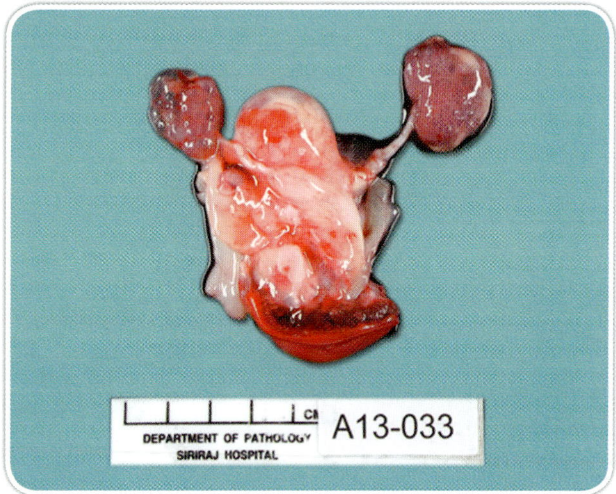

C/O Panitta Sitthinamsuwan, MD

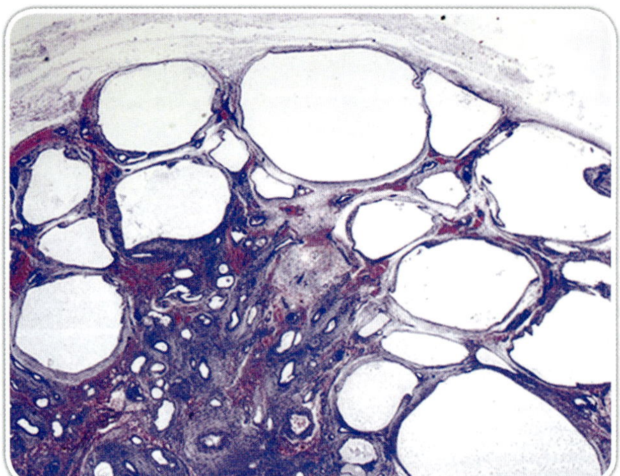

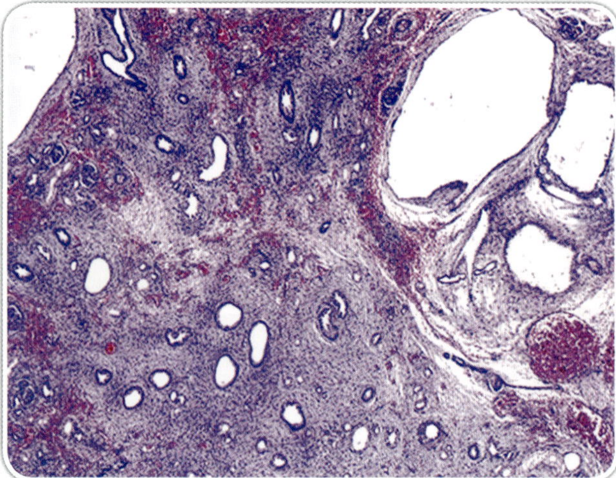

Cystic changes at renal cortex

C/O Panitta Sitthinamsuwan, MD

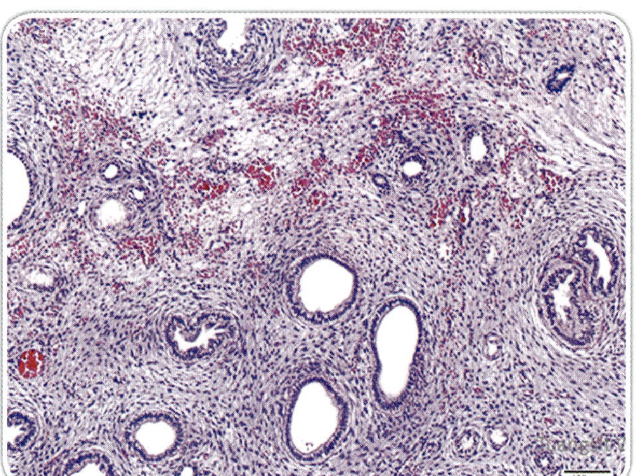

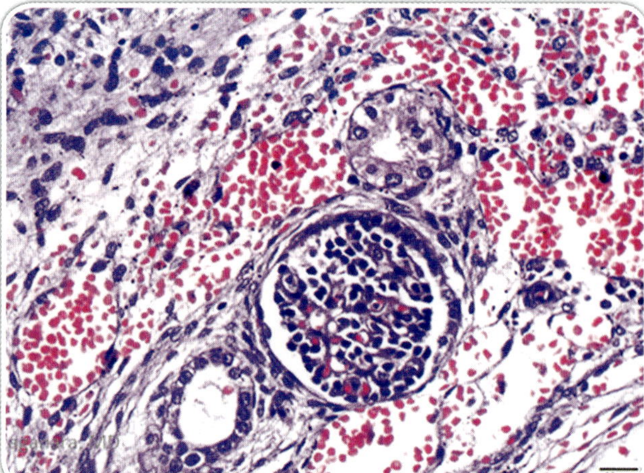

Interstitial and glomerular damages

Fetal Intervention in LUTO

- Criteria to offer interventions
  - Intact renal function: urine electrolytes, sonographic OR MRI appearances
  - No associated major malformations
  - No associated fetal aneuploidies

(LUTO = lower urinary tract obstruction)

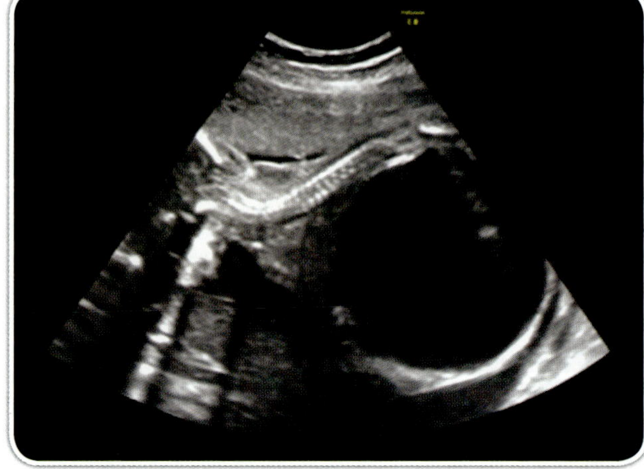

FETAL MRI IN POSTERIOR URETHRAL VALVE

Renal Damages from Posterior Urethral Valve Seen from MRI

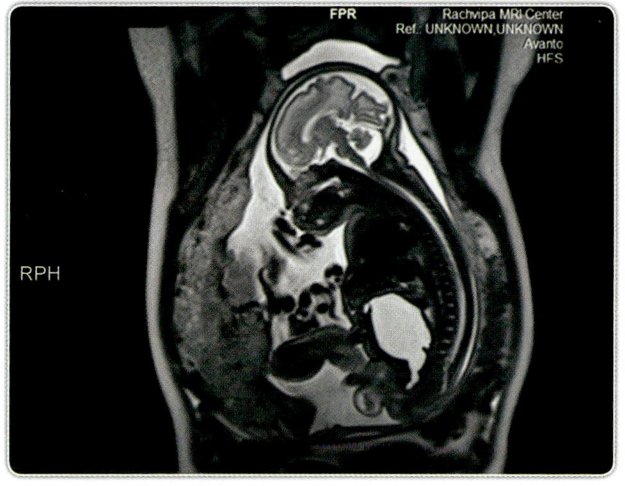

PUV in male fetus with near-normal liquor volume

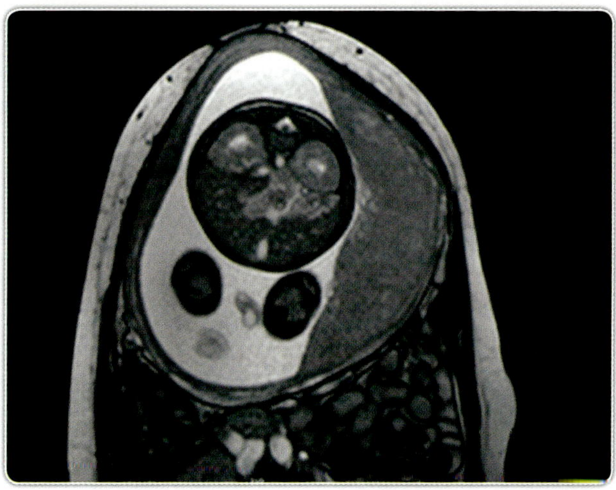

Normal MRI signaling of intact renal cortex

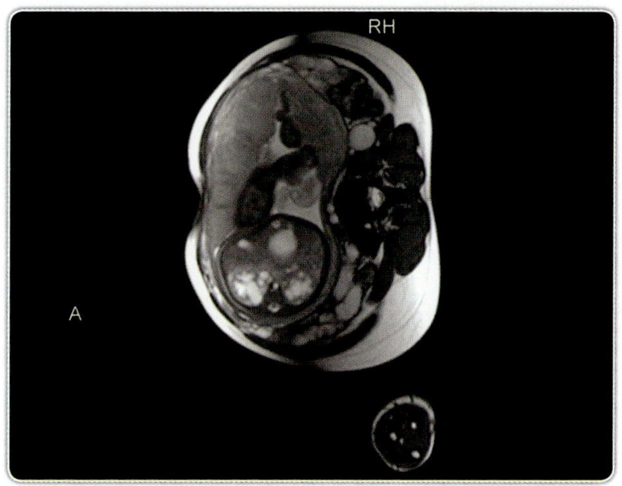

- Marked hydronephrosis
- Normal MRI signaling of renal cortex

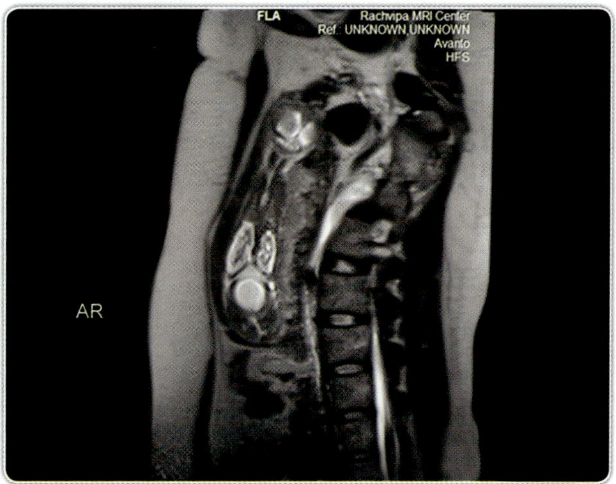

Scarring of renal cortex

Treatment Options for LUTO

No interventions	Interventions
• Termination of pregnancy	Single/serial vesicocentesis
	Percutaneous vesico-amniotic shunting
	Fetal cystoscopy with laser ablation of posterior urethral valve
• Expectant management	Open fetal surgery for vesicotomy

Vesicocentesis in LUTO

- Outpatient procedure
- Local anesthetic with maternal/fetal sedation
- ± prophylactic antibiotics
- ± ambulatory tocolysis (oral nifedipine 20–40 mg/day)
- Urine for karyotype studies and electrolytes.

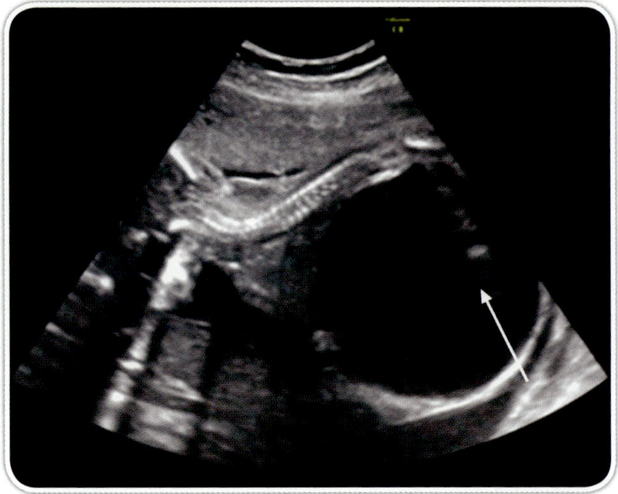

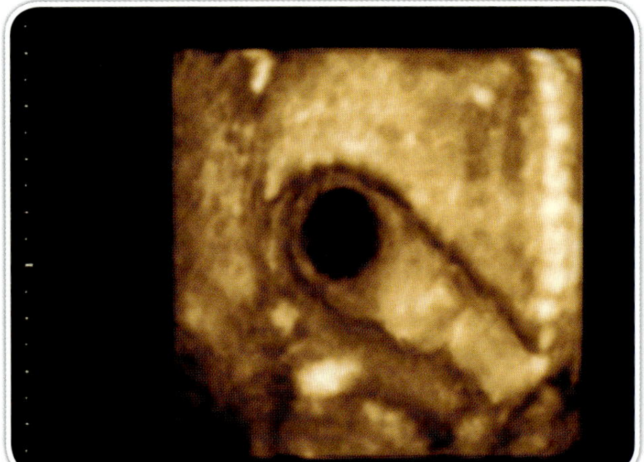

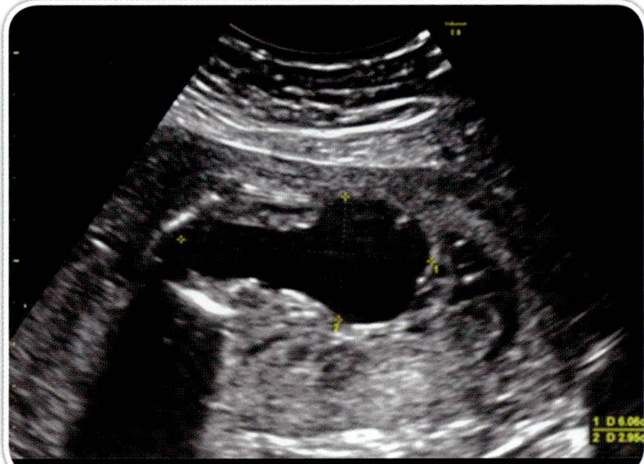

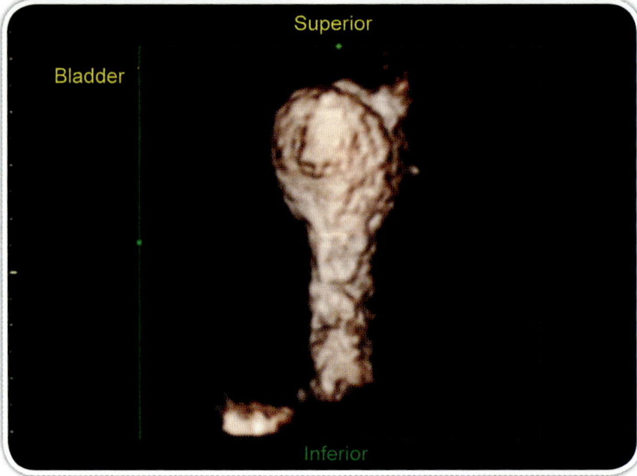

Urinary bladder refill immediately after vesicocentesis

Fetal Urine Electrolytes

Bad prognosis	Sensitivity (%)	Specificity (%)	Positive Predictive Value (%)	Negative Predictive Value (%)
Sodium < 100 mg/DL	56	64	56	88
Calcium < 8 mEq/L	100	27	43	100
Osmolality < 200 mOsm/L	83	82	71	90
β2-microglobulin < 4 mg/L	17	36	100	44
Total protein < 20 mg/dL	67	91	80	83

(Johnson et al. 1994)

Vesico-amniotic Shunting in LUTO

- Shunting should be offered only when fetal urine electrolytes are reassuring on serial vesicocentesis
- Shunting procedure yields approximately 50% survival
- It is frequently dislodged
- Some fetal death occurred as a direct consequence of shunt placement.

(Agarwal and Fisk 2001)

Fetal Cystoscopy with Laser Ablation of Posterior Urethral Valve

- Semirigid fetoscopic lens and curved sheath are used
- Pedriatrics urologist scrubbed in every surgery.

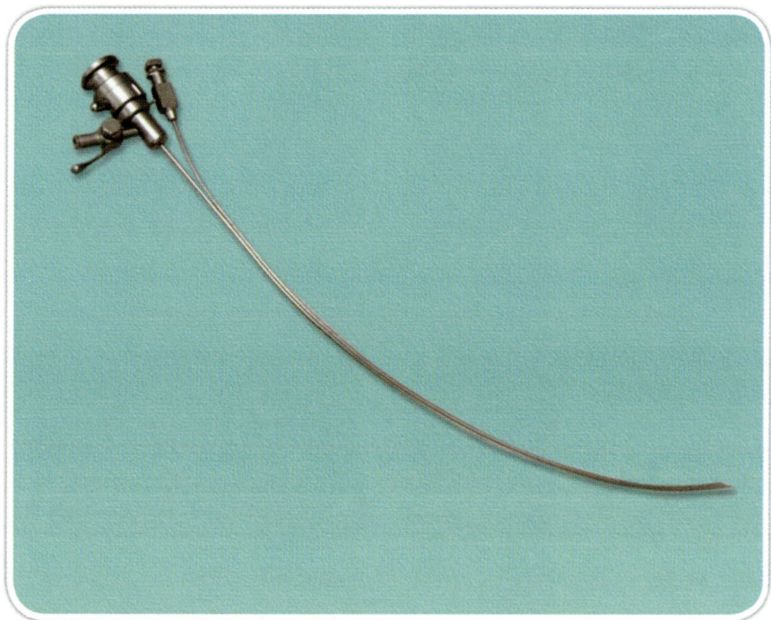

- Proximal urethra was accessed under real-time ultrasound guidance

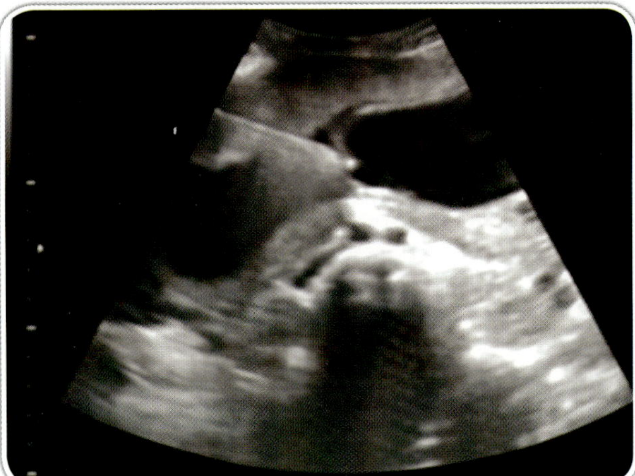

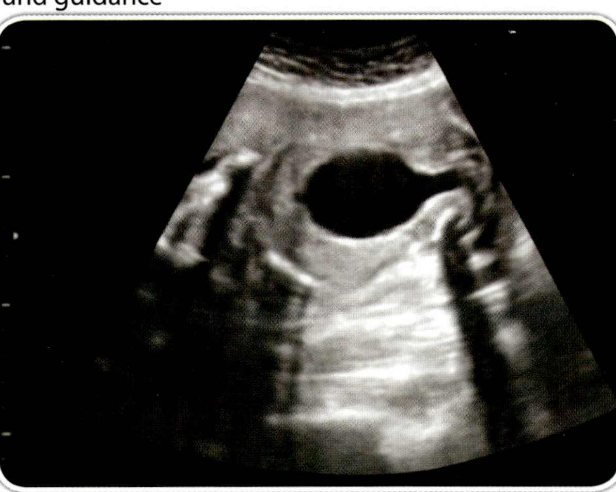

Division of Maternal Fetal Medicine, Faculty of Medicine Siriraj Hospital

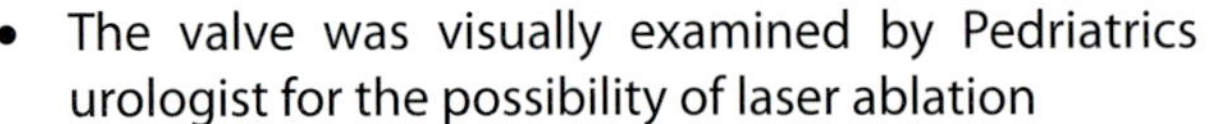

- The valve was visually examined by Pedriatrics urologist for the possibility of laser ablation
- The valve was dissected and ablated with Nd-YAG laser fiber.

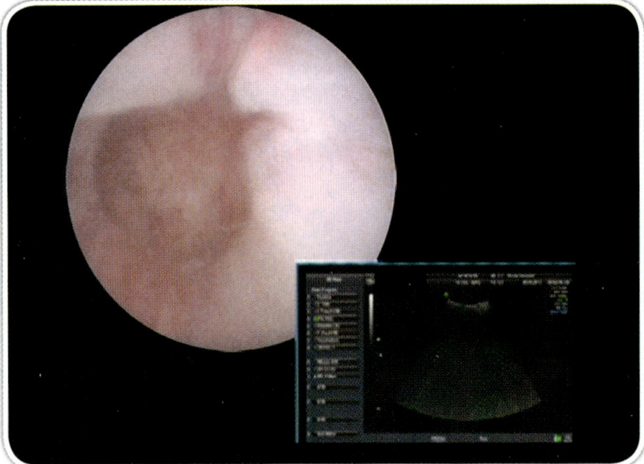

- US is performed on the day after the surgery
- The success is determined by collapse of the urinary bladder and hydronephrosis, and increased liquor volume.

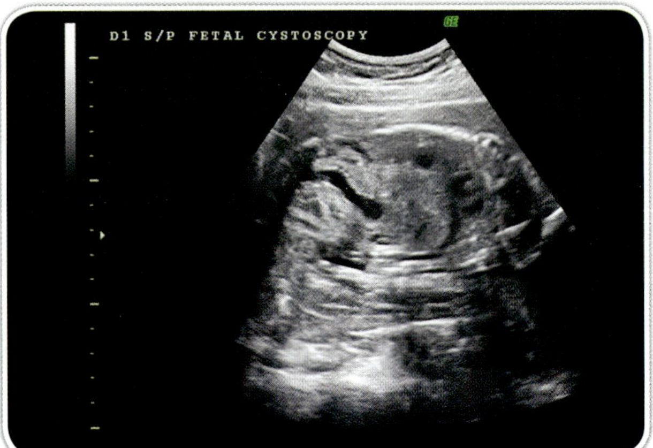

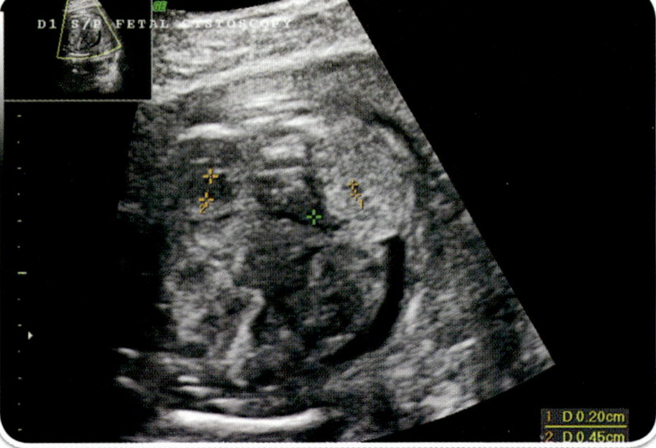

Note the thickness of the urinary bladder as a result of prolonged obstruction

CONGENITAL DIAPHRAGMATIC HERNIA

Treatment options: Fetal balloon tracheal occlusion
Postnatal surgical correction

- Congenital defect of the diaphragm
- Bochdalek is more common than Morgagni hernia.

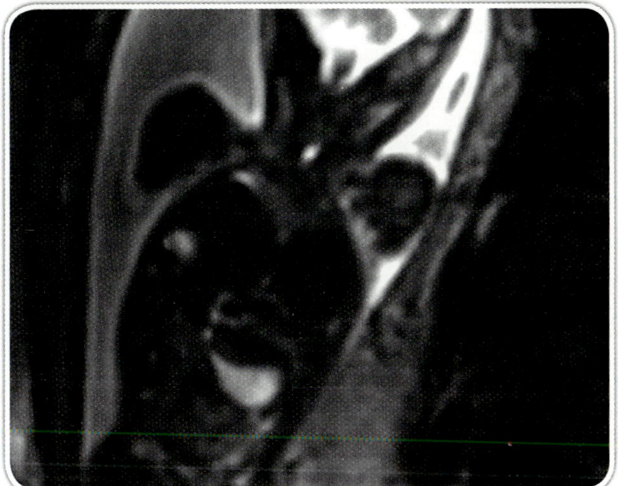

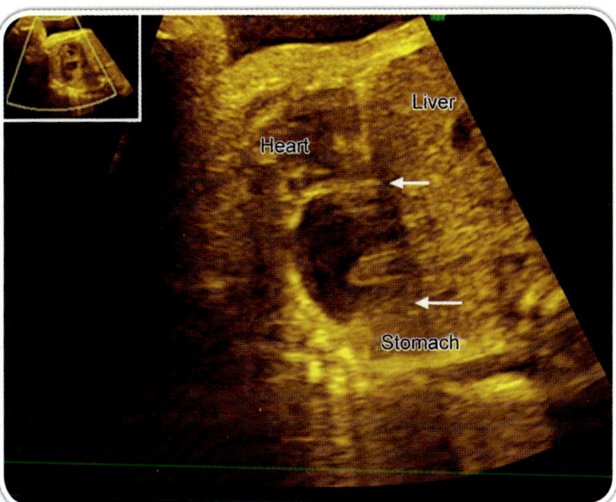

- Abdominal organs are pushed into the chest, hindering proper lung formation
- The baby can have severe respiratory distress at birth as a result of pulmonary hypoplasia and pulmonary hypertension.

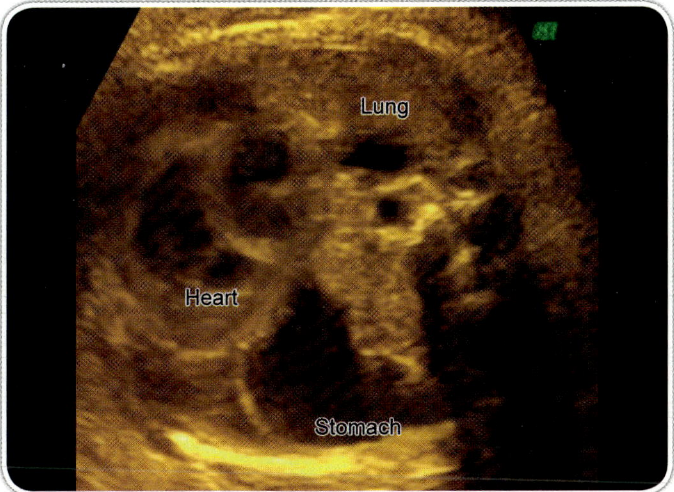

Factors Determining Neonatal Survival

- Intrathoracic liver herniation
- Residual lung volume
  - Observed/Expected Lung-to-Head Ratio (O/E LHR): **Ultrasound**
  - Fetal lung volume: **MRI**

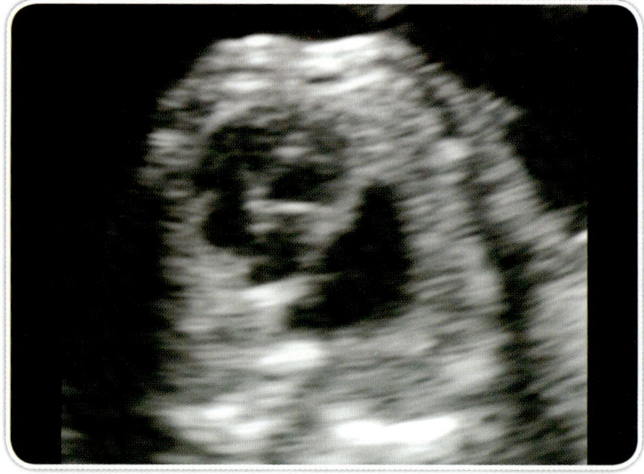

Left CDH

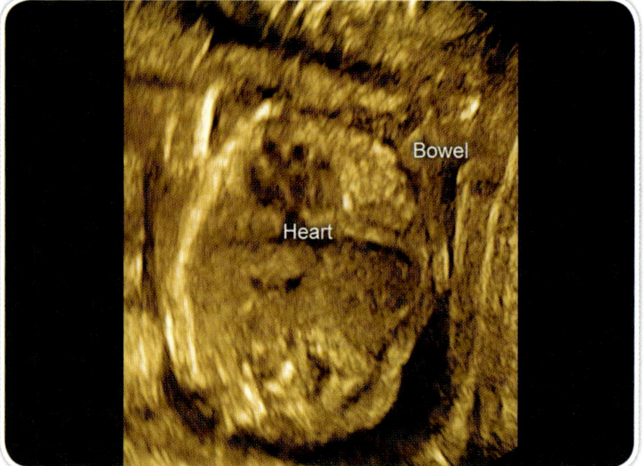

Right CDH

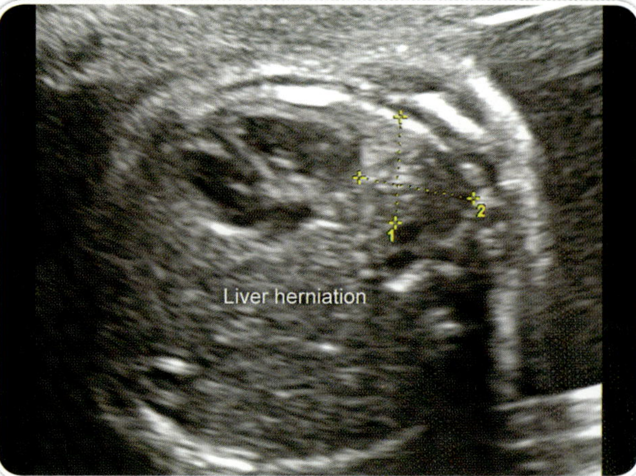

Observed-Expected Lung-Head Ratio (O/E LHR)

Ultrasound

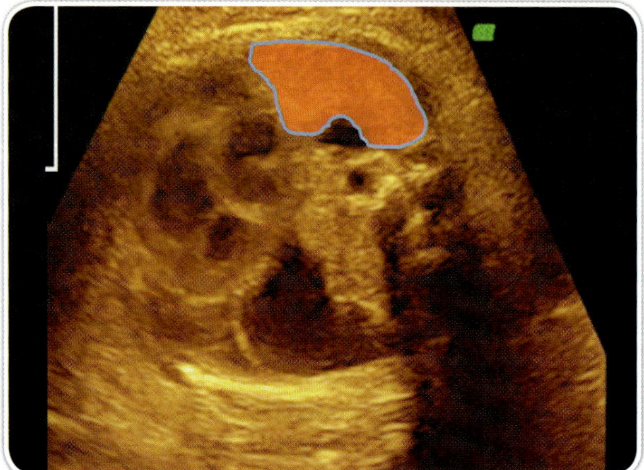

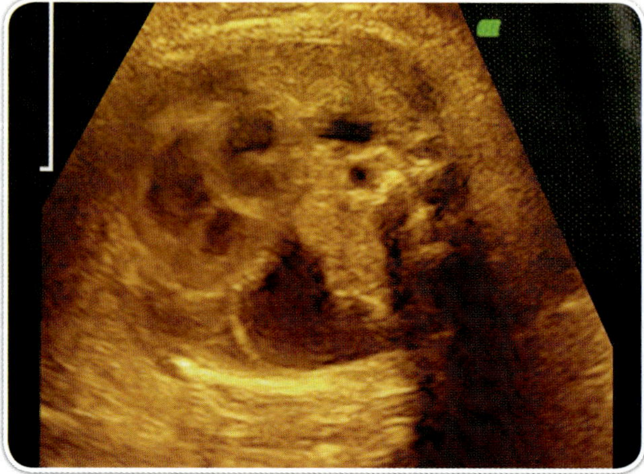

Fetal Lung Volume Assessment
MRI: Area and Slice Thickness

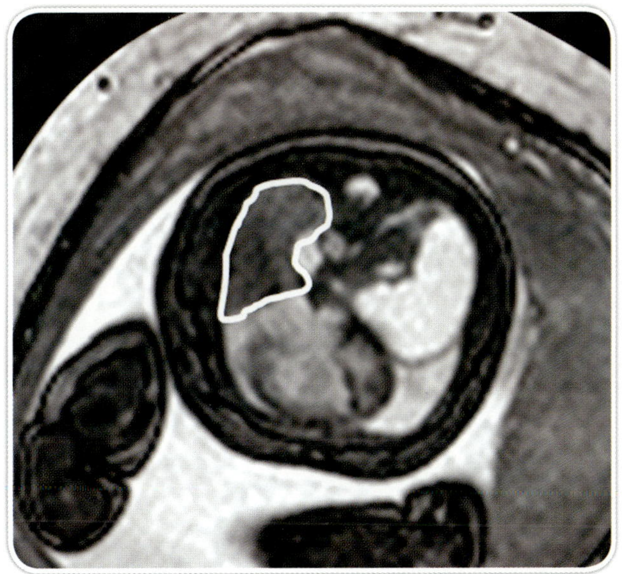

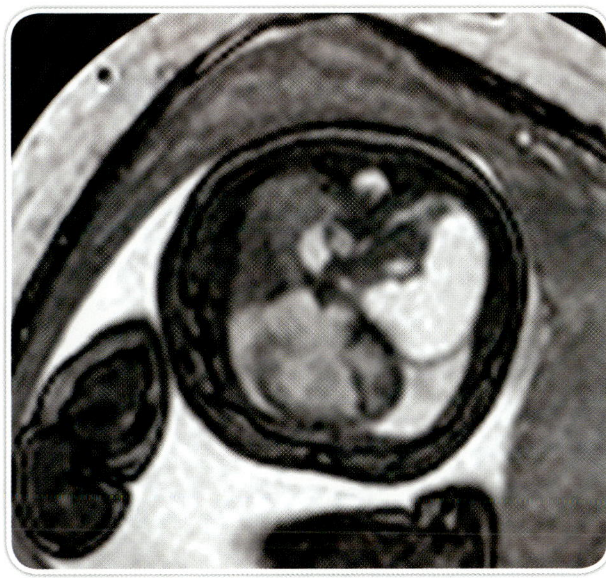

MRI to Determine Liver Position

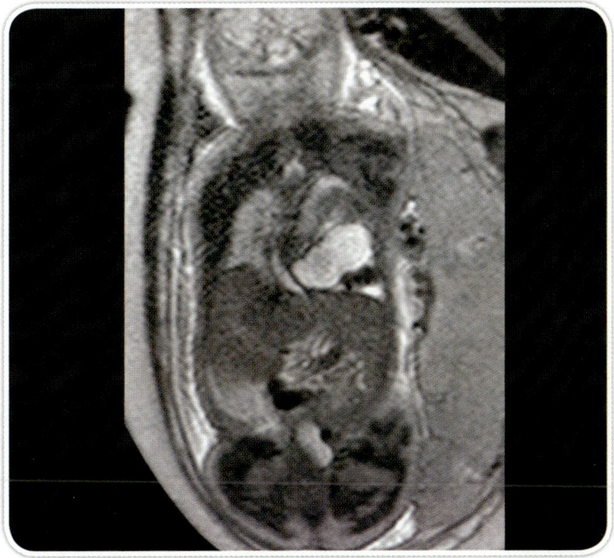

Liver down: Better prognosis

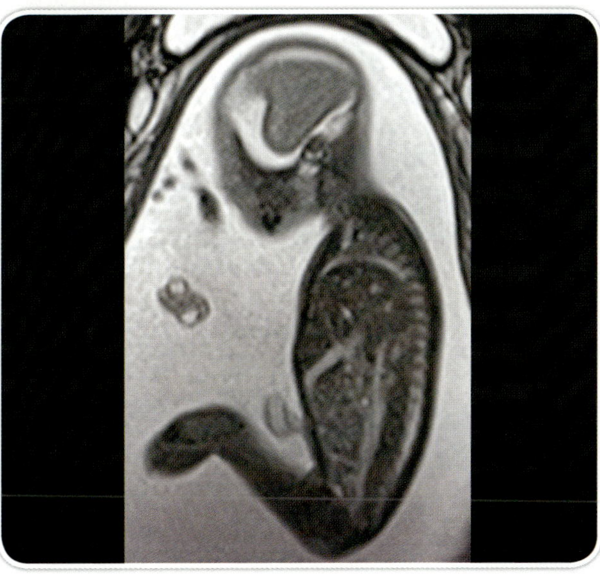

Liver up: Poorer prognosis

Fetoscopic Balloon Tracheal Occlusion

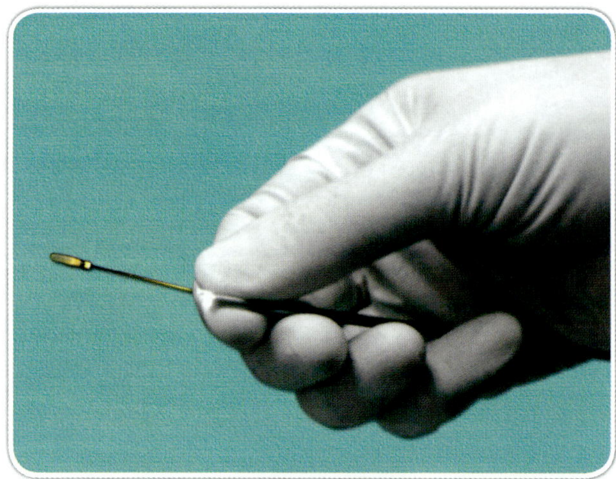

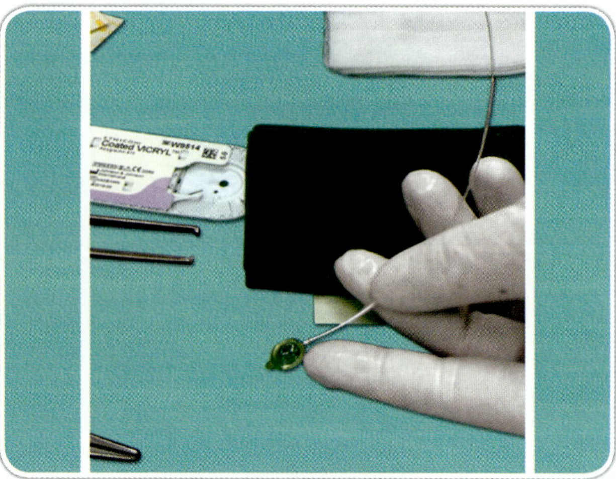

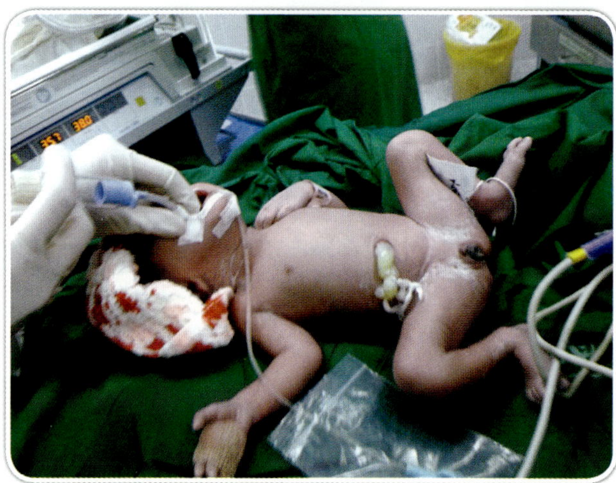

Immediately after birth

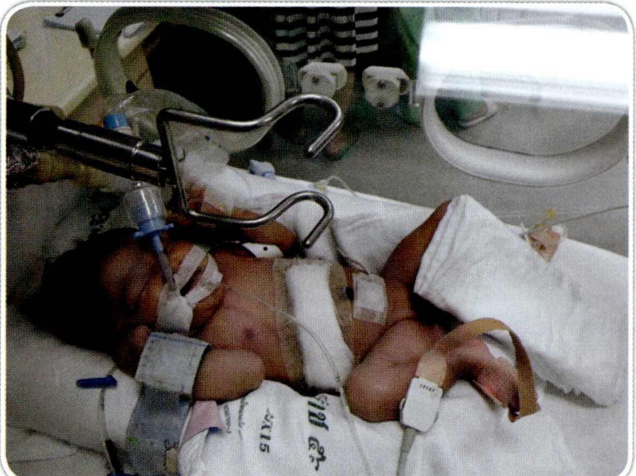

After surgical repair of diaphragmatic defect

Congenital Pulmonary Airway Malformation (CPAM)

Treatment options: Sclerotherapy
Shunting
Open fetal surgery (resection)

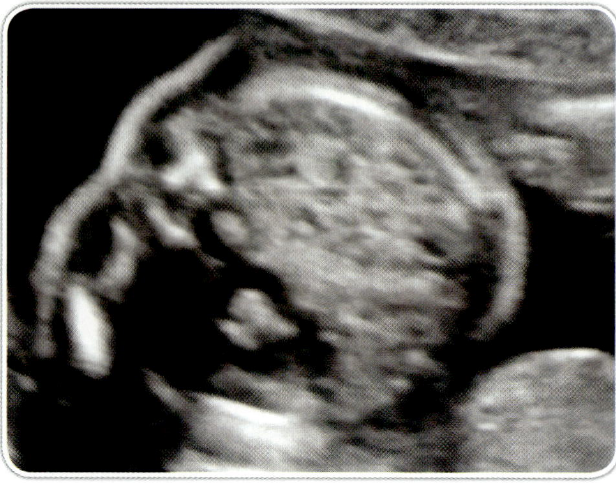

- Multicystic mass from proliferation of bronchial structures
- Incidence 1:10,000 to 1:35,000 of live births
- Macrocystic and Microcystic types can cause fetal hydrops.

(Duncombe et al. 2002)

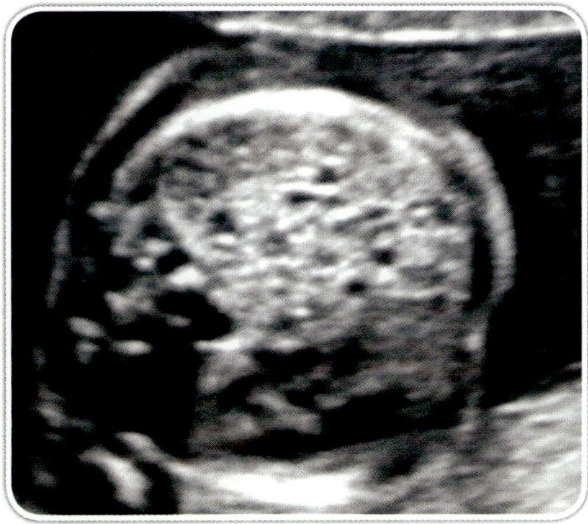

Treatment Options

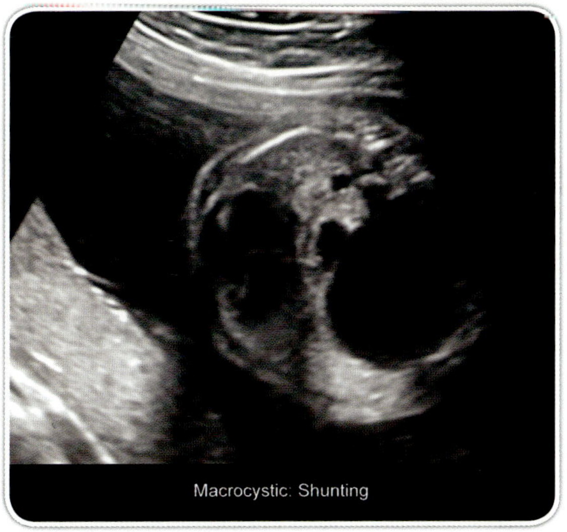

Macrocystic CPAM, can be conveniently treated with fetal shunting

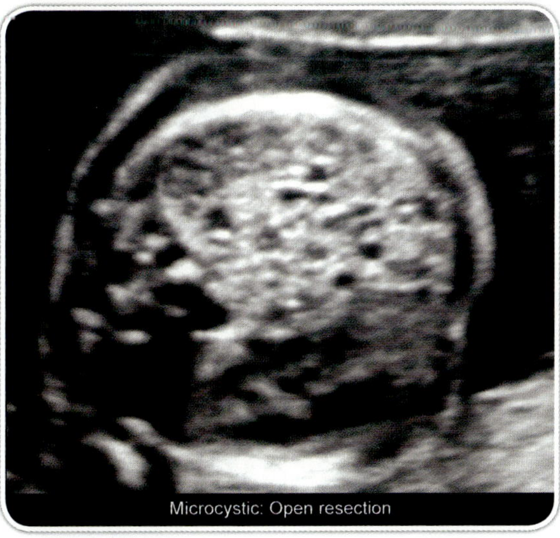

Microcystic CPAM, open fetal surgery for resection used to be the only fetal treatment option (aside from steroids)

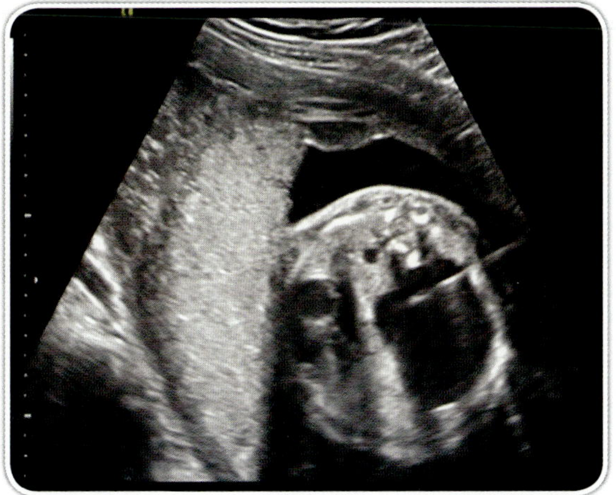

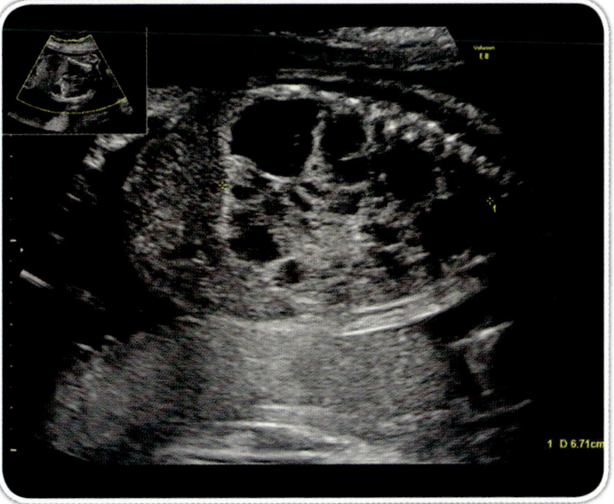

Microcystic CPAM

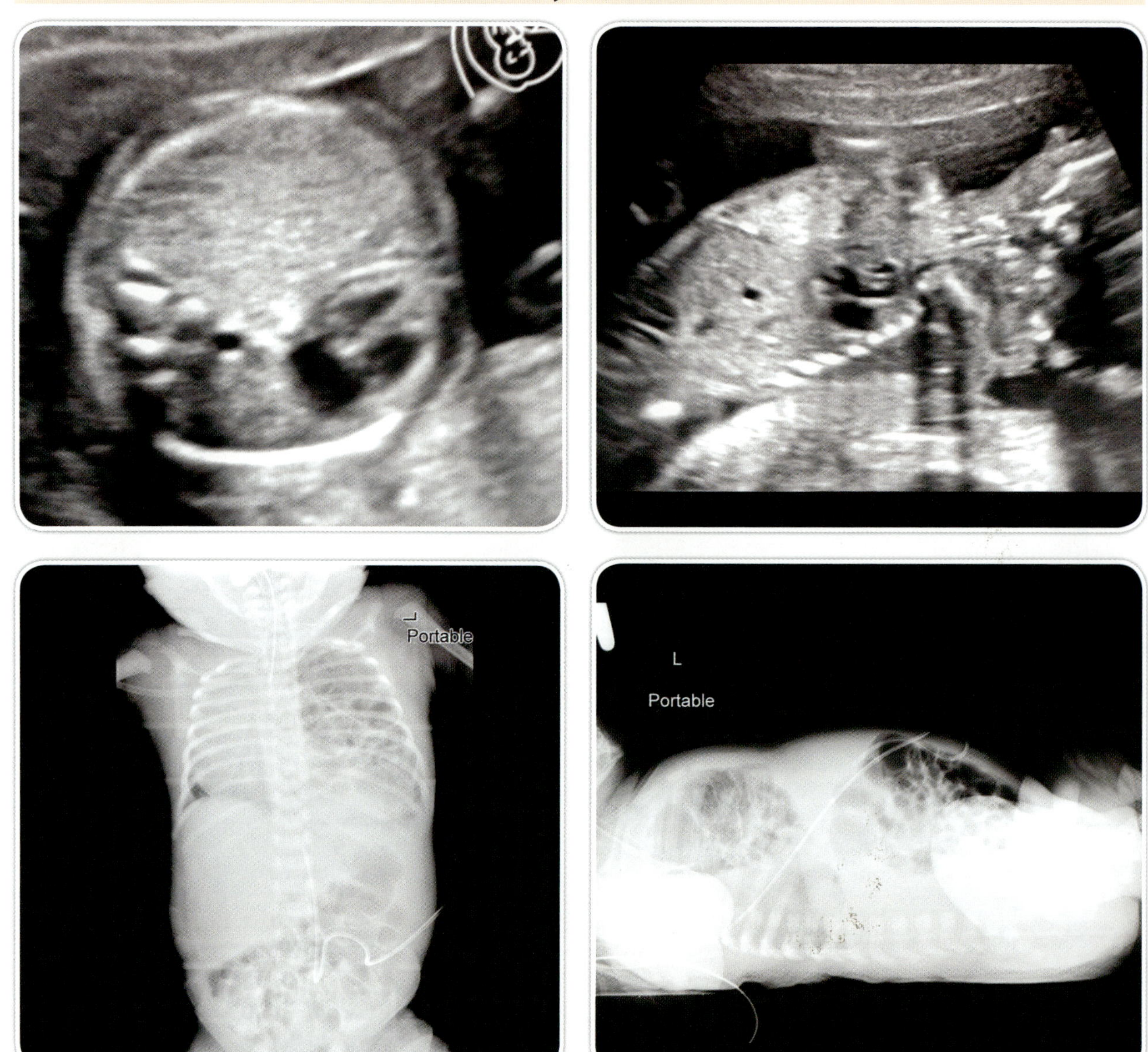

Postnatal radiograph of CPAM *(Siriraj NICU)*

Large CPAM with Mediastinal Compression, Resulting in Hydrops and Polyhydramnios

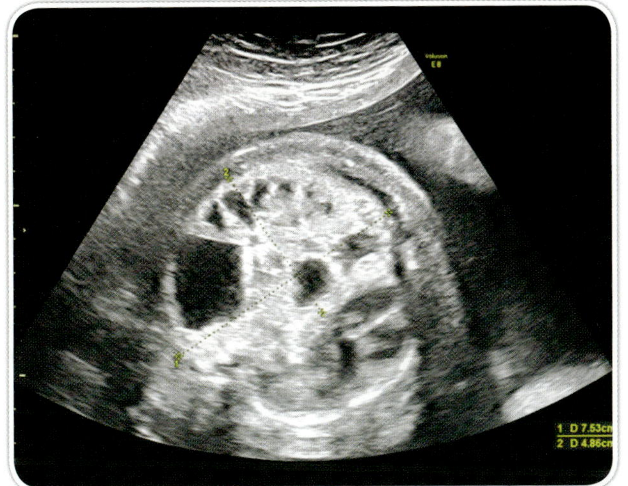

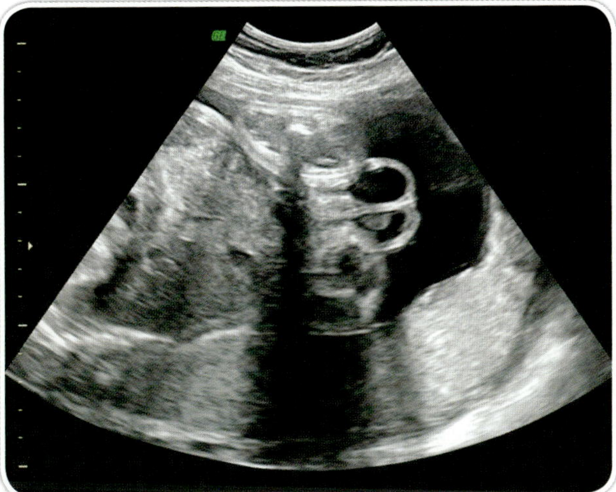

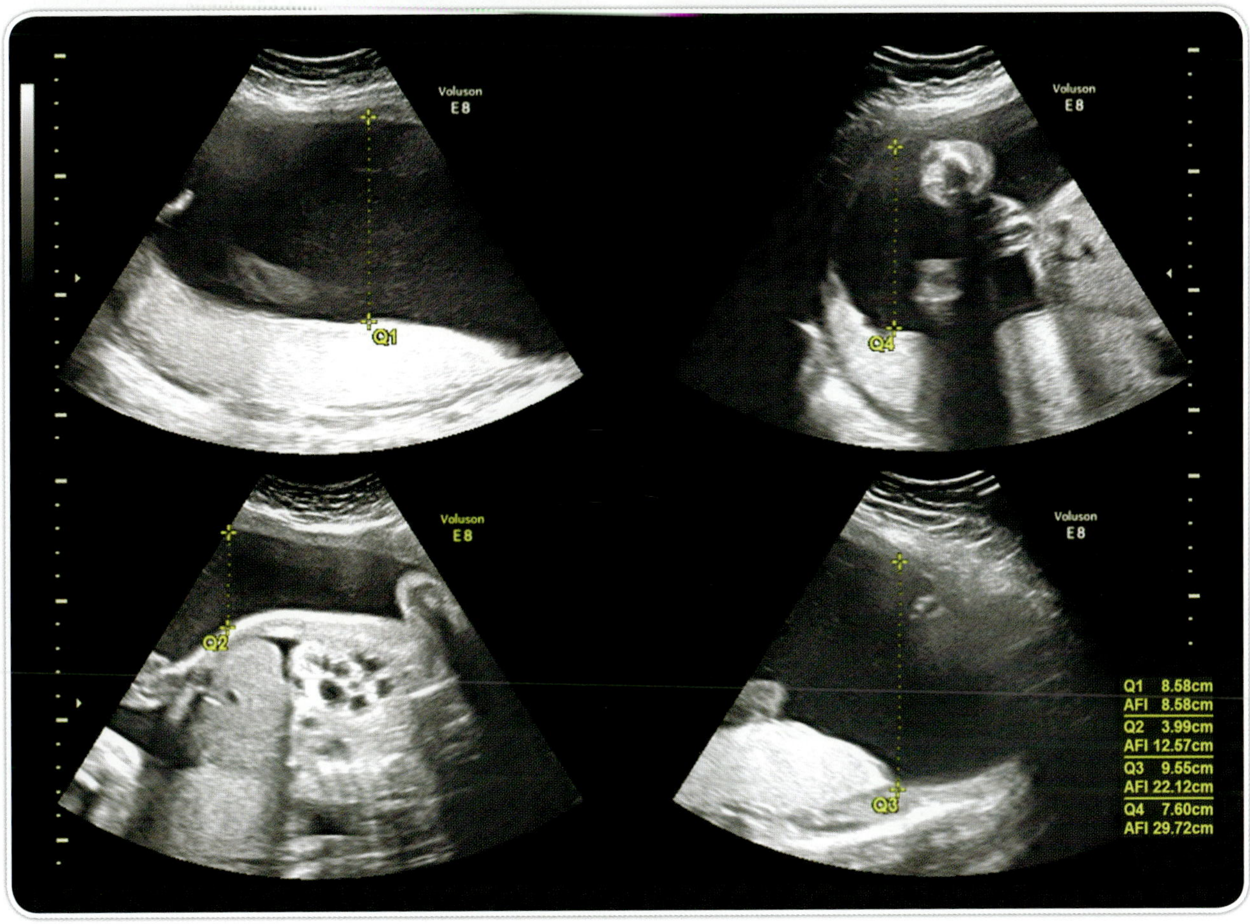

PERCUTANEOUS SCLEROTHERAPY

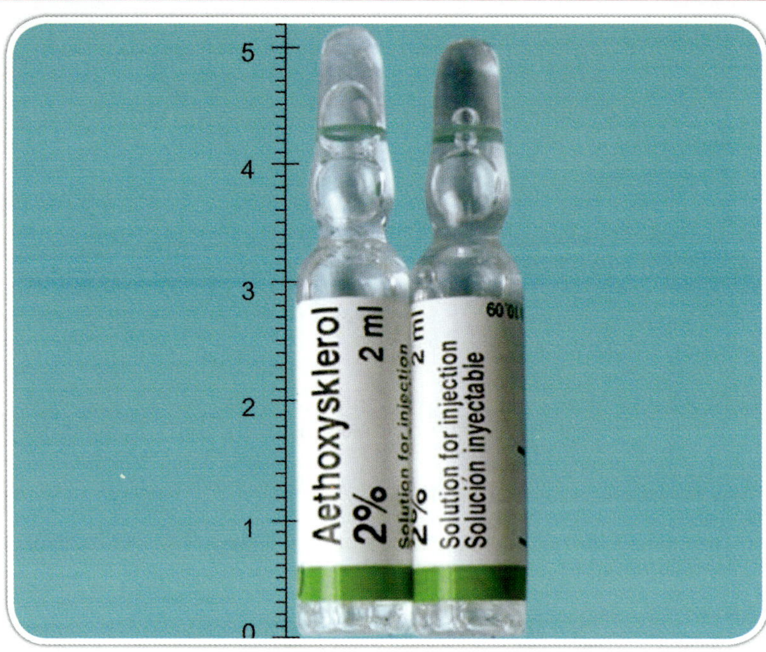

Response of Fetal Hydrops from CPAM after Percutaneous Sclerotherapy

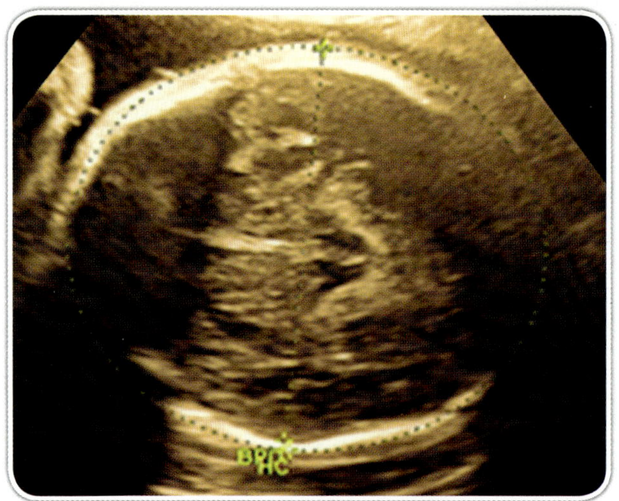

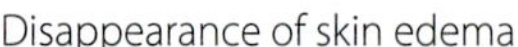
Disappearance of skin edema

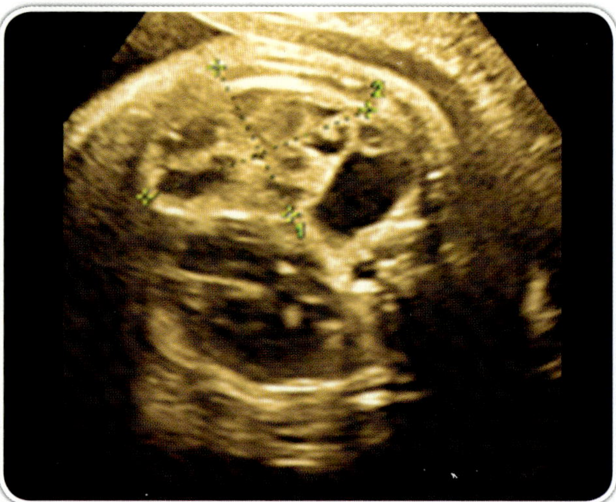

Decrease in size of the CPAM

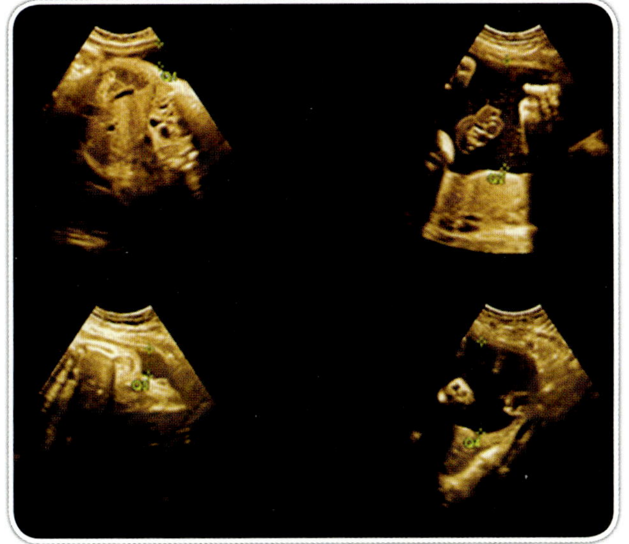

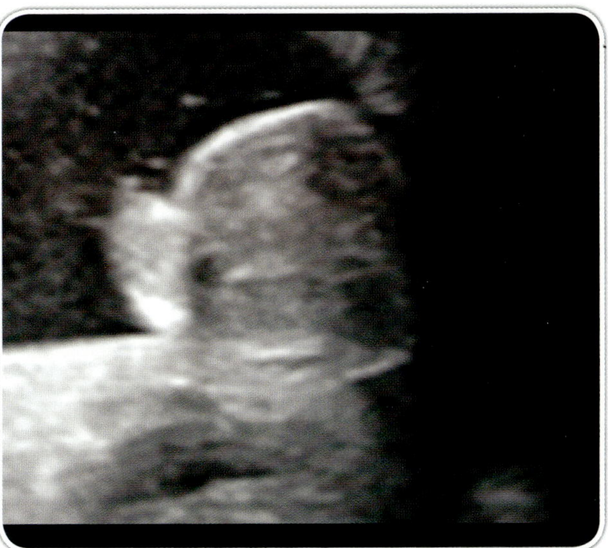

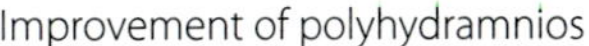

Improvement of polyhydramnios

Disappearance of ascites and hydrocele

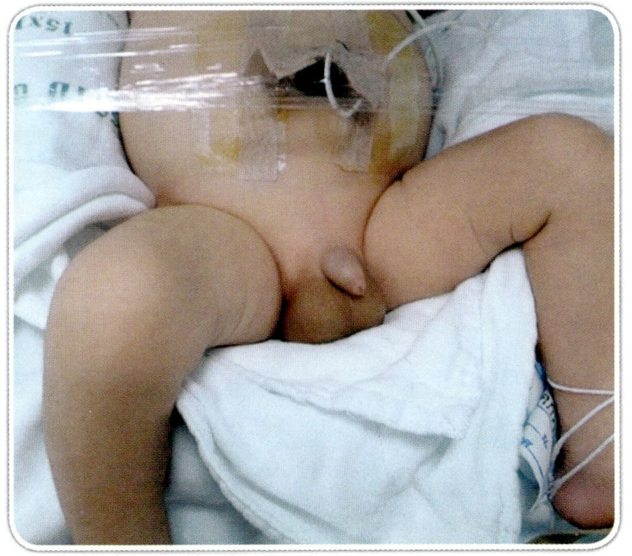

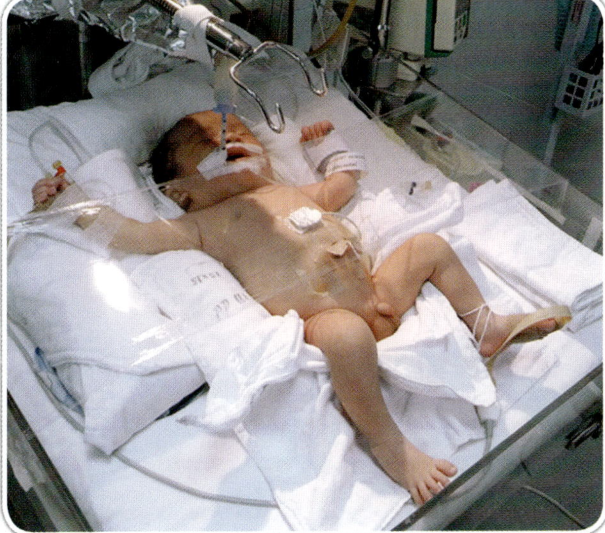

EX UTERO INTRAPARTUM TREATMENT EXIT

Large Fetal Neck Mass

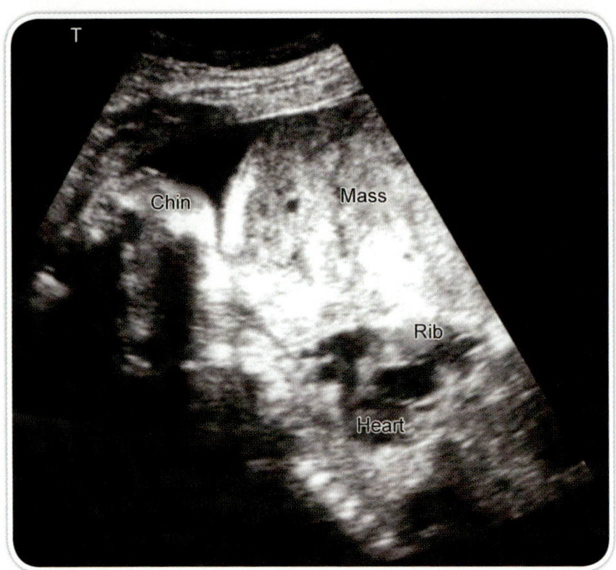

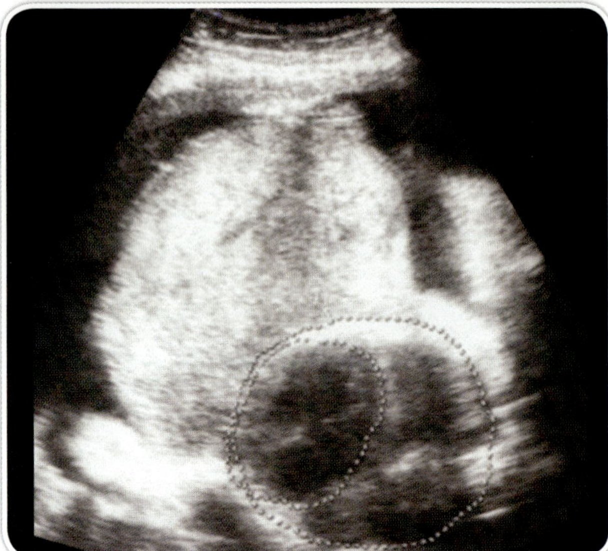

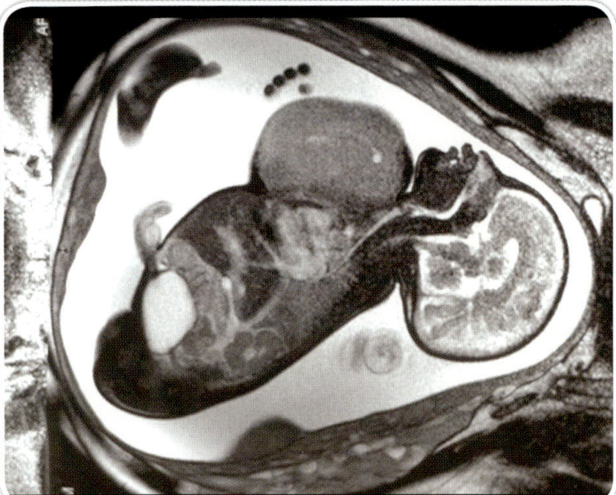

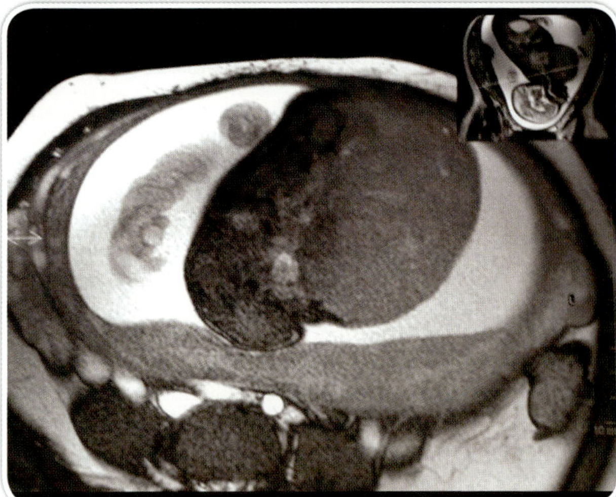

(Wataganara et al. 2007)

EXIT Procedure

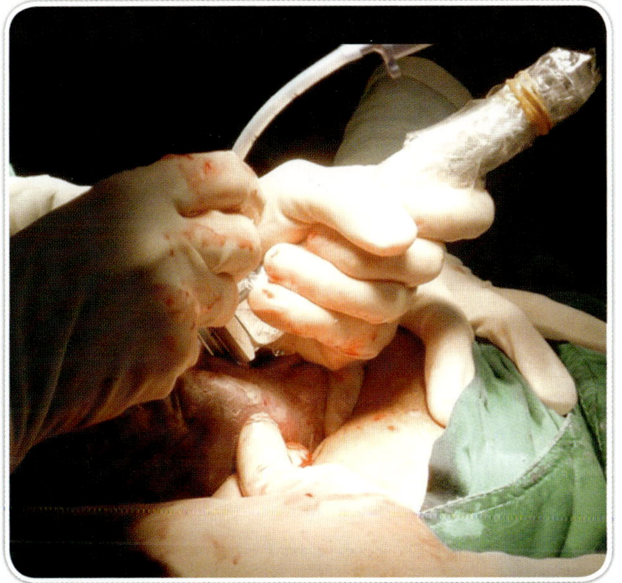

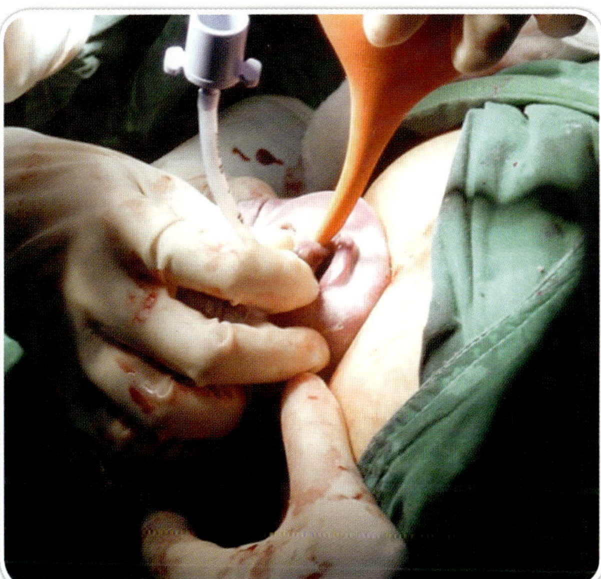

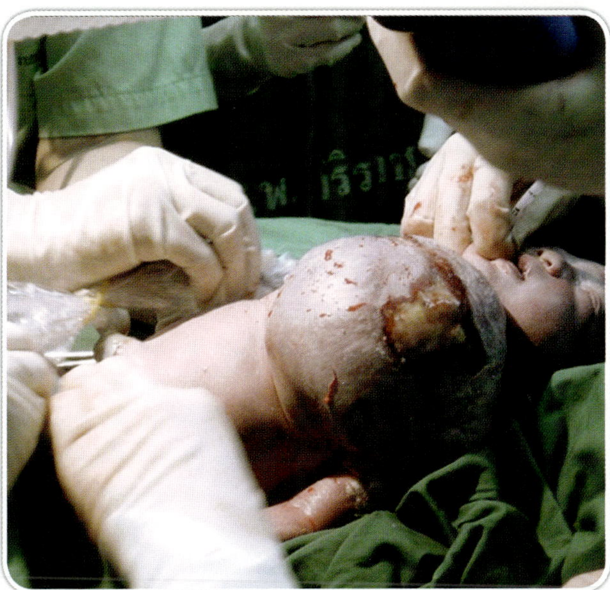

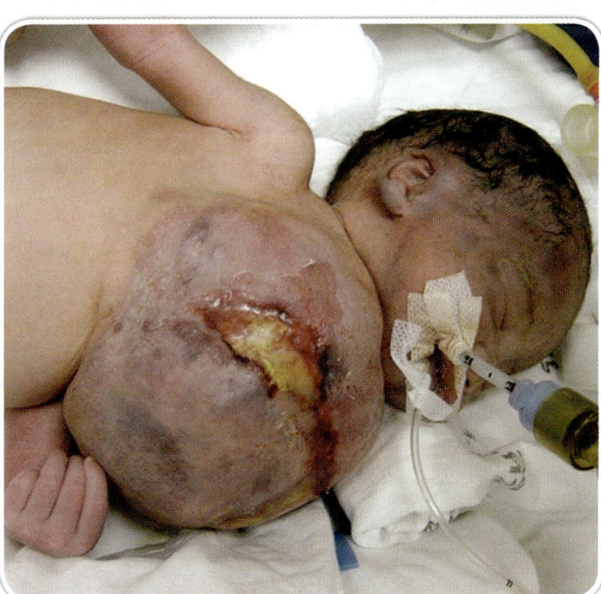

(Wataganara et al. 2007)

PLACENTAL CHORIOANGIOMA

Treatment options: Amnioreduction
Laser devascularization

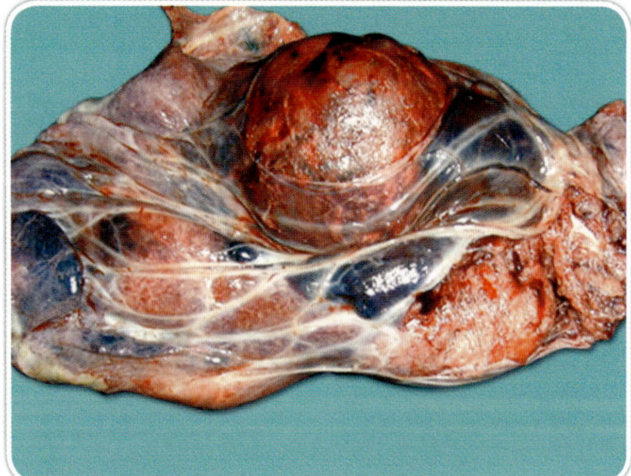

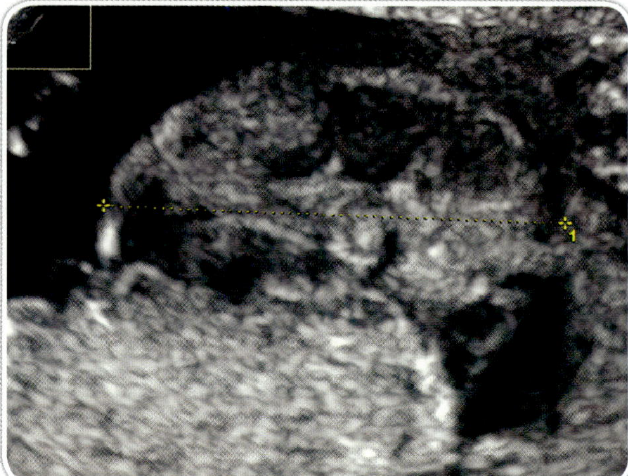

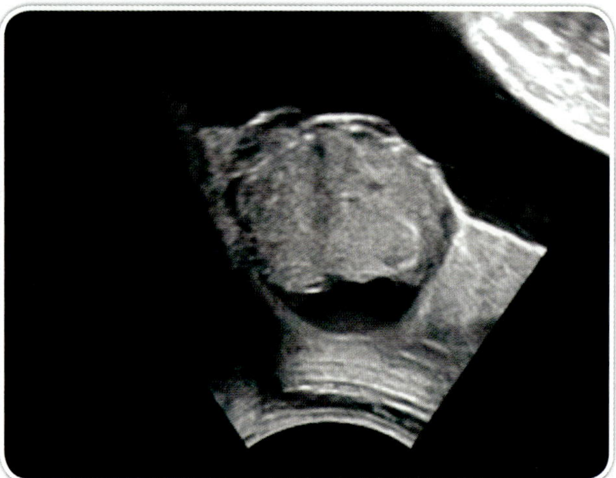

US findings

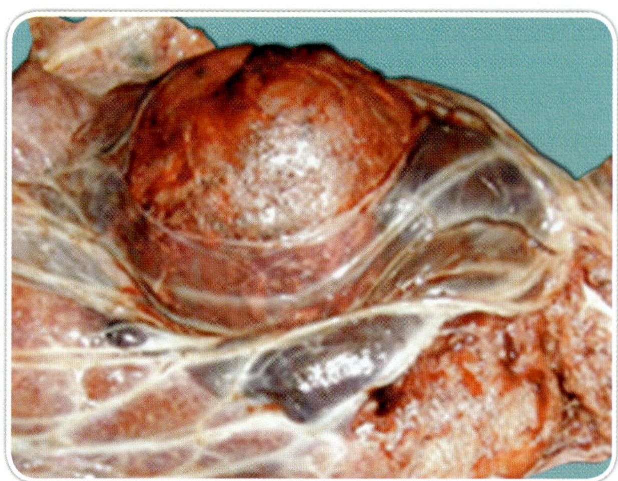

Gross appearance

- Incidence 1% of pregnancy
- Most common tumor of the placenta
- Benign nature, and often asymptomatic

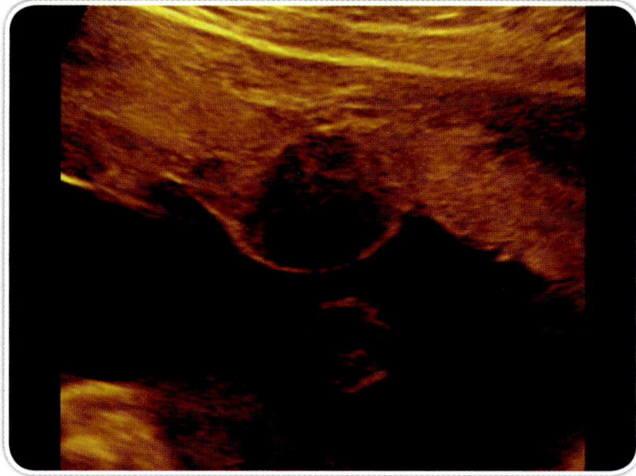

- Large tumor can cause fetal heart failure, hydrop fetalis, fetal thrombocytopenia, and polyhydramnios.
- **Ultrasound:** Hypoechoic round mass near cord insertion, distinctly separate from normal placenta.
- **Doppler:** Pulsatile flow within the anechoic areas, representing vascular channels.

(Hadi et al. 1993)

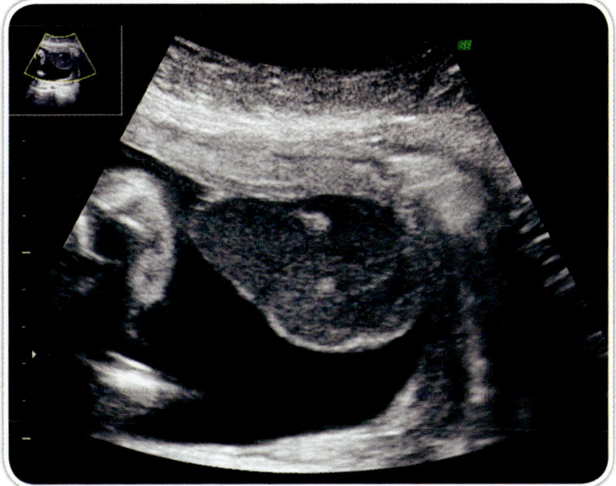

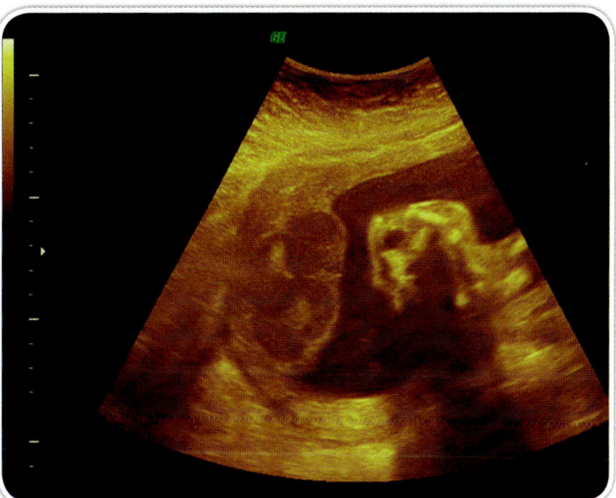

Sequelae of Placental Chorioangioma

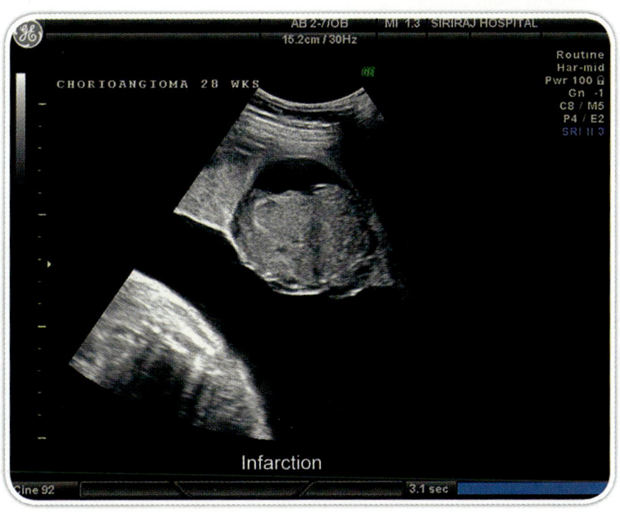

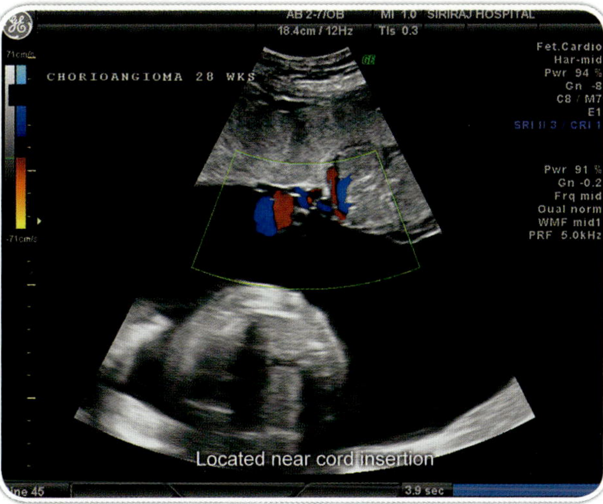

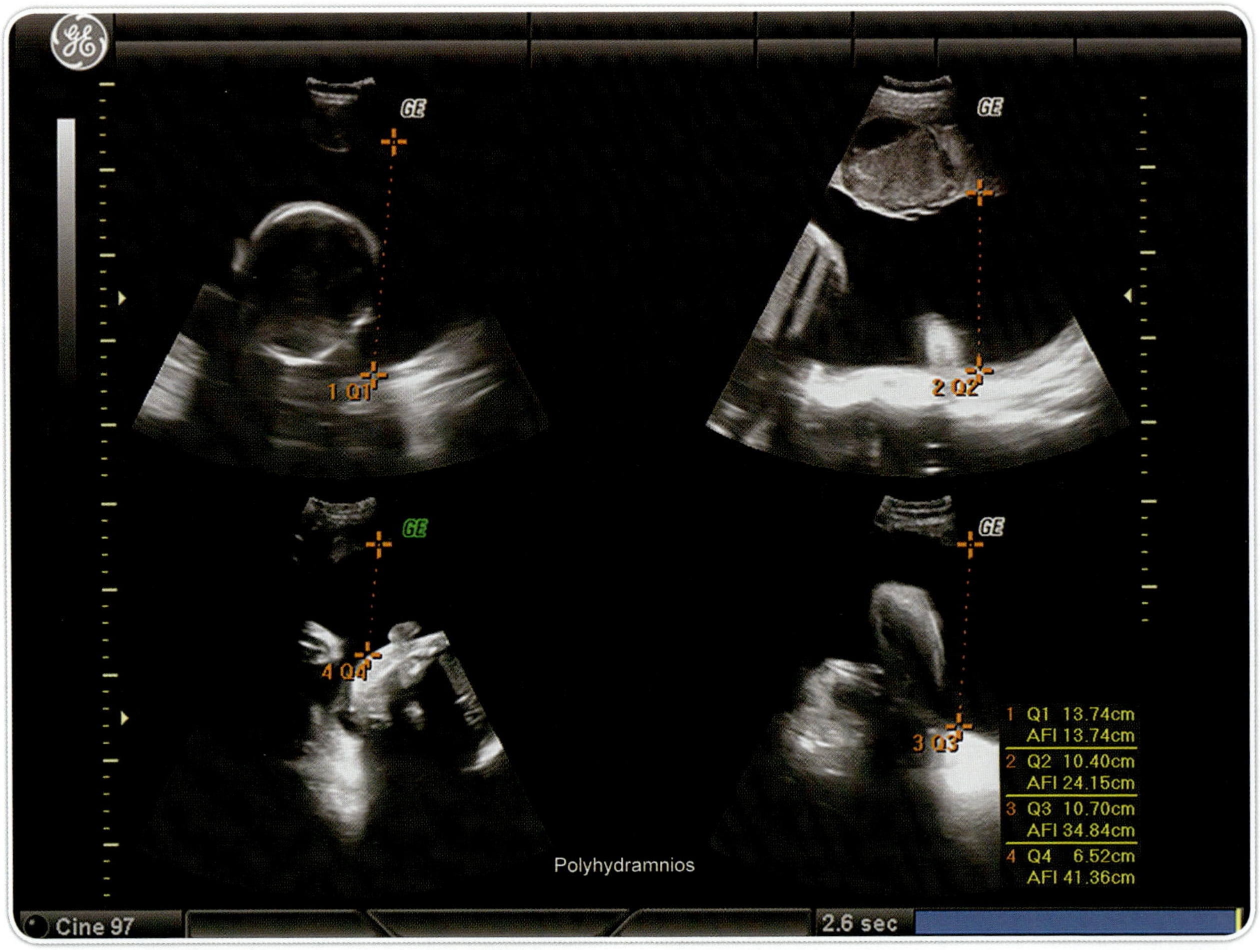

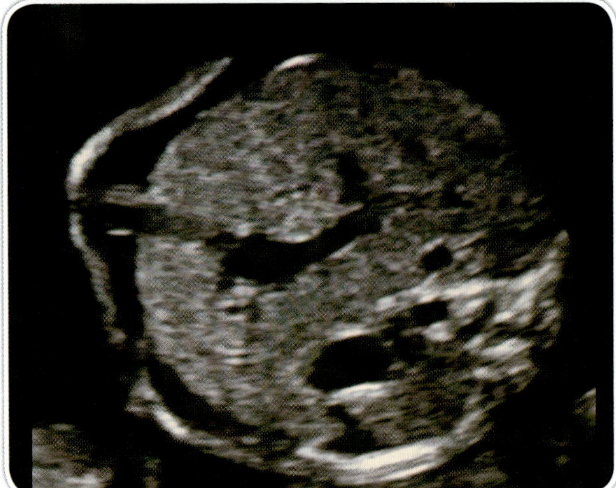

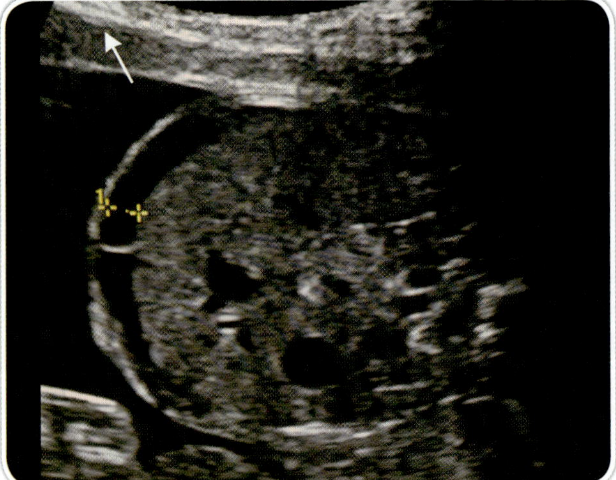

Hydrop fetalis from high-output cardiac failure

Fetal Complications from Placental Chorioangioma

- Anemia
- Congestive cardiac failure
- Hydrops
- Polyhydramnios.

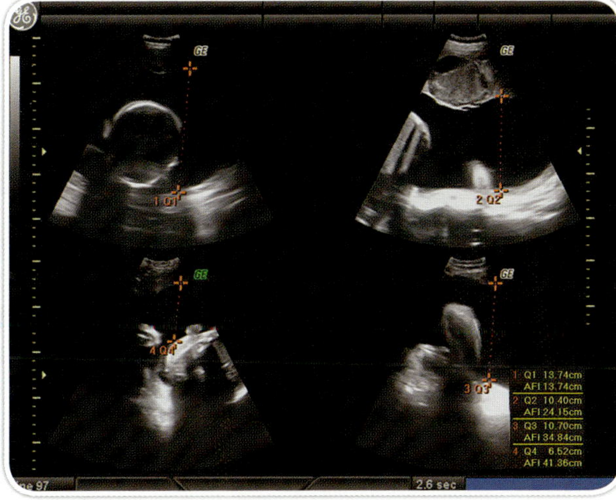

Therapeutic Amnioreduction

- Most placental chorioangiomas are treated expectantly
- Therapeutic amnioreduction is indicated in maternal discomfort from polyhydramnios.

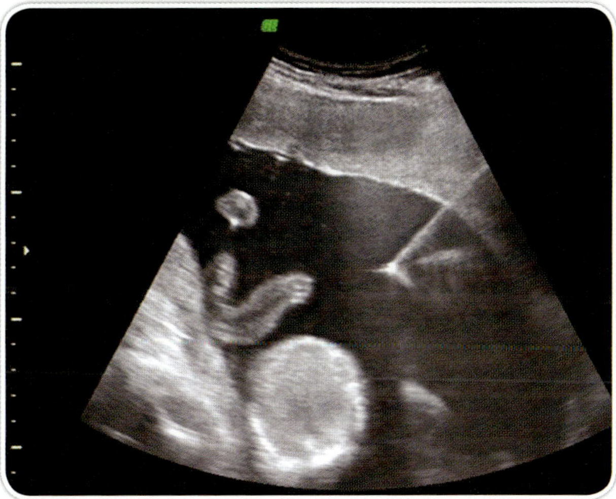

Prenatal Treatment of placental Chorioangioma

- Laser devascularization
- Alcohol ablation
- Interstitial laser ablation.

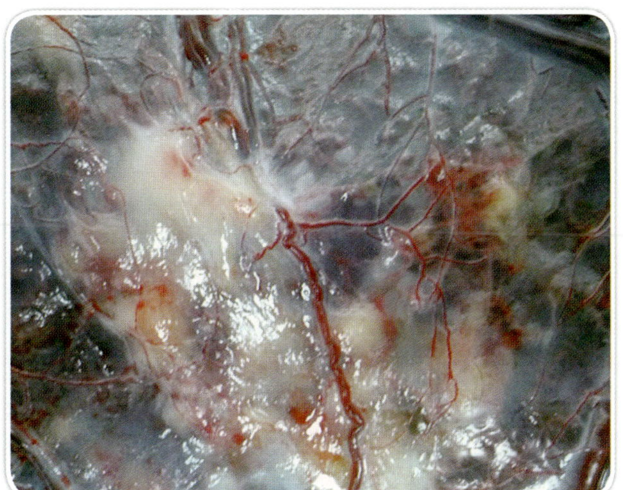

(Amer and Heller 2010)

Limitations of Currently Available Treatment

- Bleeding complications from the treatment are not uncommon
- Rich vascular supply and juxtaposition of the umbilical cord to the tumor.

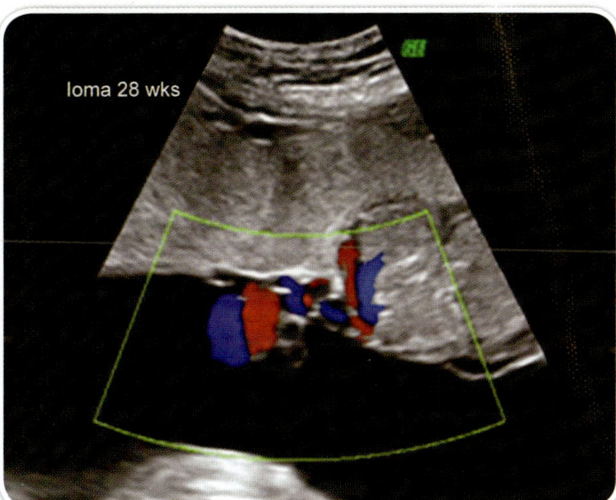

Alternative Treatment Option Radiofrequency Therapy

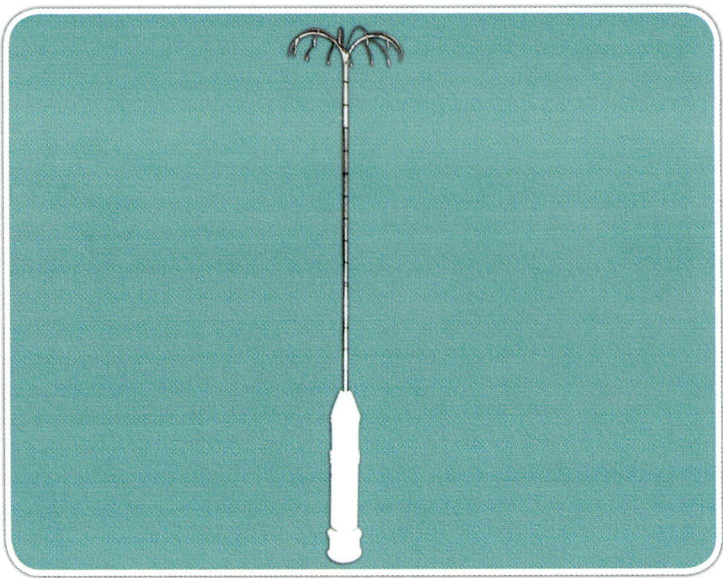

Fetal Diagnosis and Therapy

Original Paper

Fetal Diagn Ther
DOI: 10.1159/000368602

Received: April 22, 20
Accepted after revisic
Published online:

Effects of Power and Time on Ablation Size Produced by Radiofrequency Ablation: In vitro Study in Fresh Human Placenta

Pornsak Sataporntera[a] Manasanan Raveesunthornkiat[d] Sanya Sukpanichnant[b]
Trongtum Tongdee[c] Saowanee Homsud[c] Tuangsit Wataganara[a]

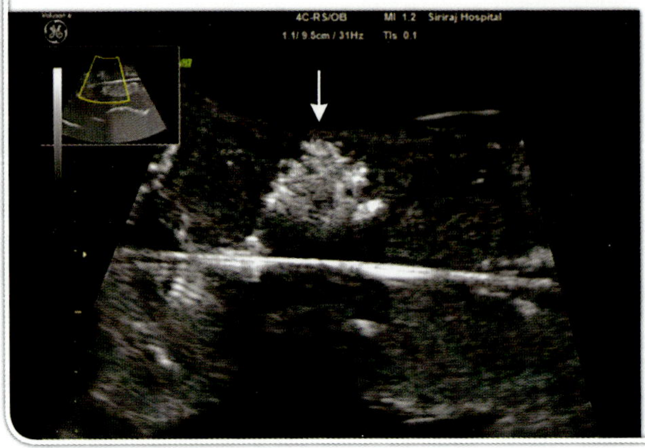

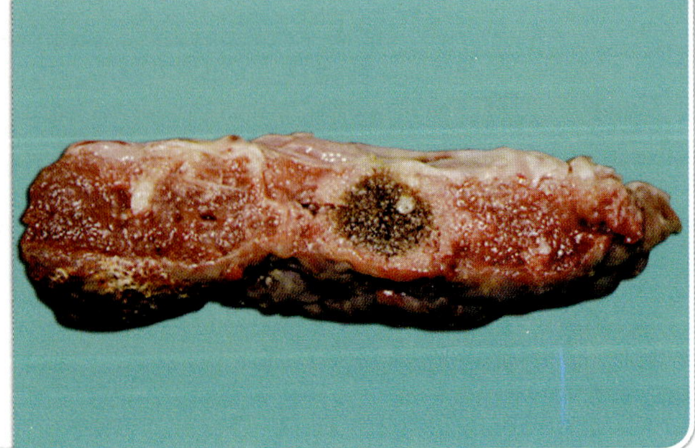

DIFFERENTIAL DIAGNOSES OF PLACENTAL MASS

Placental Cyst

- Sonolucent areas seen by ultrasound
- Isolated from the placental circulation and contain a gelatinous fluid.
- These cysts are located
  - Within the placental tissue (septal cysts)
  - OR under the fetal plate (subchorionic cyst).

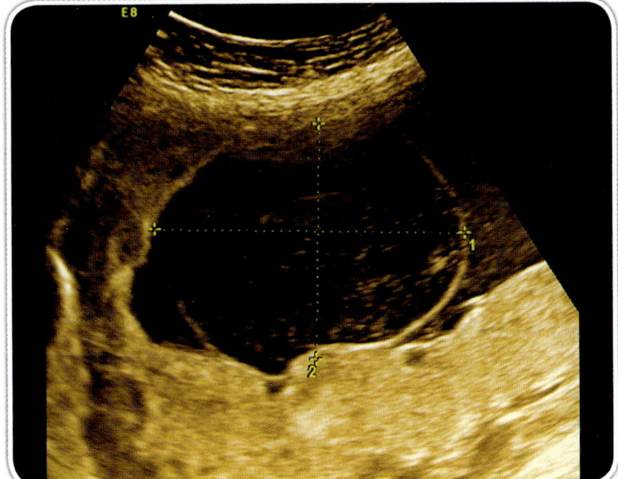

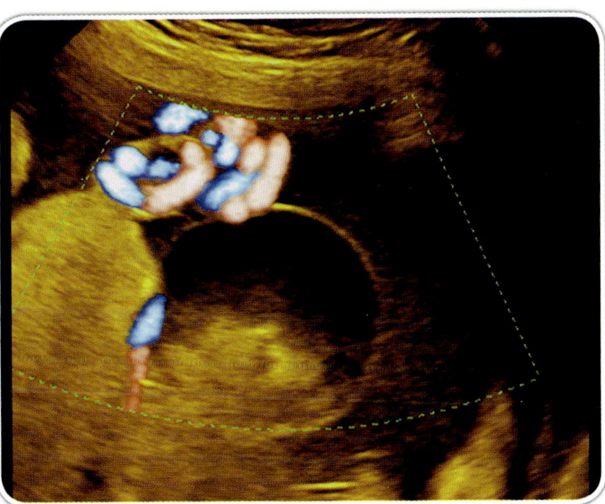

Placental Chorionic Hematoma

Spontaneous Rupture of Chorionic Vessels

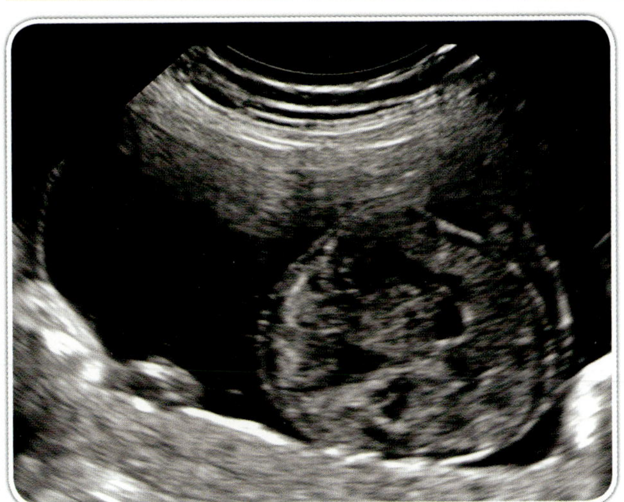

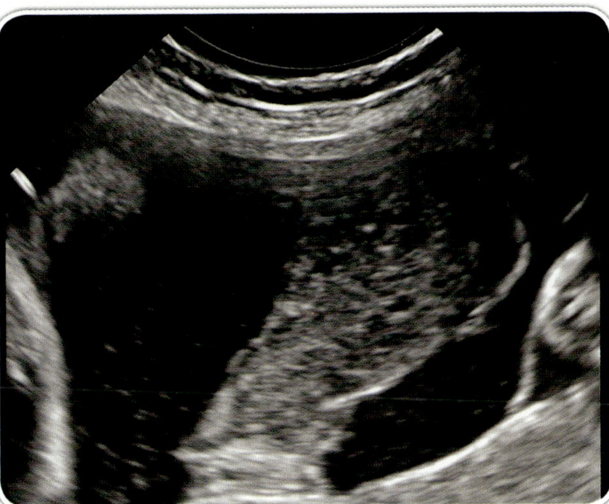

Check for fetal anemia (MCA PSV)

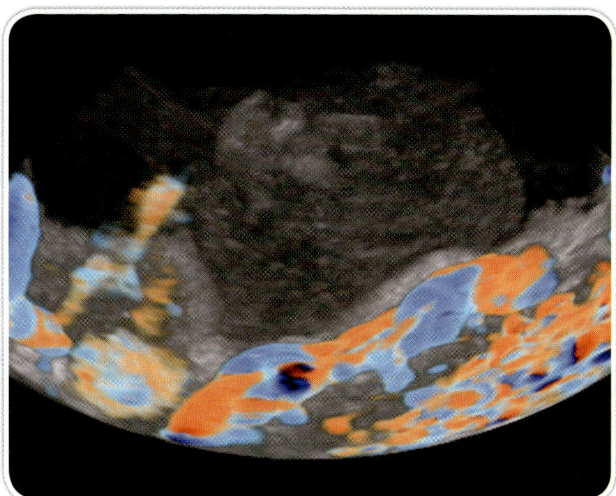

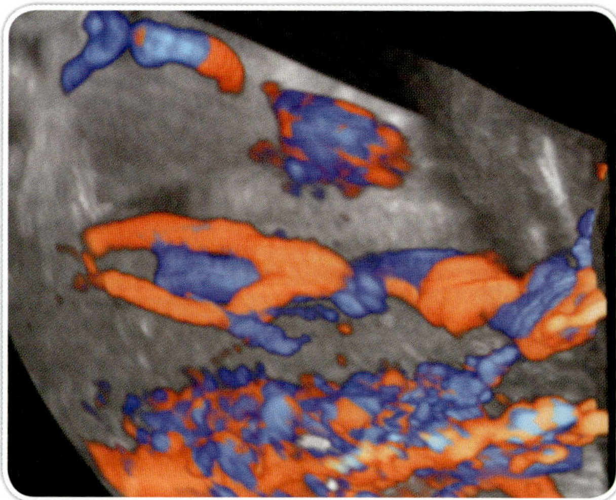

Challenges in Fetal Surgery

- Damage to the uterus or the fetus could cause premature delivery or lead to need of immediate delivery (Cesarean section)
- Massive bleeding from flaccid uterus under anesthesia
- Perioperative risk, such as infection
- Future fertility.

SUGGESTED READING

1. Agarwal SK, Fisk NM. In utero therapy for lower urinary tract obstruction. Prenat Diagn. 2001;21(11):970-6.
2. Amer HZ, Heller DS. Chorangioma and related vascular lesions of the placenta--a review. Fetal Pediat Pathol. 2010;29(4):199-206.
3. Anuwutnavin S, Wanitpongpan P, Chungsomprasong P, Soongswang J, Srisantiroj N, Wataganara T. Fetal long QT syndrome manifested as atrioventricular block and ventricular tachycardia: a case report and a review of the literature. Pediatr Cardiol. 2013;34(8):1955-62.
4. Hadi HA, Finley J, Strickland D. Placental chorioangioma: prenatal diagnosis and clinical significance. Am J Perinat. 1993;10(2):146-9.
5. Haeri S, Ruano SH, Farah LM, Joffe R, Ruano R. Prenatal cytogenetic diagnosis from fetal urine in lower urinary tract obstruction. Congenit Anom. 2013;53(2):89-91.
6. Johnson MP, Bukowski TP, Reitleman C, Isada NB, Pryde PG, Evans MI. In utero surgical treatment of fetal obstructive uropathy: a new comprehensive approach to identify appropriate candidates for vesicoamniotic shunt therapy. Am J Obstet Gynecol. 1994;170(6): 1770-6; discussion 6-9.
7. Moise KJ, Jr., Dorman K, Lamvu G, Saade GR, Fisk NM, Dickinson JE, et al. A randomized trial of amnioreduction versus septostomy in the treatment of twin-twin transfusion syndrome. Am J Obstet Gynecol. 2005;193(3 Pt 1):701-7.
8. Nicolaides KH, Azar GB. Thoraco-amniotic shunting. Fetal Diagn Ther. 1990;5(3-4):153-64.
9. Satapornteera P, Raveesunthornkiat M, Sukpanichnant S, Tongdee T, Homsud S, Wataganara T. Effects of Power and Time on Ablation Size Produced by Radiofrequency Ablation: In vitro Study in Fresh Human Placenta. Fetal Diagn Ther. 2015.
10. Touraine JL, Raudrant D, Royo C, Rebaud A, Roncarolo MG, Souillet G, et al. In-utero transplantation of stem cells in bare lymphocyte syndrome. Lancet. 1989;1(8651):1382.
11. Ville Y. Fetal therapy: practical ethical considerations. Prenat Diagn. 2011;31(7):621-7.
12. Wataganara T, Kanokpongsakdi S. Changing landscapes of In Utero minimally invasive surgical interventions. Sirjraj Med J. 2008;60.368-70.
13. Wataganara T, Ngerncham S, Kitsommart R, Fuangtharnthip P. Fetal neck myofibroma. J Med Assoc Thai. 2007;90(2):376-80.
14. Wataganara T, Sutanthavibool A, Limwongse C. Real-time three dimensional sonographic features of an early third trimester fetus with achondrogenesis. Journal of the Medical Association of Thailand = Chotmaihet thangphaet. 2006;89(10):1762-5.
15. Wataganara T, Triyasunant N, Viboonchart S,. Fetal therapy in 2011: A review. Sirjraj Med J. 2011;63:97-101.
16. Wataganara T, Uschararattanasopon, P, Phatihattakorn, C, Limwongse, C, Viboonchart, S, Nawapan, K. In utero bipolar diathermy to salvage a phenotypically normal fetus in 45,X/46,XY heterokaryotypic monochorionic twins. Surgical Science. 2012;3:100-3.
17. Wataganara T, Wiwanichayakul B, Ruengwuttilert P, Sunsaneevithayakul P, Viboonchart S, Wantanasiri C. Noninvasive diagnosis of fetal anemia and fetal intravascular transfusion therapy: experiences at Siriraj Hospital. J Med Assoc Thai. 2006;89(7):1036-43.

Chapter

12

Ultrasound Diagnosis of Fetal Tumors

Vincenzo D'Addario

LEARNING OBJECTIVES

- To evaluate the possible mechanisms of tumor development in the fetus
- To classify fetal tumors in according to the fetal anatomical sites
- To evaluate the sonographic findings and the differential diagnosis of the various fetal tumors.

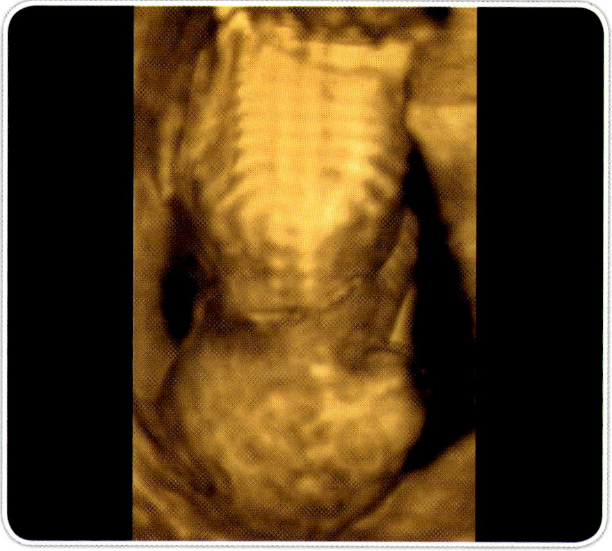

Sacrococcygeal teratoma

Fetal tumors originate from a defect in the integrated control of cellular differentiation and proliferation.

"Rest Cell" Theory

(Durante E Cohnheim)

- During embryogenesis more cells are produced than are required for the formation of an organ or tissue
- The origin of embryonic tumors could rest in developmental errors in these surplus embryonic rudiments
- Both genetic mutations and environmental factors could be responsible for the abnormal cell proliferation and tumor development.

SONOGRAPHIC PATTERNS OF FETAL TUMORS

- General signs
- Tumor specific signs
- Organ specific signs

Sonographic General Signs

- Disruption of contour, shape, location, sonographic texture or size of a normal anatomic structure
- Presence of an abnormal structure
- Abnormal fetal biometry
- Abnormal fetal motion
- Polyhydramnios
- Hydrops.

Polyhydramnios

- Present in almost 50% of the cases
- Possible mechanisms:
  - Interference with swallowing of amniotic fluid (intestinal tumors, goiter, mediastinal masses)
  - Hyperproduction of amniotic fluid (sacrococcygeal teratoma)
  - Decreased reabsorption of amniotic fluid (lung tumors)
  - Altered central control (brain tumors).

Tumor Specific Signs

Pathologic changes within the tumor mass may display specific sonographic findings

Mainly solid

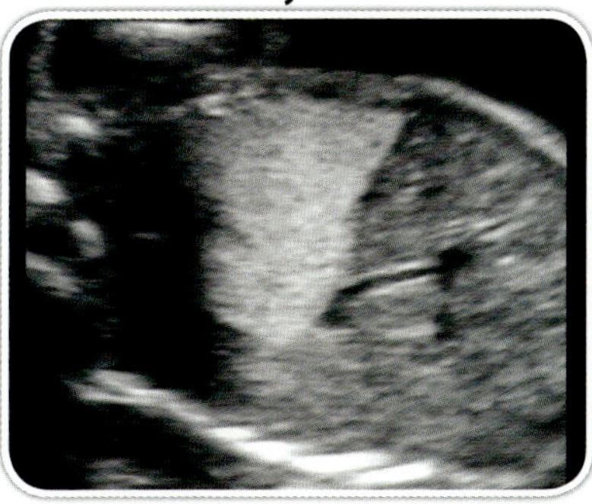

CCAM type III

Mainly cystic

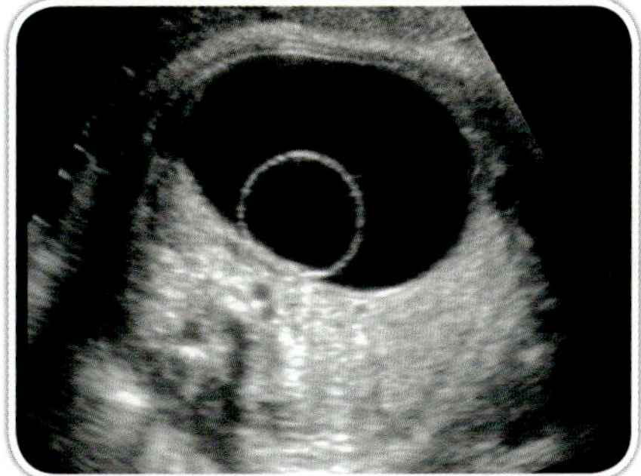

Ovarian cyst

Complex

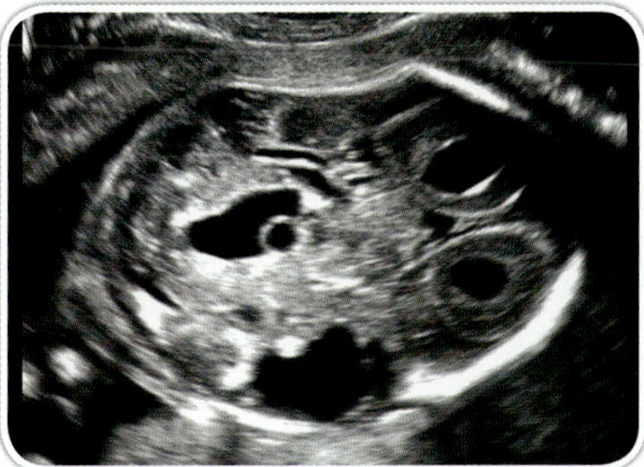

Brain teratoma

For complete presentation, please refer the accompanying CD-ROM...

SUGGESTED READING

1. D'Addario V, Capuano G, Volpe G. Late onset brain anomalies: tumors, cysts and hemorrhages. Donald School Journal of Ultrasound in Obstetrics and Gynecology. 2013;7:484-91.
2. Gucciardo L, Uyttebroek A, De Wever I, Renard M, Claus F, Devlieger R, et al.: Prenatal assessment and management of sacrococcygeal teratoma. Prenat Diagn. 2011;31:678-88.
3. Isaacs H Jr. Fetal and neonatal cardiac tumors. Pediatr Cardiol. 2004;25:252-73.
4. Kamil D, Tepelmann J, Berg C, Heep A, Axt-Fliedner R, Gembruch U. Spectrum and outcome of prenatally diagnosed fetal tumors. Ultrasound Obstet Gynecol. 2008;31:296-302.
5. MacArthur CJ. Prenatal diagnosis of fetal cervicofacial anomalies. Curr Opin Otolaryngol Head Neck Surg. 2012;20:482-90.
6. Ozyuncu O, Canpolat FE, Ciftci AO, Yurdakok M, Onderoglu LS, Deren O. Perinatal outcomes of fetal abdominal cysts and comparison of prenatal and postnatal diagnoses. Fetal Diagn Ther. 2010;28:153-9.
7. Wilson RD, Hedrick HL, Liechty KW, Flake AW, Johnson MP, Bebbington M, et al. Cystic adenomatoid malformation of the lung: review of genetics, prenatal diagnosis, in utero treatment. Am J Med Genet A. 2006;140:151-5.

Chapter 13

Invasive Prenatal Procedures

Giovanni Monni

Serious birth defects, often genetically determined, complicate and threaten the lives of 3% of newborn infants

VA McKusick 1990

PRE-CONCEPTION GENETIC CONSULTATION

- **Previous pregnancy history:**
  - Fetal demise, recurrent pregnancy loss
- **Previous child with a genetic disorder:**
  - Chromosomal: Down's syndrome
  - Structural: Dwarfism, neural tube defects
  - Metabolic: Neonatal or early childhood death, ambiguous genitalia
  - Hematologic: Anemia, bleeding disorder
  - Mental retardation
- **Family history of a genetic disorder**
  - Bleeding disorders: Hemophilia
  - Neurologic diseases: Muscular dystrophy, myotonic dystrophy
  - Mental retardation: Fragile X syndrome, cystic fibrosis
- **Ethnic origin from population at high risk of genetic disorder:**
  - Ashkenazi Jewish and French-Canadian: Tay-Sach disease
  - African-American: Sickle cell anemia
  - Mediterranean: β-thalassemia
  - Oriental: α-Thalassemia and β-Thalassemia
- **Maternal medications:**
  - Anticonvulsants, Lithium, Accutane, any chronically used medications
- **Socially used drugs:**
  - Alcohol, Cocaine.

Pre-Test Counseling: Invasive Prenatal Diagnosis

- Genetic risk
- Prognosis, availability of treatments
- Limits of diagnosis
- Invasive procedure techniques
- Therapeutic options.
- Possibility of screening, diagnosis
- Risks of invasive prenatal diagnosis
- Gestational age to obtain diagnosis
- Diagnostic problems

Prenatal and Pre-Implantation Genetic Diagnosis

In vitro

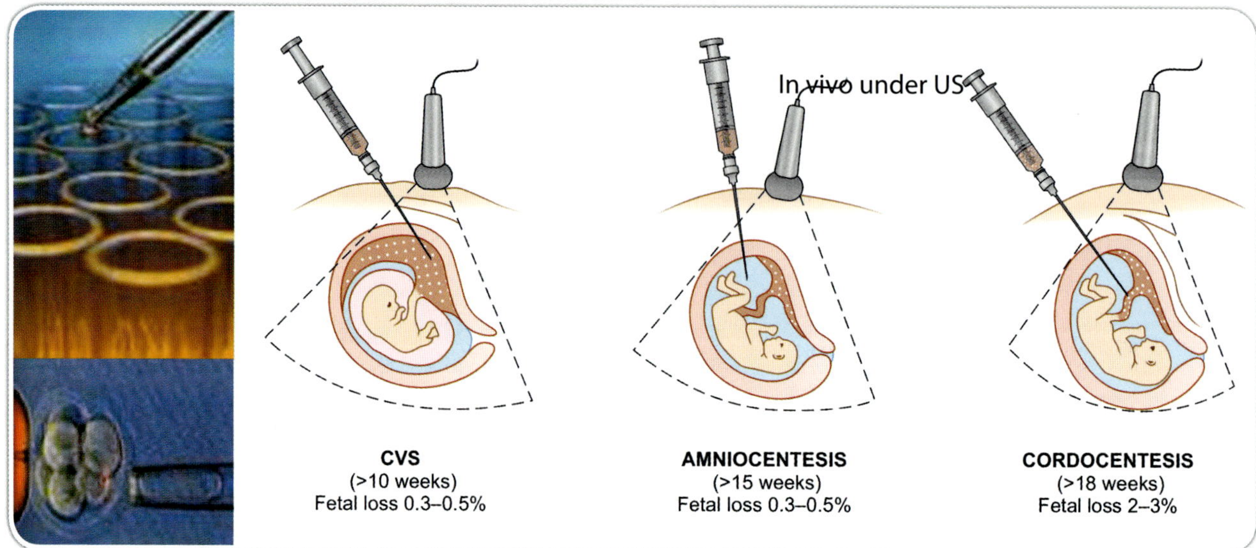

In Cagliari Centre since 1977 > 60,000 invasive procedures

Changes in Our PND Approach (35,127 Cases, 1977–2004)

Table 1. Invasive prenatal diagnosis for β-thalassemia

	PC	PS	CoC	CaC	AC	TC-CVS	TA-CVS	Total	PGD
1977–1981	949 (100%)	0	0	0	0	0	0	949	0
1982–1985	32 (3.2%)	67 (6.7%)	120 (12.0%)	6 (0.6%)	203 (20.3%)	572 (57.2%)	0	1,000	0
1986–1993	0	0	0	0	0	0	2,011(100%)	2,011	0
1994–1999	0	0	0	0	0	0	1,477(100%)	1,477	0
2000–2004	0	0	0	0	0	0	1,110(100%)	1,110	42
Total	**981**	**67**	**120**	**6**	**203**	**572**	**4,598**	**6,547**	**42**

PC = Placentacentesis; FS = fetoscopy; CoC = cordocentesis; CaC = cardiocentesis; AC = amniocentesis; TA-CVS = transabdominal chorionic villi sampling; TC-CVS = transcervical chorionic villi sampling; PGD = preimplantation genetic diagnosis

Monni, Fetal Diagn Ther 2006

For complete presentation, please refer the accompanying CD-ROM...

SUGGESTED READING

1. Bang J, Bock JE, Trolle D. Ultrasound-guided fetal intravenous transfusion for severe rhesus haemolytic disease. Br Med J (Clin Res Ed). `982;284(6313):373-4.
2. Cao A, Cossu P, Monni G, Rosatelli MC. Chorionic villus sampling and acceptance rate of prenatal diagnosis. Prenat Diagn. 1987;7(7): 531-533.
3. Daffos F, Capella-Pavlovsky M, Forestier F. "A new procedure for fetal blood sampling in utero: preliminary results of fifty-three cases." Am J Obstet Gynecol. 1983;146(8):985-987.
4. Eddleman KA, Malone FD, Sullivan L, Dukes K, Berkowitz RL, Kharbutli Y, et al. Pregnancy loss rates after midtrimester amniocentesis. Obstet Gynecol. 2006;108(5):1067-72.
5. Liebaers I, Sermon K, Staessen C, Joris H,. Lissens W, Assche EV, et al. "Clinical experience with preimplantation genetic diagnosis and intracytoplasmic sperm injection." Hum Reprod. 1998;13 (Suppl 1):186-95.
6. McKusick VA. The morbid anatomy of the human genome: the role of gene mapping in clinical medicine. Acta Paediatr Jpn. 1990;32(3): 234-41.
7. Monni G, Cau G, Usai V, Perra G, Lai R, Ibba V, et al. Preimplantation genetic diagnosis for beta-thalassaemia: the Sardinian experience. Prenat Diagn. 2004;24(12): 949-54.
8. Monni G, Olla G, Cao A. Patient's choice between transcervical and transabdominal chorionic villus sampling. Lancet. 1988;1(8593): 1057.
9. Monni G, Olla G, Rosatelli C, Cao A. Second-trimester placental biopsy versus amniocentesis for prenatal diagnosis of beta-thalassemia. N Engl J Med. 1990, 322(1): 60-61.
10. Monni G, Zoppi MA. Improved first-trimester aneuploidy risk assessment: an evolving challenge of training in invasive prenatal diagnosis. Ultrasound Obstet Gynecol. 2013;41(5):486-8.
11. Monni G, Zoppi MA, Axiana C, Ibba RM. Changes in the approach for invasive prenatal diagnosis in 35,127 cases at a single center from 1977 to 2004. Fetal Diagn Ther. 2006;21(4):348-54.
12. Monni G, Zoppi MA, Iuculano A, Piras A, Arras M. Invasive or non-invasive prenatal genetic diagnosis? J Perinat Med. 2014;42(5): 545-8.
13. Morgan S, Delbarre A, Ward P. Impact of introducing a national policy for prenatal Down syndrome screening on the diagnostic invasive procedure rate in England. Ultrasound Obstet Gynecol. 2013;41(5):526-9.
14. Novelli A, Grati FR, Ballarati L, Bernardini L, Bizzoco D, Camurri L, et al. Microarray application in prenatal diagnosis: a position statement from the cytogenetics working group of the Italian Society of Human Genetics (SIGU).November 2011. Ultrasound Obstet Gynecol. 2012;39(4):384-8.
15. Saltvedt S, Almstrom H, Kublickas M, Valentin L, Bottinga R, Bui TH, et al. Screening for Down syndrome based on maternal age or fetal nuchal translucency: a randomized controlled trial in 39,572 pregnancies. Ultrasound Obstet Gynecol 2005;25(6): 537-45.
16. Tabor A, Alfirevic Z. Update on procedure-related risks for prenatal diagnosis techniques. Fetal Diagn Ther 2010;27(1):1-7.
17. Tabor A, Philip J, Madsen M, Bang J, Obel EB, Norgaard-Pedersen B. Randomised controlled trial of genetic amniocentesis in 4606 low-risk women. Lancet. 1986;1(8493):1287-93.
18. Zoppi MA, Ibba RM, Putzolu M, Floris M, Monni G. Nuchal translucency and the acceptance of invasive prenatal chromosomal diagnosis in women aged 35 and older. Obstet Gynecol. 2001;97(6):916-20.

Chapter 14

Basics in Fetal Echocardiography

Gwang Jun Kim

Importance of Fetal Echocardiography?

- Congenital heart disease (CHD): Most common congenital malformation: 4–13/1,000 live births
- Major CHD: 2-4/1,000 births
- 20% of still birth, 42% of infant deaths related with cardiac defects
- Prenatal detection rate vary widely
- Diagnostic rate doubled after 2 years of training.

(Lin et al. 2014)

Contents

- Cardiac anatomy
- Guidelines for fetal heart screening
- Method for fetal cardiac evaluation
- Basic views for fetal cardiac evaluation.

Anatomy of the Fetal Heart

- In the chest, right ventricle (RV) is located most front and PA (pulmonary artery) originates from it.
- Aorta (Ao) arises just next to the left side of PA.

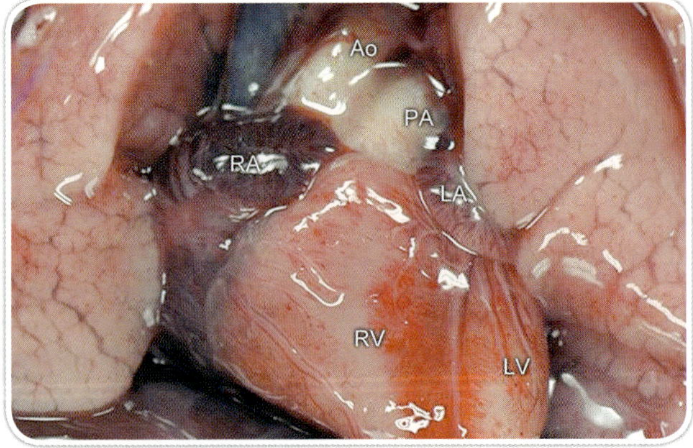

Anterior Anatomy of the Fetal Heart

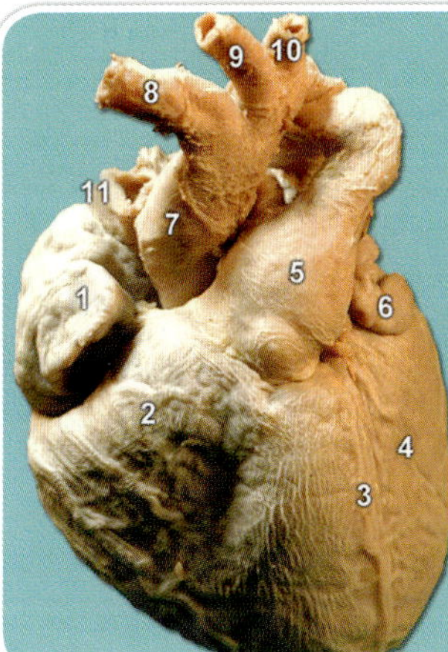

1. Right auricle
2. Right ventricle
3. Anterior interventricular artery
4. Left ventricle
5. Pulmonary trunk
6. Left auricle
7. Ascending aorta
8. Brachiocephalic artery
9. Left common carotid artery
10. Left subclavian artery
11. Superior vena cava

Posterior Anatomy of the Fetal Heart

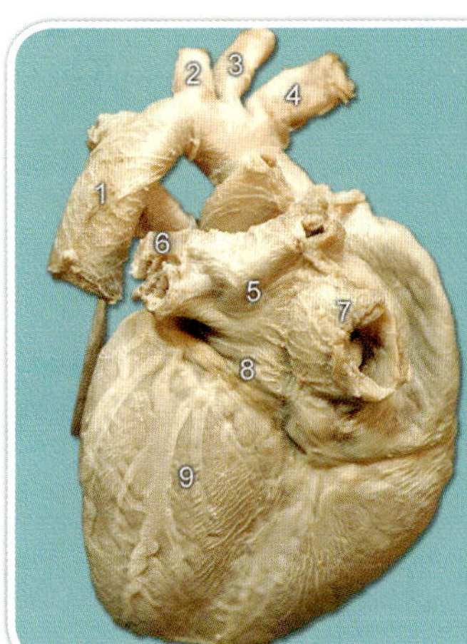

1. Descending aorta
2. Left subclavian artery
3. Left common carotid artery
4. Brachiocephalic artery
5. Left atrium
6. Left pulmonary veins
7. Inferior vena cava
8. Coronary sinus
9. Left ventricle

Inside of the Right Atrium

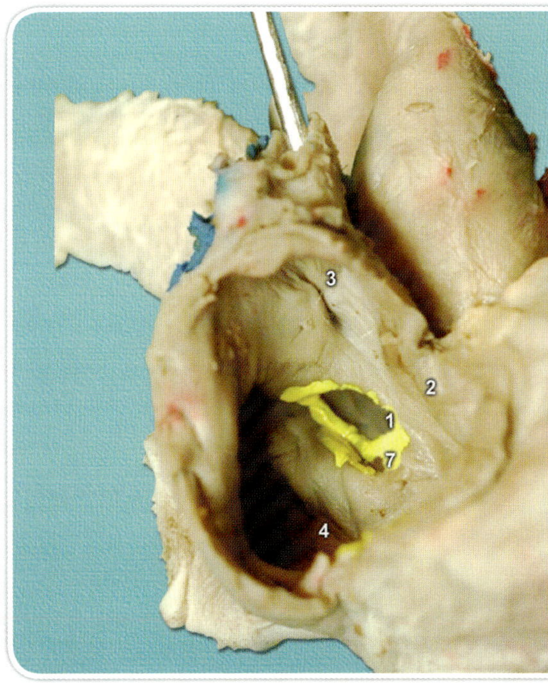

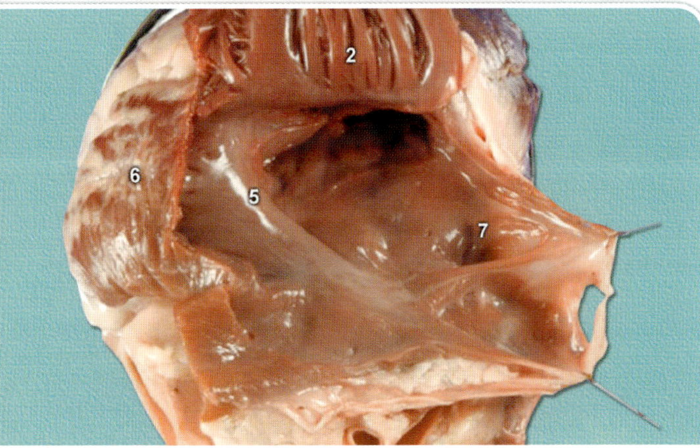

1. Foramen ovale
2. Pectinate muscle
3. Superior vena cava
4. Inferior vena cava
5. Pectinate muscle
6. Auricle
7. Orifice of coronary sinus

For complete presentation, please refer the accompanying CD-ROM…

SUGGESTED READING

1. Carvalho JS, et al. ISUOG Practice Guidelines (updated): sonographic screening examination of the fetal heart. Ultrasound Obstet Gynecol: the official journal of the International Society of Ultrasound in Obstetrics and Gynecology. 2013;41:348-59.
2. Lin CH, Hegde S, Marshall AC, et al. Incidence and management of life-threatening adverse events during cardiac catheterization for congenital heart disease. Pediatric Cardiology. 2014;35:140-8.

Chapter 15

High Definition 3D Ultrasound: From Beginning to Birth

Tuangsit Wataganara

OBJECTIVES

- To demonstrate the additional benefits of 3-dimensional high-definition (3DHD) ultrasound for the assessment of normal and abnormal fetal anatomy
- To demonstrate embryologic and fetal development using 3DHD.

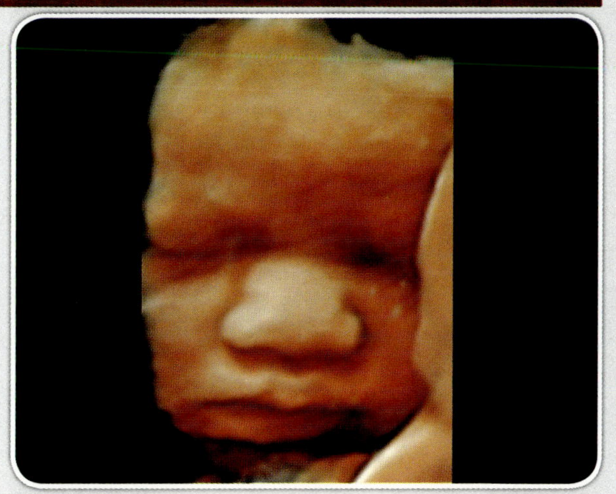

What is 3DHD?

- 3DHD is a new surface rendered mode with 'computerized' adjustable light source.
- The operator can create lighting and shadowing effects to increase depth perception.

(Kagan et al. 2011)

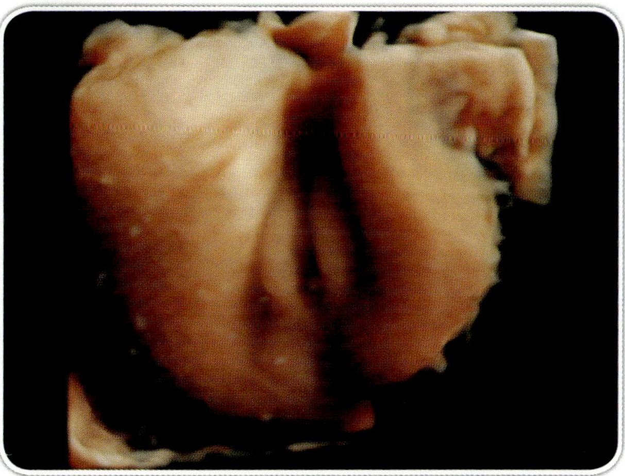

Comparison between Standard 3D and 3DHD

Adjustable Lighting and Skin-like Color Lead to a more Natural Appearance

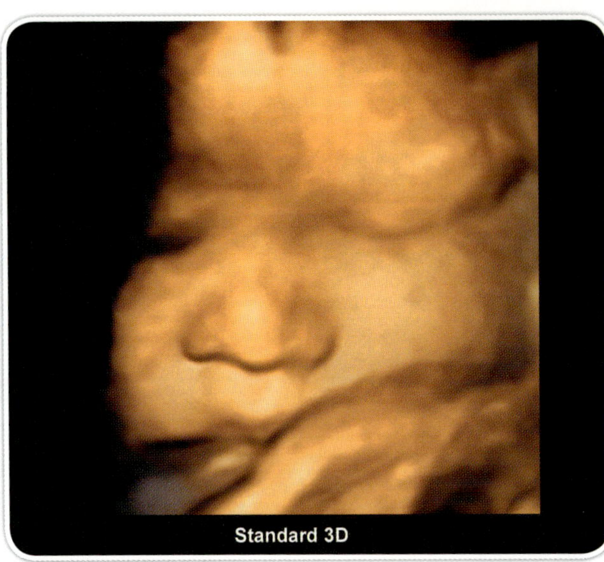

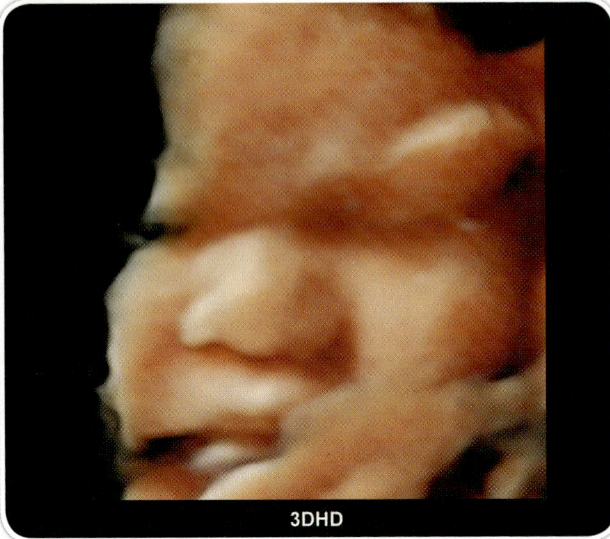

"Backlight" Mode Allows for a Better Interrogation in Early Pregnancy

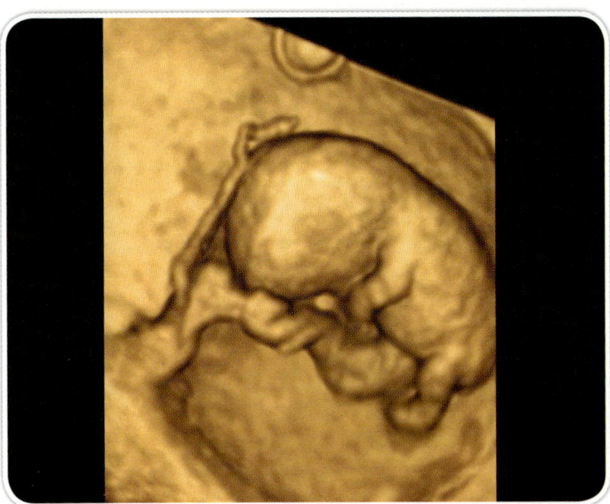

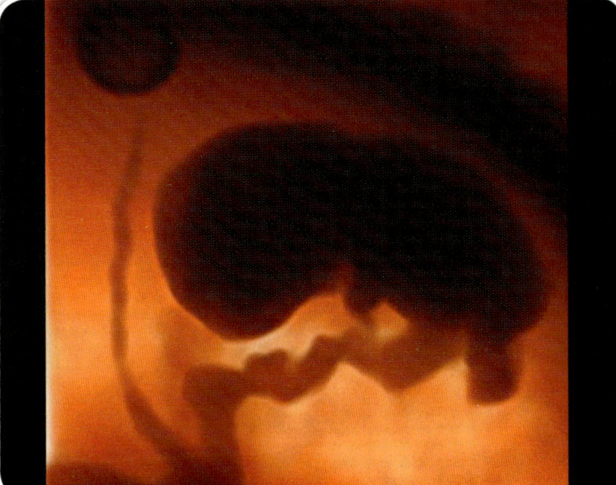

Early Yolk Sac from 3DHD Backlight Mode

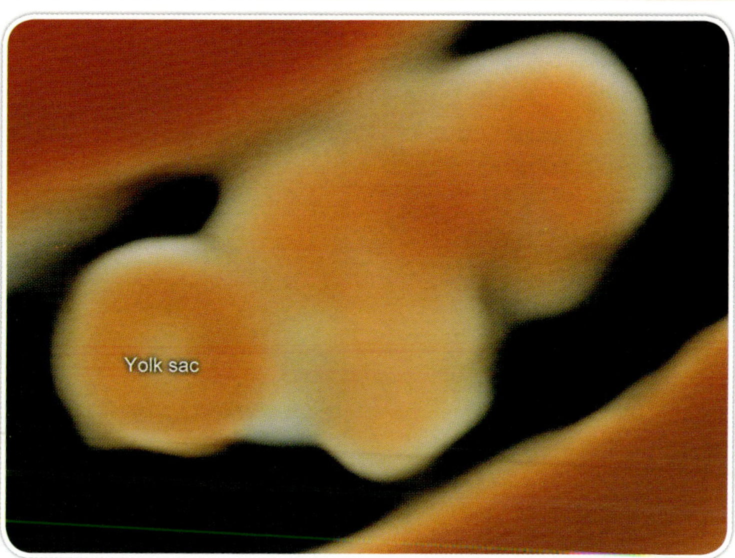

Static 3D Fetal Images in the Past (Siriraj Hospital, 2002)

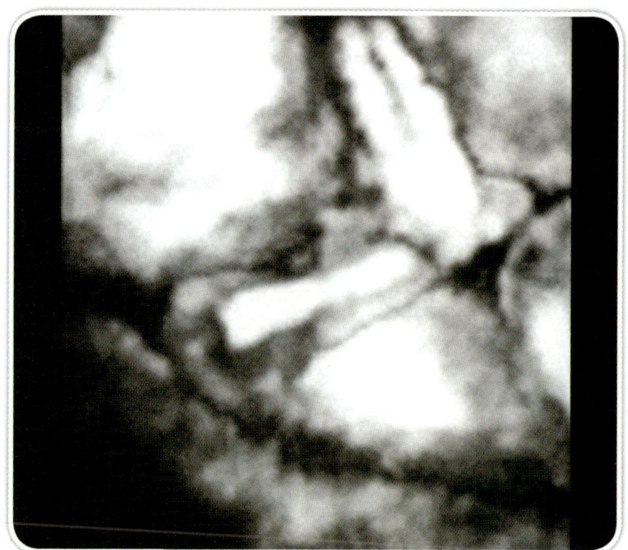

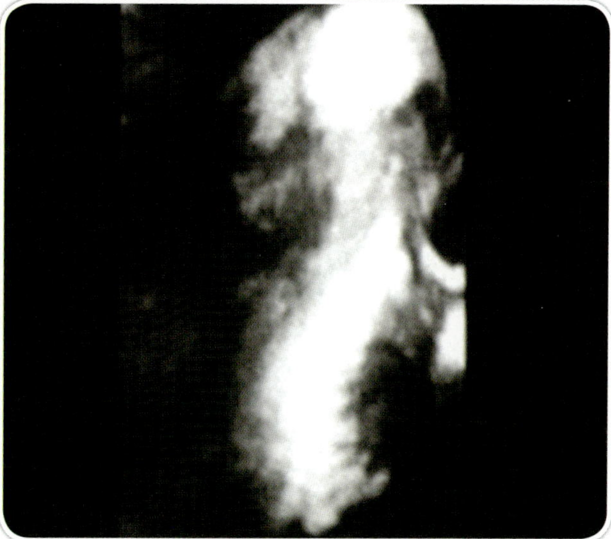

Note the grainy quality of the image

Development of 3D Fetal Ultrasound

- First report on a 3D ultrasound was from Japan in 1984
- Continuous developments and breakthroughs have been achieved in the past 30 years
- With the power of 3DHD, most pictures will be self explanatory.

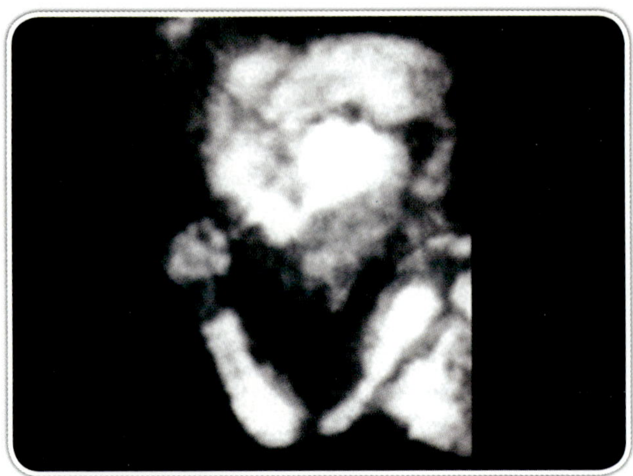

(Siriraj Hospital, 2002)

Advantage of 3DHD: Effects of "Lighting"

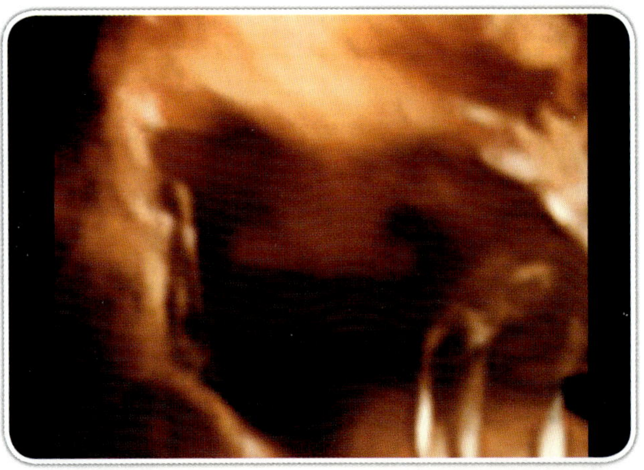

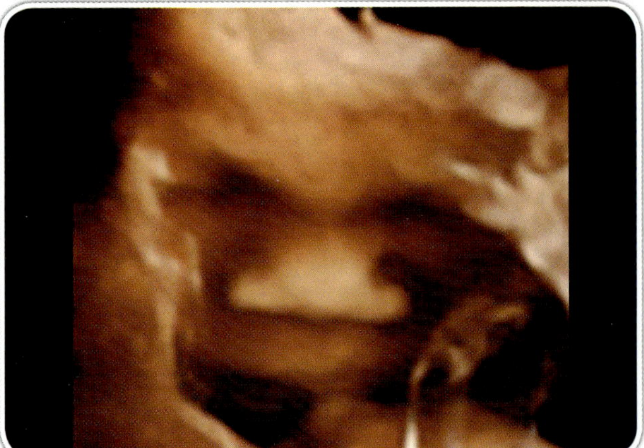

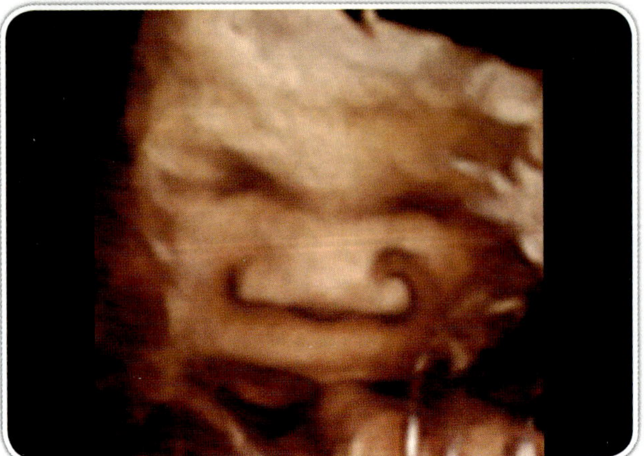

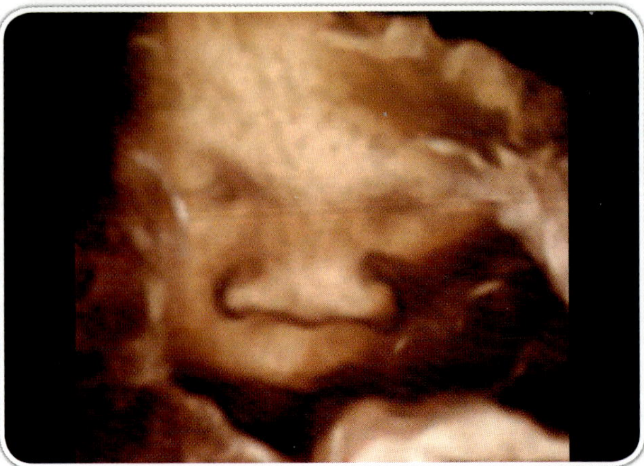

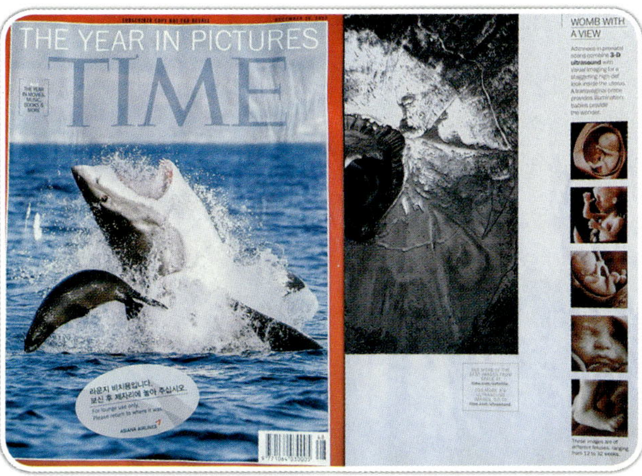

Public attention of fetal 3DHD
Time Magazine, December 2013

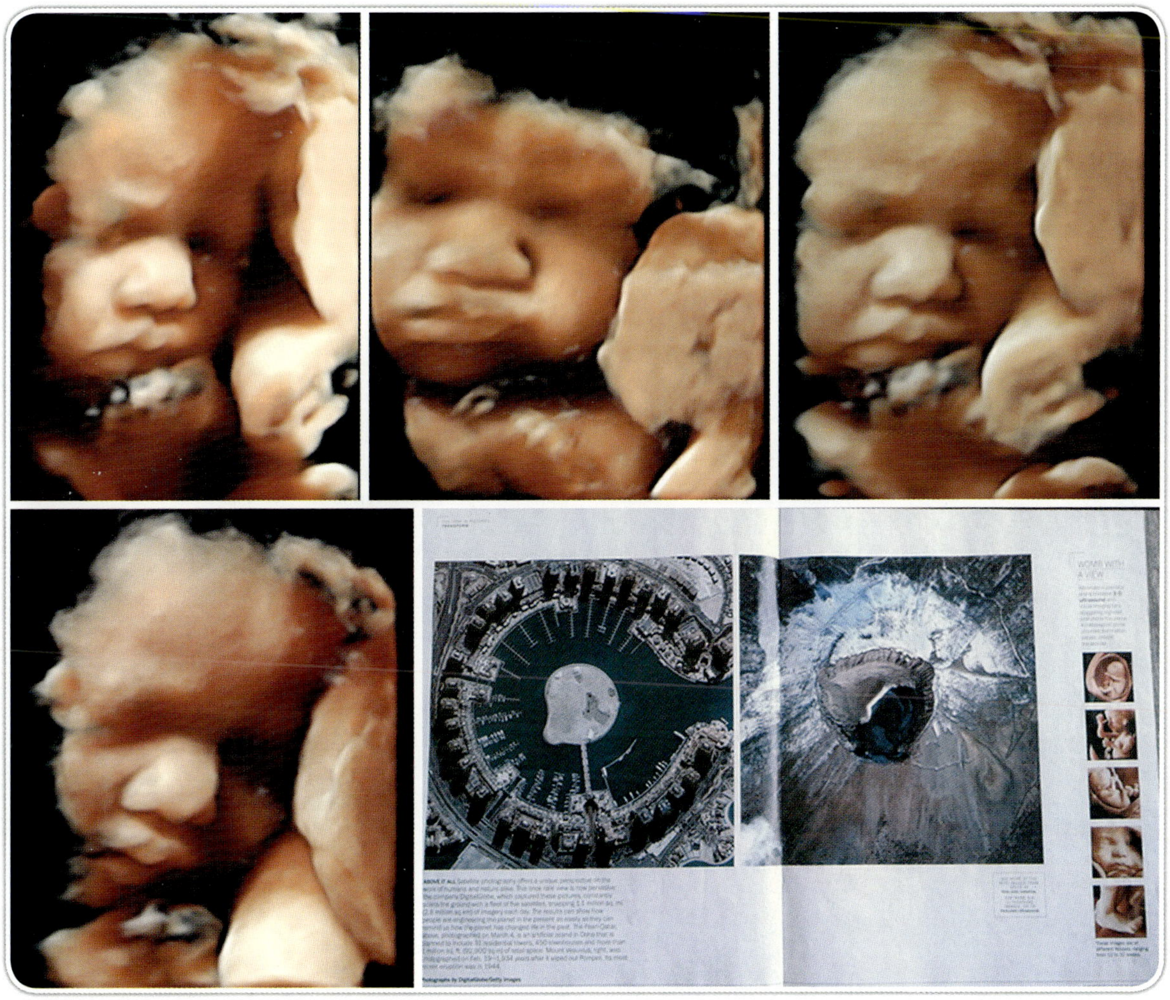

Public attention of fetal 3DHD
Time Magazine, December 2013

Where the life begins...
Uterine Cavity during Proliferative Phase

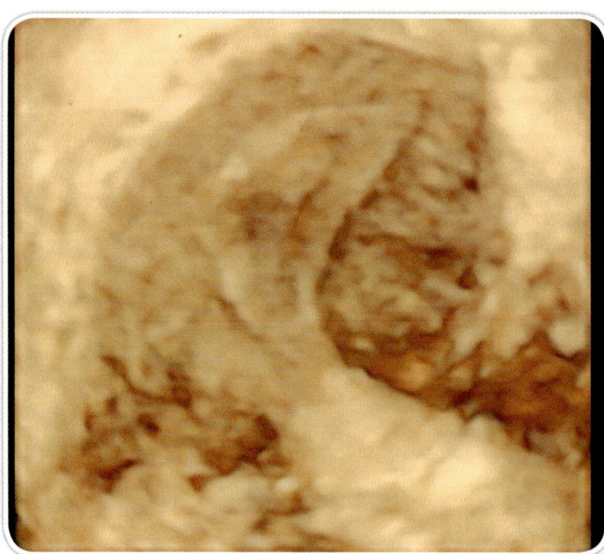

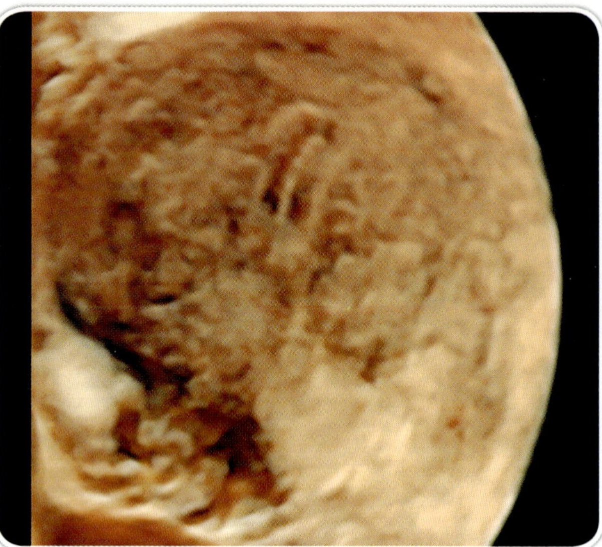

- Note the triple layer appearance, indicating the mid-cycle of ovulation
- Endometrial appearance can reflect its receptivity to conception.

Uterine Cavity during Secretory Phase

Note the change in the shape of uterine cavity from proliferative to secretory phase

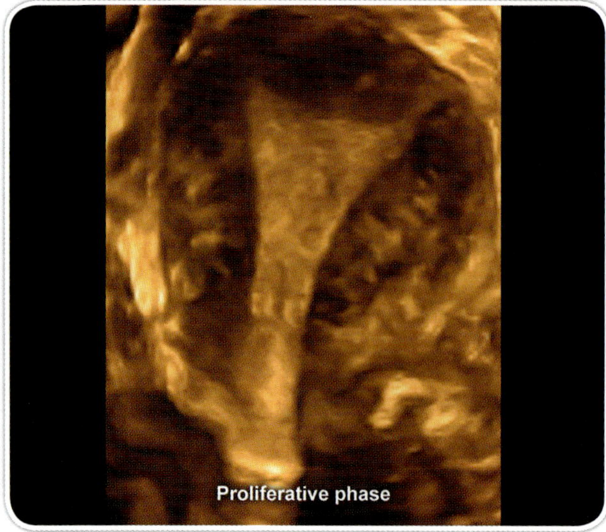

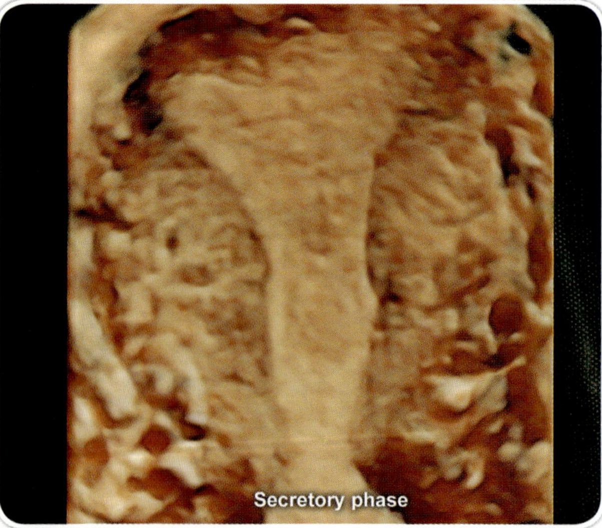

Abnormal Uterine Cavity: Arcuate Uterus

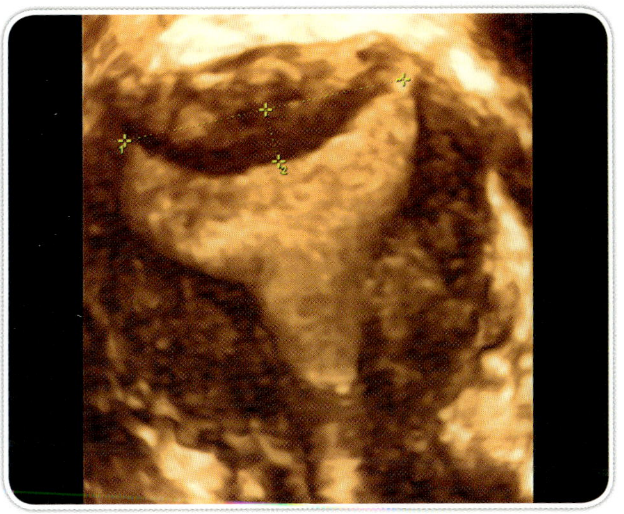

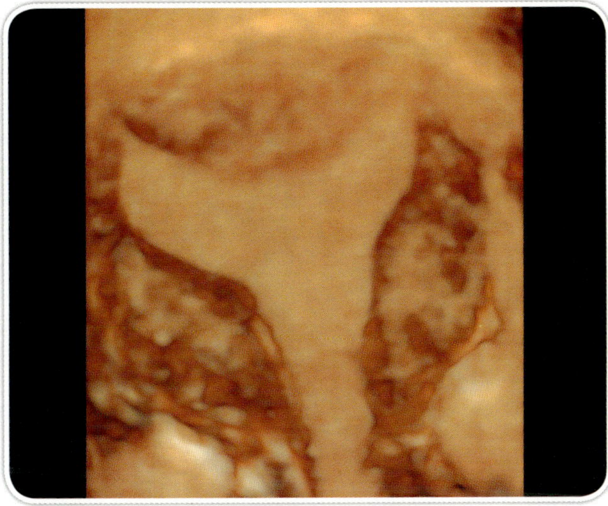

Arcuate Uterus

- Müllerian anomaly
- Concave contour of fundal part of the uterine cavity
- May have a higher risk for miscarriage, premature birth, and malpresentation.

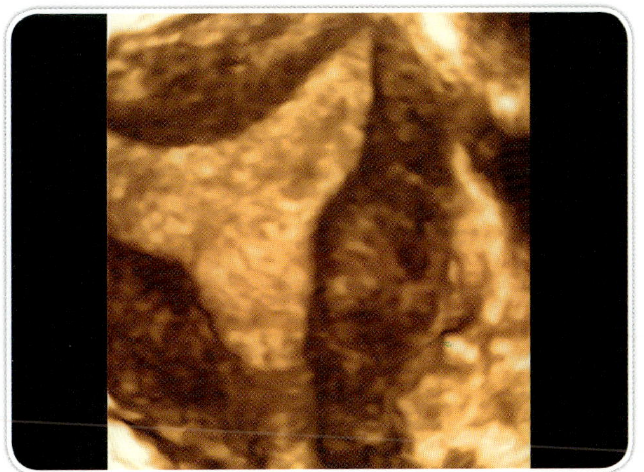

Early Intrauterine Pregnancy

- Early intrauterine gestational sac by 2D scan

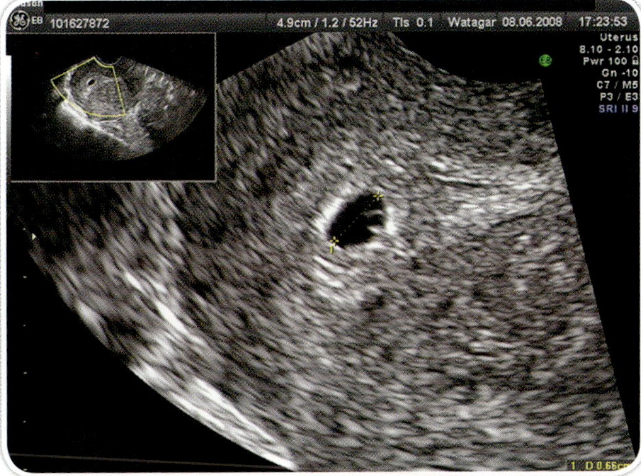

- Note the 'puffiness of the endometrium' as a result of decidualization
- The uterine cavity is asymmetrical in early intrauterine pregnancy.

(Rempen et al. 1998)

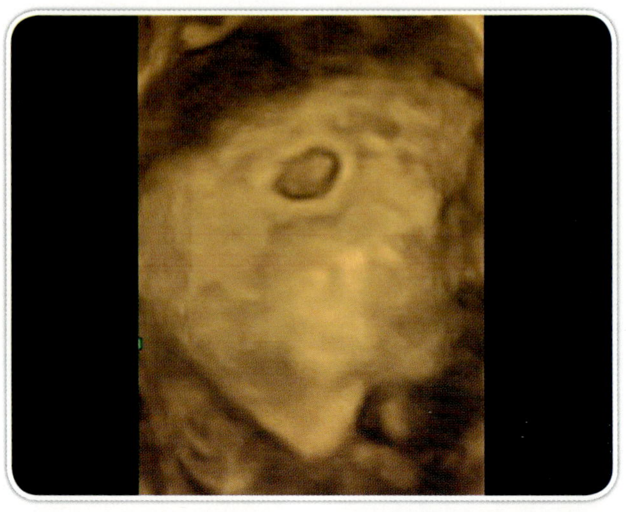

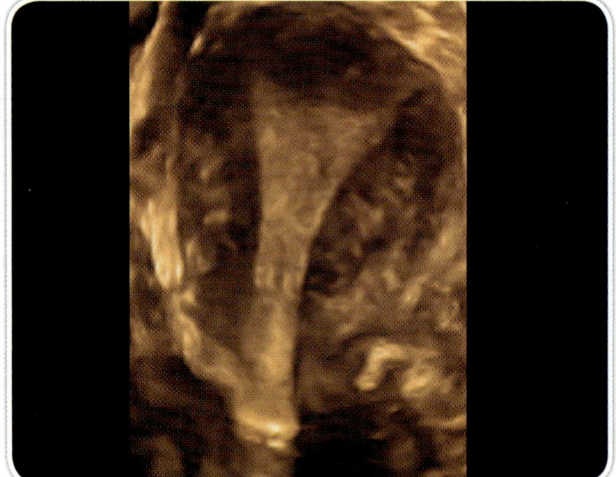

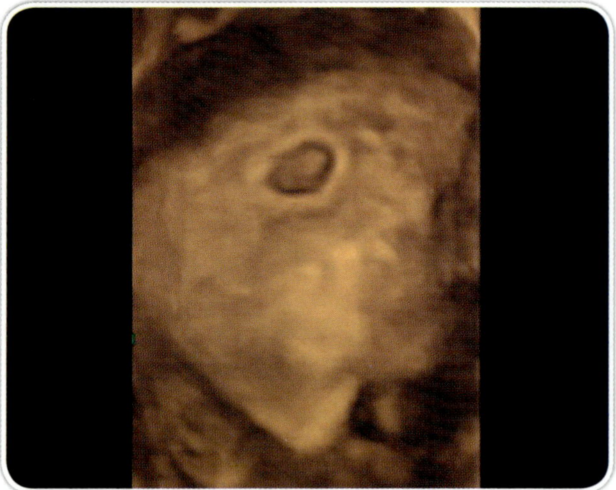

Note the endometrial thickening as a result of decidualization

Gestational Sac in 3DHD

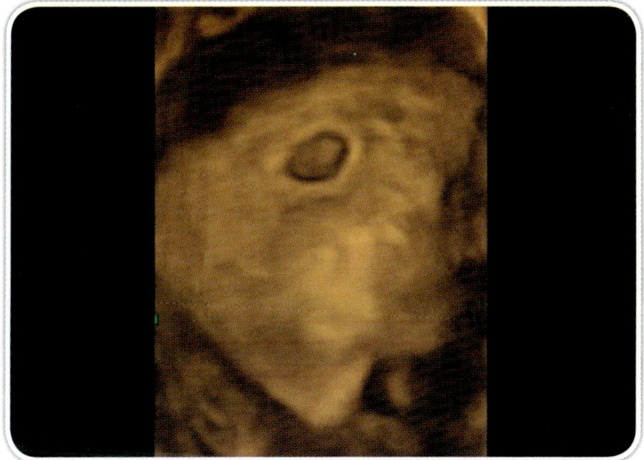

Gestational sac 3D

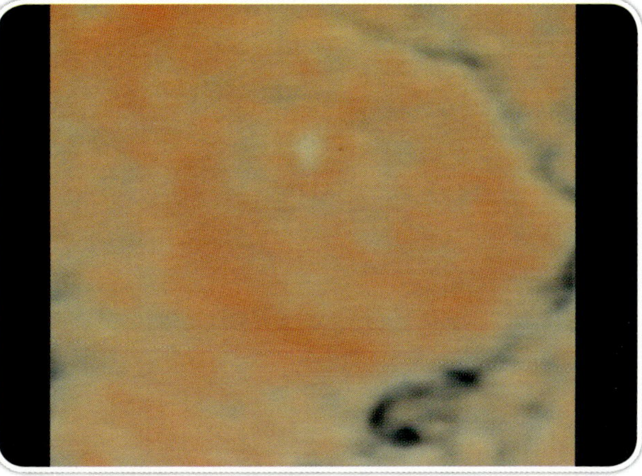

Gestational sac 3DHD
Note the echogenic rim (choriodecidual reaction)

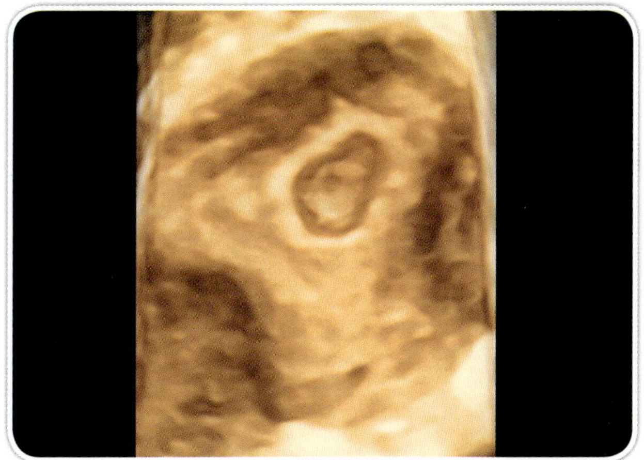

Gestational sac 3D

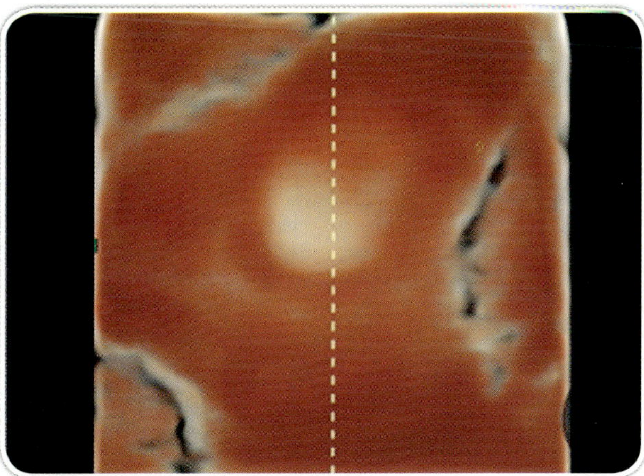

Gestational sac 3DHD

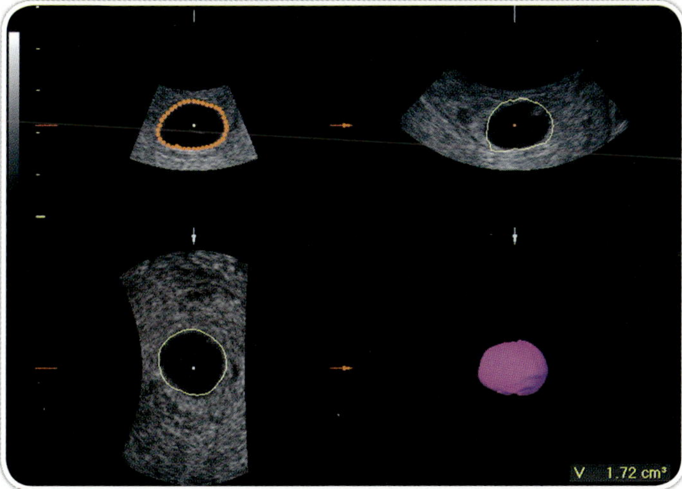

Volume measurement of the gestational sac

Volume of Gestational Sac

- Gestational sac volume (GSV) in anembryonic pregnancy is smaller than that of normal pregnancy.

(Odeh et al. 2010)

Laterality of Gestational Sac

- Eccentric location of the gestational sac is more reassuring for the diagnosis of intrauterine pregnancy
- Pseudogestational sac, which is a fluid collection in the endometrial cavity, is usually centrally located.

(Doubilet 2014)

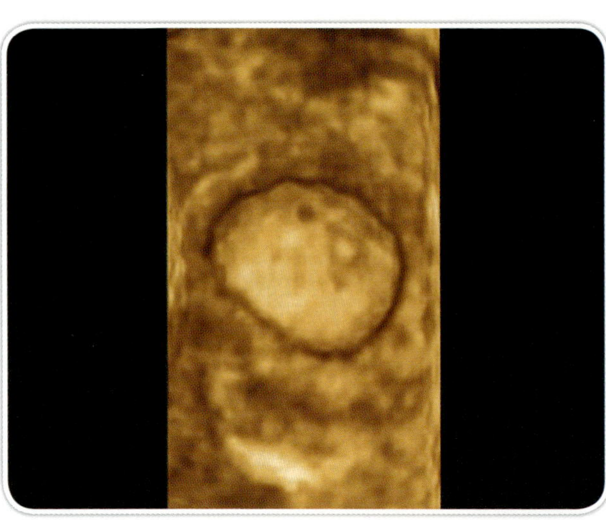

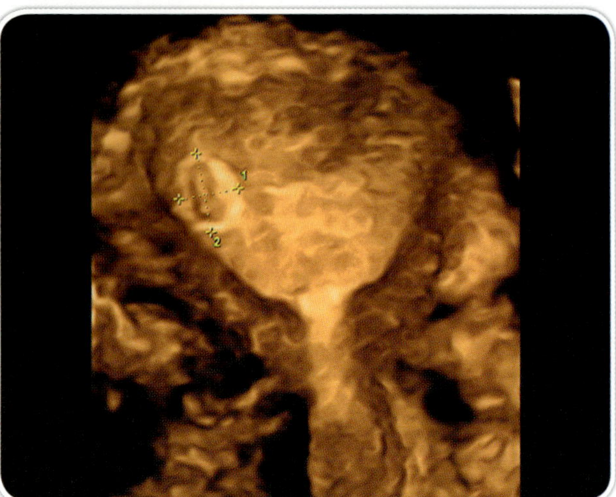

3D US for Pregnancy Localization

- Early pregnancy with sudden onset of pelvic pain and vaginal bleeding may be signs of cornual/interstitial pregnancy
- Eccentric location of the gestational sac or mass at the cornu can be visualized from the US.

(Doubilet 2014)

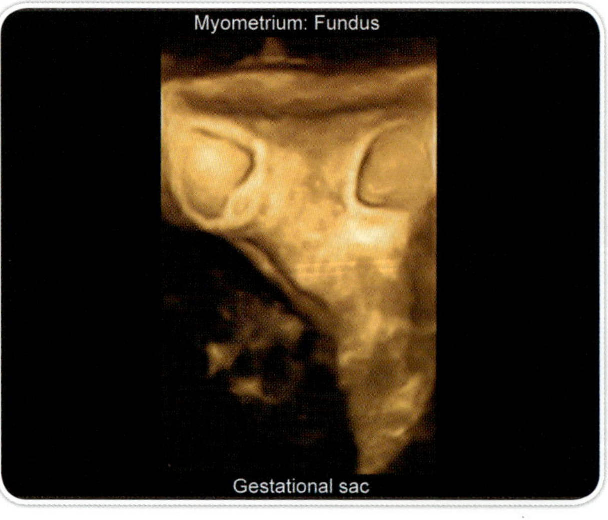

Early Pregnancy Failure

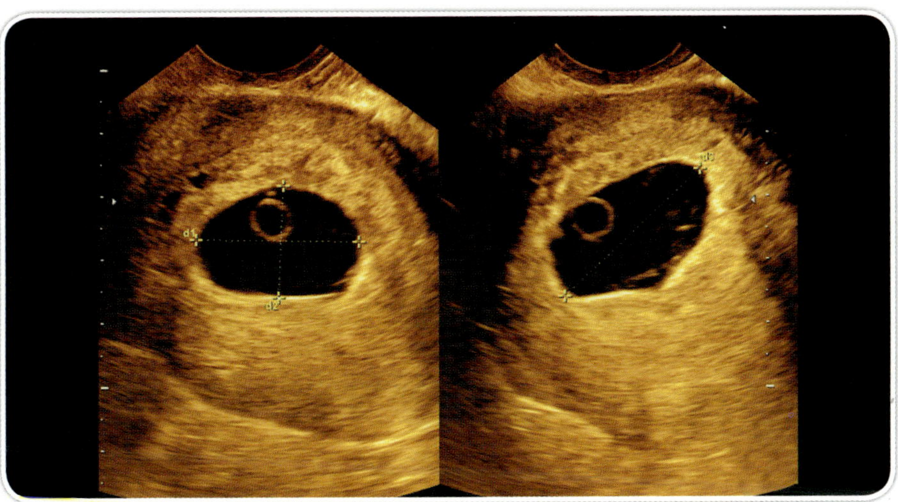

Only yolk sac is visible, but not fetal pole

Blighted Ovum: Anembryonic Pregnancy

- Mean sac diameter (MSD) ≥ 25 mm without fetal pole (by RCOG criteria)
- If the MSD is too small, a follow up scan in 2 weeks' should be recommended.
- Absent yolk sac when MSD >8 mm
- Poor decidual reaction (<2 mm)
- Irregular gestational sac shape
- Abnormally low sac position.

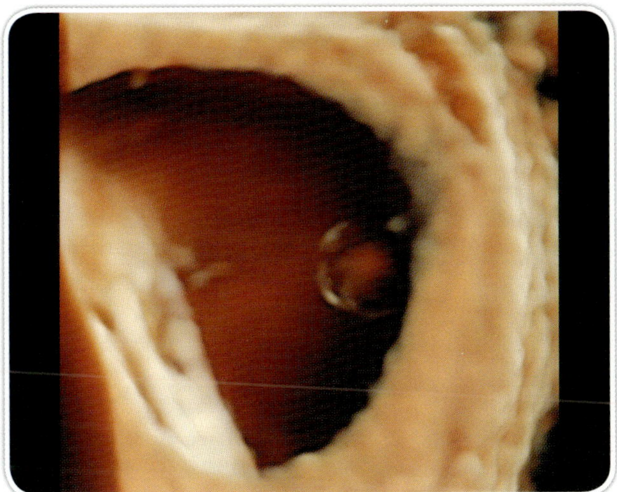

Yolk sac without fetal pole

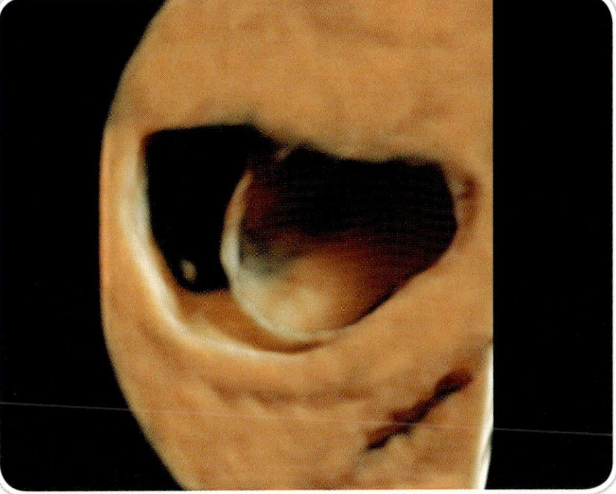

Amniotic sac without either fetal pole or yolk sac

6 Weeks': Fetal Pole and Yolk Sac

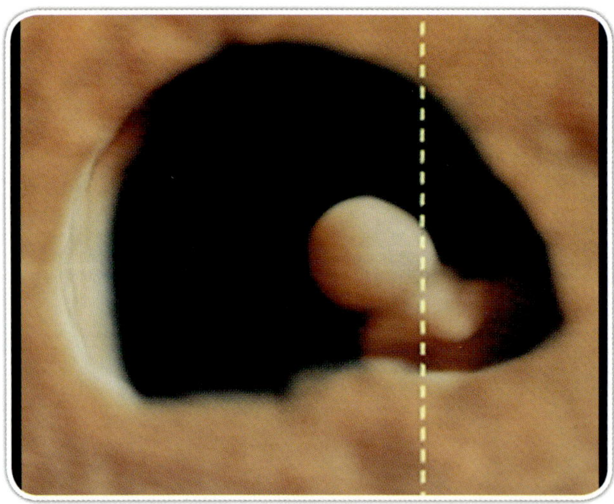

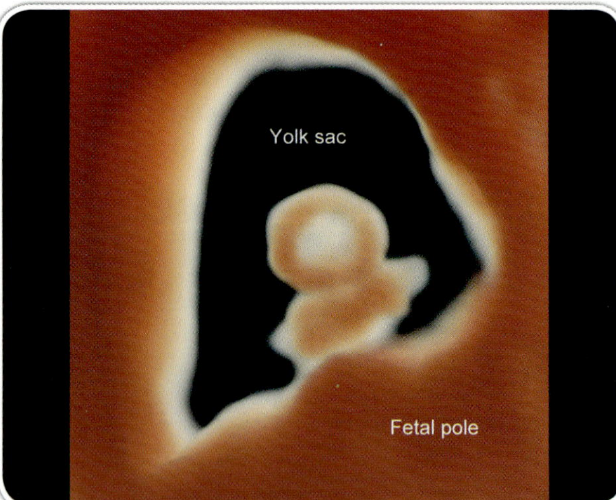

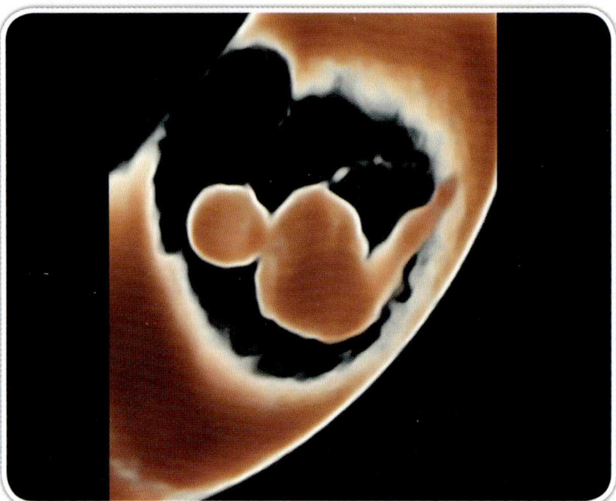

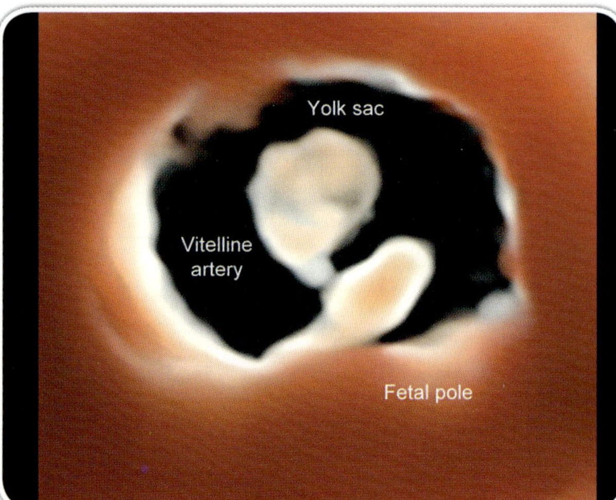

Vitelline artery connects yolk sac and the embryo

Embryology of 6 Weeks'

- The embryo measures 4 mm in length
- The heart beats in a regular rhythm
- Yolk sac is clearly visible.

(William 2001)

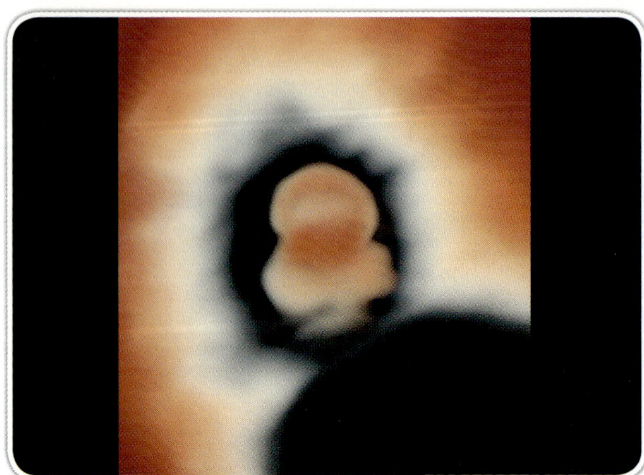

7 Weeks'

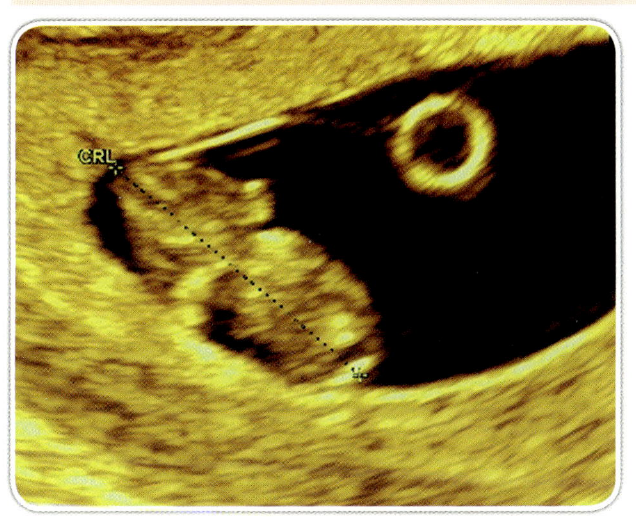

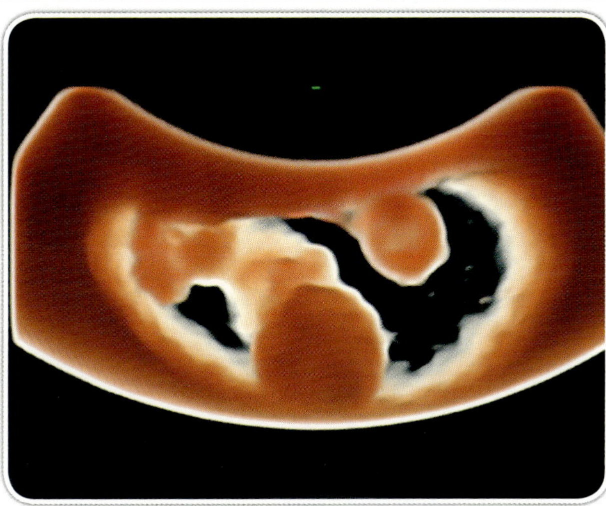

Embryology of 7 Weeks'

- The embryo measures 9 mm in length
- Development of eyes, ear pits, and brain
- Leg and hand buds
- Blood flow through yolk sac (vitelline artery).

(William 2001)

7 Weeks' Vitelline Duct

- Vitelline (or omphalomesenteric) duct connects yolk sac and midgut
- Yolk sac and Vitelline duct are extra-amniotic structures, which is clearly appreciated by 3DHD.

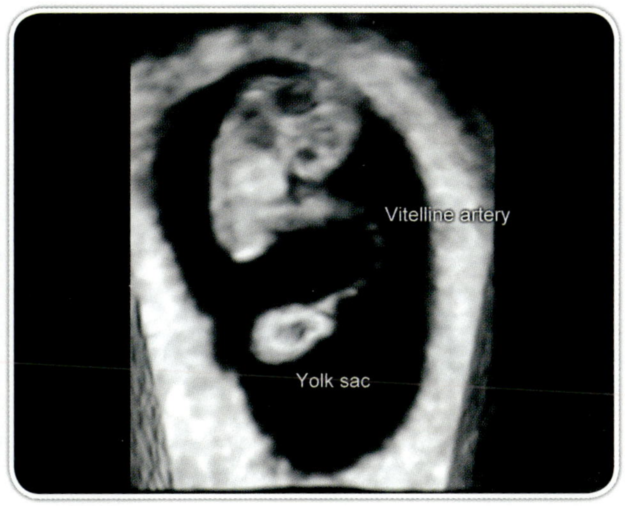

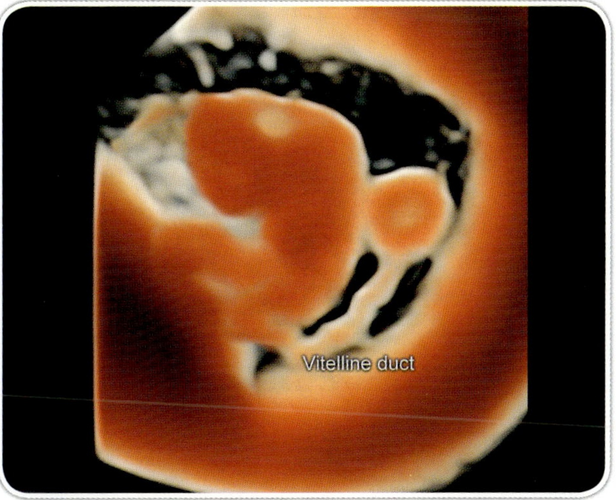

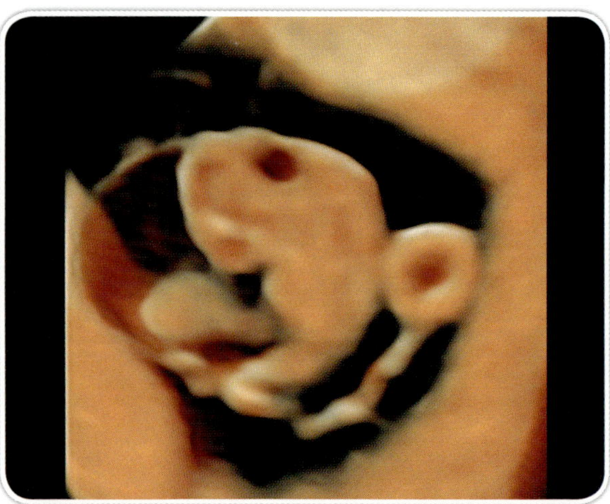

- Vitelline duct should be completely obliterated by the end of 9th menstrual weeks'.
- Complete and partial failure of obliteration will result in vitelline fistula and Meckel's diverticulum, respectively.

7 Weeks': Embryonic Demise

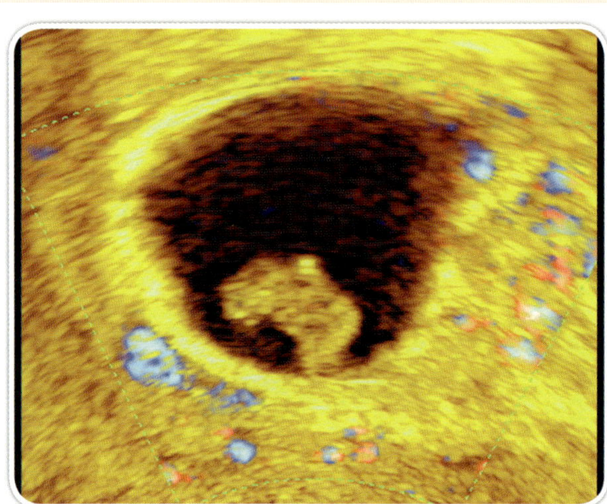

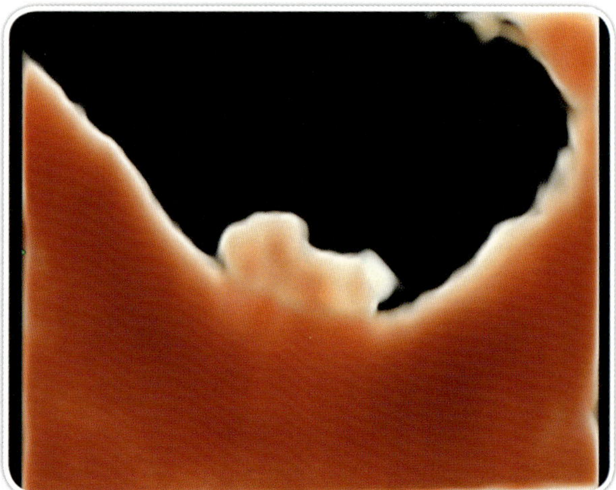

From 3DHD, note how 'lifeless' the fetus is

Subchorionic Hemorrhage: 2D

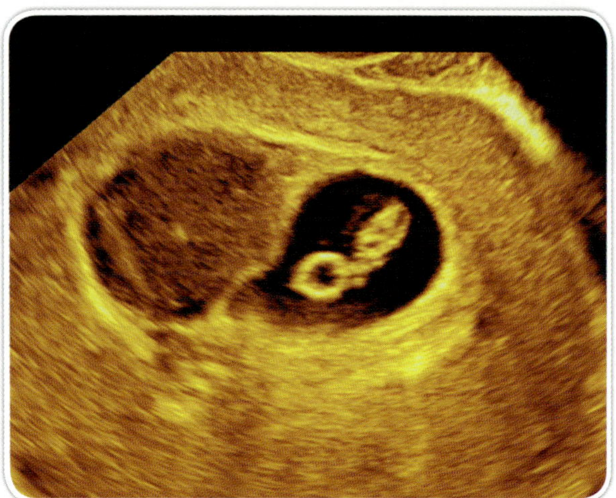

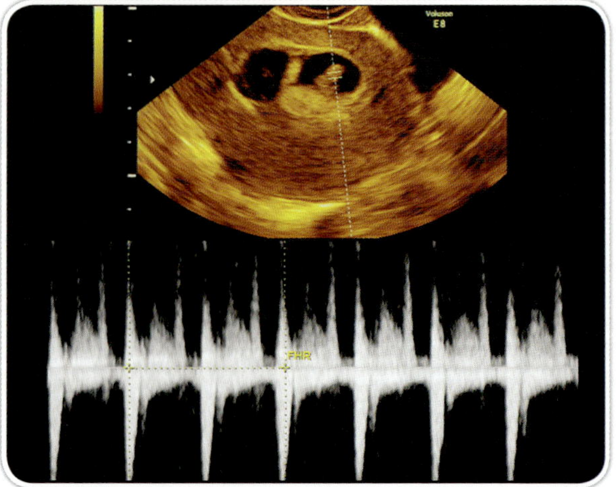

Subchorionic Hemorrhage: 3DHD

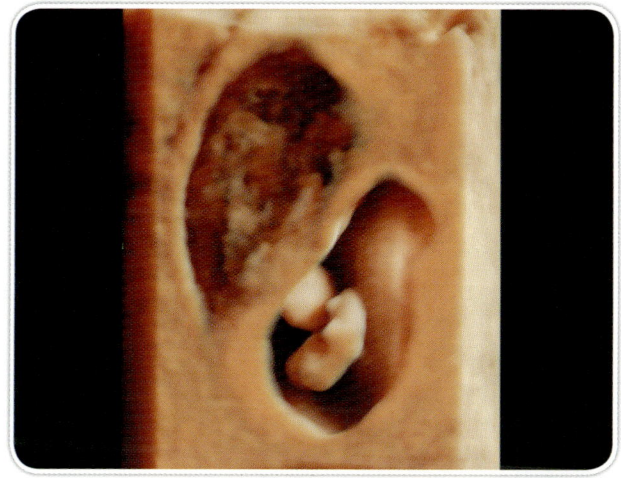

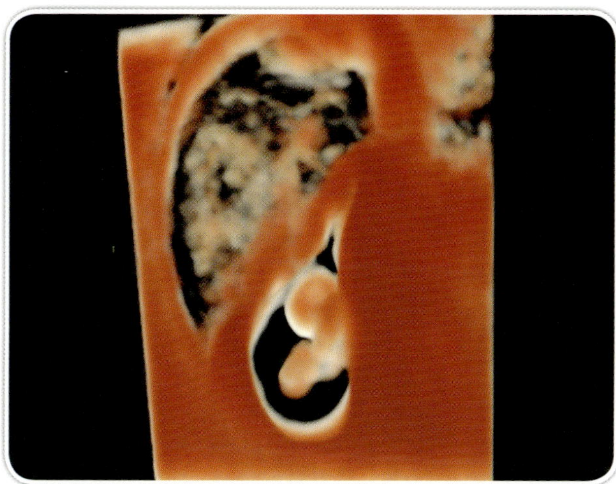

8 Weeks': Yolk Sac and Umbilical Cord

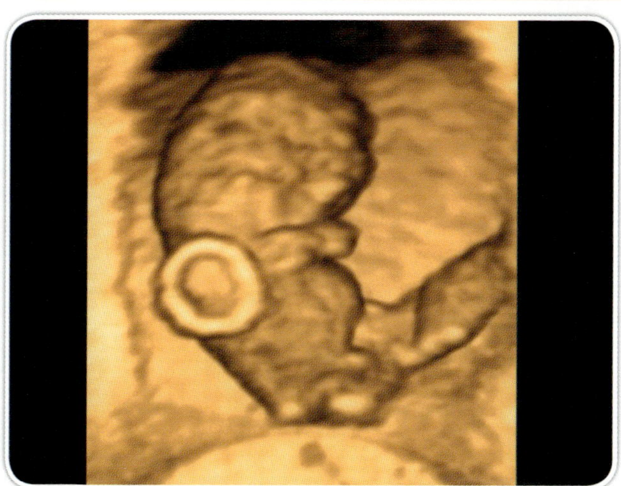

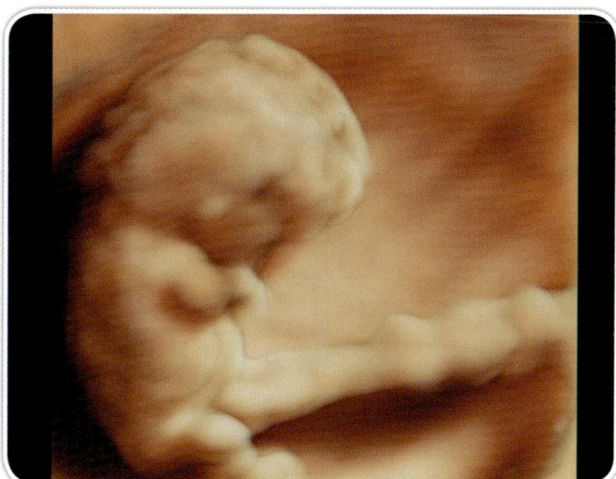

8 Weeks': Amnion can be demonstrated with optimal setting

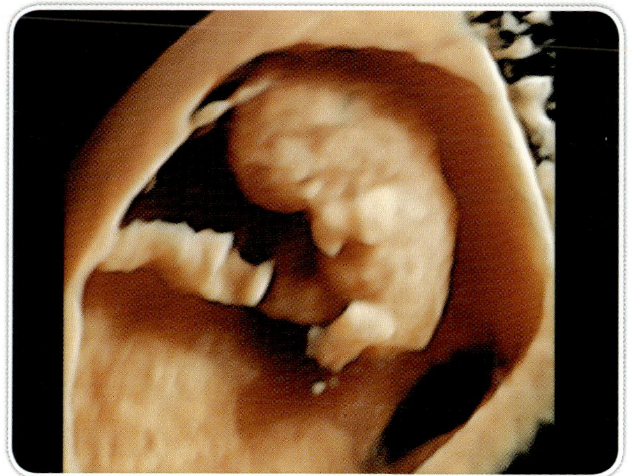

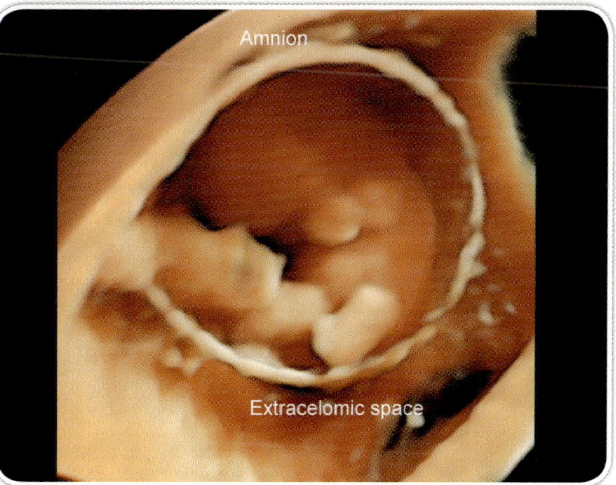

Embryology of 8 Weeks'

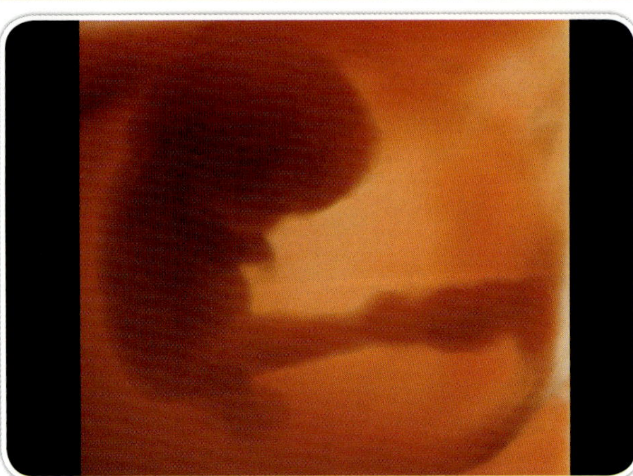

- The embryo measures 13 mm in length
- Arms and legs are lengthened with hands and feet clearly distinguished
- Lungs and brain are developed.

(William 2001)

8 Weeks'

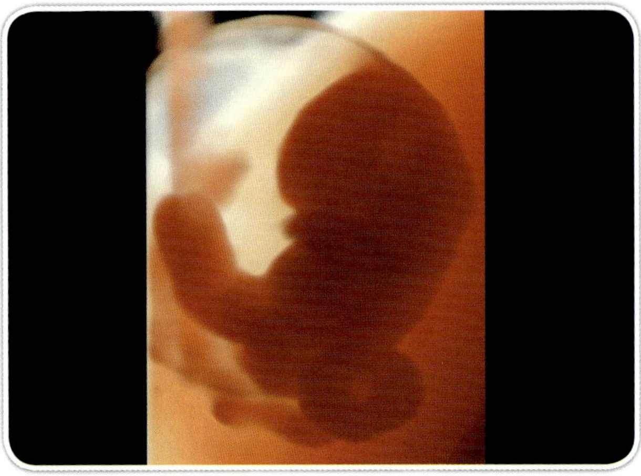

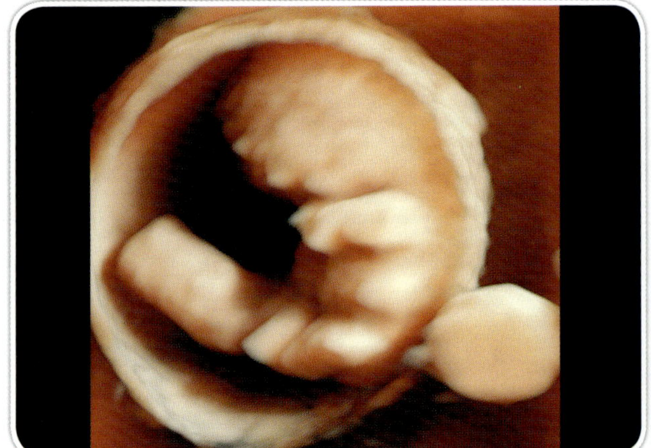

Amnion: 9 Weeks'

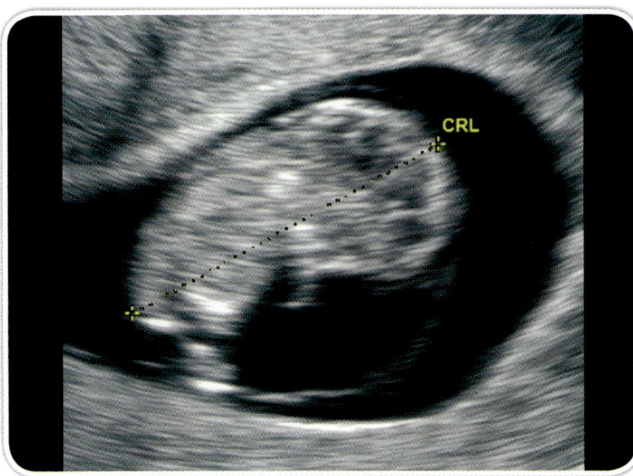

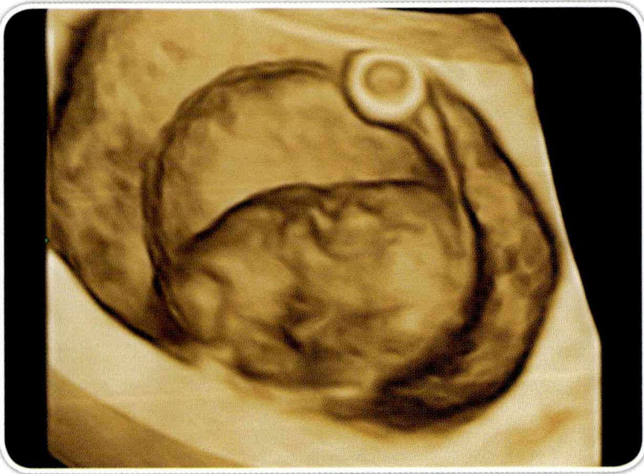

With optimal rendering: amnion, yolk sac, and vitelline duct can be appreciated

Body Stalk and Amnion

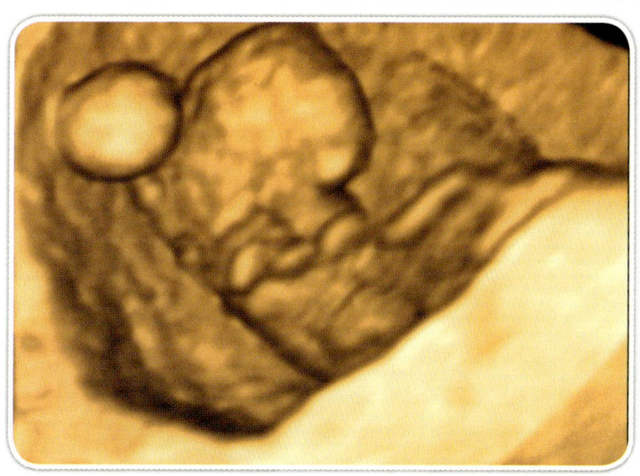

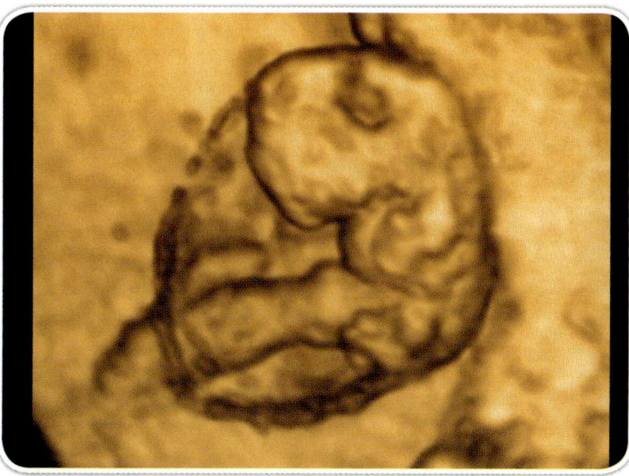

Amnion: 9 Weeks' 3DHD

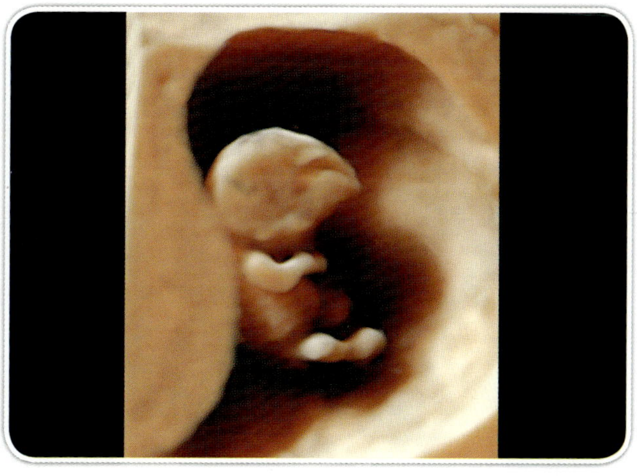

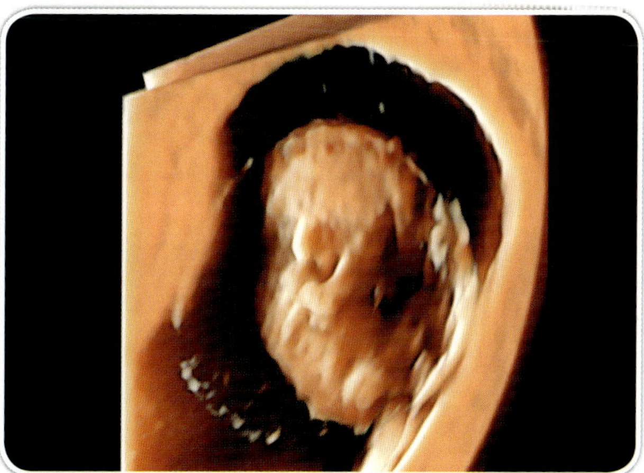

The thinness of amnion can be appreciated with proper adjustment

Embryology of 9 Weeks'

- The embryo measures 18 mm in length
- The elbows and toes are visible
- Spontaneous limb movements may be detected
- All essential organs at least begun.

(William 2001)

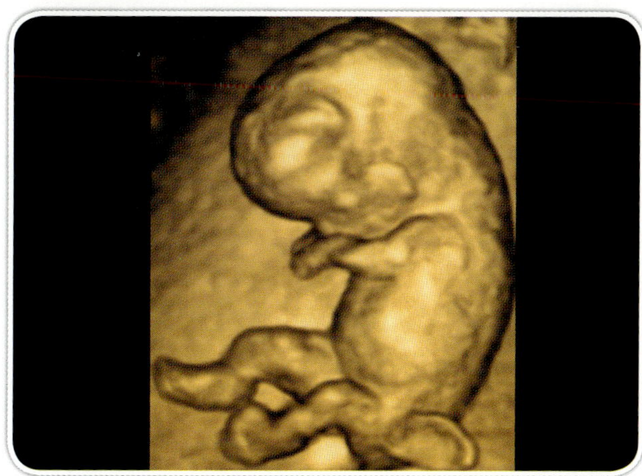

9 Weeks': Comparison between Surface Rendered and Backlight 3D HD

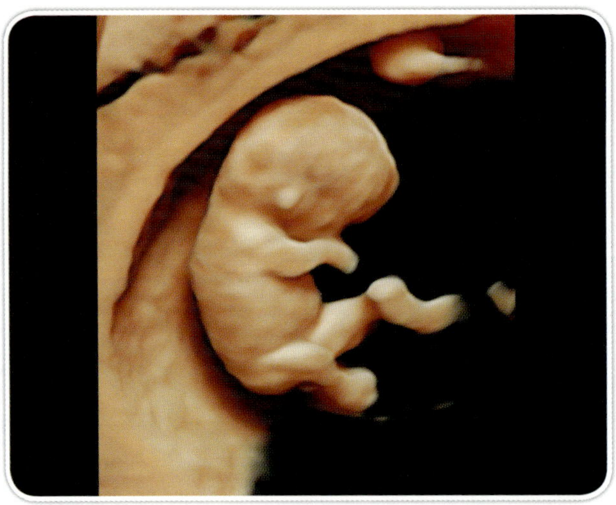

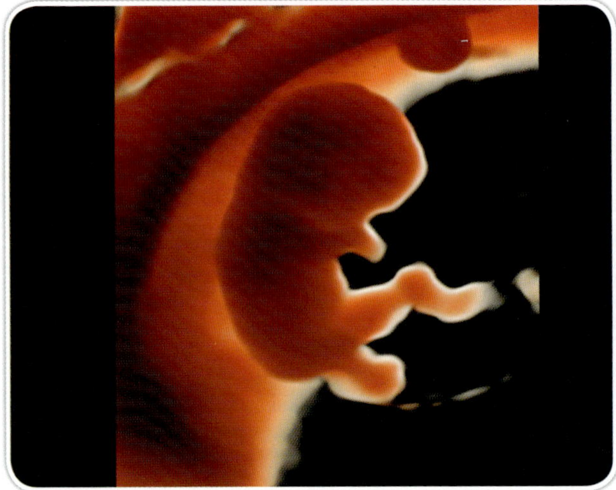

Embryology of 9 Weeks': HDLive Silhouette Mode

- HDLive Silhouette is the new 3D ultrasound rendering software
- It outlines the structure, make it transparent, so that surrounding structures are visible at the same time.
- The image obtained from this software is artistic.
- The diagnostic roles remain to be proven.

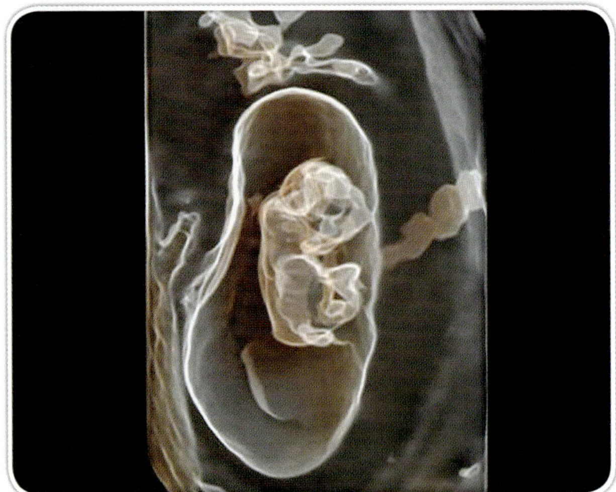

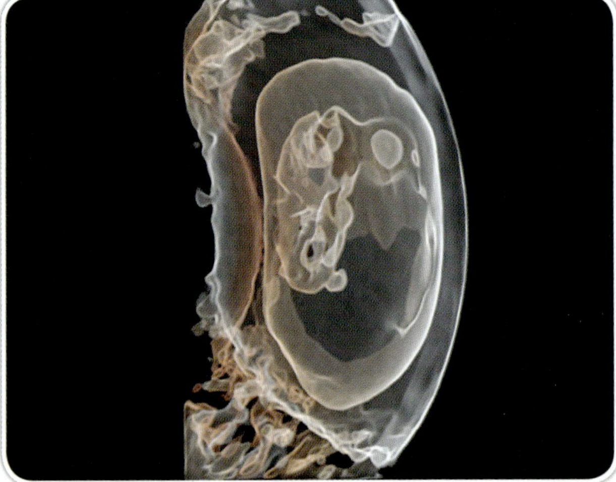

- HDLive Silhouette can be combined with other 3D HD modalities to create 'more surreal' images
- Picture on this slide demonstrate a combination of HDLive Silhouette and 3DHD backlight.

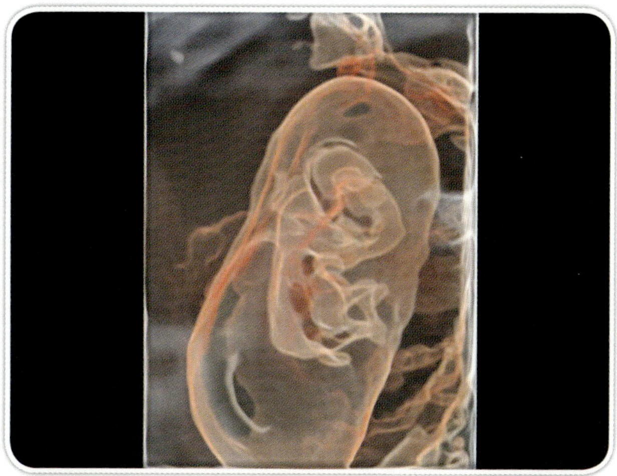

Embryology of 9 Weeks': Umbilical Cord Insertion

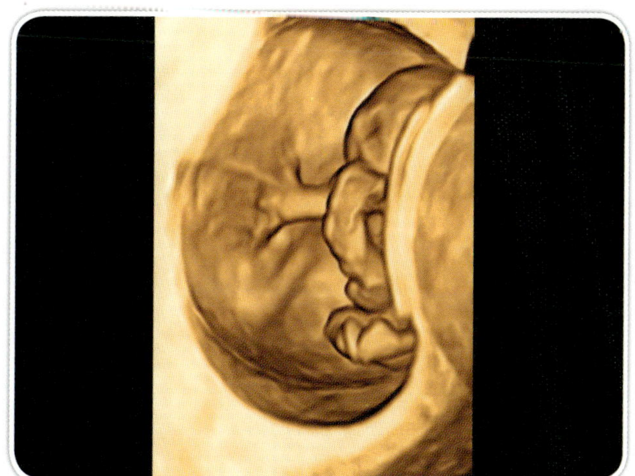

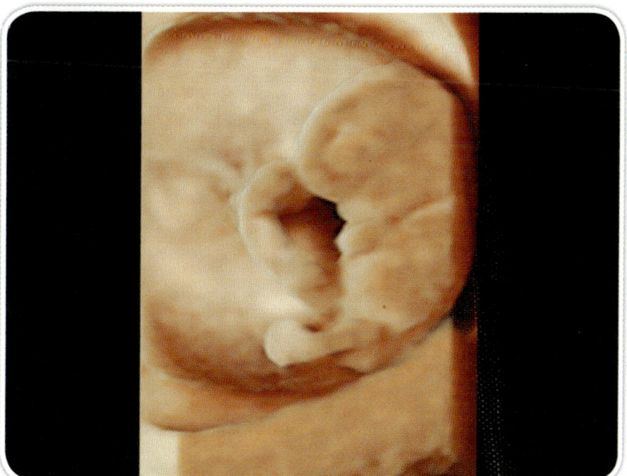

Dichorionic Diamniotic Twins 9 Weeks'

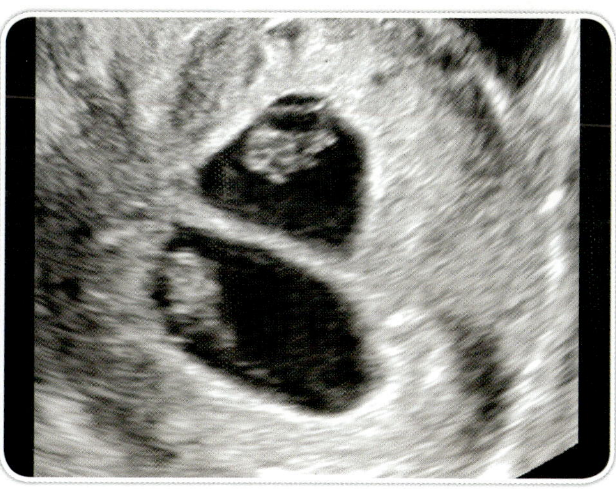

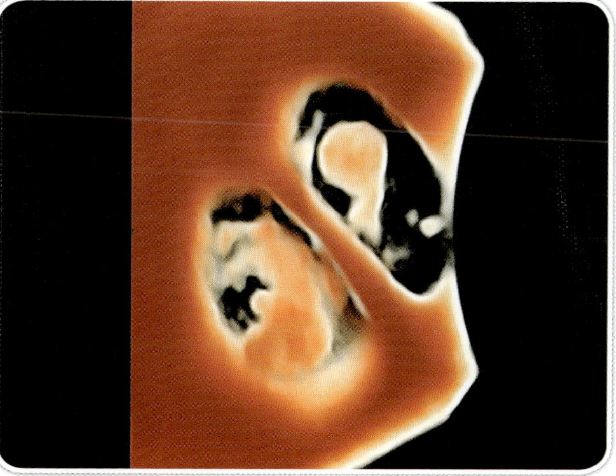

Note the thickness of intertwin membranes from standard 2D and 3DHD

Dichorionic Diamniotic Twins 7 Weeks': HDLive Silhouette Mode

- Note the thick intertwin membranes
- "Lambda sign", which is the interposing chorion, is appreciated from this 3D image.
- Diagnosis of 'twins' is not enough
- It is 'chorionicity' that predict the perinatal outcomes
- Up to 20% of monochorionic (MC) twins have complications, i.e. twin-twin transfusion syndrome (TTTS).

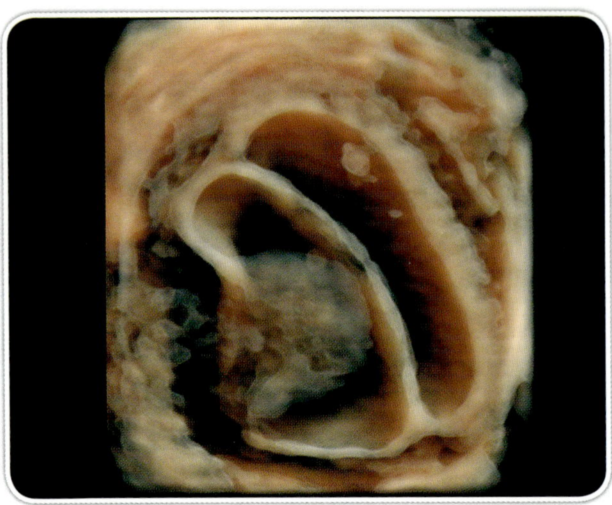

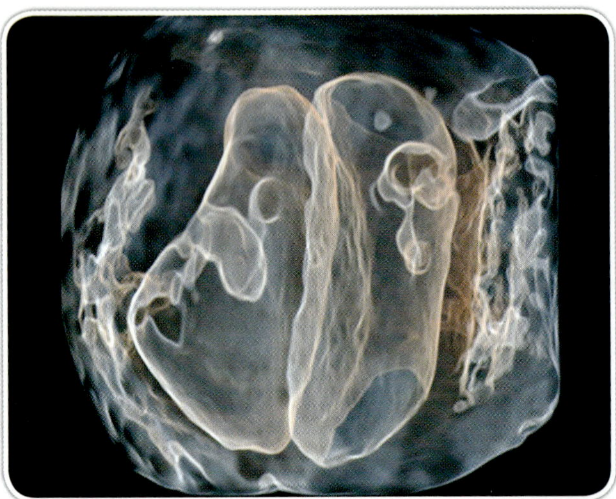

Indications of US in Twins

- Dating
- Chorionicity
- Nuchal translucency
- Anatomical survey
- Placental evaluation
- Cervical length assessment.

(Simpson 2013)

- Fetal growth
- Liquor volume
- Complicated MC twins, i.e. TTTS
- Diagnostic or therapeutic interventions

(Simpson 2013)

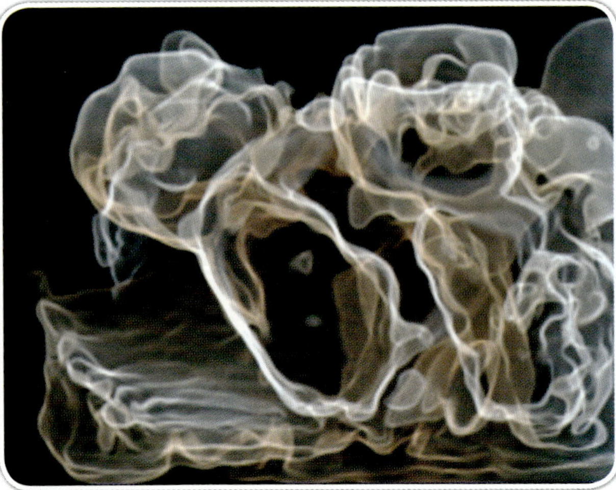

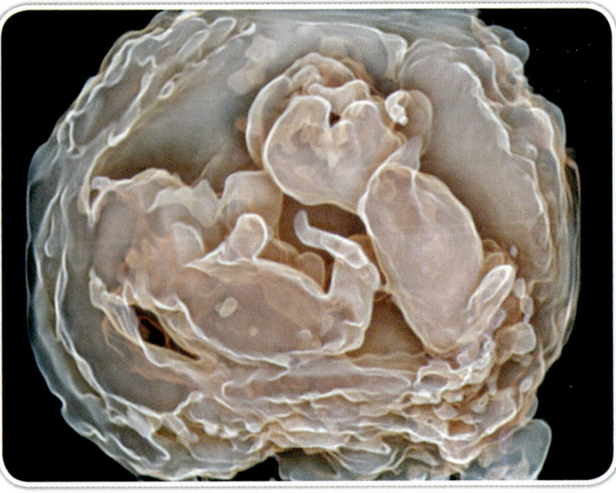

Dichorionic diamniotic twins 7 weeks': HDLive Silhouette Mode

Complicated MC Twins: TTTS

- Incidence 5.5–17.5% of MC twins
- Serious, perinatal mortality > 90%
- Long-term neurological sequelae of the surviving twin ≈ 25%

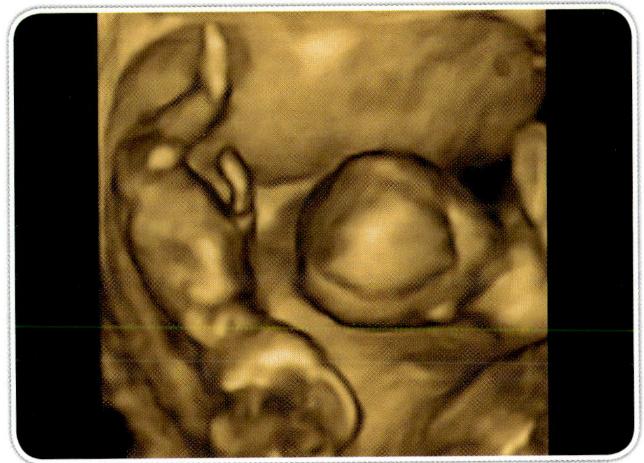

Complicated MC twins: Acardiac Twin

- Incidence 1:100 of MC twins
- Associated with twins reversed arterial perfusion sequence (TRAPS)
- Non-viable fetus
- The 'pump twin' can suffer from high-output cardiac failure.

(Moore et al. 1990)

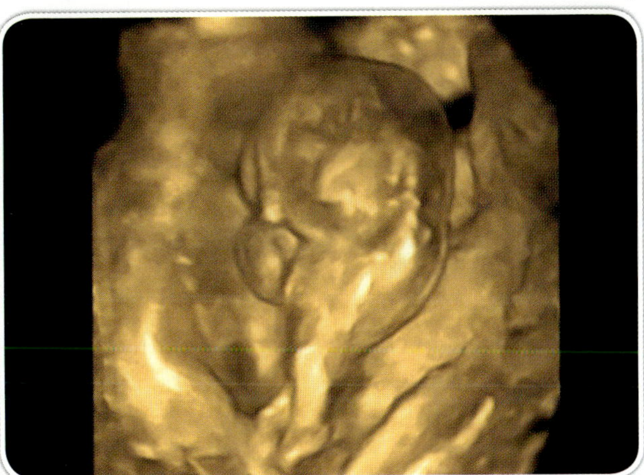

Complicated MC Twins: Cord Entanglement

- Incidence 70% of monoamniotic twins
- May impair blood flow in the umbilical cord
  - ↑ resistance indices of umbilical artery
  - Absent end-diastolic flow of umbilical artery
  - Pulsatile Doppler umbilical vein.

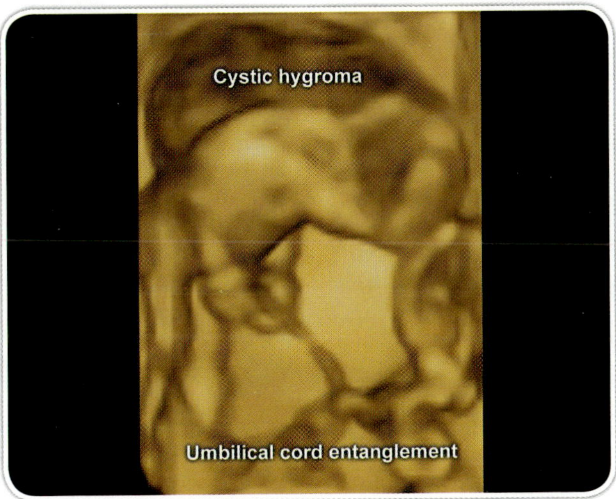

Complicated MC Twins: Conjoined Twins

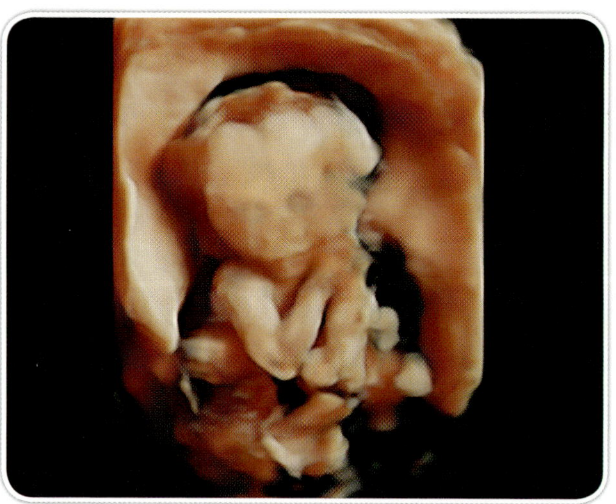

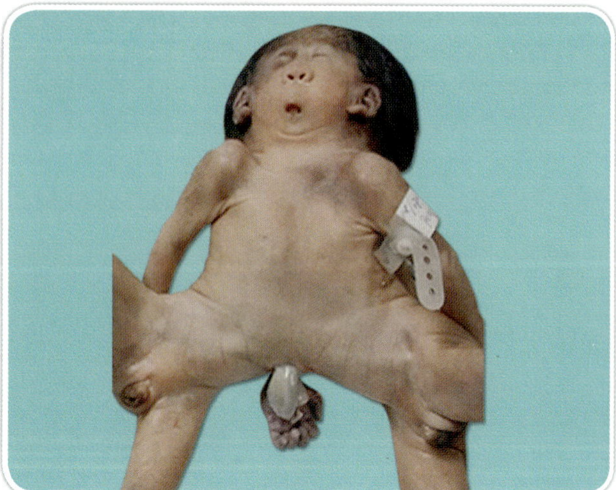

"Janiceps"

Embryology of 10 to 12 Weeks'

- Embryo measures 30 to 80 mm in length
- Facial features continue to develop
- The external ear begin to form final shape
- The head comprises nearly half of the fetus' size.
- The face is well formed
- The eyelids close
- The limbs are long and thin
- The fetus can make a fist
- Genital organ is well differentiated.

(William 2001)

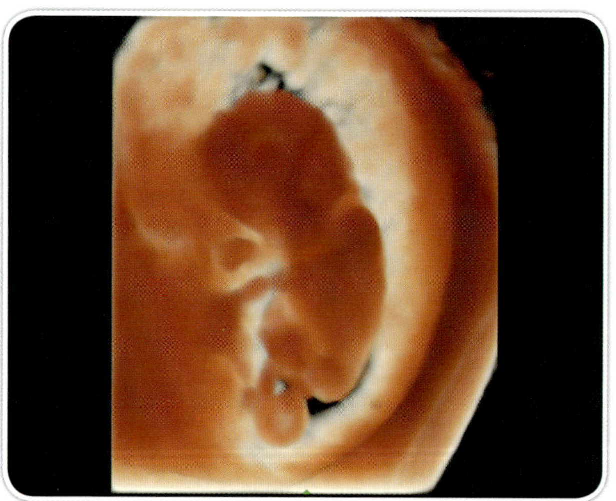

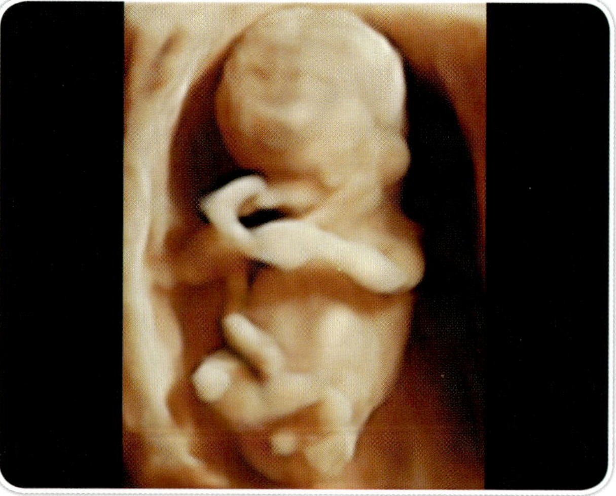

Different Rendering:11 Weeks'

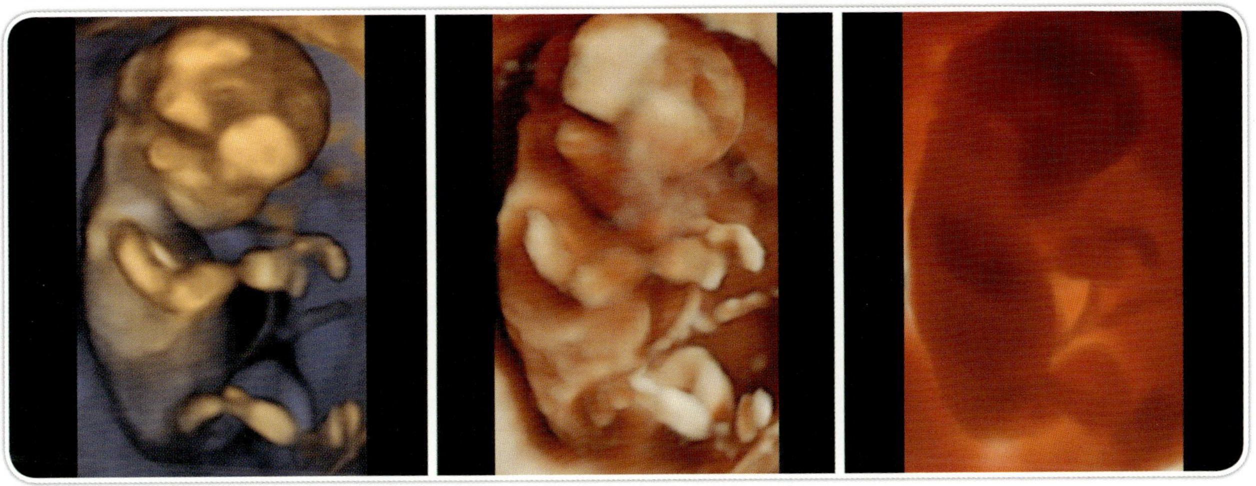

Dichorionic Diamniotic Twins 12 Weeks'

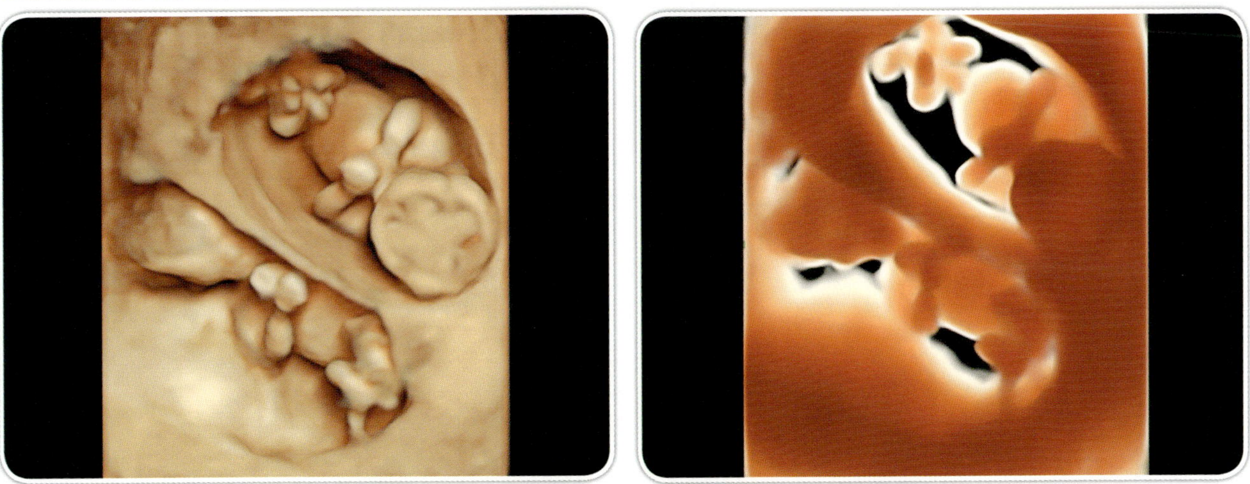

Note the thickness of intertwin membranes

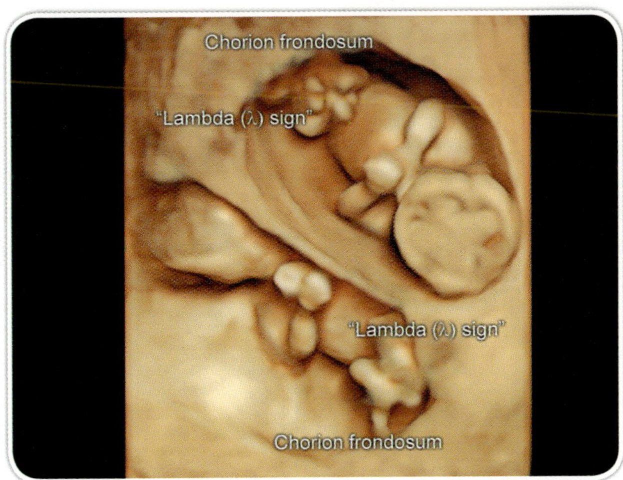

Nuchal edema 10 Weeks'

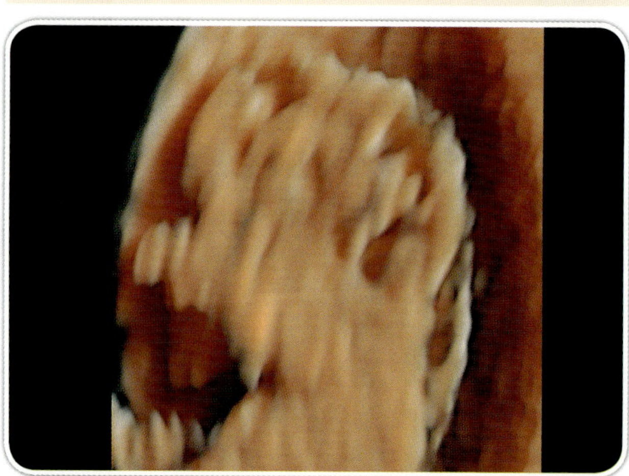

- Concerns
  - Fetal aneuploidies
  - Fetal cardiac anomalies
  - Syndromes
- Additional US markers
- Non-invasive prenatal testing (NIPT)
- Biochemical screening
- Invasive diagnostic procedures.

Cystic Hygroma: 3D Surface Rendered

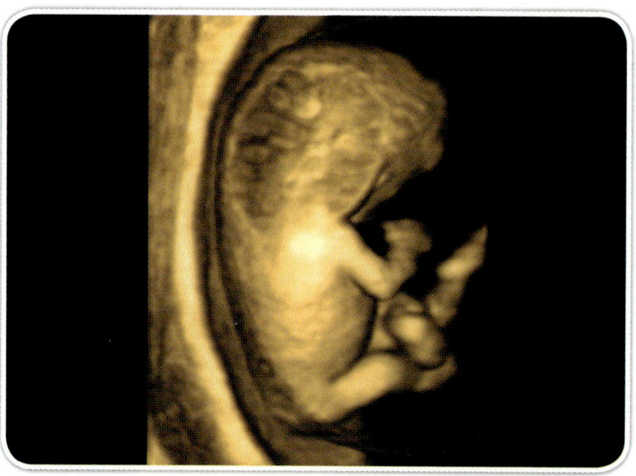

- Well-circumscribed nuchal cysts or fluid density
- Increased risk of fetal aneuploidies, and invasive prenatal diagnostic procedure is warranted.

Cystic Hygroma: HDLive Silhouette Mode

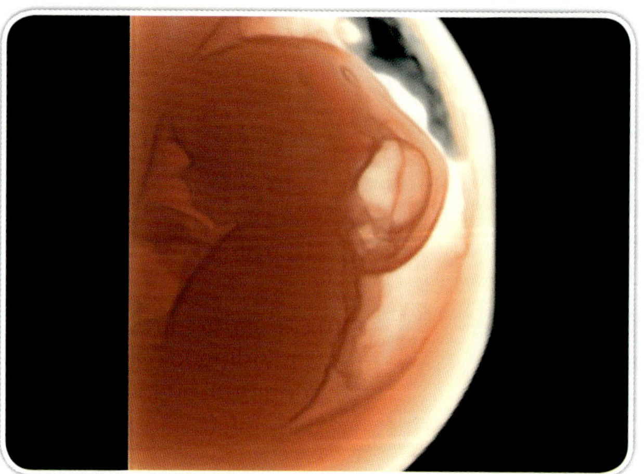

- Cystic hygroma is also known as congenital lymphangioma
- Delayed development of the lymphatic channels connecting to venous system of the neck
- Commonly associated with other anomalies and hydrops.

Fetal Hydrops: 13 Weeks'

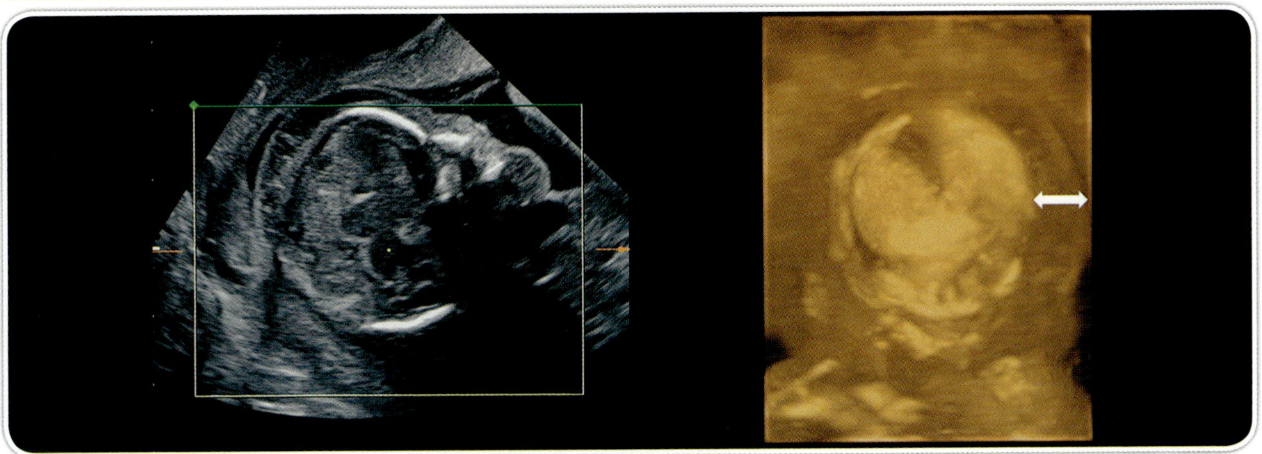

Subcutaneous fluid collection can be appreciated from skeletal 3D mode

Fetal Hydrops: 1st Trimester

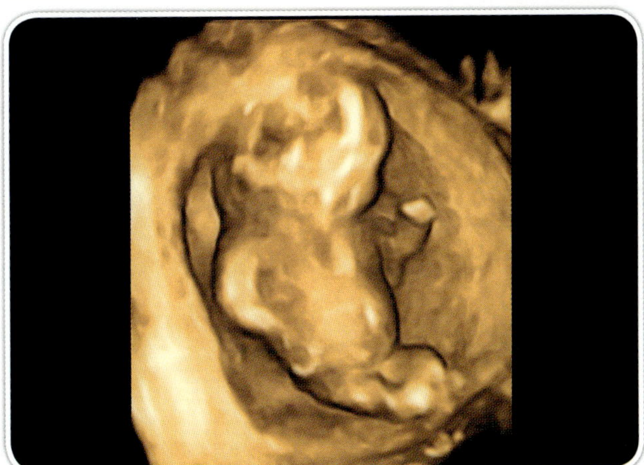

- Chromosomal defects
- Subchromosomal deletions/duplications
- Serious congenital malformations: cardiac, lymphatic
- Congenital infection and anemic hydrops (i.e. Bart's hydrops) are less likely at < 16 wks'.

(Wataganara et al. 2006)

Monochorionic Diamniotic Twins 19 Weeks'

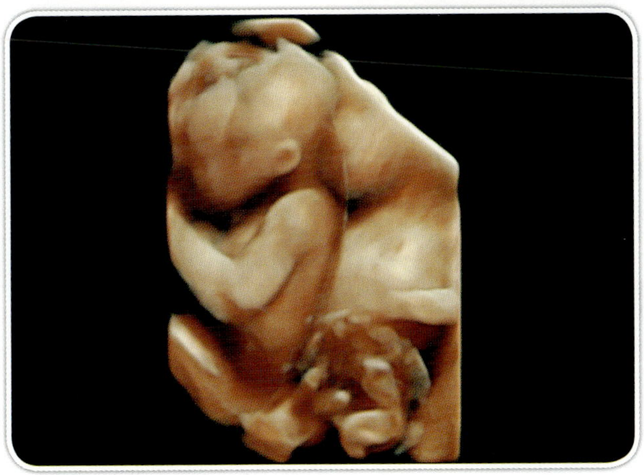

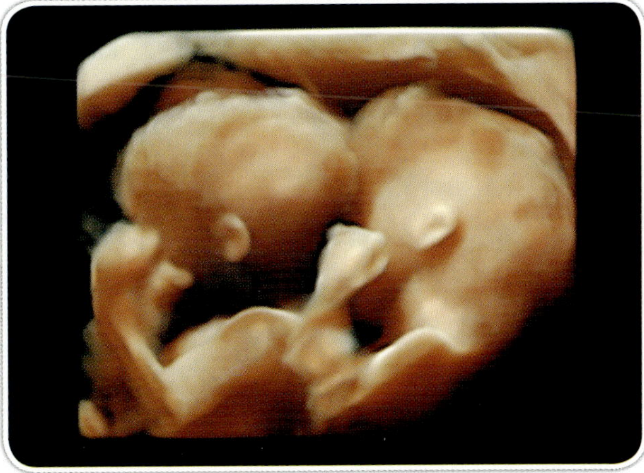

Note the thin intertwin membranes

Iatrogenic Septostomy

- Can occur following diagnostic or therapeutic fetal interventions:
  - ↑ preterm delivery < 32 wks'
  - ↑ preterm premature rupture of the membranes < 32 wks'
  - ↑ fetal demises
  - ↑ pseudoamniotic band syndrome.

(Wataganara and Kanokpongsakdi, 2008)

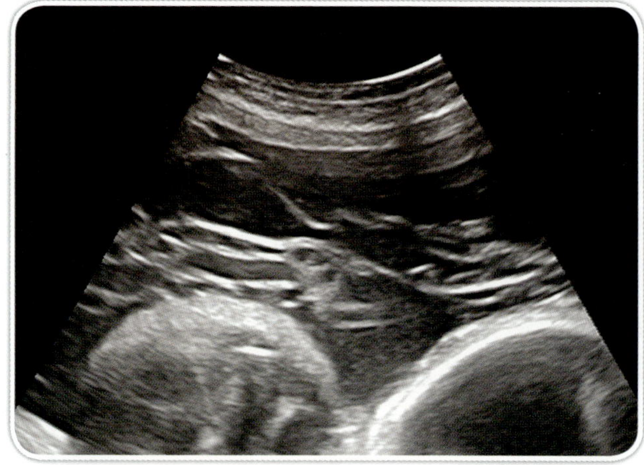

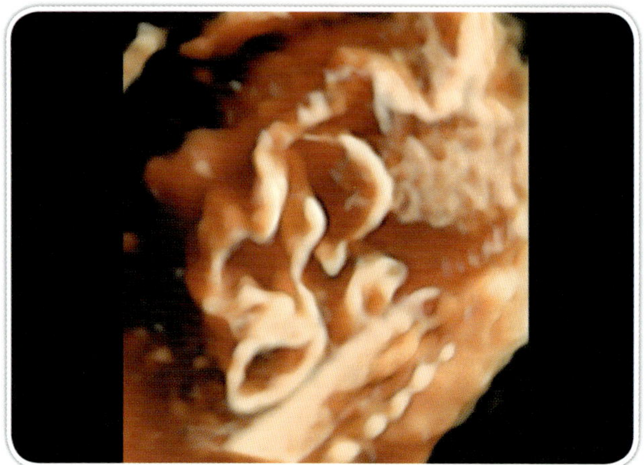

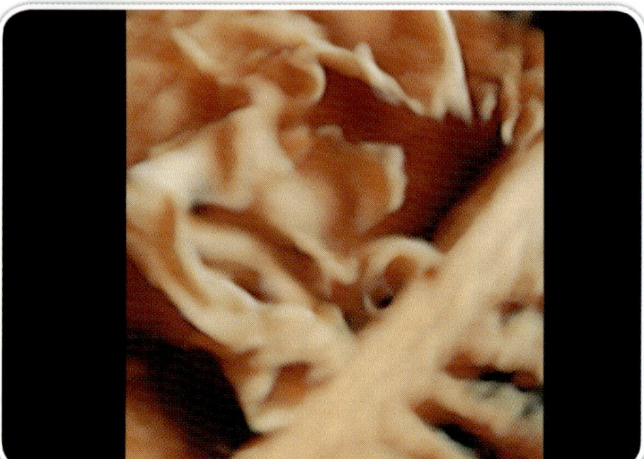

Facial Expression

- Fetal facial expression can be visible as early as 20 weeks'
- Mouthing is the most common movement.

(Sato et al. 2014)

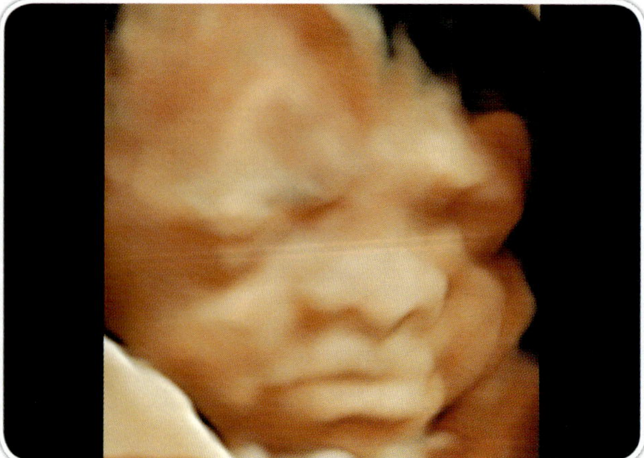

26 Weeks': Fetal Mouthing 3D

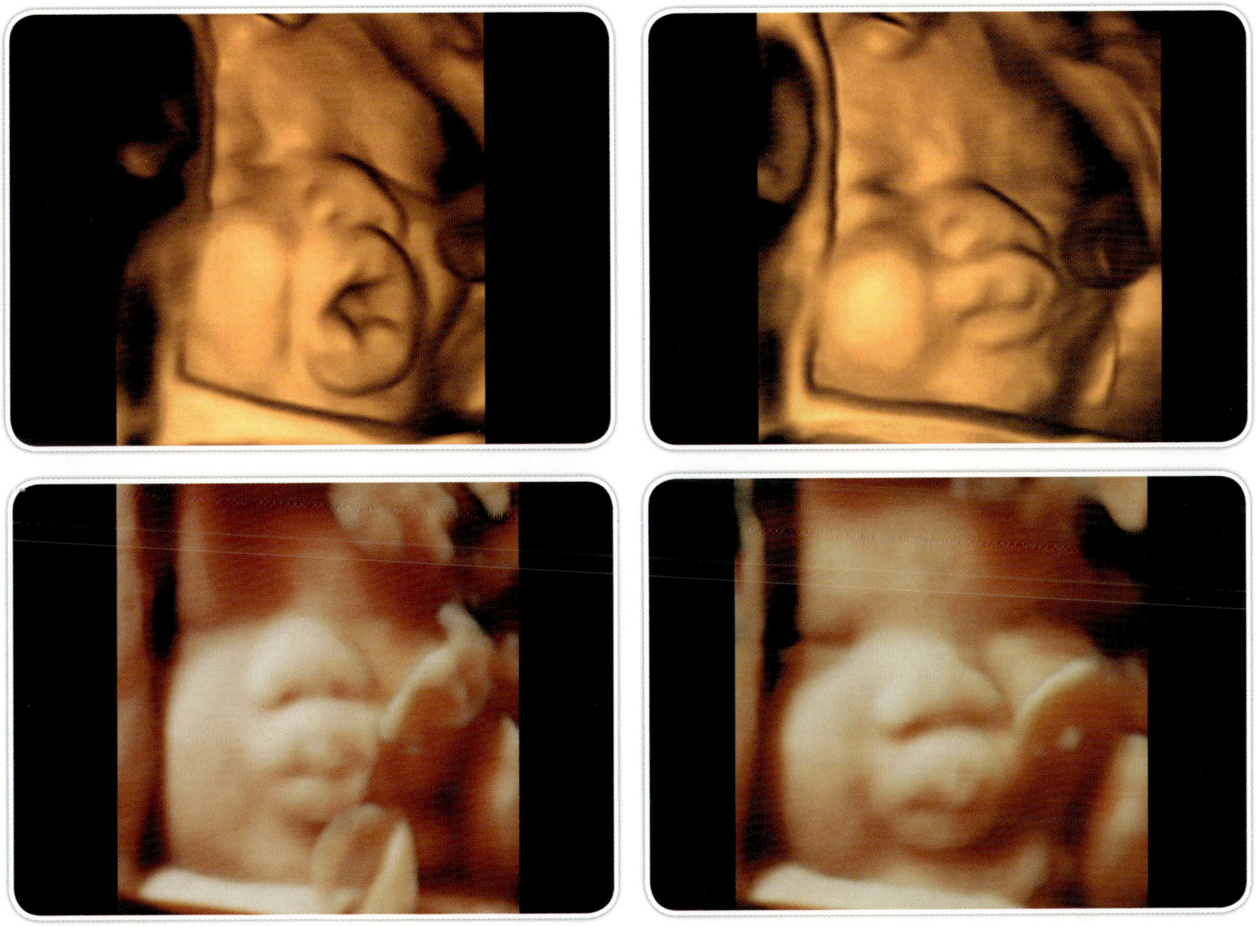

Facial Expression: 26 Weeks'

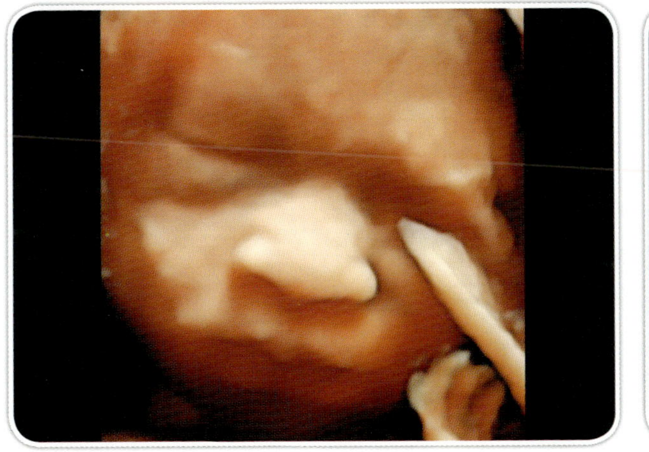

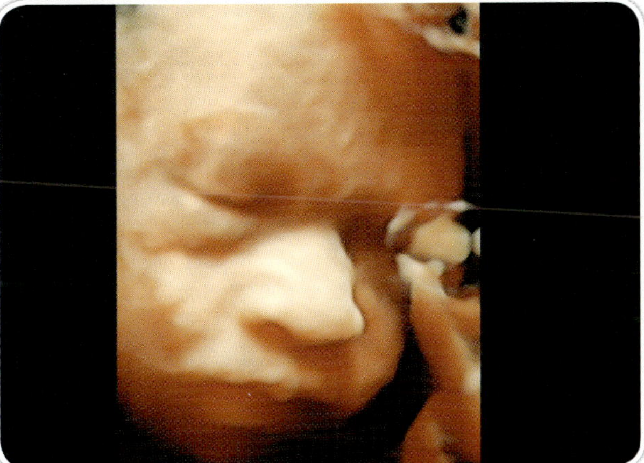

Eye Opening 28 Weeks'

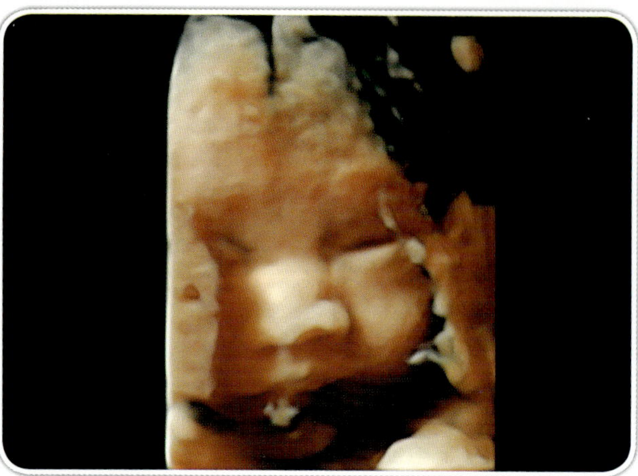

- At 28 weeks', eyes start to open.

(William 2001)

Grimace 29 Weeks'

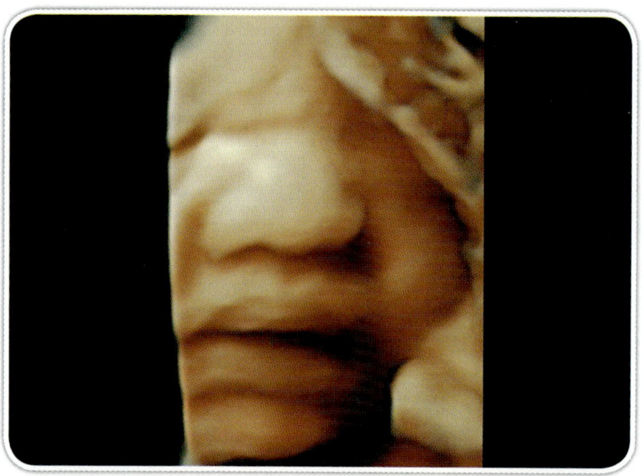

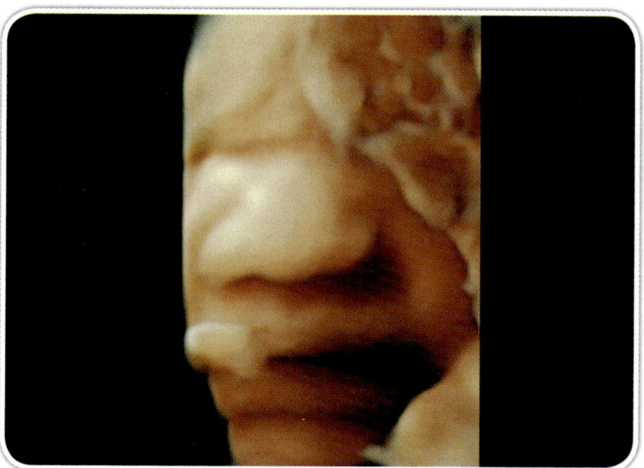

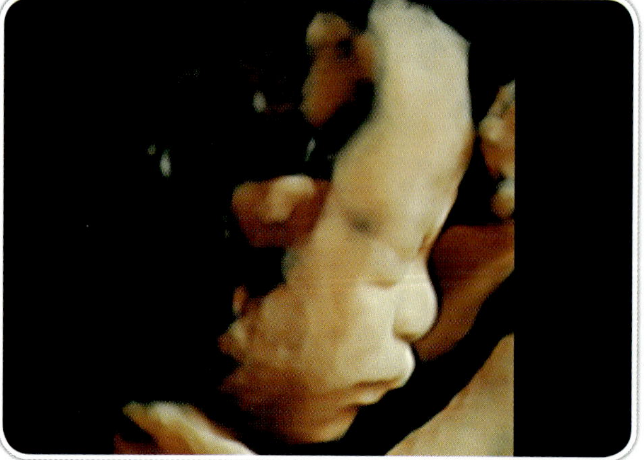

- Details of facial profile and expression.

Facial Expression

- More complex facial expression can be appreciated when the gestational age is advancing
- 3D for facial expression can help with maternal-fetal bonding.

(de Jong-Pleij et al. 2013)

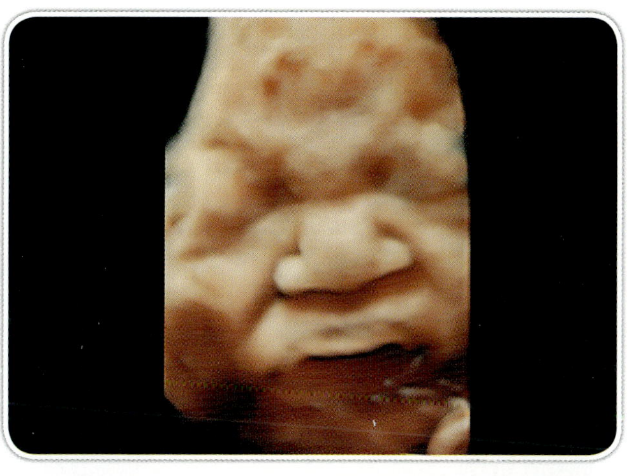

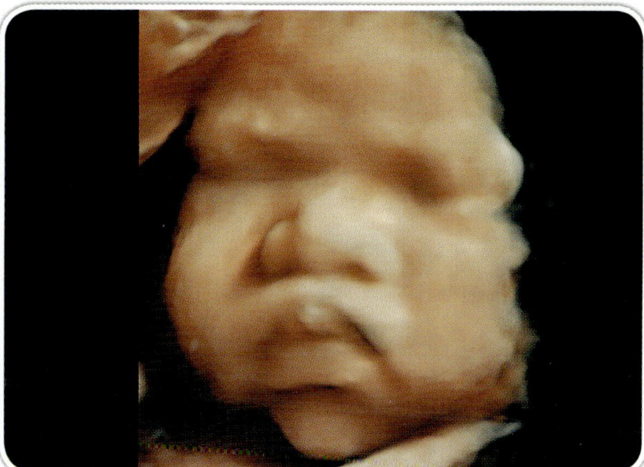

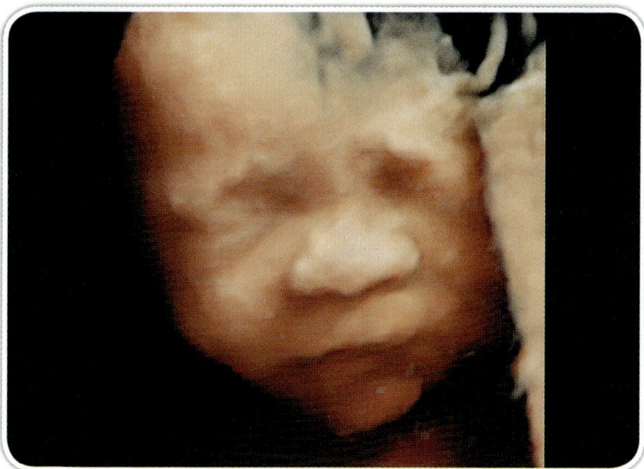

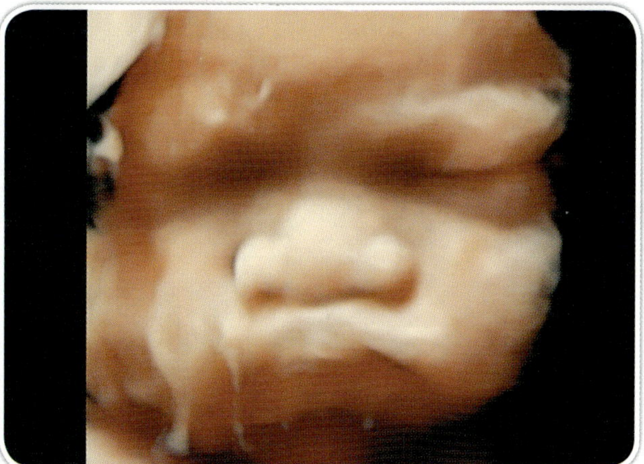

Low-set Ear

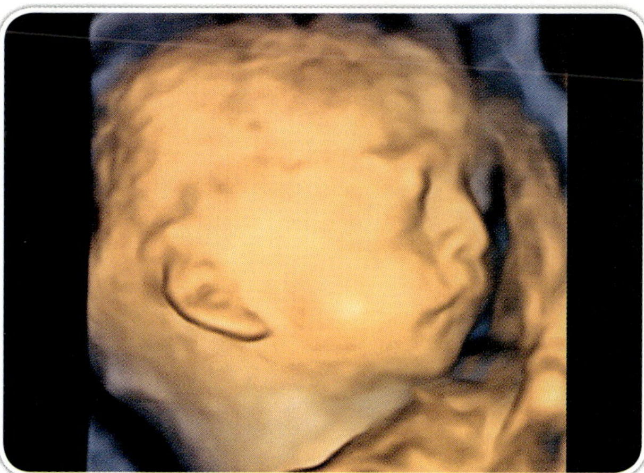

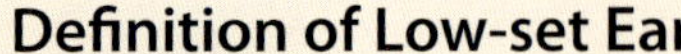

Definition of Low-set Ear

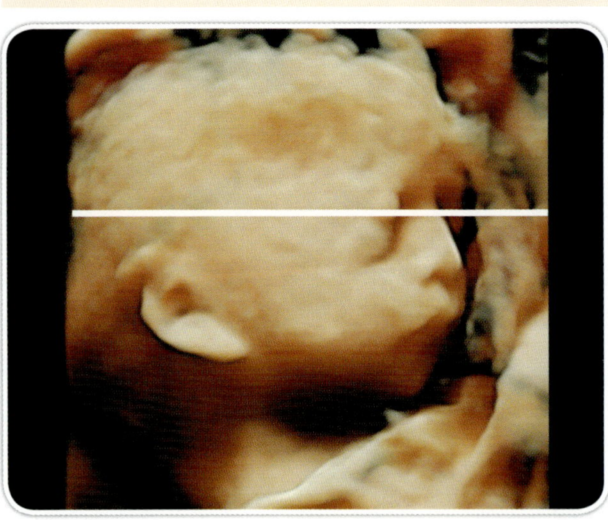

- The helix is at a level below a horizontal plane with the corner of the orbit.

Clinical Significance of Fetal Low-set Ear

Chromosomal syndrome
- Trisomy 18
- Jacobsen syndrome

Non-chromosomal syndrome
- Fetal valproate syndrome
- Freeman-Sheldon syndrome
- Fryns syndrome
- Noonan syndrome
- Potter sequence.

Unilateral Cleft Lip

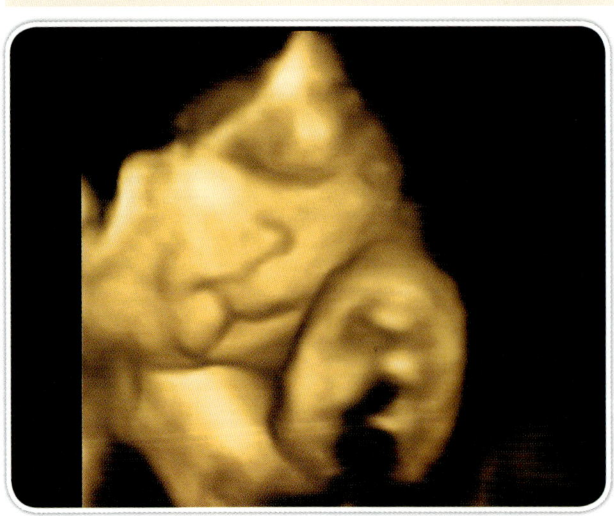

- Cleft lip and/or palate can be associated with numerous fetal syndromes
- Definitive diagnosis can be linked to successful postnatal surgical correction.

(Burnell et al. 2014)

Craniofacial Abnormalities in Fetal Trisomy 13

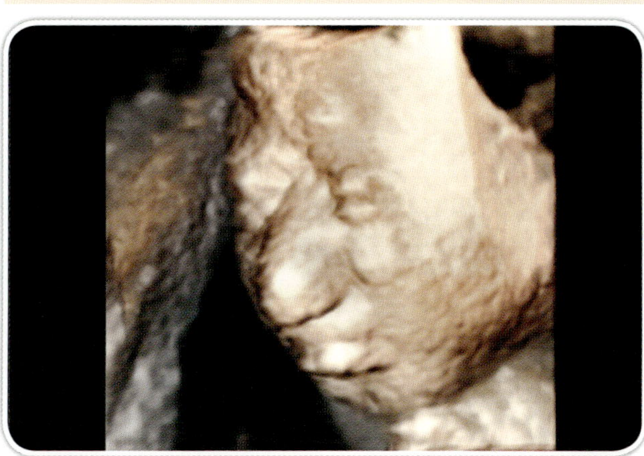

- Holoprosencephaly
- Ventriculomegaly
- Microcephaly
- Cleft lip and palate
- Midface hypoplasia
- Cyclopia
- Microphthalmia
- Hypotelorism.

Achondrogenesis

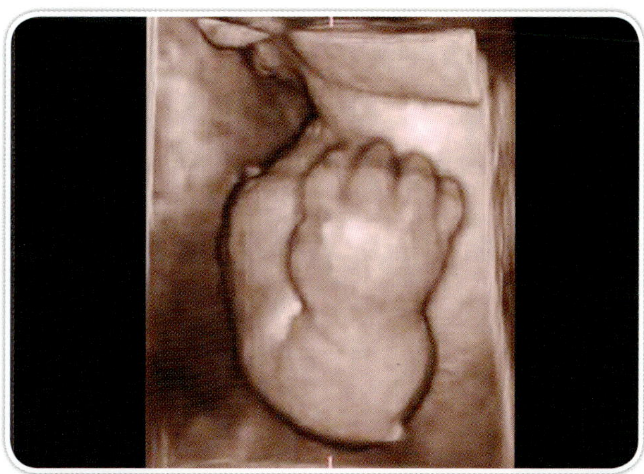

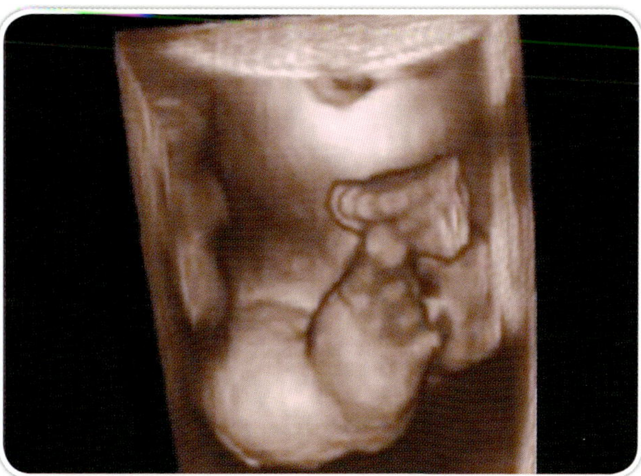

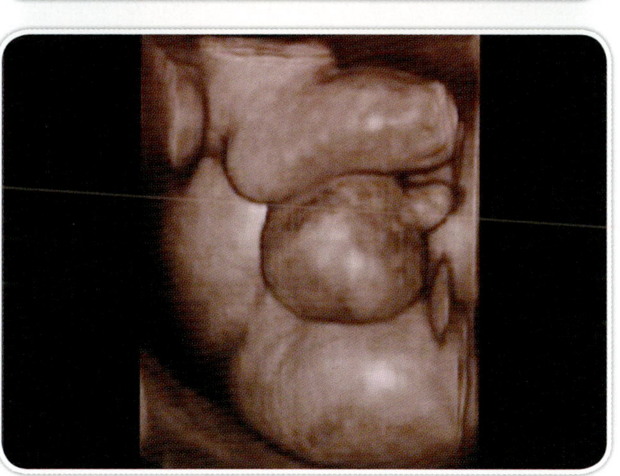

Bilateral hydrocele

- Generalized shortening of fetal long bones
- Lethal skeletal dysplasia
- 3D US allows for a better understanding for the parents and the family

(Wataganara et al. 2006)

Facial Profiles in Fetal Trisomy 13

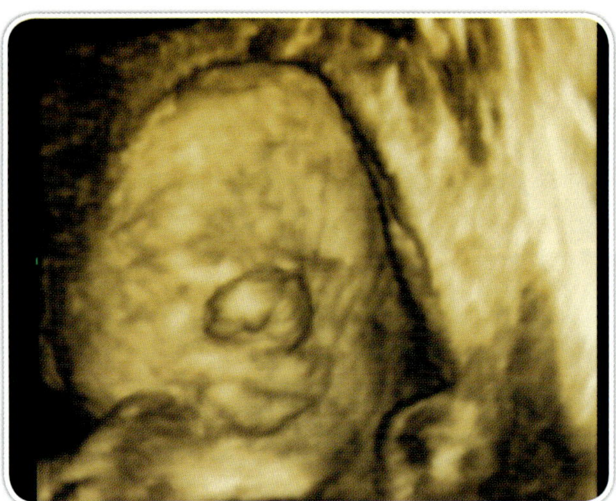

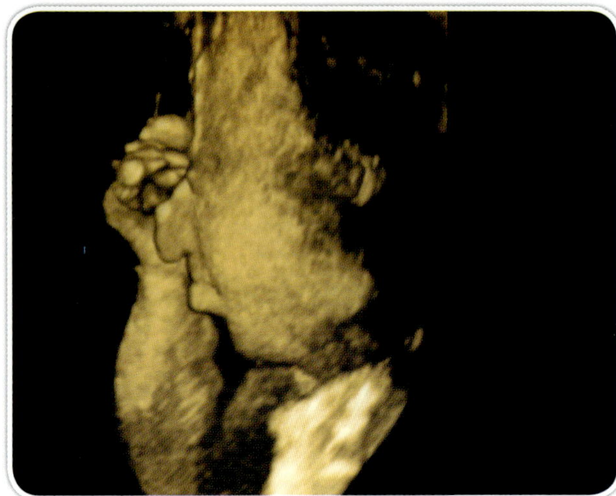

Proboscis and hypotelorism in fetal trisomy 13

Male Genitalia

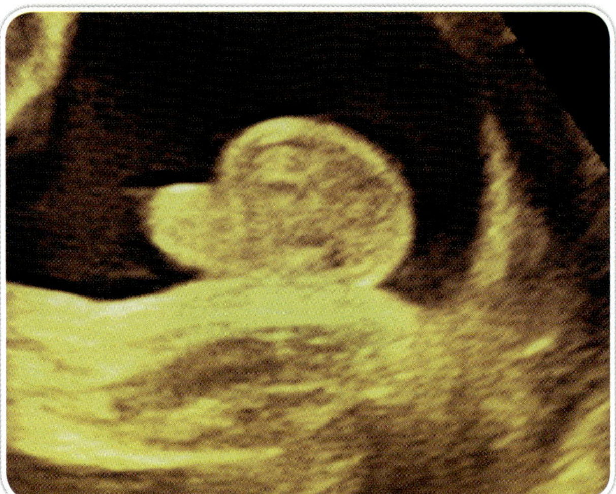

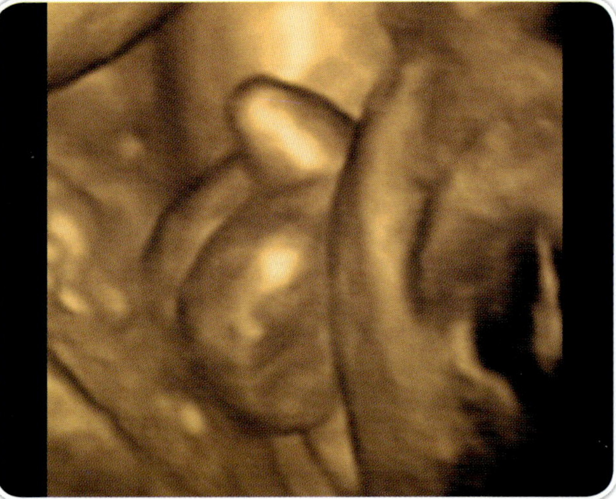

Penis 29 Weeks'

Taken from the same 2D data

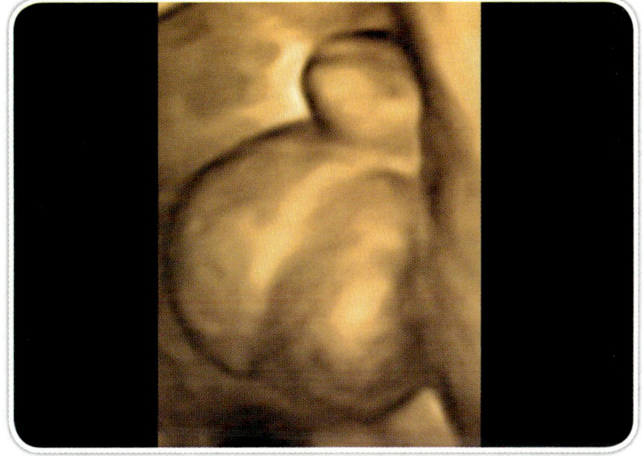

3D surface-rendered

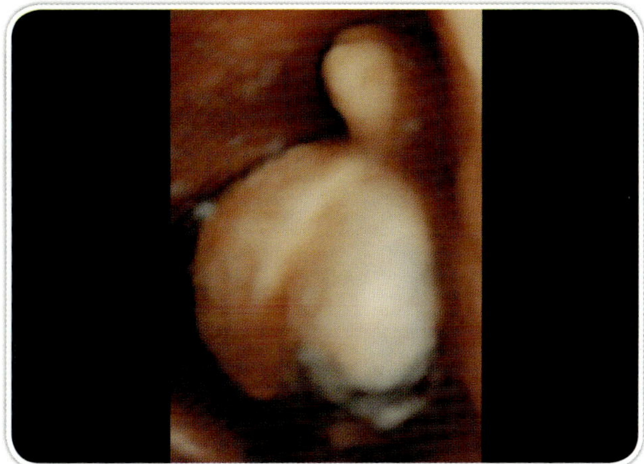

3DHD surface-rendered

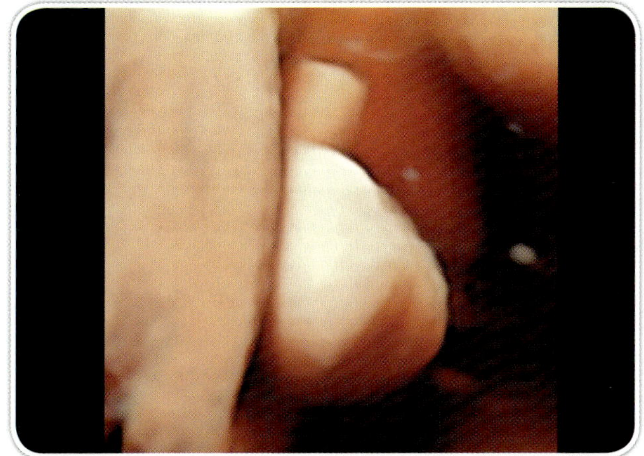

More Apparent Labia Minora at Younger Gestational Age

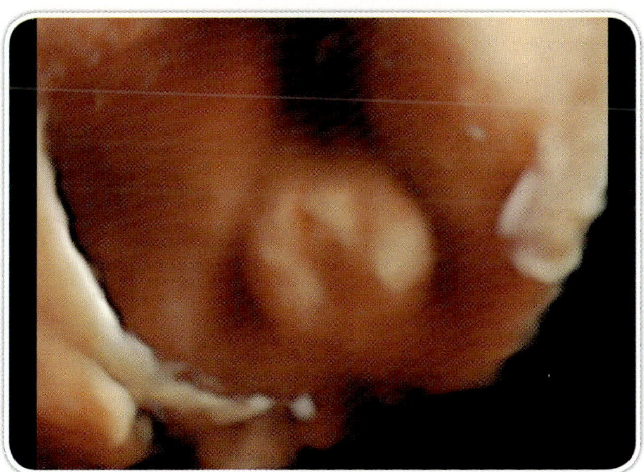

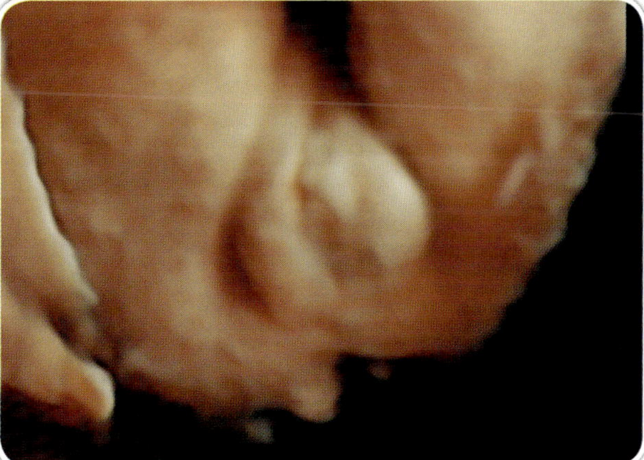

More Mature Female Genitalia

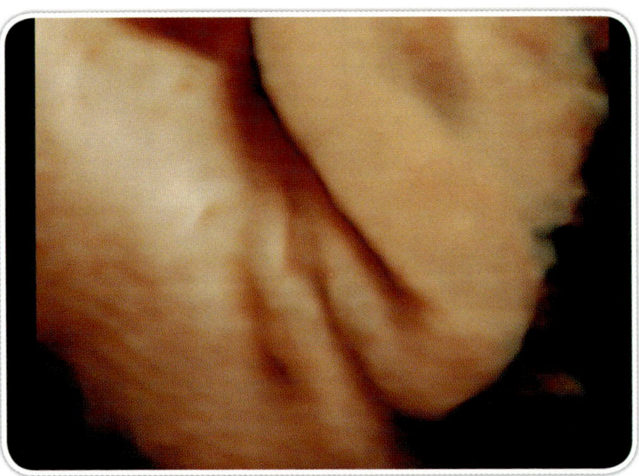

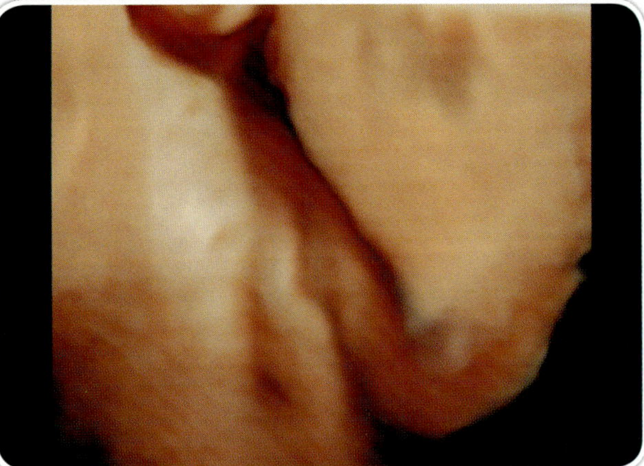

Compare Female Genitalia at 24 and 34 Weeks'

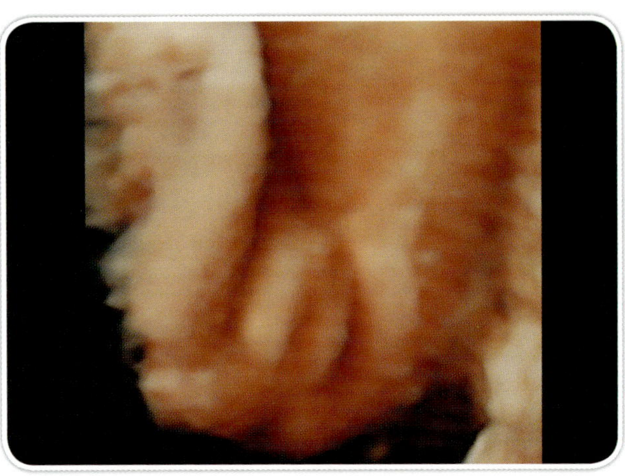

24 weeks'

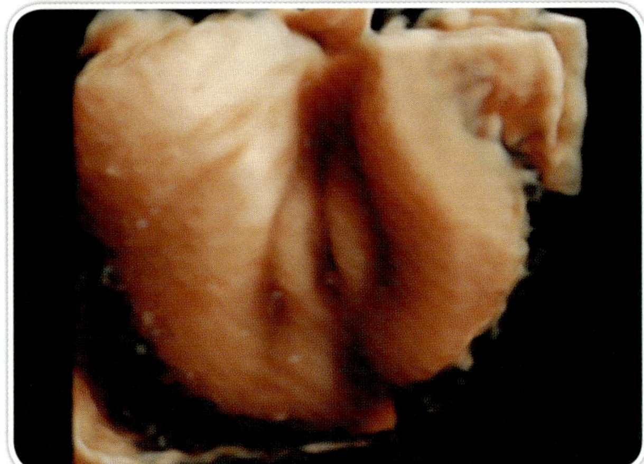

34 weeks'

Female Genitalia: 29 Weeks'

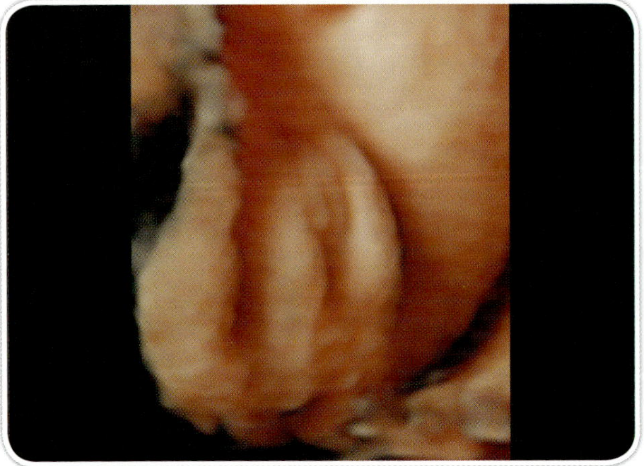

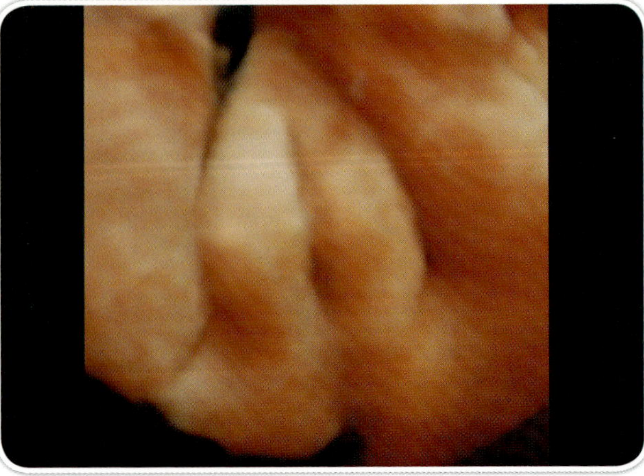

Note that labia majora is more prominent with advancing gestational age

Anus

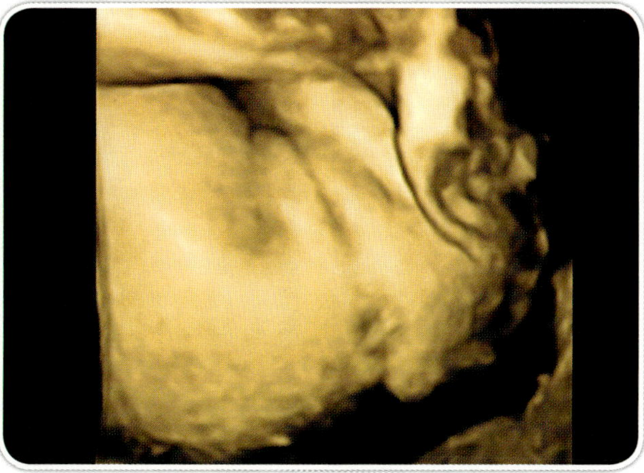

Ambiguous Genitalia

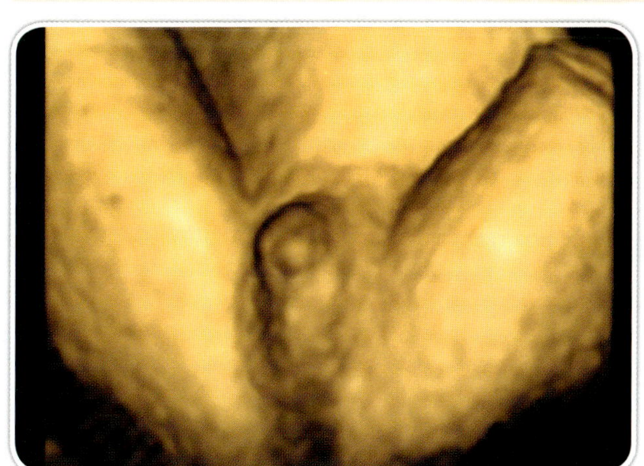

- May be related to autosomal recessive congenital adrenal hyperplasia
- Early prenatal administration of dexamethasone can prevent virilization.

(Wataganara et al. 2011)

Abnormalities of Fetal Penis

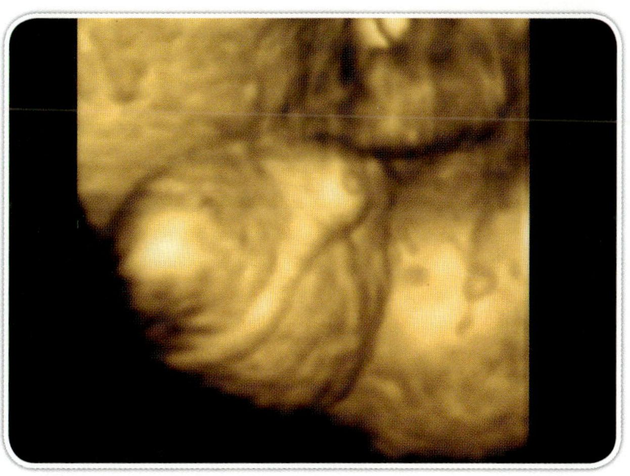

Micropenis

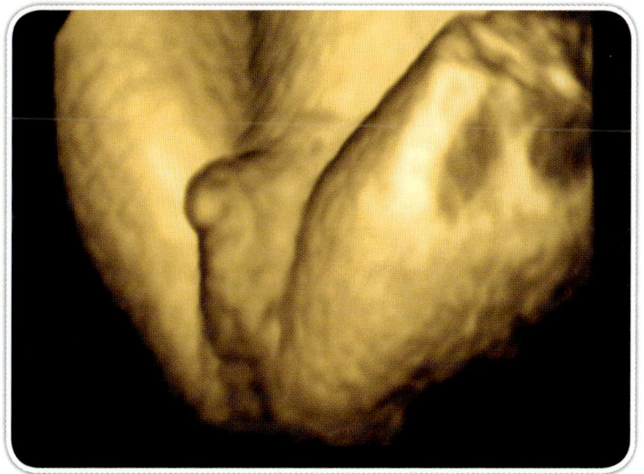

Hypospadias

Fetal Micropenis

Penile length <2.5 SD for the menstrual weeks'

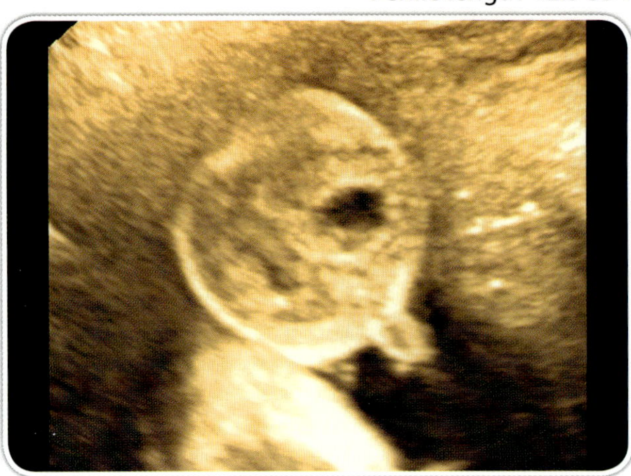

Conventional 2D

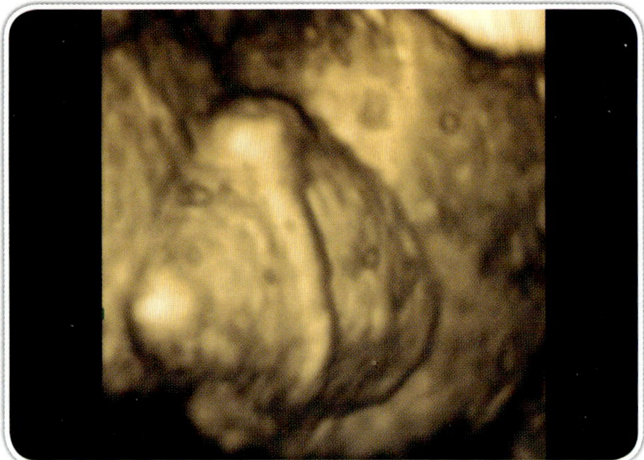

3D surface renolered

Fetal Micropenis Clinical Relevance

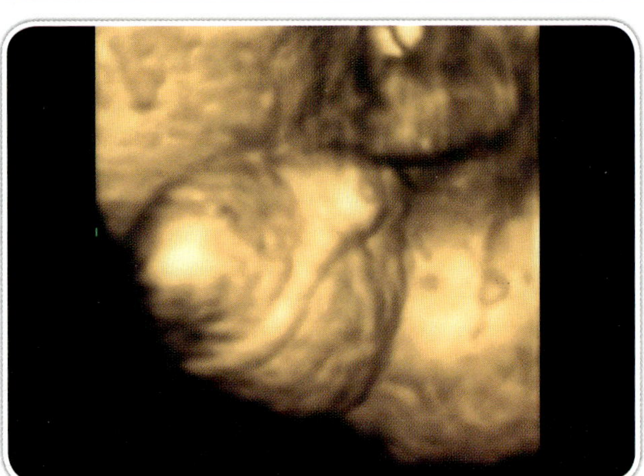

- Idiopathic
- Hypogonadotropic hypogonadism (Kallmann syndrome, Prader Willi syndrome, Laurence-Moon-Biedl syndrome, Rud syndrome)
- Androgen insensitivity
- Aneuploidies
- CNS abnormalities.

Fetal Gastroschisis

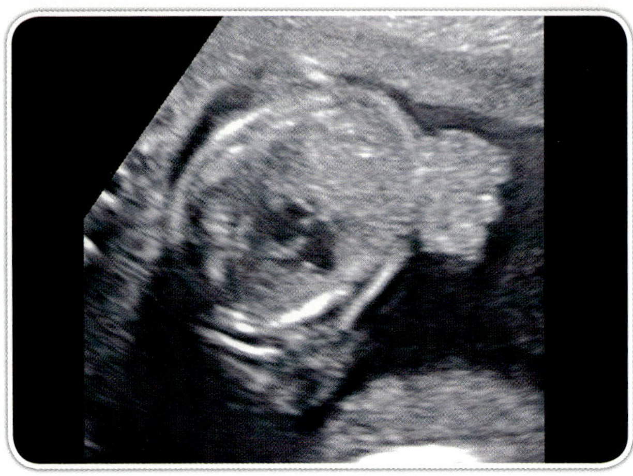

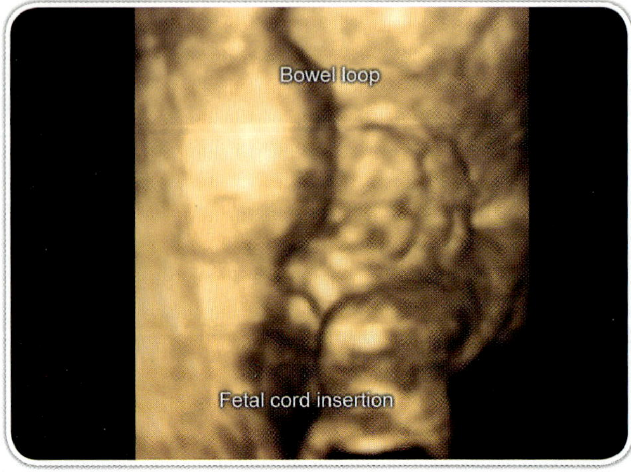

- Premature regression of the omphalomesenteric artery leading to failure of the mesodermal components of the abdominal wall.

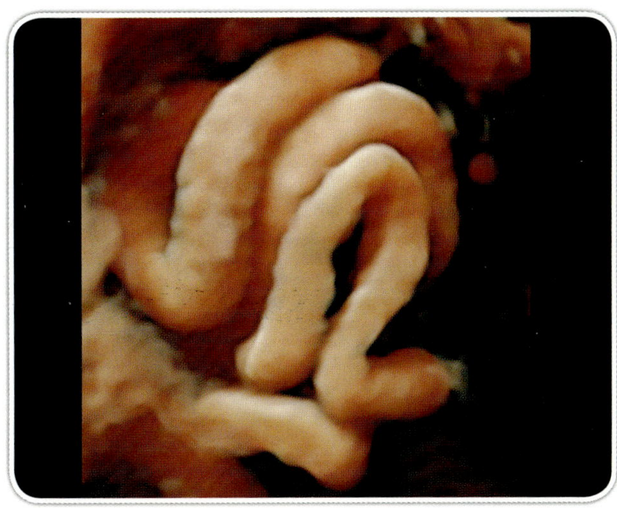

Protruded bowel loop in 3DHD

Hands: 2nd and 3rd Trimester

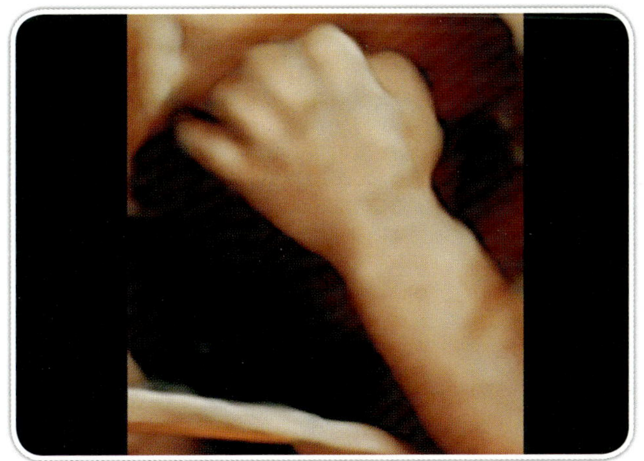

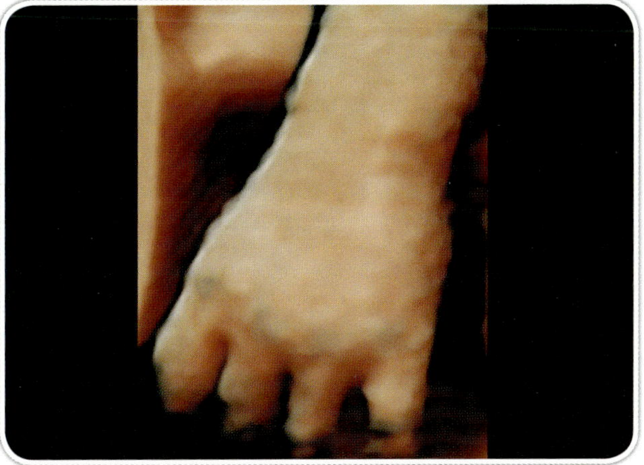

Feet

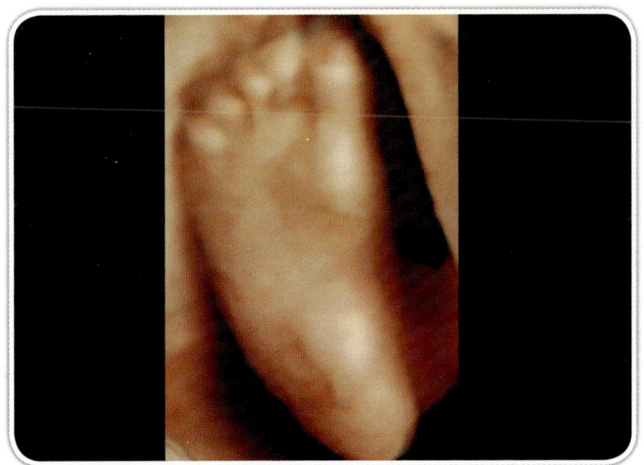

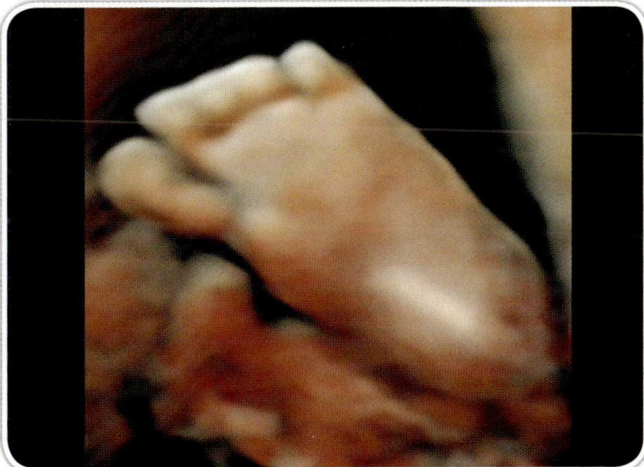

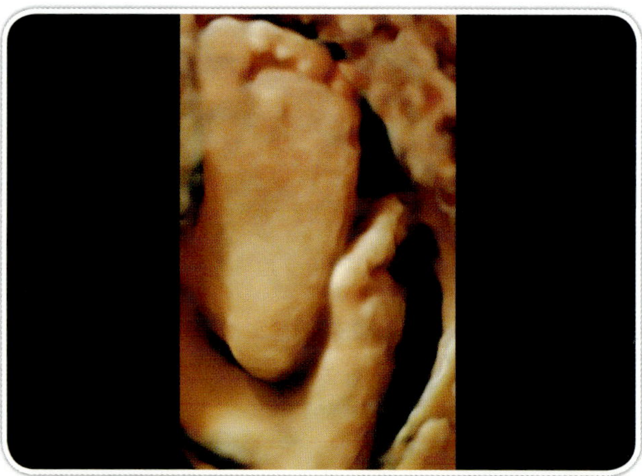

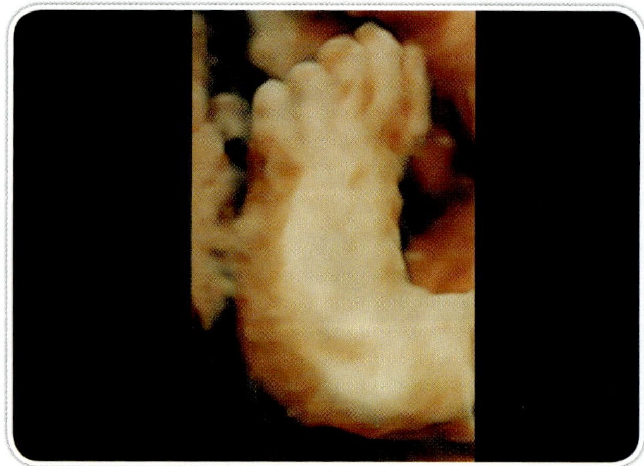

Fetal Extremities: HDLive Silhouette Mode

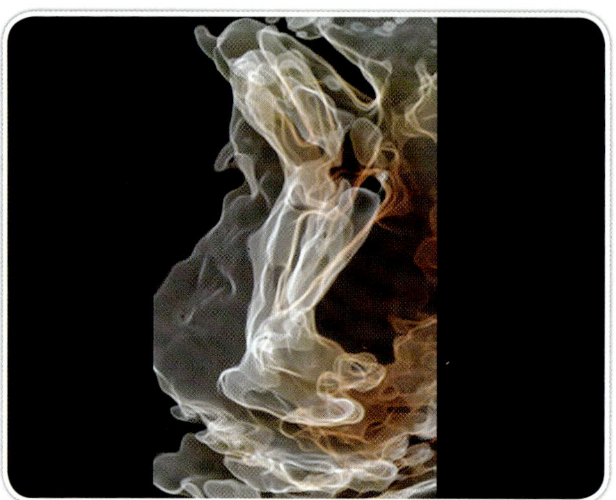

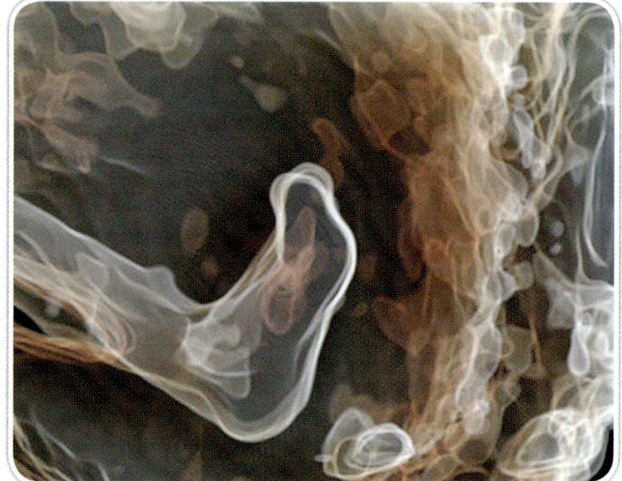

Details of the Face from Different Angles

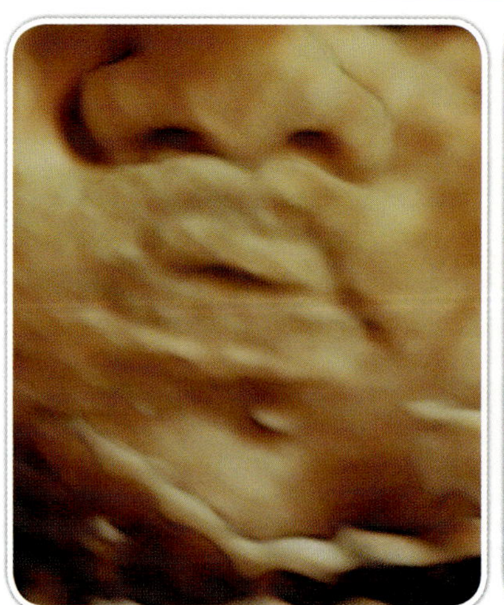

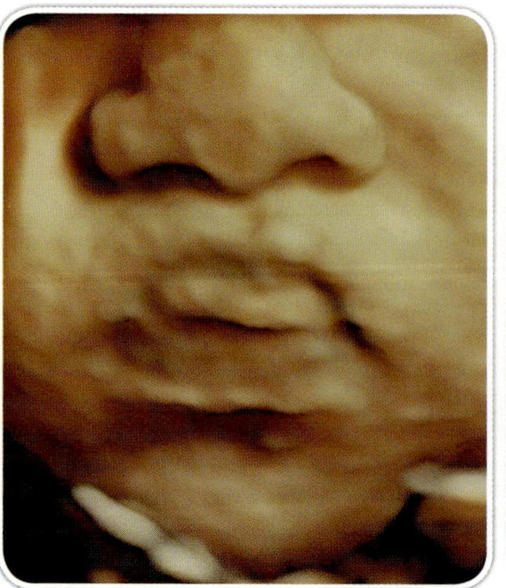

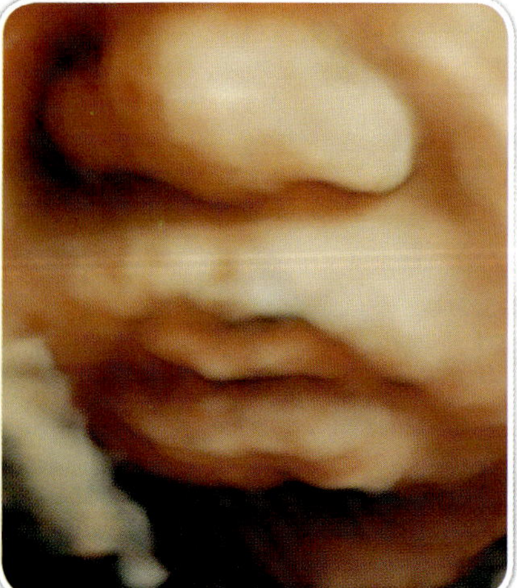

Note the differences after adjustment of lights and angles

Fetal Macrosomia

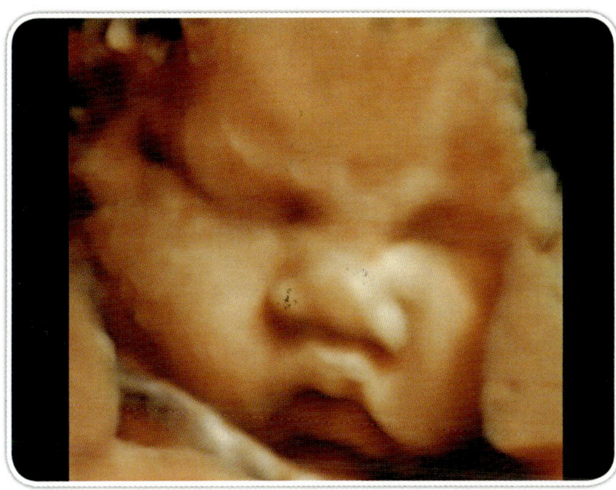

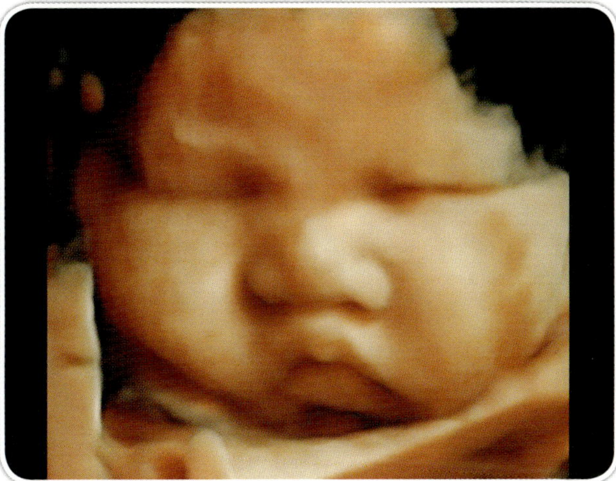

Facial Expression at Advancing Gestational Age

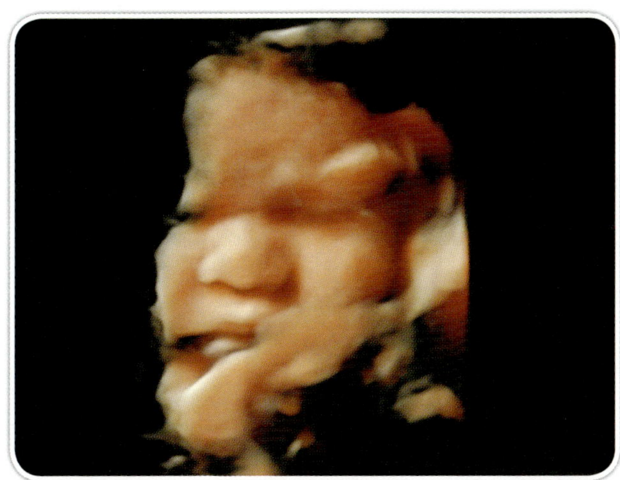

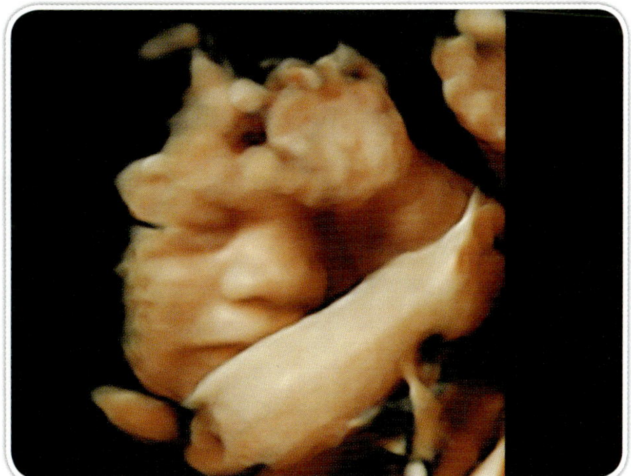

Vertebral Column

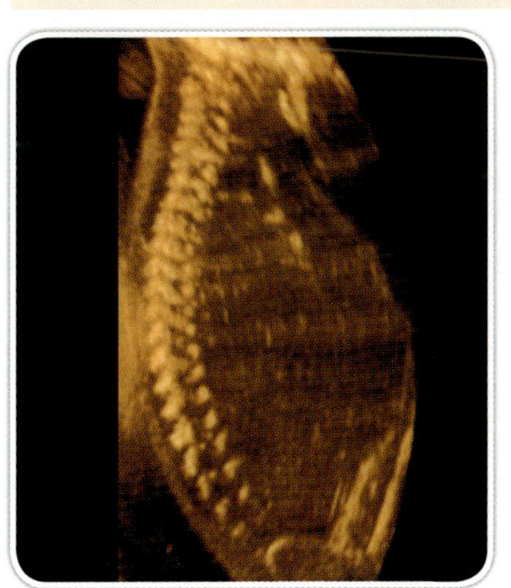

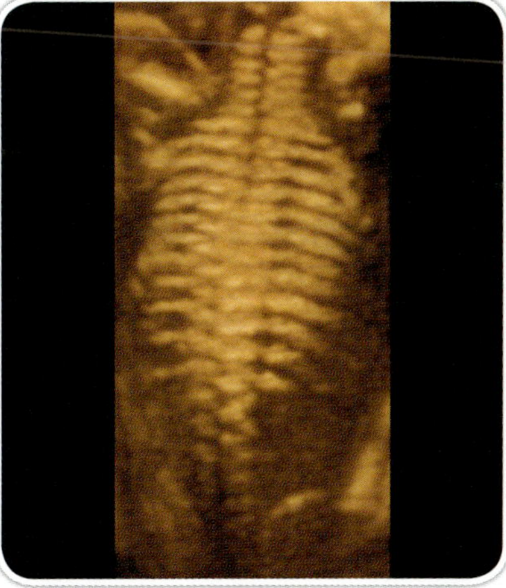

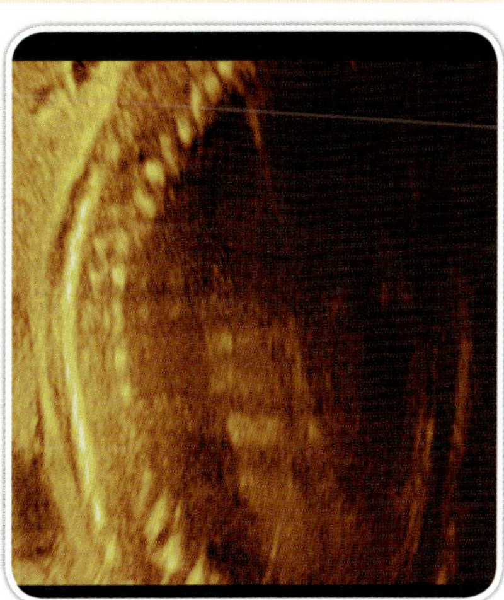

Vertebral Column: Anteroposterior View

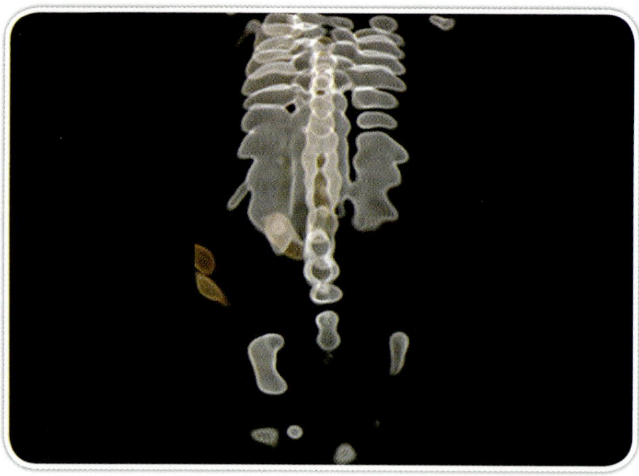
3DHD Silhouette

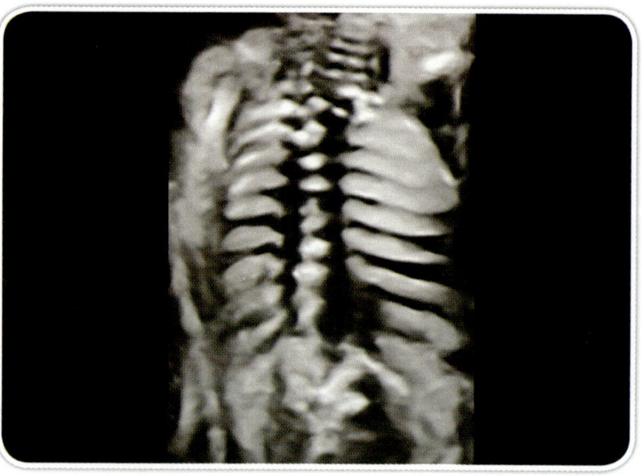
Conventional 3D max gradient (skeletal) mode

Vertebral Column: Lateral View

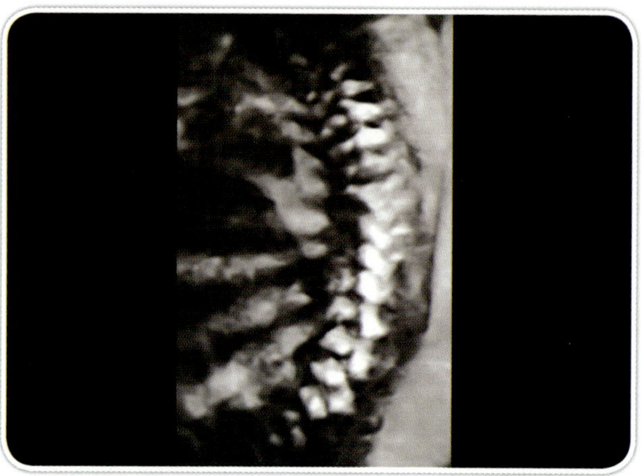
Conventional 3D max gradient (skeletal) mode

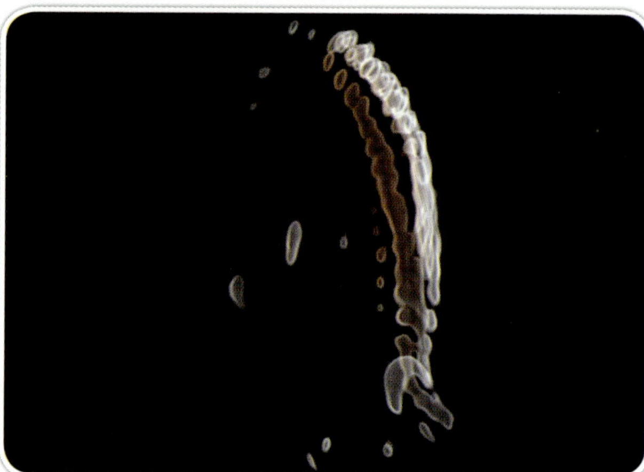
3DHD Silhouette

Vertebral Column: HDLive Silhouette Mode

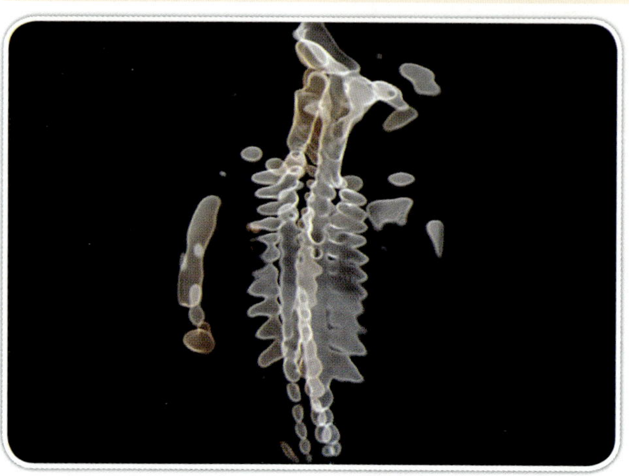

- Common vertebral anomalies
  - Hemivertebrae
  - Block vertebrae: Improper segmentation
  - Butterfly vertebrae: Sagittal cleft
  - Transitional vertebrae
  - Spina bifida: Myelomeningocele.

Cranial Vault (Skull)

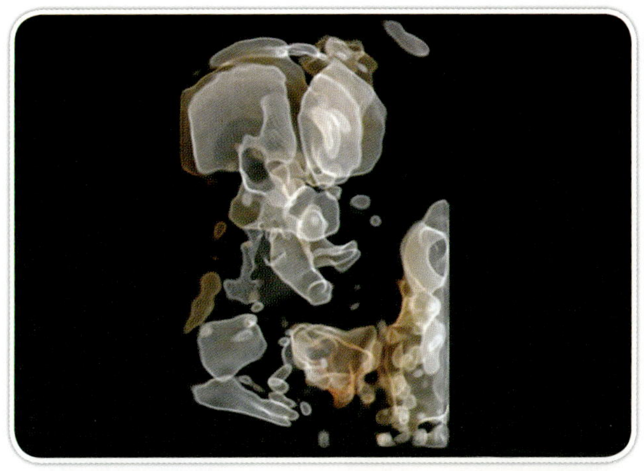
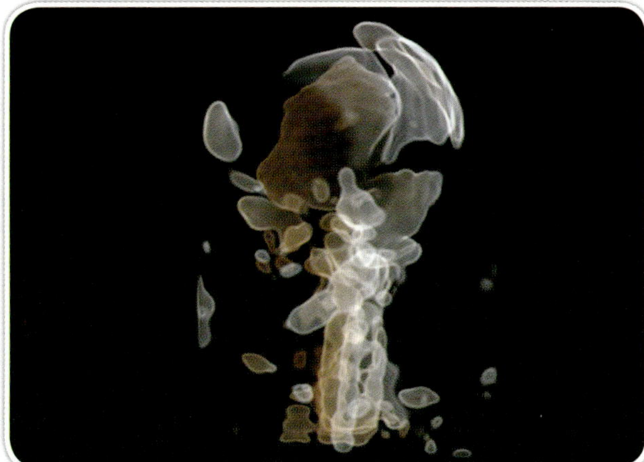
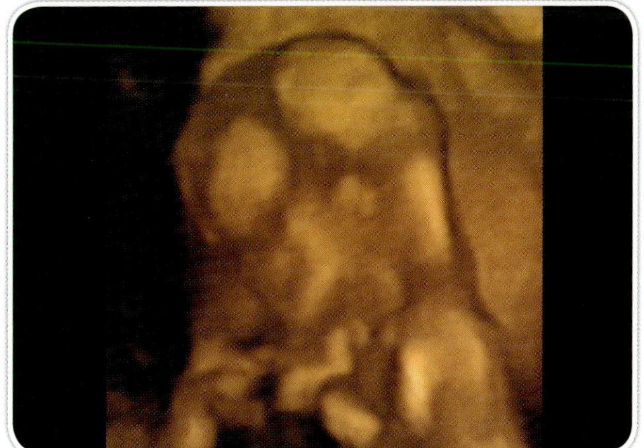
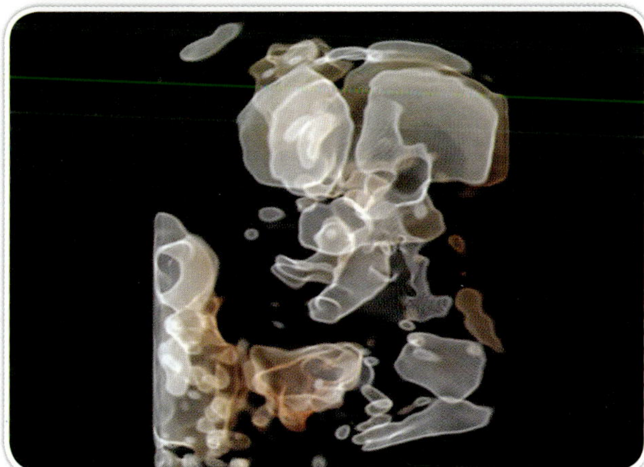

Fetal Brain and Skull Assessment

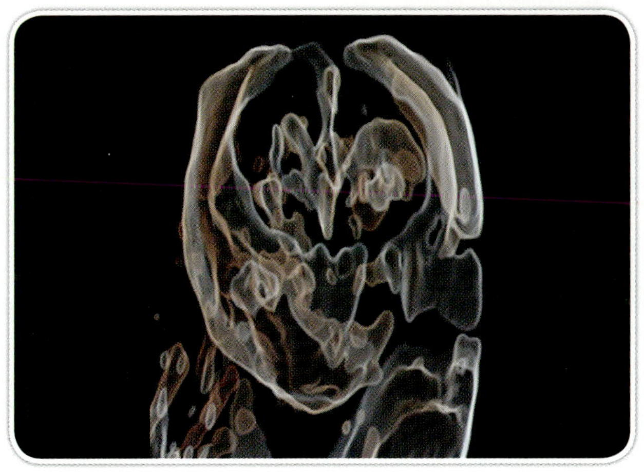
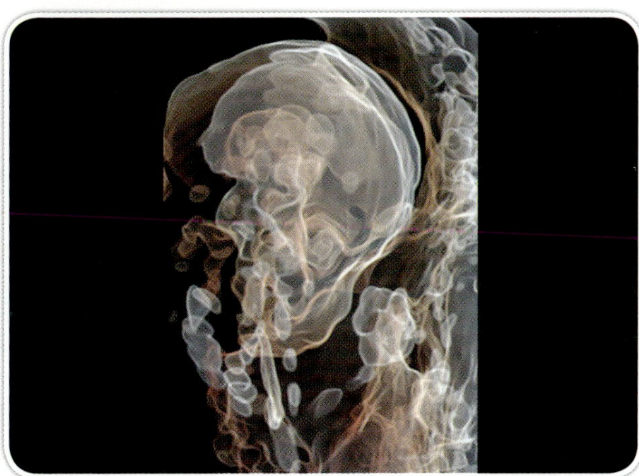

3D Sonoangiogram Intra-abdominal Blood Vessels

- 3D sonoangiogram with soft tissue subtraction
- Demonstration of intra-abdominal vessels in one of the conjoined twins at 23 wks'.

(Wataganara et al. 2008)

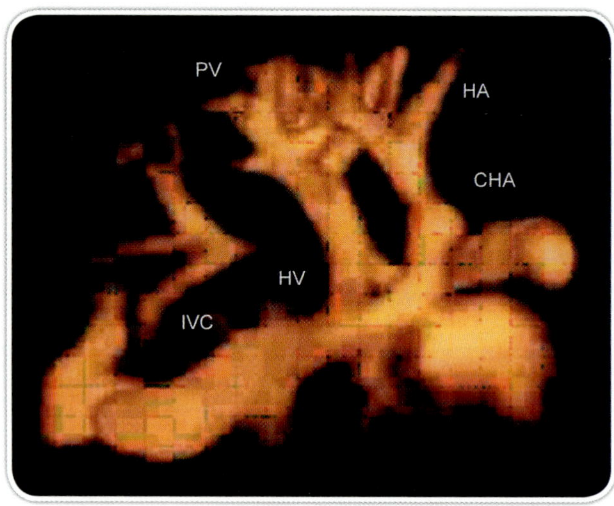

(IVC=inferior vena cava, HV=hepatic vein, PV=portal vein, CHA=common hepatic artery, HA=hepatic artery)

Umbilical Cord Entanglement

- Umbilical cord entanglement (13 wks').

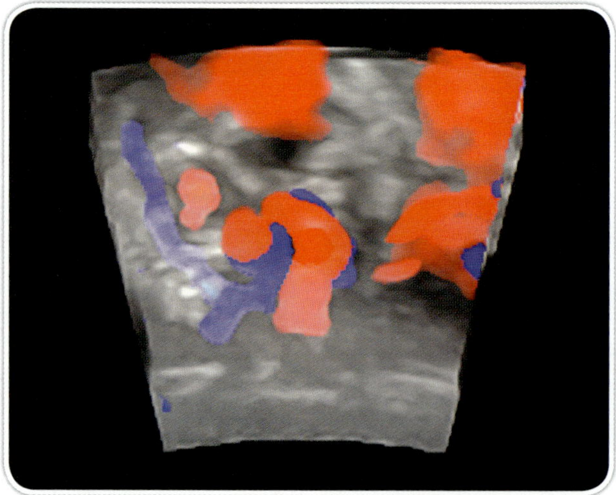

3D Sonoangiogram: Fetal Cord Insertion in Conjoined Twins

- Intertwin vascular connection determines the success of postnatal surgical separation
- The surgical separation was a success.

(Wataganara et al. 2008)

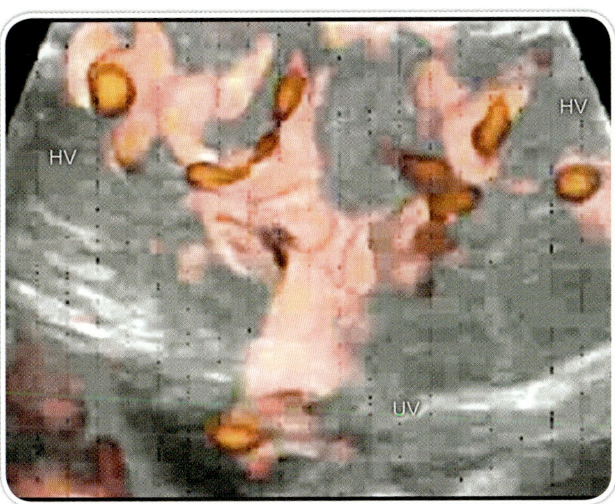

(UV=umbilical vein, HV=hepatic vein)

HDLive Flow

- HDLive Flow is a novel 3D demonstration of cardiovascular structure.

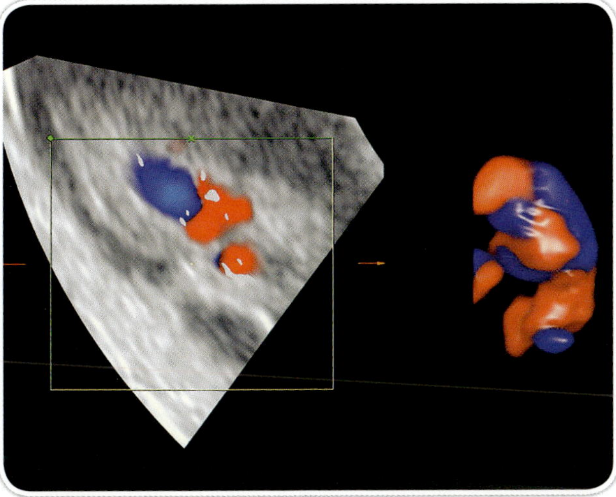

Fetal heart: 12 wks'

CONCLUSION

- The advent of 3D HD can re-define 'sonoembryology' and 'sonofetology'
- Keepsake or non-medical use of 3DHD ultrasound in Obstetrics

SUGGESTED READING

1. Burnell L, Verchere C, Pugash D, Loock C, Robertson S, Lehman A. Additional postnatal diagnoses following antenatal diagnosis of isolated cleft lip +/- palate. Archives of disease in Childhood Fetal and Neonatal Edition. 2014;99:F286-90.
2. Chen GD, Lin MT, Lee MS. Diagnosis of interstitial pregnancy with sonography. J Clin Ultrasound. 1994;22:439-42.
3. De Jong-Pleij EA, Ribbert LS, Pistorius LR, Tromp E, Mulder EJ, Bilardo CM. Three-dimensional ultrasound and maternal bonding, a third trimester study and a review. Prenatal diagnosis. 2013;33:81-8.
4. Doubilet PM. Ultrasound evaluation of the first trimester. Radiologic clinics of North America. 2014;52:1191-9.
5. Kagan KO, Pintoffl K, Hoopmann M. First-trimester ultrasound images using HDlive. Ultrasound in Obstetrics & Gynecology : the Official Journal of the International Society of Ultrasound in Obstetrics and Gynecology. 2011;38:607.
6. Moore TR, Gale S, Benirschke K. Perinatal outcome of forty-nine pregnancies complicated by acardiac twinning. American Journal of Obstetrics and Gynecology. 1990;163:907-12.
7. Odeh M, Tendler R, Kais M, Grinin V, Ophir E, Bornstein J. Gestational sac volume in missed abortion and an embryonic pregnancy compared to normal pregnancy. J Clin Ultras. 2010;38:367-71.
8. Rempen A. The shape of the endometrium evaluated with three-dimensional ultrasound: an additional predictor of extrauterine pregnancy. Human reproduction. 1998;13:450-4.
9. Sato M, Kanenishi K, Hanaoka U, Noguchi J, Marumo G, Hata T. 4D ultrasound study of fetal facial expressions at 20-24 weeks of gestation. International Journal of Gynaecology and Obstetrics: the Official Organ of the International Federation of Gynaecology and Obstetrics. 2014;126:275-9.
10. Simpson LL. Ultrasound in twins: dichorionic and monochorionic. Seminars in perinatology. 2013;37:348-58.
11. Wataganara T, Kanokpongsakdi S. Changing landscapes of In Utero minimally invasive surgical interventions. Sirjraj Med J. 2008;60:368-70.
12. Wataganara T, Sutanthavibool A, Limwongse C. Real-time three dimensional sonographic features of an early third trimester fetus with achondrogenesis. Journal of the Medical Association of Thailand (Chotmaihet thangphaet). 2006;89:1762-5.
13. Wataganara T, Triyasunant N, Viboonchart S. Fetal therapy in 2011: A review. Sirjraj Med J. 2011;63:97-101.
14. Wataganara T. Identification and management of high-risk pregnancies. Sirjraj Med J. 2006;58:982-3.
15. William J. Larsen (2001). Human embryology. Edinburgh: Churchill Livingstone.

Chapter

16

Cervical Length Measurement for Prediction of Preterm Delivery

Panos Antsaklis, Asim Kurjak

Incidence of PTD 1992–2002 (USA)

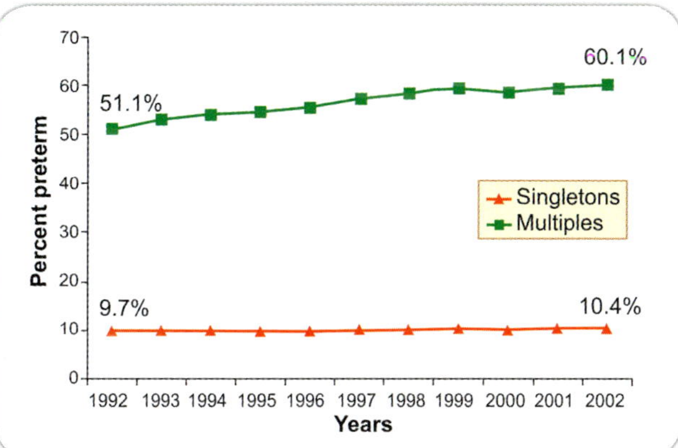

(Edward, 2005)

Preterm Delivery

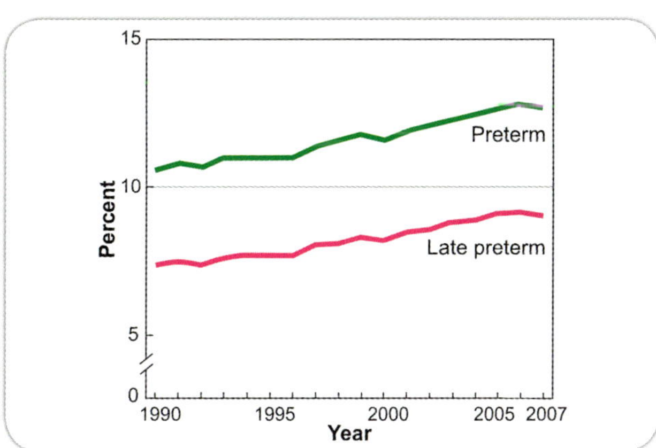

Note: *Preterm is less than 37 completed weeks of gestation. Late preterm is 34–36 completed weeks of gestation.*

Source: *CDC/NCHS, National Vital Statistics System.*

(National Vital Statistics Reports, 2009)

- Incidence of PTD (< 37 weeks)
  - USA ~ 12%
  - WHO ~ 9.6%
  - Range ~ 5–15%
- Incidence of PTD (< 34 weeks) 2.9 - 3.6%
- Incidence of PTD (< 32 weeks) 1–2%

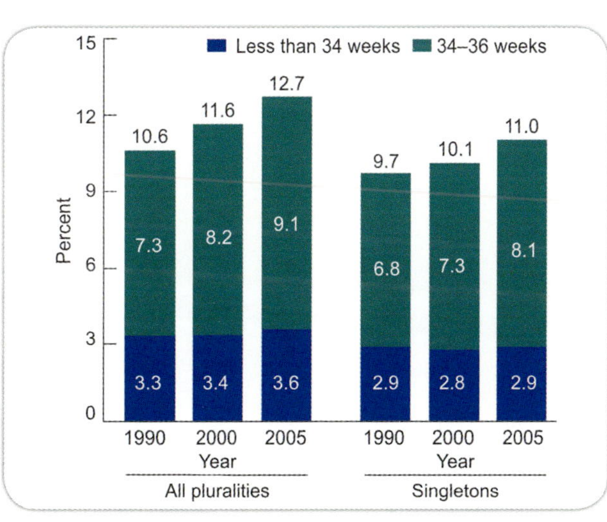

(National Vital Statistics Reports, 2009)

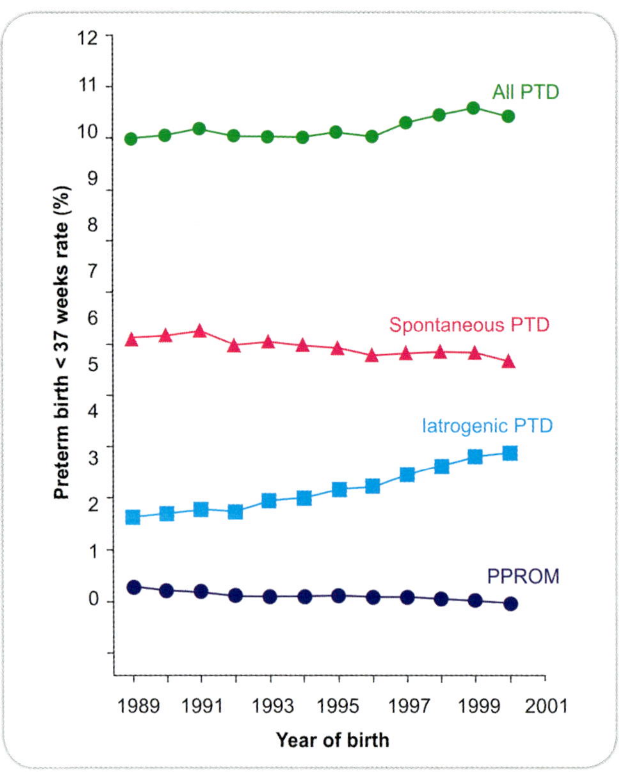

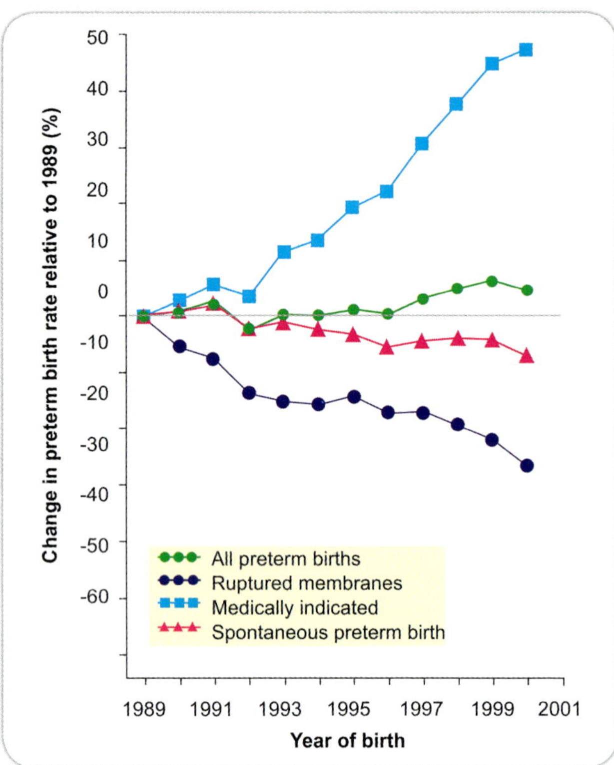

(Ananth et al. 2005)

Preterm Neonates-Mortality

Probability of mortality

1988-90

1993-94

1998-99

Gestation (weeks)

Mortality of neonates < 32 weeks

Parry et al. Lancet 2003

For complete presentation, please refer the accompanying CD-ROM…

SUGGESTED READING

1. Ananth et al. 2005.
2. Antsaklis et al. 2010.
3. Berghella and Bega, BJOG. 2009.
4. Berghella BJOG. 2009.
5. Berghella et al. Obstet Gynecol. 2007.
6. Burger et al. Ultrasound Obstet Gynecol. 1997.
7. Callen PW. Ultrasonography in Obstetrics and Gynaecology. 4th ed.
8. Carlan et al. Obstet Gynecol. 1997.
9. Celik et al. Ultrasound Obstet Gynecol. 2008.
10. Duta et al. Ultrasound Obstet Gynecol. 2003.
11. Edward R. Newton: Clin Perinatol. 32 (2005).
12. Goldberg et al. Am J Obstet Gynecol. 1997.
13. Gomez et al. Am J Obstet Gynecol. 1994.
14. Greco et al. 2012.
15. Hassan et al. Am J Obs & Gyne. 2000.
16. Heath et al. Ultrasound Obstet Gynecol. 1998.
17. Iams et al. Am J Obstet Gynecol. 1995.
18. Iams et al. New Engl J Med. 1996.
19. Krebs-Jimenez et al. J Ultrasound Med. 2002.
20. Matijevic et al. Acta Obstet Gynecol Scand. 2006.
21. National Vital Statistics Reports. 57 (12); 2009.
22. Parry et al. Lancet. 2003.
23. Romero R, Espinoza J, Kusanovic JP, Gotsch F, Hassan S, Erez O et al. The preterm parturition syndrome. BJOG. 2006;113 (Suppl 3):17-42. Review. Erratum in: BJOG. 2008;115(5):674-5.
24. Romero. Ultrasound Obstet Gynecol. 2007.
25. Souka et al. 2011.
26. Tabor et al. 2010.
27. To et al. Ultrasound Obstet Gynecol. 2006.

Chapter 17

Gestational Diabetes Mellitus

Panos Antsaklis, Eleni Anastasiou, Asim Kurjak

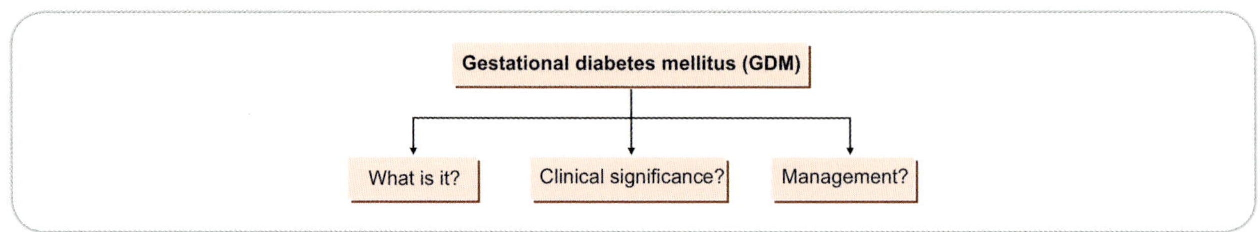

GDM - General

Diabetes in pregnancy

Pre-existing diabetes

Gestational diabetes

IDDM (Type 1)

NIDDM (Type 2)

Pre-existing diabetes

True GDM

Diabetes in pregnancy

Pre-existing diabetes

Gestational diabetes

IDDM (Type 1)

NIDDM (Type 2)

Pre-existing diabetes

True GDM

- TRUE GDM → 3rd TRIMESTER problem
- PRE-EXISTING GDM → 1st TRIMESTER problem

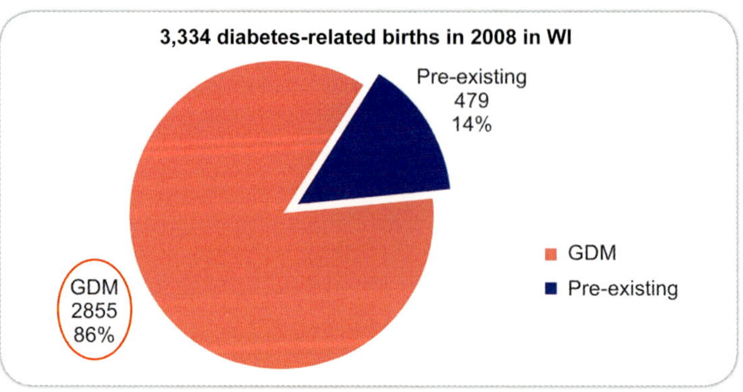

GDM: Definition (ADA 2011)

- **Abnormal glucose metabolism that is identified during the *present pregnancy***
- *From this definition the cases of DM type 2 that are diagnosed at the beginning of pregnancy are exempted.*

GDM: Epidemiology

- **GDM** is a quite frequent complication of pregnancy
- **GDM** affects around **5-15%** of all pregnancies
- The incidence of **GDM** has increased: from 14.5 (1991) → to 47.9 cases/1000 pregnancies (2003) ***X3 times*** ↑
- ↑ of incidence of **DM2** in young people
- **87%** of DM cases in PREGNANCY are due to **GDM.**

Screening Rates are Unacceptably Low

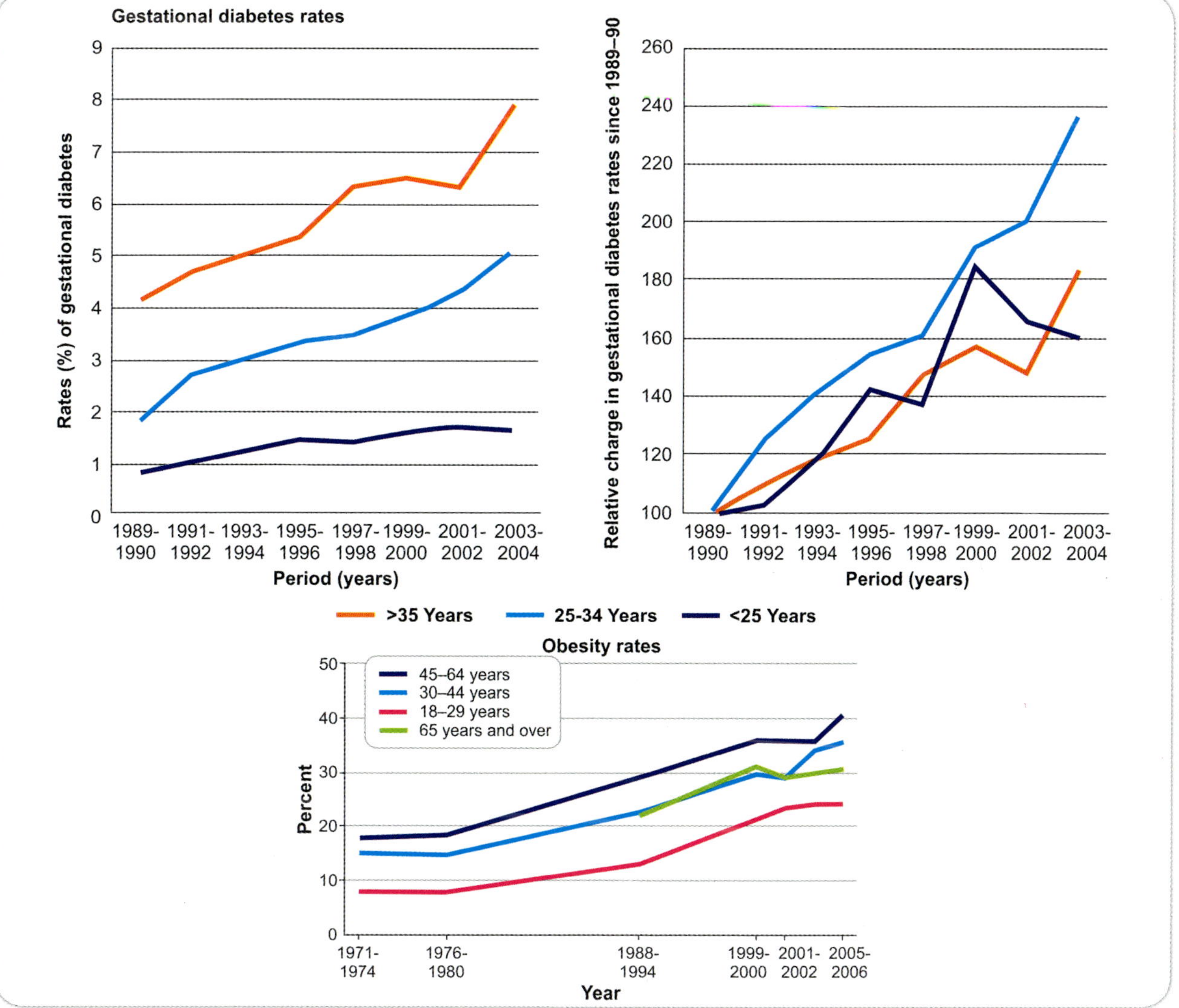

Source: *Getahun D, Nath C, Ananth CV, et al. Gestational diabetes in the United States: temporal trends 1989 through 2004. Am J Obstet Gynecol. 2008;198:525.1l-525.e5.*

For complete presentation, please refer the accompanying CD-ROM...

SUGGESTED READING

1. ACOG
2. ADA, Pregnancy Complicated by Diabetes, 2009
3. ADA Guidelines 2011
4. Anastasiou et al. 2013
5. Annath et al. Am J Obstet Gyn. 2008;198:525
6. Antsaklis P et al 2013
7. Bellamy L, Lancet, 2009
8. Bell R, BJOG 2008
9. Ben-Haroush et al 2004
10. Best & Pressman 2002
11. Best et al 2002
12. Buchanan T, Diabetes Care,2007
13. Catalano P Diabetes Care, 2012
14. CDA CPG 2008
15. Coetzee et al D.Care,2007, p2978-2982
16. Consensus Statement, ADA 2008
17. Diabetes Care, 2010
18. Ferreira et al 2011
19. Gui J, Liu Q, Feng L (2013
20. Gunderson EP, Diabetes Care, 2012
21. http://dhs.wisconsin.gov/births/pdf/08births.pdf
22. IOM 2009
23. Kerssen et al 2007
24. Khalil et al 2012
25. Landon et al N Engl J Med 2009
26. Langer 1996
27. Lawrence JM, Diabetes Care. 2008
28. Lowe LP, Diabetes Care, 2012
29. Makgoba et al 2011
30. Metzger B.E., D.Care Suppl 2,2007
31. Metzger et al N Engl J Med 2008
32. Mongelli et al 2005
33. Moyer et al, Annals of internal medicine, 2014
34. Nanda et al 2011
35. Nice guidelines 2008
36. Papaioannou et al 2012
37. Rowan JA, N Engl J Med 2008
38. Sacks DA, Diabetes Care, 2012
39. Savvidou et al 2010
40. Savvidou et al 2012
41. Savvidou et al 2013
42. Shah B R, Diabetes Care, 2008
43. UPSTF
44. Wong et al 2002
45. IDF Global Guideline ,2009

Doppler in Intrauterine Fetal Growth Restriction

Ivica Zalud

OBJECTIVES

- Discuss IUGR antenatal natural history
- Present controversies in antepartum and intrapartum management (Doppler and optimal delivery).

IUGR

- *American Congress of Obstetricians and Gynecologists (ACOG)*: IUGR is one of the most common and complex problems in obstetrics
- *Problems*:
  - Inconsistent definitions
  - Poor detection rate
  - Limited preventive and treatment options
  - Multiple associated morbidities
  - Increased likelihood of perinatal mortality
  - Impaired intellectual development, hypertension and obesity in adulthood.

IUGR: So What!

- *2nd leading* contributor to *perinatal mortality!!!*
- Perinatal mortality: x6–10
- Intrapartum asphyxia: up to 50%
- As many as 40% stillborns are IUGR
- A portion of perinatal complications is *preventable* (morbidity and mortality)
- Association with *multiple sequelae* (short-and long-term morbidity).

The Doppler Effect

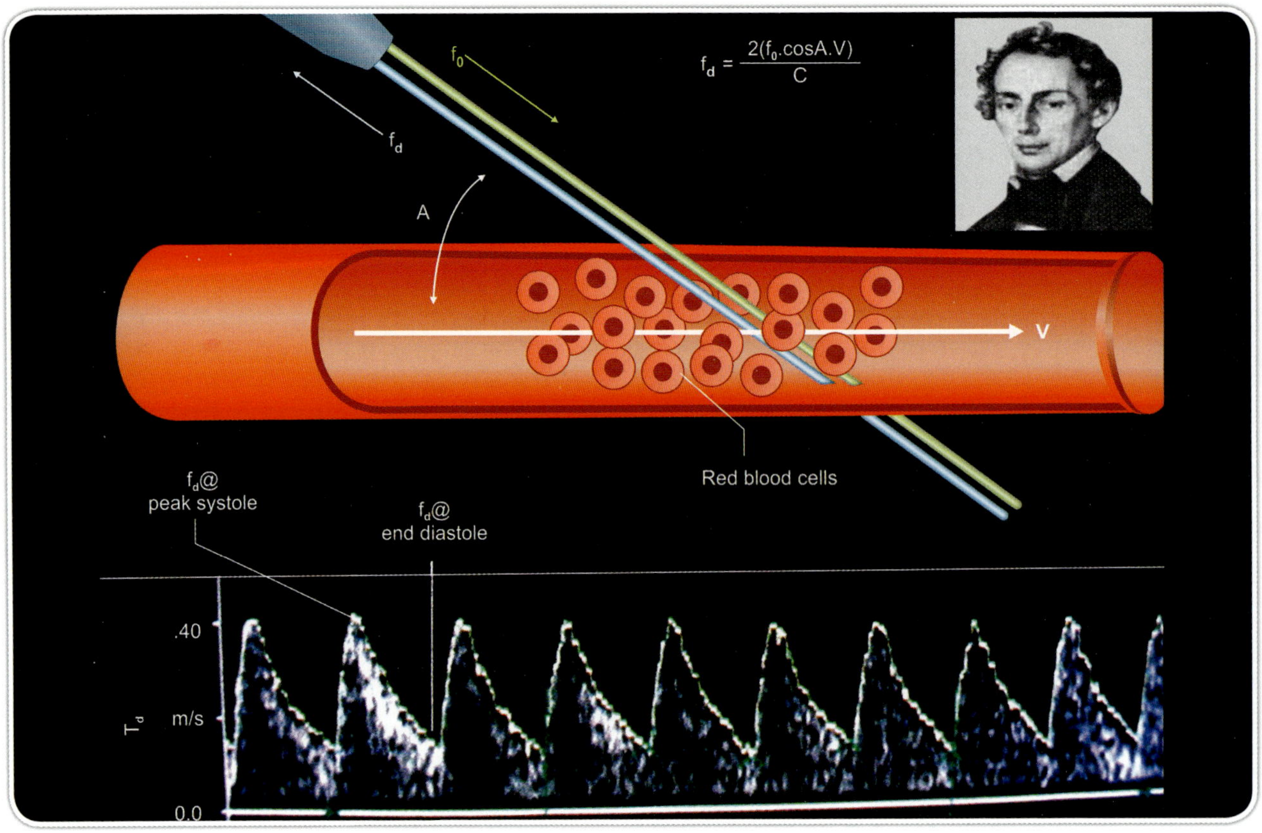

Umbilical Artery (UA) Doppler—Reversed end-diastolic flow (EDF)

This is an advanced stage of fetal compromise, associated with increased perinatal morbidity and mortality.

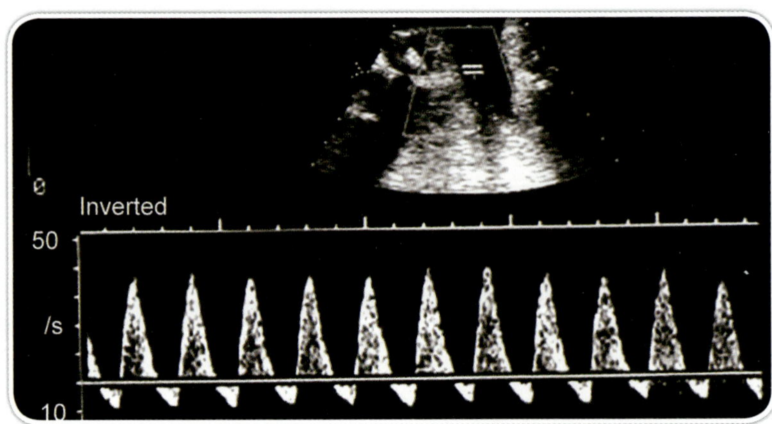

For complete presentation, please refer the accompanying CD-ROM...

SUGGESTED READING

1. Alfirevic Z, Neilson JP. Doppler ultrasonography in high-risk pregnancies: systematic review with meta-analysis. Am J Obs and Gynec. 1995;172:1379-87.
2. Baschat AA, Cosmi E, Bilardo CM, et al. Predictors of neonatal outcome in early-onset placental dysfunction. Obs and Gynec. 2007;109:253-61.
3. Boers KE, Vijgen SM, Bijlenga D, et al. Induction versus expectant monitoring for intrauterine growth restriction at term: randomised equivalence trial (DIGITAT). BMJ. 2010;341:c7087.
4. Ghidini A. Doppler of the ductus venosus in severe preterm fetal growth restriction: a test in search of a purpose? Obs and Gynec. 2007;109:250-2.
5. Group GS. A randomised trial of timed delivery for the compromised preterm fetus: short term outcomes and Bayesian interpretation. BJOG :An international journal of obstetrics and gynaecology. 2003;110:27-32.
6. Society for maternal-fetal medicine publications, Berkley E, Chauhan SP, Abuhamad A. Doppler assessment of the fetus with intrauterine growth restriction. Am J Obs and Gynec. 2012;206:300-8.
7. Spong CY, Mercer BM, D'Alton M, Kilpatrick S, Blackwell S, Saade G. Timing of indicated late-preterm and early-term birth. Obs and Gynec. 2011;118:323-33.
8. Thornton JG, Hornbuckle J, Vail A, Spiegelhalter DJ, Levene M, Group GS. Infant wellbeing at 2 years of age in the growth restriction intervention trial (GRIT): multicentred randomised controlled trial. Lancet. 2004;364:513-20.
9. Walker DM, Marlow N, Upstone L, et al. The growth restriction intervention trial: long-term outcomes in a randomized trial of timing of delivery in fetal growth restriction. Am J Obs and Gynec. 2011;204:34:e1-9.

Chapter 19

Clinical Application of KANET Test

Panos Antsaklis, Asim Kurjak

FETAL NEUROLOGY—INTRODUCTION

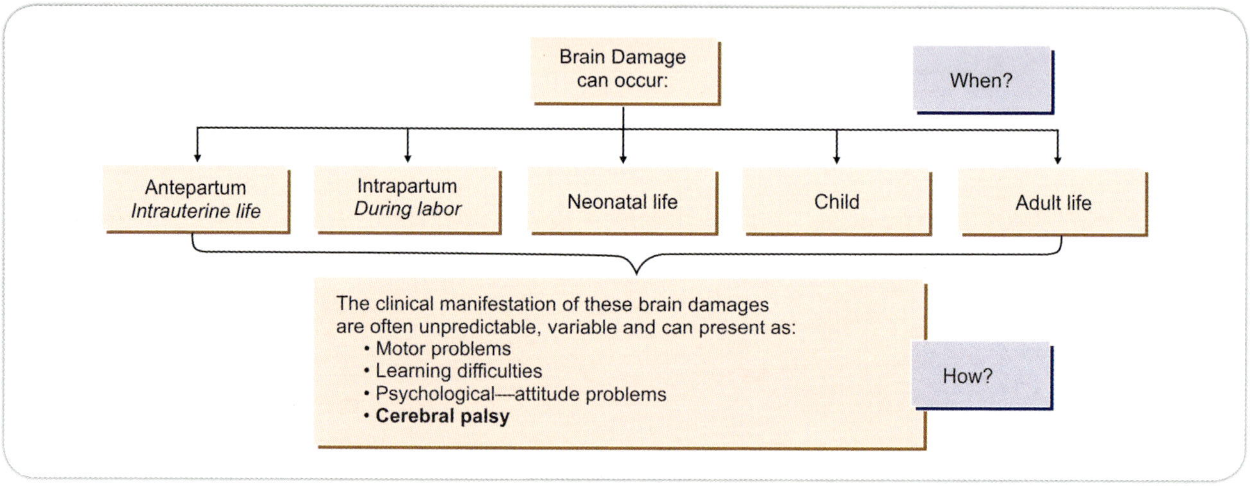

Brain Damage can occur:

When?

Antepartum *Intrauterine life*

Intrapartum *During labor*

Neonatal life

Child

Adult life

The clinical manifestation of these brain damages are often unpredictable, variable and can present as:

- Motor problems
- Learning difficulties
- Psychological—attitude problems
- **Cerebral palsy**

How?

- It is well-established that fetal behavioral patterns are directly reflecting developmental and maturational processes of fetal central nervous system
- The assessment of fetal behavior and developmental processes in different periods of gestation may make possible the distinction between normal and abnormal brain development
- Early diagnosis of various structural and functional abnormalities is possible
- The innovation in fetal imaging, which enabled the study of fetal activity in explicit detail, was made by the introduction of high quality 3D and 4D ultrasound
- It allows real time observation of the fetus, with sufficient dynamics and good image resolution
- Evaluation of the face and small anatomic parts of the fetus, and especially the movements of the mouth, eyes (facial expressions) and fingers is possible.

Fetal Neurology—KANET

- The first test that succeeded to combine all these parameters and form a scoring system that would assess the fetus in a comprehensive and systematic approach
- It is in the same way that neonatologists perform a neurological assessment in newborns, in order to determine their neurological status during the first days of their life.
- This is the **Kurjak antenatal neurodevelopmental test (KANET).**

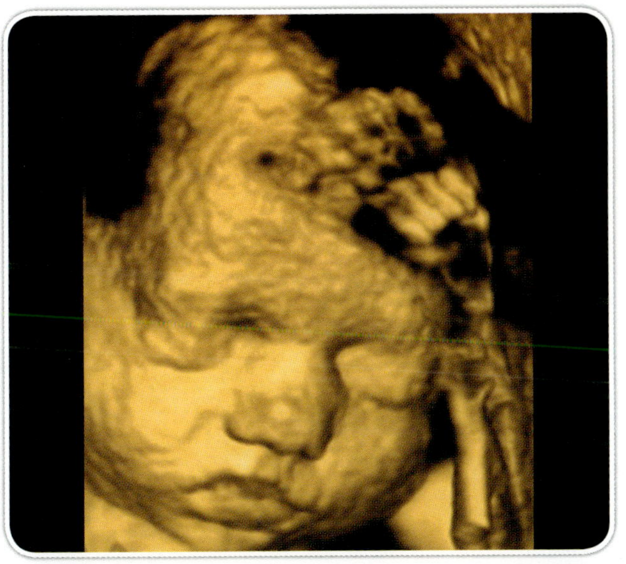

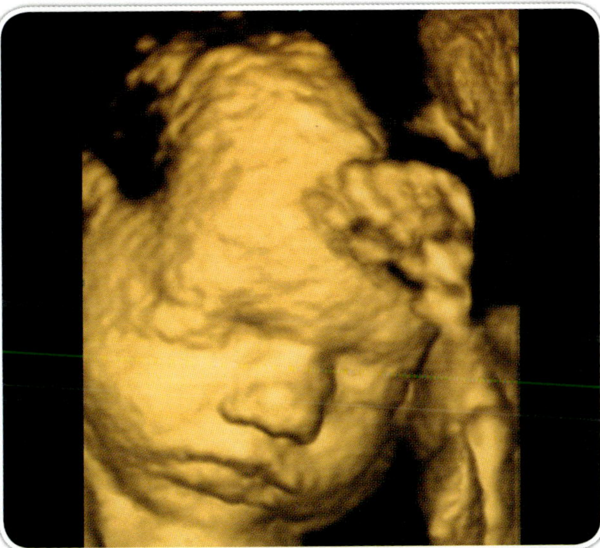

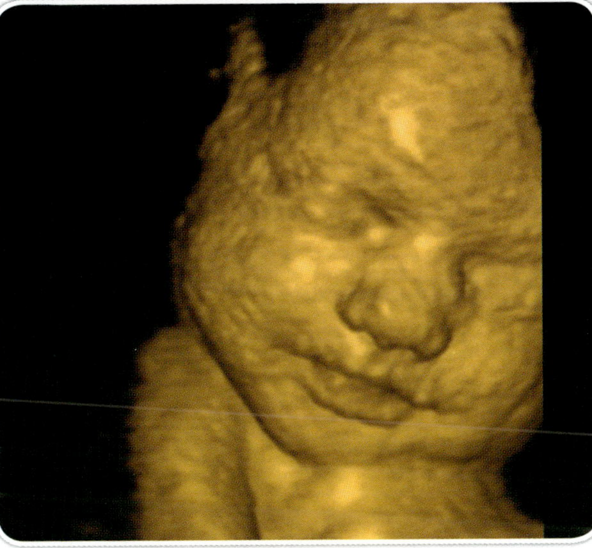

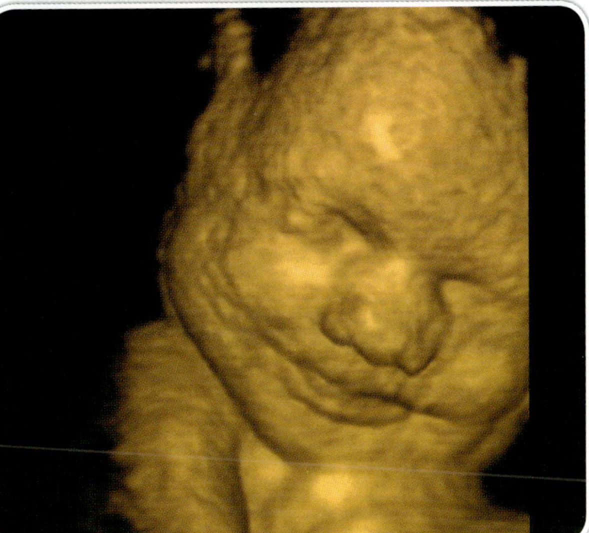

For complete presentation, please refer the accompanying CD-ROM...

SUGGESTED READING

1. Antsaklis et al. DSJUOG 2012
2. FMF, www.fetalmedicine.org
3. Kurjak et al. 2004
4. Mulder et al. 1991
5. Nicolaides et al. BJOG 1992
6. Stanojevic et al. DSJUOG 2011
7. Stanojevic et al. Seminars in Fetal & Neonatal Medicine 2012
8. Yeoshoua et al. 2012

Chapter

20

Fetal Magnetic Resonance Imaging

Tuangsit Wataganara

FETAL IMAGINGS

- Radiogram
- Amniogram
- Ultrasound (US)
- High-resolution US
- 3- or 4-dimensional US
- Ultrafast magnetic resonance imaging (MRI)
- Diagnostic embryo-fetoscopy.

History of Fetal MRI

(Smith et al. 1983)

- First MRI in pregnant woman in 1983
- Initial indications were placental abnormalities
- Fetal indications were primarily volumetric measurements
- Nowadays, the applications are expanding.

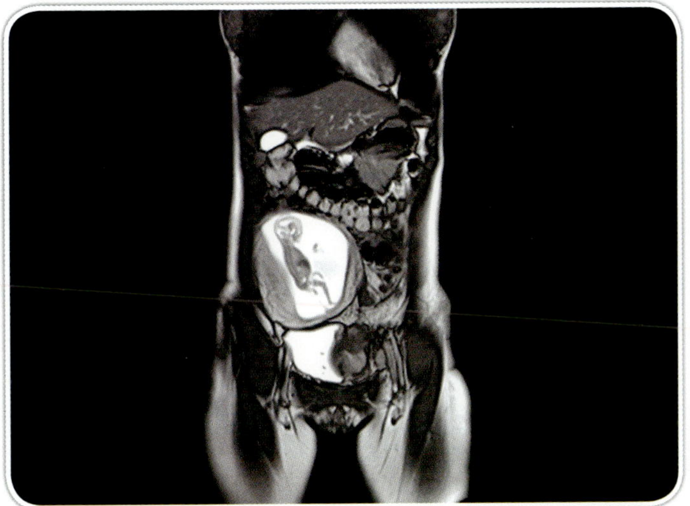

Image Creation with MRI

- MRI machine creates powerful magnetic field
- The magnetism aligns proton of intracellular water with the direction of the field
- After the electromagnetic field is turned off, relaxation of protons release radiofrequency signal that can be measured
- Computerized interpretation of electromagnetic signal can accurately delineate types of soft tissue in the field
- The soft tissue quality is defined as "increased or decreased signaling", which is not equivalent to "hypoechoic or hyperechoic density" from US.

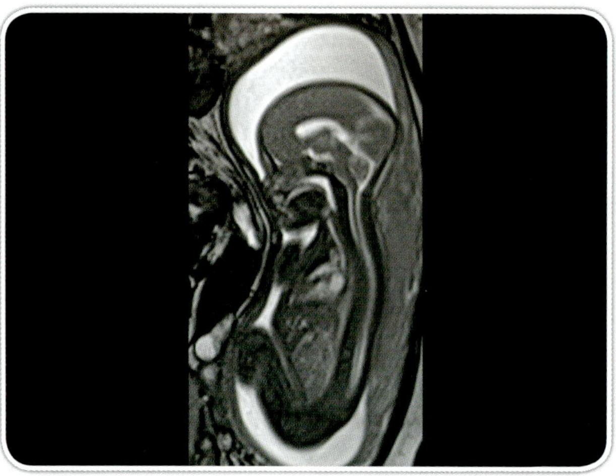

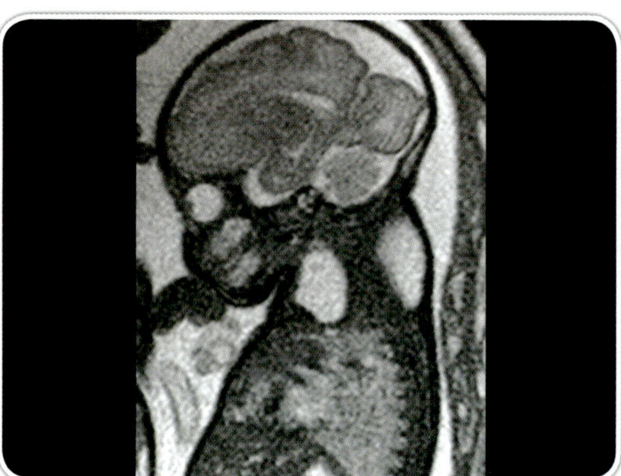

SAFETY OF FETAL MRI

- Noninvasive, nonionizing imaging system
- No known fetal effect

(Stecco et al. 2007)

- Should be avoided in the first half of pregnancy; unknown effect to the fetal development and excessive movement of small fetus.

(Glenn et al. 2006)

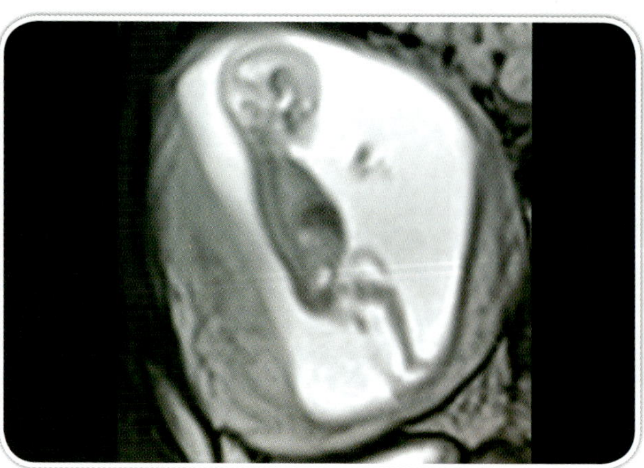

Indications of Fetal MRI

- Fetal lesions encased in bony structures, such as intracranial or intrathoracic lesions
- Some fetal tissues that may not show echoic difference on US, such as developing brain.

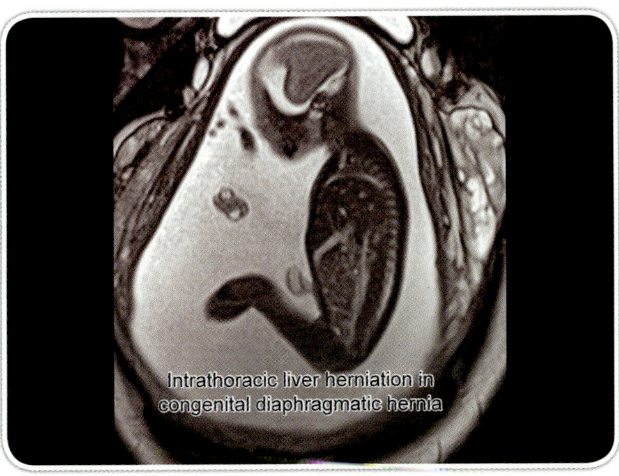

Fetal US: Advantages

- Convenient and widely available
- Affordable
- Real-time interpretation by perinatologist
- Better for calcified lesion.

Fetal US: Disadvantages

- Operator dependent
- Obstructed view
  - Fetal position
  - Oligohydramnios
  - Maternal obesity and pelvic bone
- Limited field view
- Detect the more serious changes.

Fetal MRI: Advantages

- Excellent tissue contrast for subtle changes
- Large field of view
- Not limited by fetal position or maternal structures
- Off-line interpretation by pediatric neurologists.

Fetal MRI: Disadvantages

- Expensive and not widely available
- Higher false positive and nonspecific findings
- Not suitable for first-trimester fetus
- Gadolinium contrast should be avoided.

(Garcia-Bournissen et al. 2006)

Rationale of Using Fetal MRI

- US remains the primary tool of fetal imaging
- MRI is indicated when it may provide additional information, and that specific information can lead to change in fetal care.

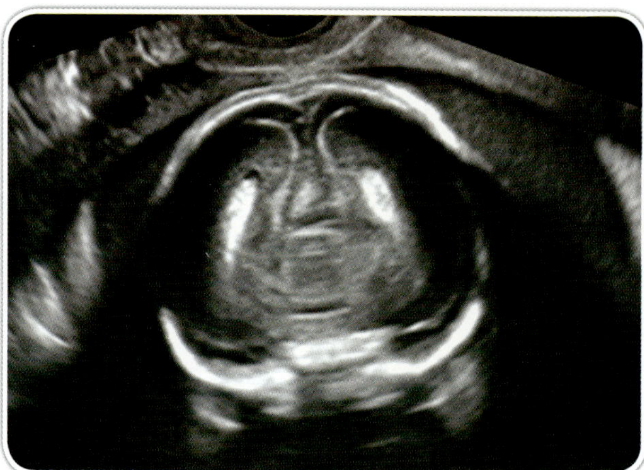

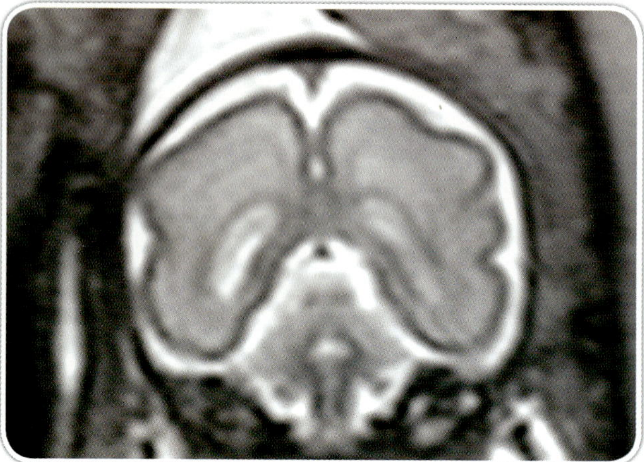

Benefits of MRI: Obstructed View

- Fetal brain US is a challenge, because the view is obstructed by 2 bony plates: fetal skull and maternal pelvis
- MRI can produce a good image quality through the fetal and maternal bony structures

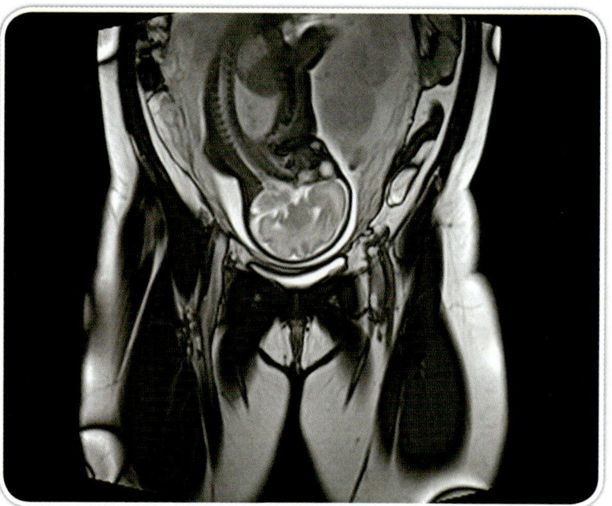

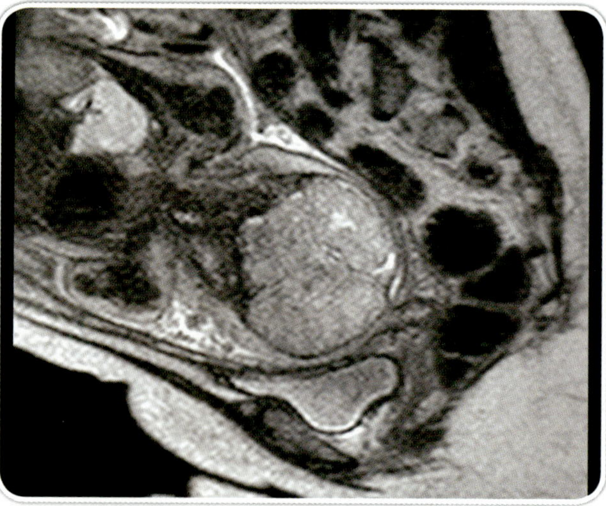

Surrounding maternal bones do not affect MRI image quality

Benefits of MRI: Large Field of View

- Large field of view allows for a simultaneous evaluation of the whole fetal anatomy, as well as its relationship with maternal structures.

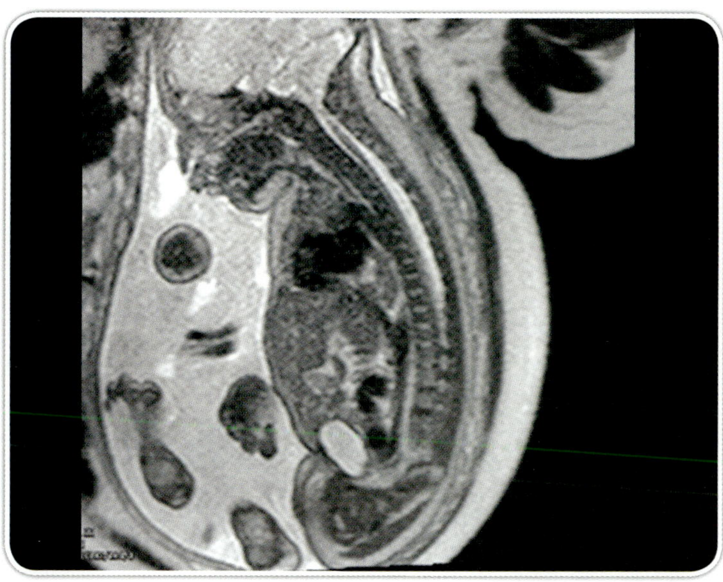

Benefits of MRI: Maternal Anatomy

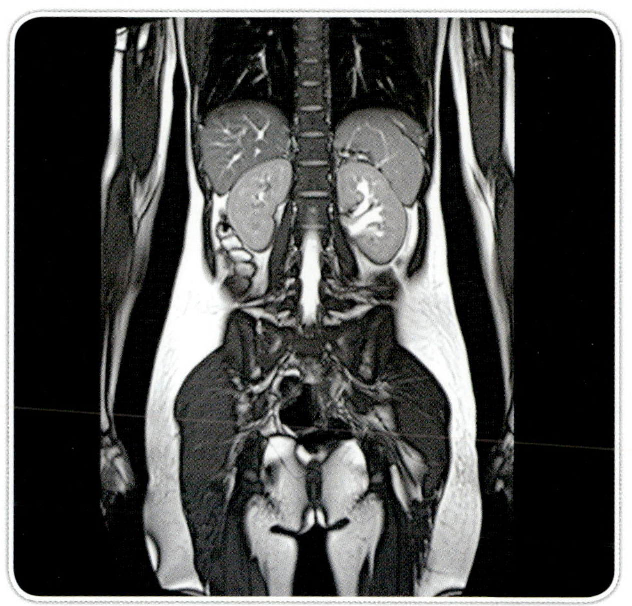

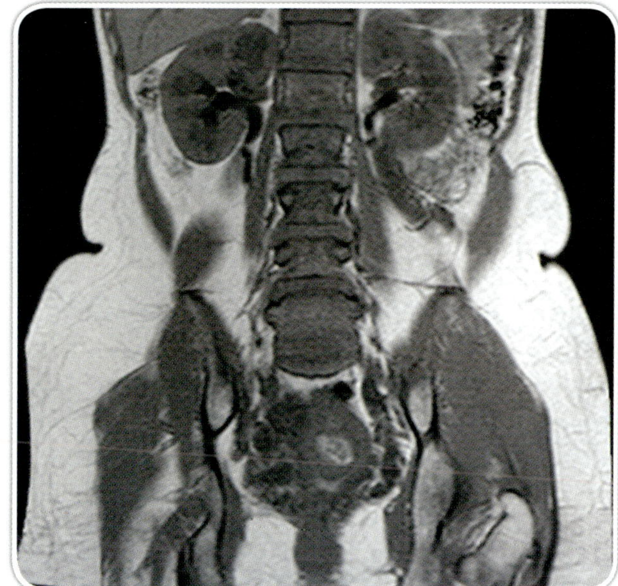

Prenatal MRI: Evaluation of Placenta

- Understanding the MRI image of the placenta requires basic knowledge of placental anatomy
- *Fetal surface:* Chorionic plate, chorionic vessels, umbilical cord insertion
- *Maternal surface:* Cotyledon, placental septa and clefts, as shown in the figure.

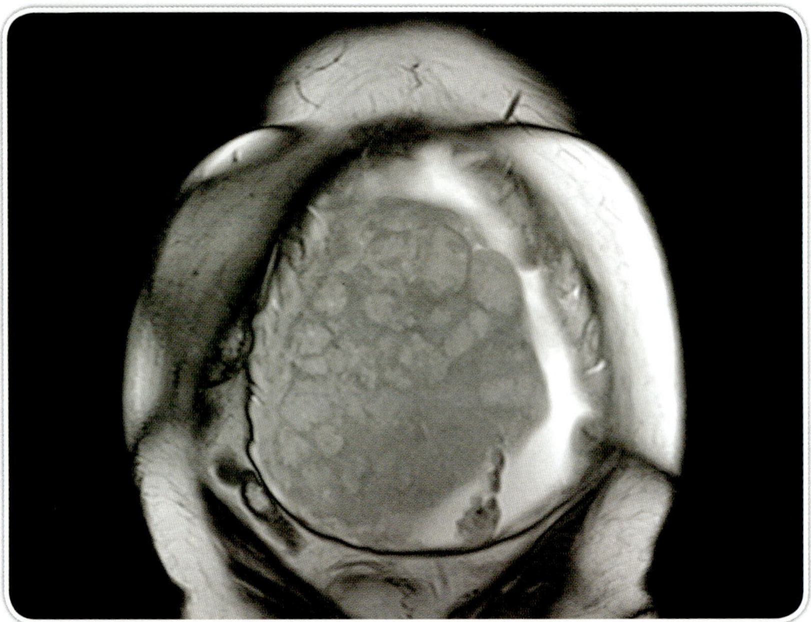

US PLACENTA ACCRETA: GRAY SCALE

- Obliteration of retroplacental sonolucent line (sensitivity 44%, specificity 95%)

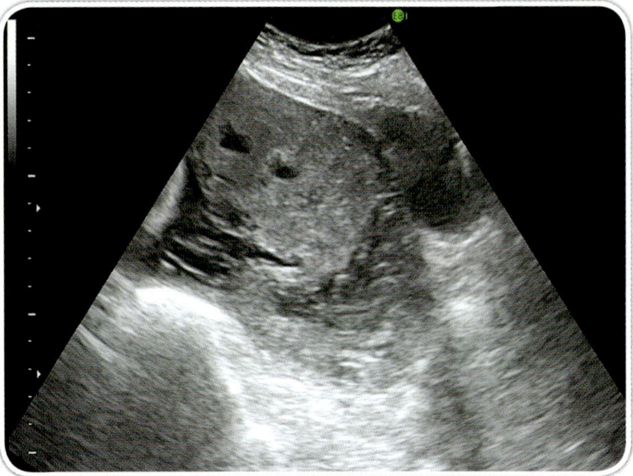

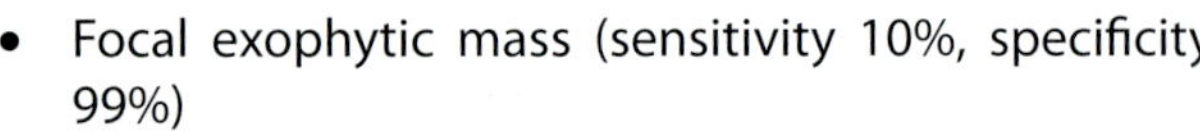

- Focal exophytic mass (sensitivity 10%, specificity 99%)

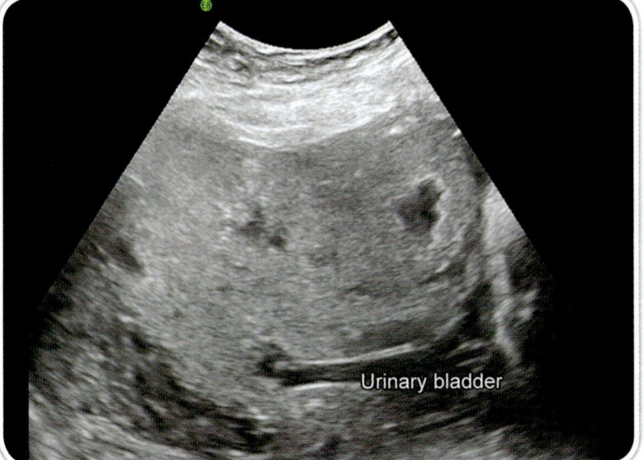

- Disruption of hyperechoic uterine serosa/bladder interface (sensitivity 18%, specificity 100%)

- Prominent placental lacunae (sensitivity 54%, sensitivity 85%).

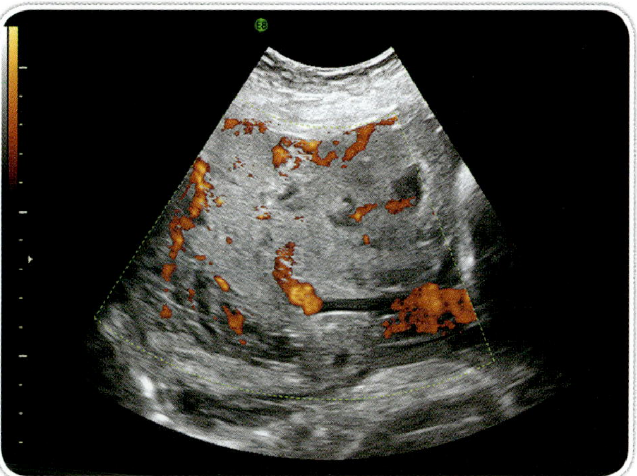

(Shih et al. 2009)

US PLACENTA ACCRETA: COLOR DOPPLER

- Increased vascularity of uterine serosa/bladder interface (sensitivity 77%, specificity 79%)

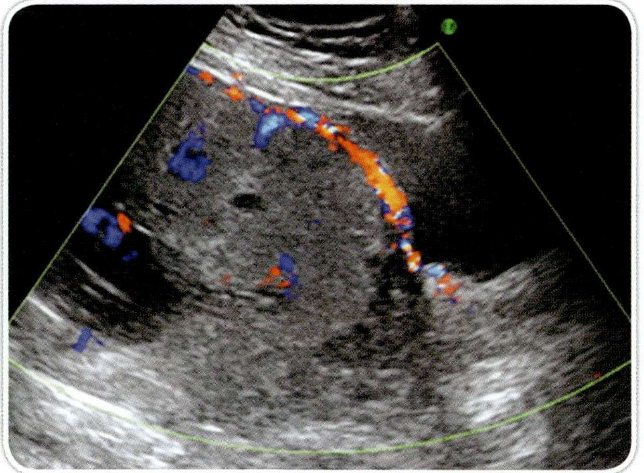

- Note the LOW SENSITIVITY for ultrasound used to detect placenta accreta.

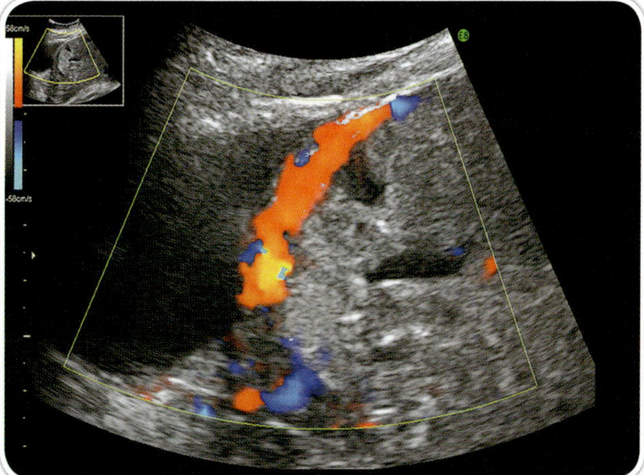

(Shih et al. 2009)

US PLACENTA ACCRETA: 3D POWER DOPPLER

- Intraplacental hypervascularity (sensitivity 90%, specificity 89%, PPV 70%)
- Inseparable cotyledon and intervillous circulations (sensitivity 90%, specificity 89%, PPV 70%)
- Tortuous and chaotic branching
- Multiple coherent vessels at the uterine serosa-bladder interface coherent vessels (sensitivity 97%, specificity 92%, PPV 77%).

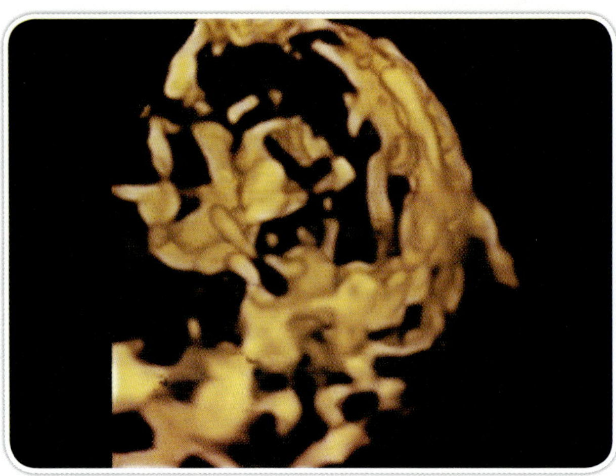

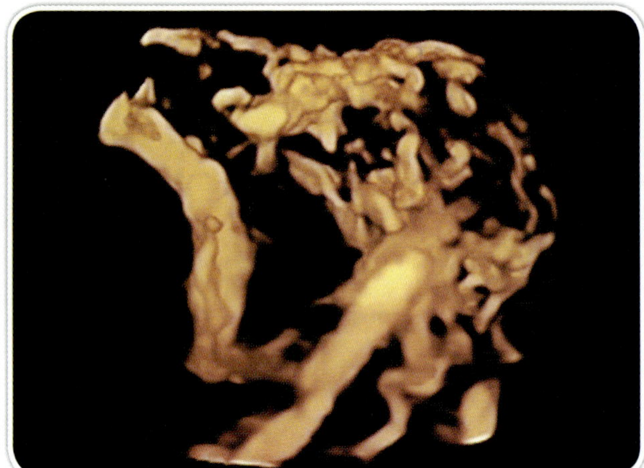

(Shih et al. 2009)

MRI DIAGNOSIS OF PLACENTA ACCRETA

- Intraplacental dark bands on T2-weighted HASTE and T2-weighted true FISP images

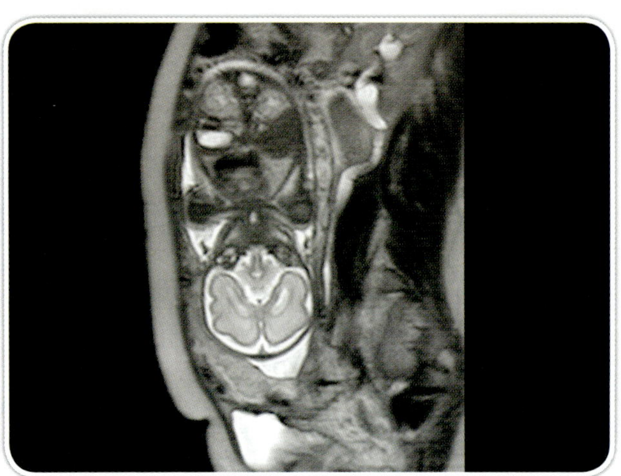

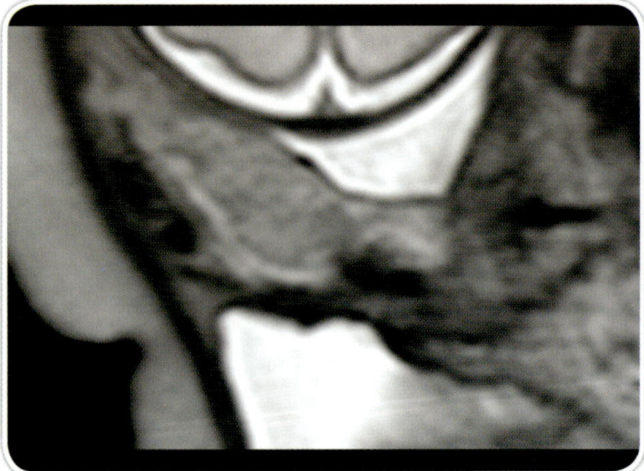

- Markedly heterogeneous placenta
- Disorganized abnormal placental vascularity.

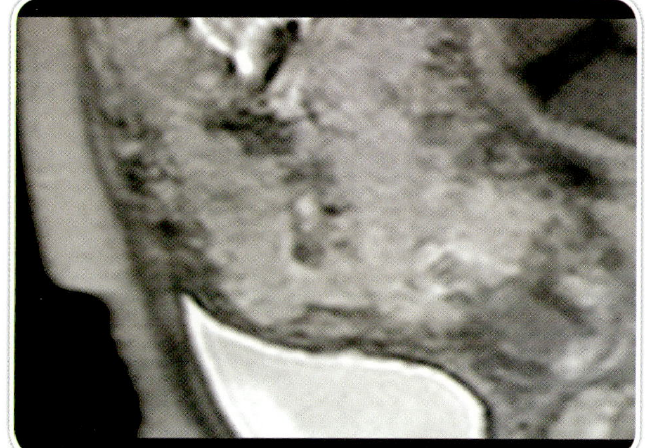

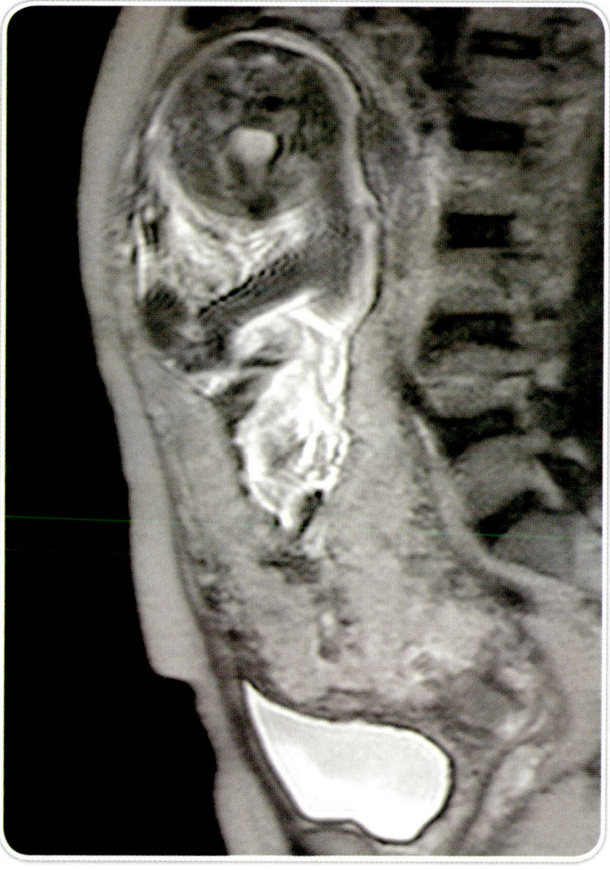

(Derman et al. 2011)

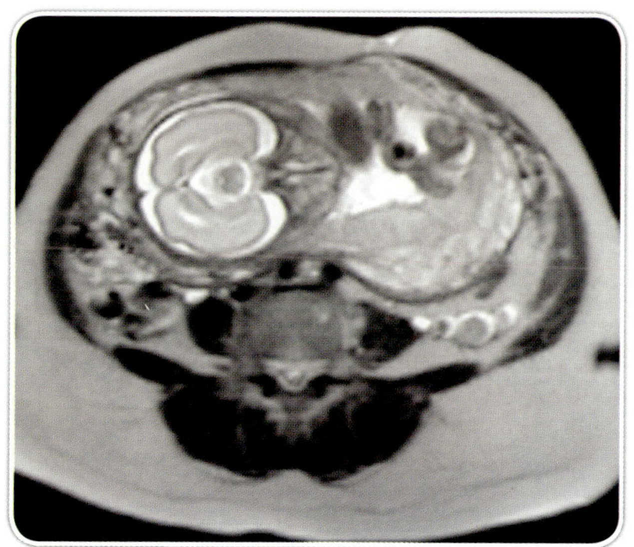

Invasion of the placenta through the myometrium.

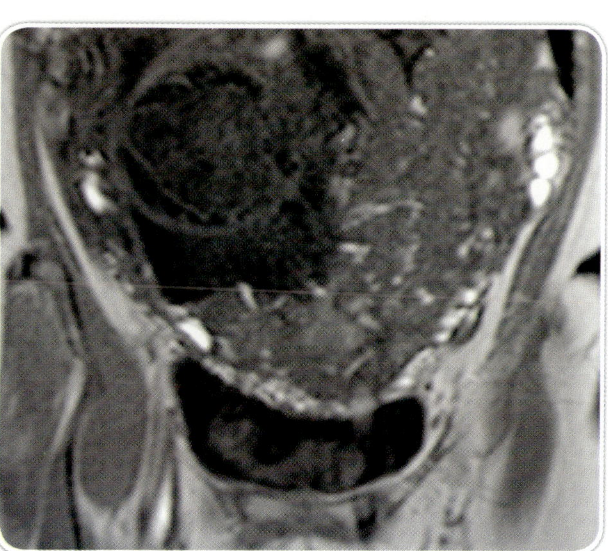

Disorganized abnormal placental vascularity

GROSS SPECIMEN OF PLACENTA ACCRETA

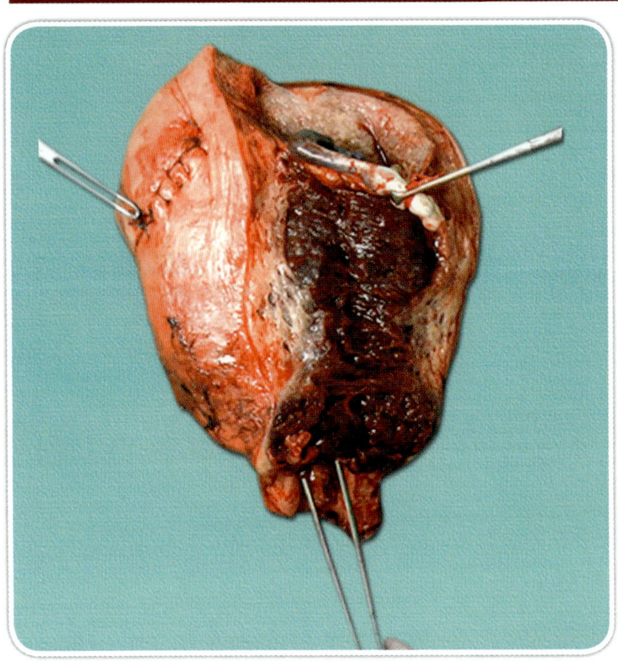

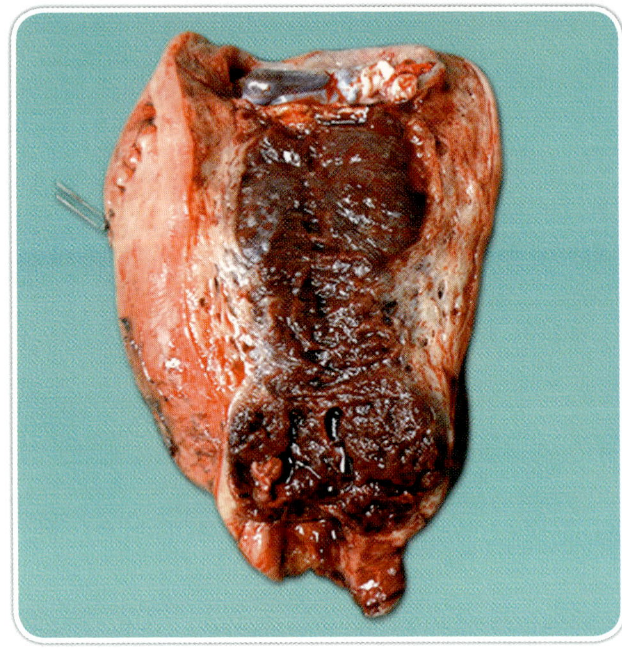

PLACENTA ACCRETA MRI AND GROSS SPECIMEN

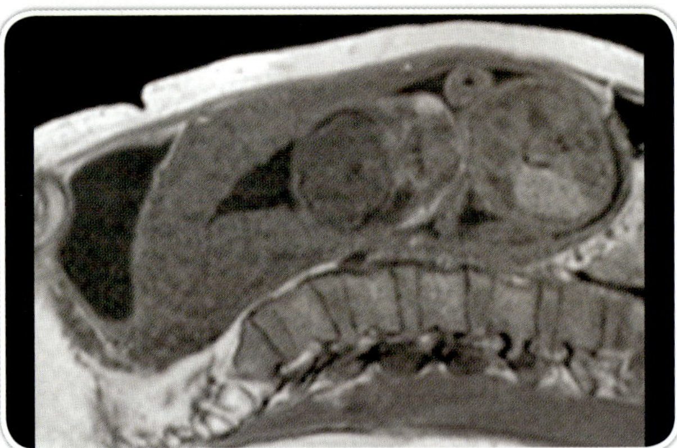

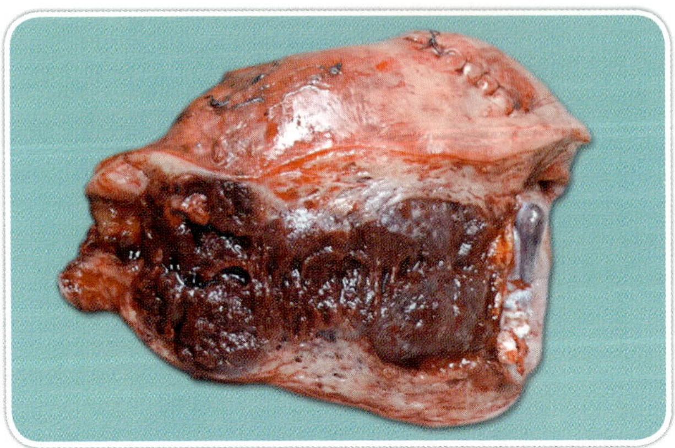

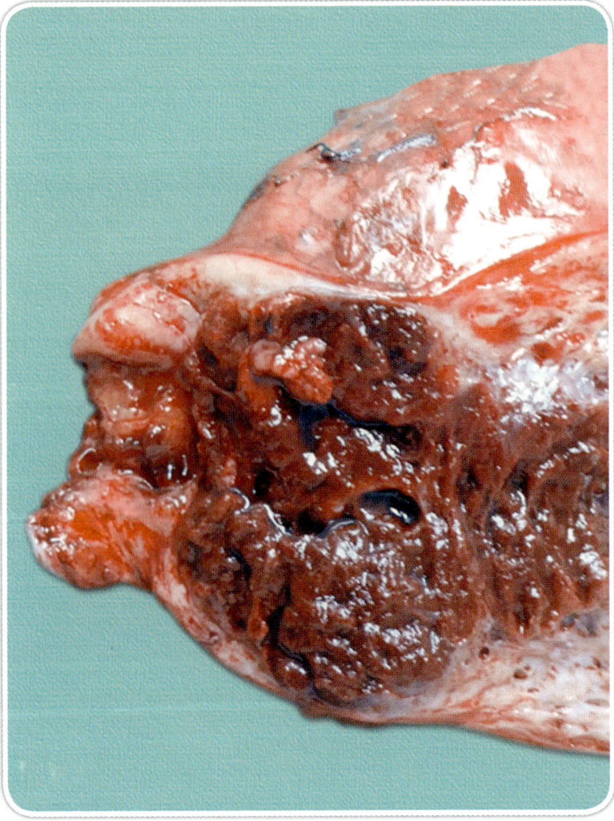

ABDOMINAL PREGNANCY

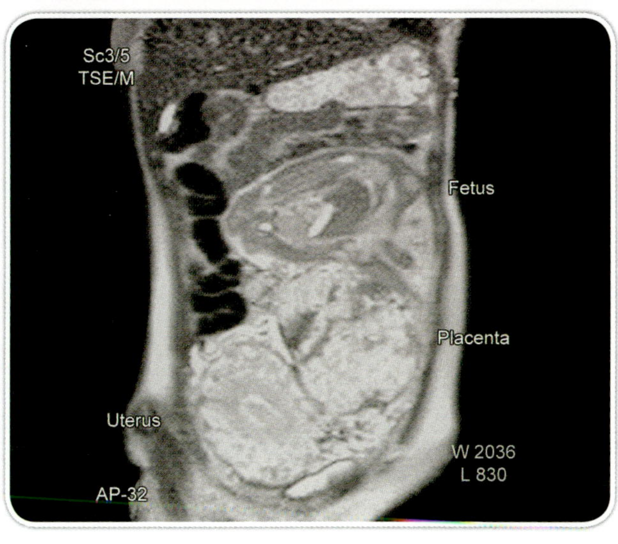

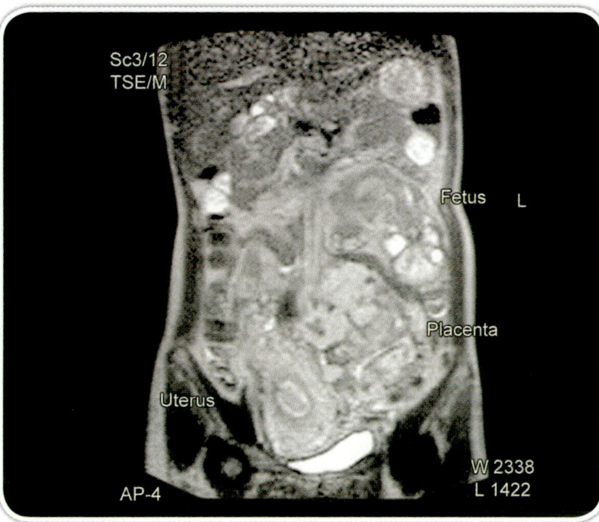

MRI has been used to identify maternal visceral organ relationship to the extrauterine fetus and placenta

- After surgical evacuation, sequential gray-scale, 3D, and Doppler US have been used to monitor the regression of placental mass.

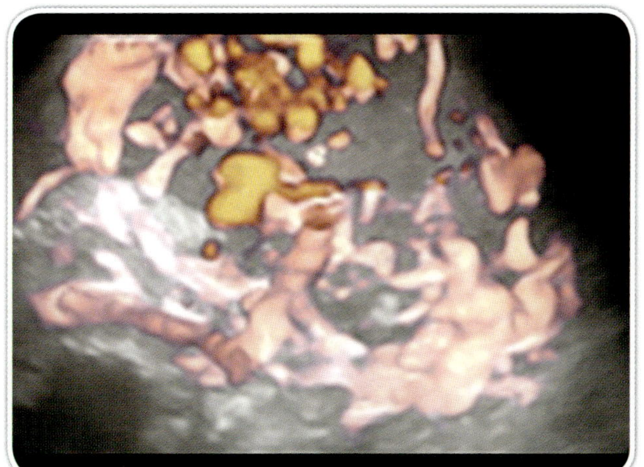

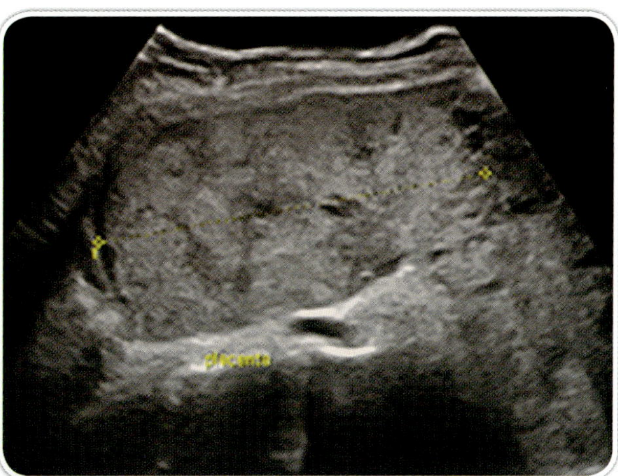

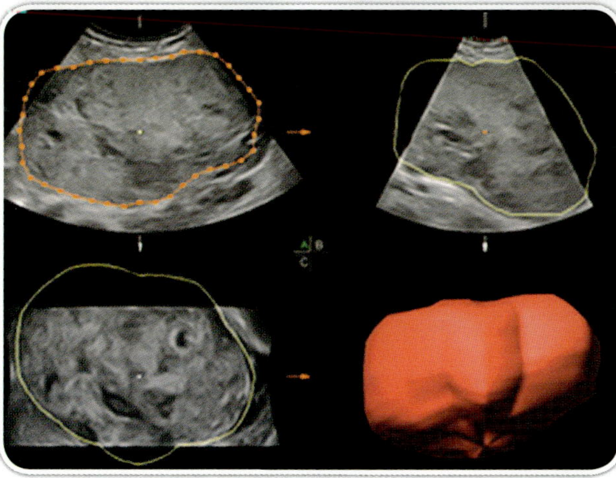

Fetal Congenital Diaphragmatic Hernia (CDH)

- Failure of septum transversum, pleuroperitoneal membranes, dorsal mesentery of the esophagus, and body wall to fuse results in diaphragmatic hernia.

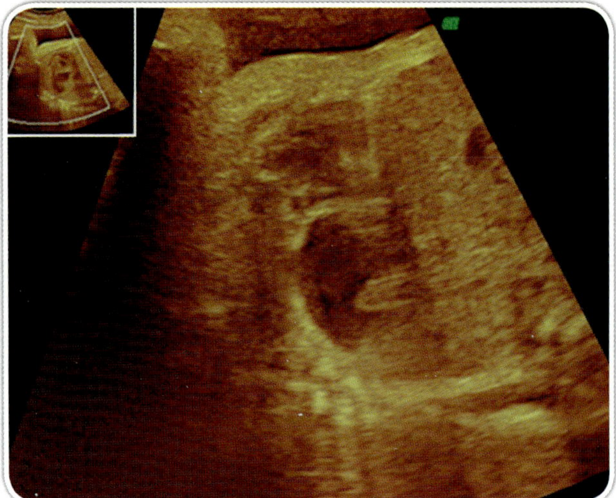

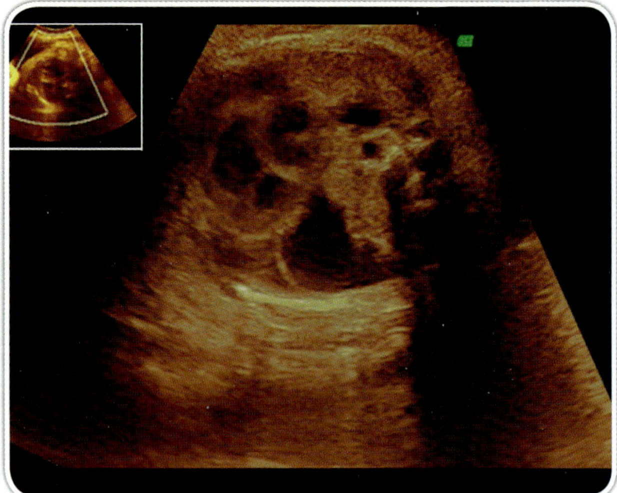

(Wenstrom 2003)

Fetal CDH

- High neonatal mortality from lung hypoplasia is expected in left-sided diaphragmatic defect with liver herniation and lung-to-head ratio < 1.4.
- MRI may help assessing the hernia content and fetal lung volume.

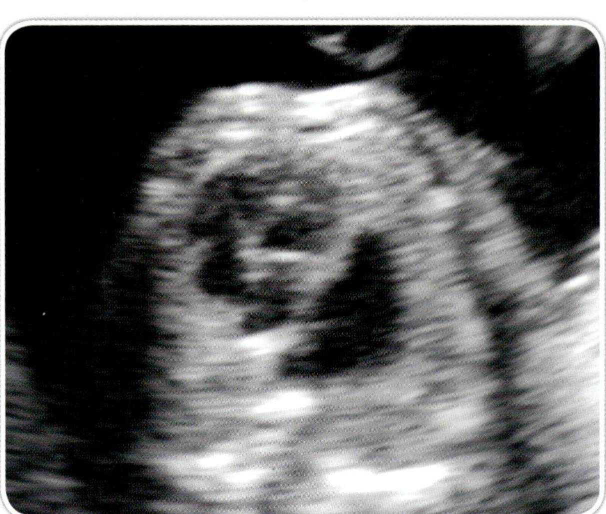

(Harrison 2011)

(Kilian et al. 2009)

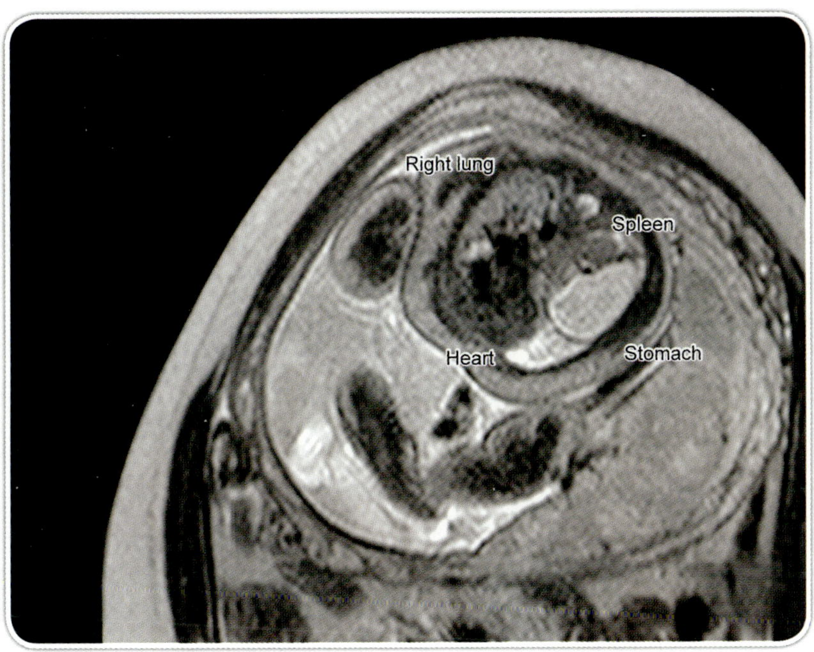

Left-sided Fetal CDH: Liver Down

- Note the intrathoracic herniation of stomach and spleen, but not liver.
- Contralateral lung was still intact (good prognosis).

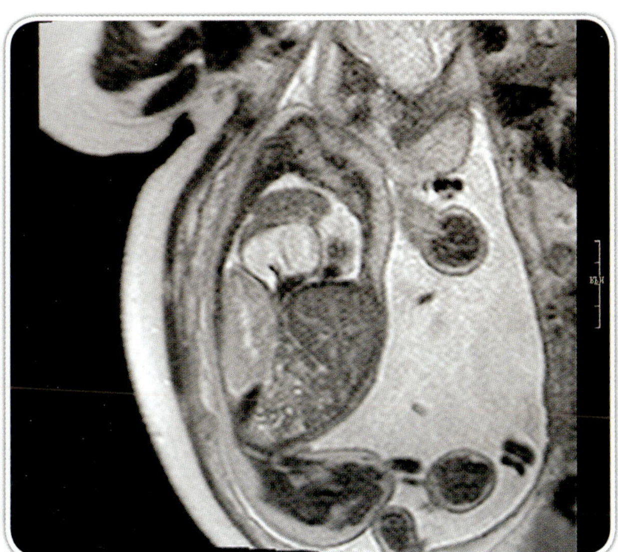

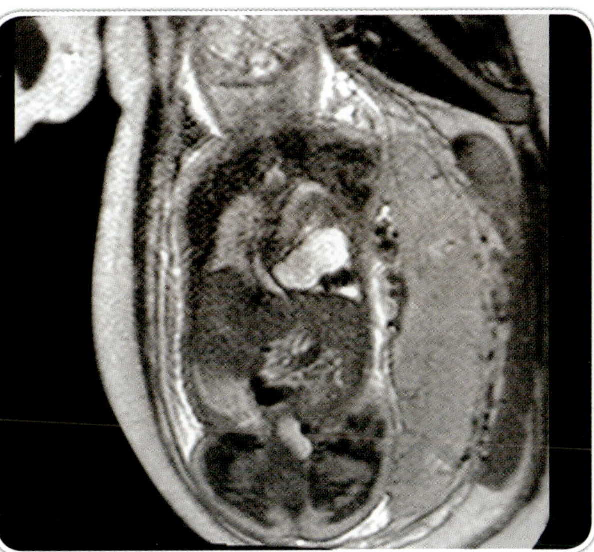

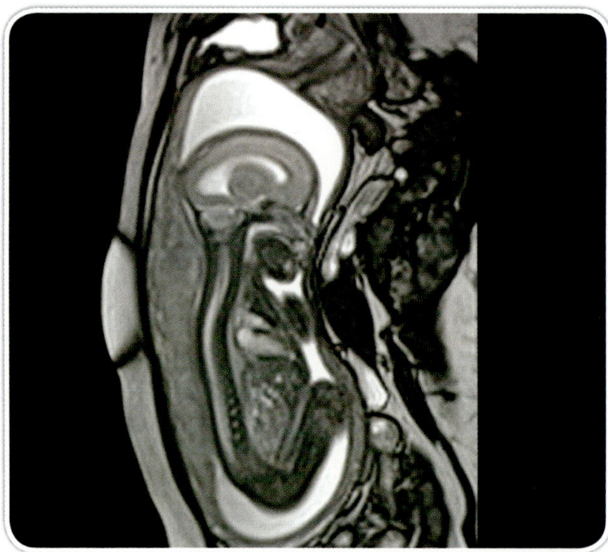

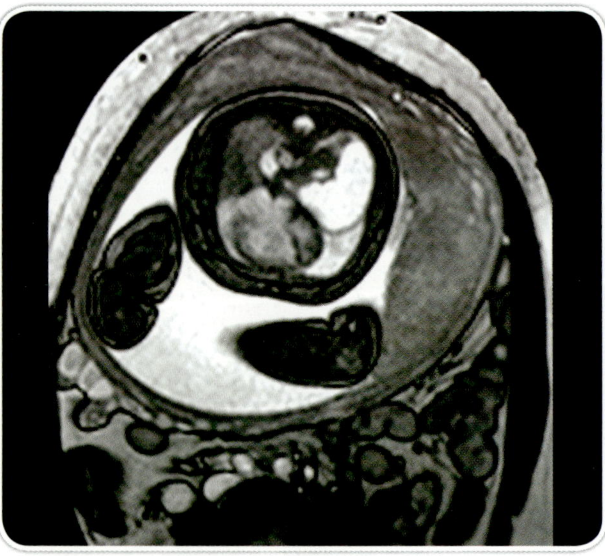

Measurement of Contralateral Lung Area with MRI

- Prediction of neonatal survival
  - **US:** Observed/Expected (O/E) lung-to-head ratio (LHR)
  - **MRI:** Total lung volume
- These parameters may help optimizing fetal/neonatal managements.

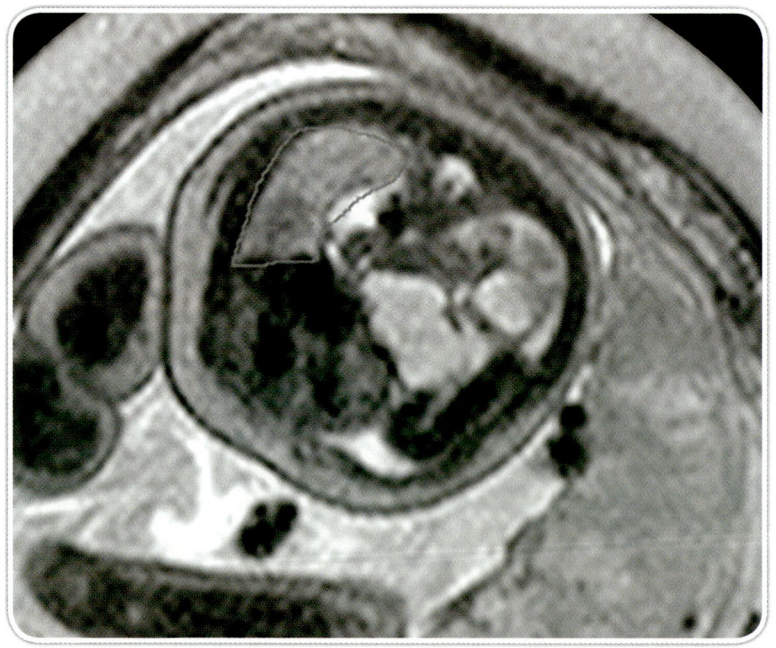

(Alfaraj et al. 2011)

LIVER POSITION IN CDH

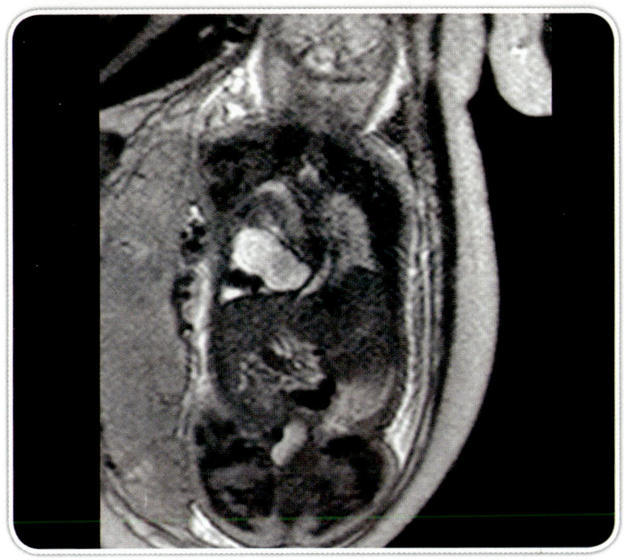

Liver down: Better prognosis

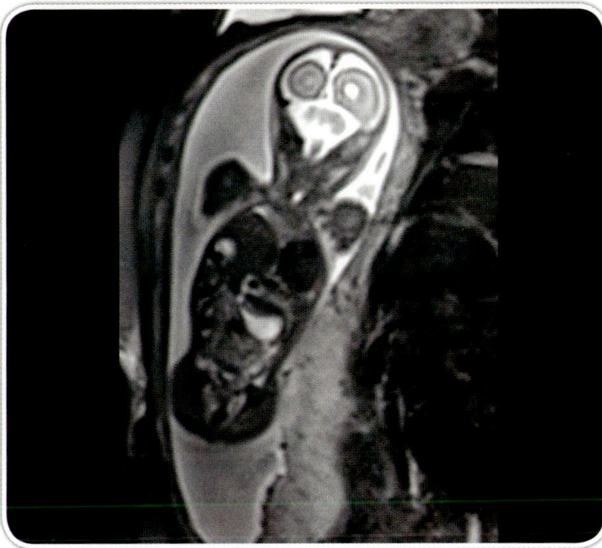

Liver up: Worse prognosis

Prognosis of Fetal CDH with 'Liver-up'

- The liver-up CDH more often requires extracorporeal membrane oxygenation (ECMO) (53%) compared with the liver-down (19%)
- The liver-up has lower postnatal survival (43%) compared with the liver-down (93%).

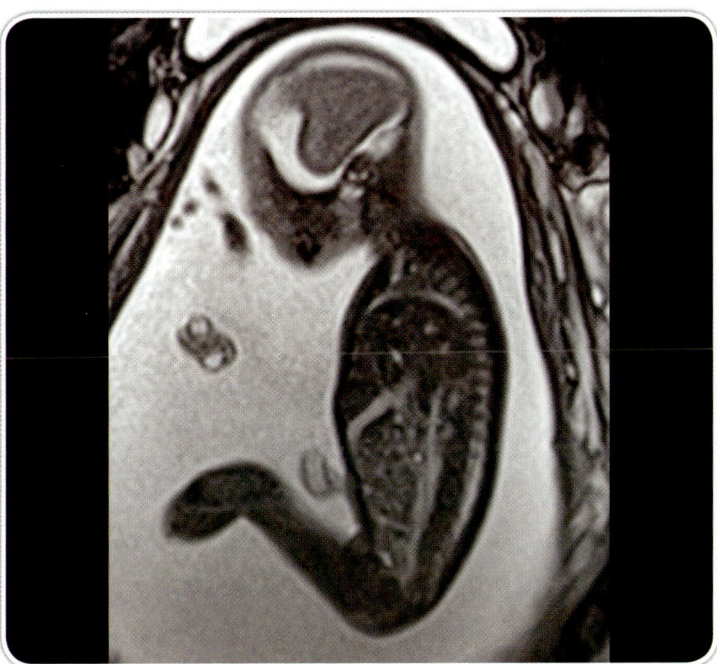

(Albanese et al. 1998)

Associated Anomalies can Worsen the Prognosis in CDH Baby

- Associated anomalies, such as esophageal atresia can be occasionally (0.5%) found with CDH
- Neonatal survival is significantly lower than in cases with isolated CDH.

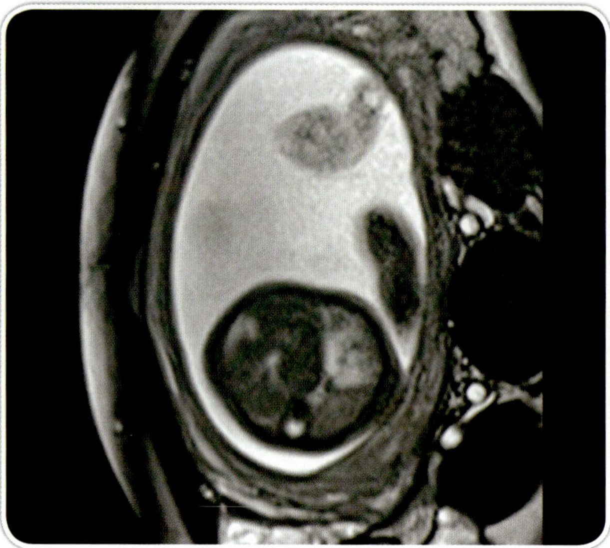

(Ben-Ishay et al. 2013)

BRONCHOPULMONARY SEQUESTRATION

- Rare form of lower respiratory tract malformation

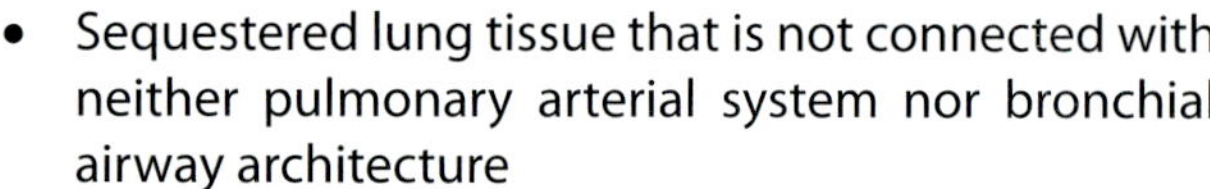

- Sequestered lung tissue that is not connected with neither pulmonary arterial system nor bronchial airway architecture

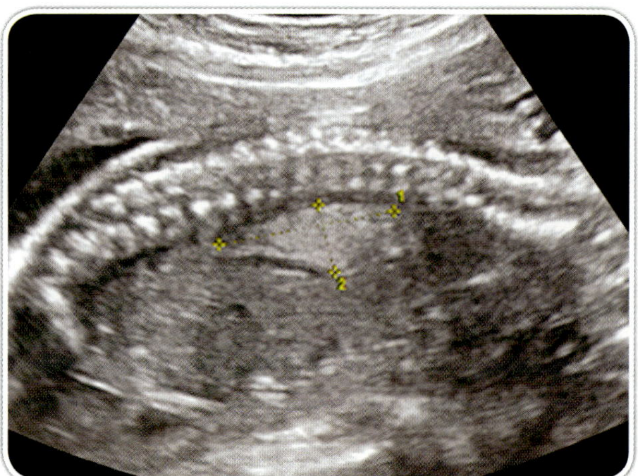

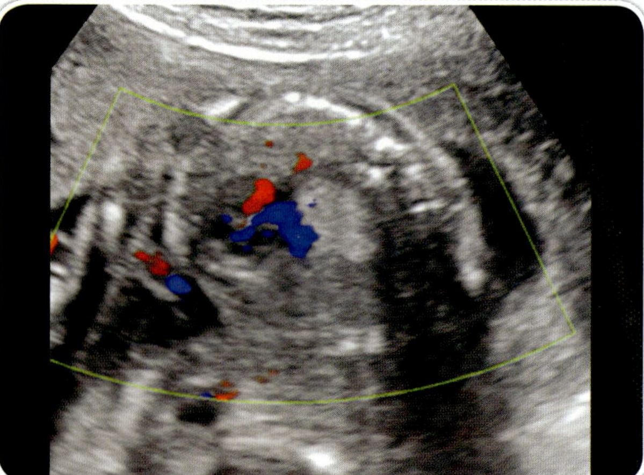

- Most of the time, the prognosis is excellent. It may cause hydrops in some cases
- It is related to recurrent lung infection in childhood period.

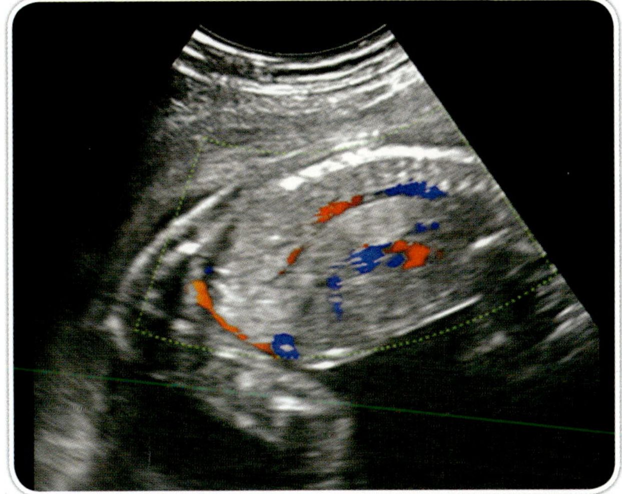

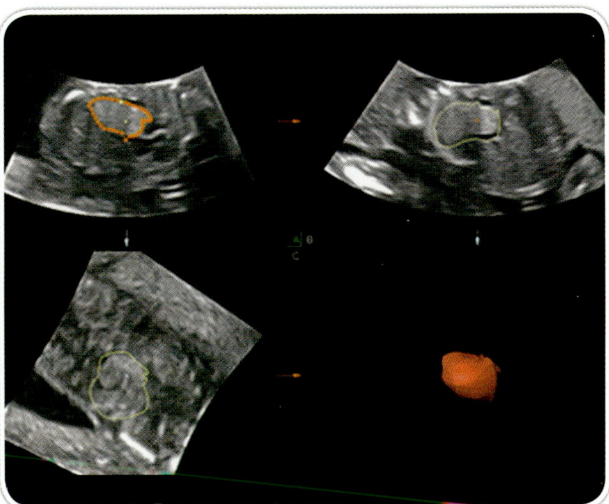

(Zhang et al. 2014)

MRI Aids in Diagnosis of Rare Form of Bronchopulmonary Sequestration: Subdiaphragmatic Type

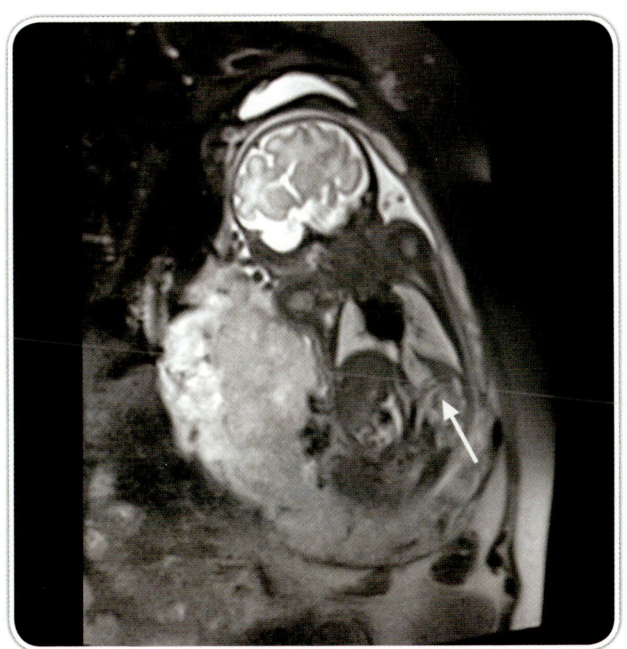

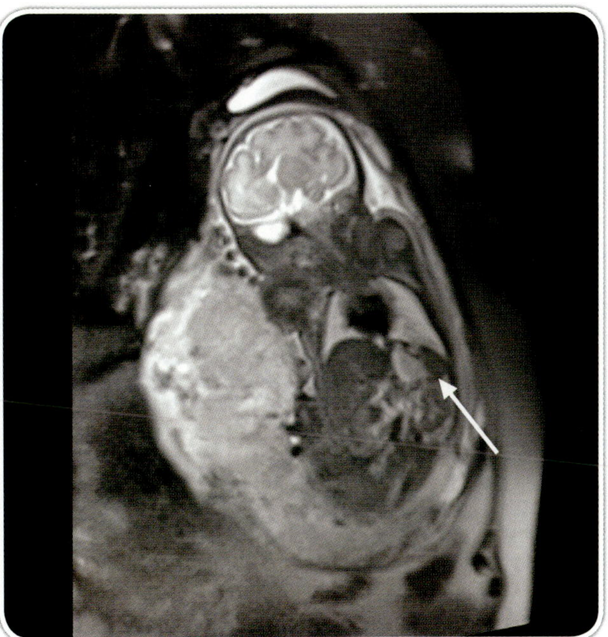

CONGENITAL HIGH AIRWAY OBSTRUCTION (CHAOS)

- Obstruction of fetal airway (laryngeal/tracheal atresia, subglottic stenosis, laryngeal cyst/web.)

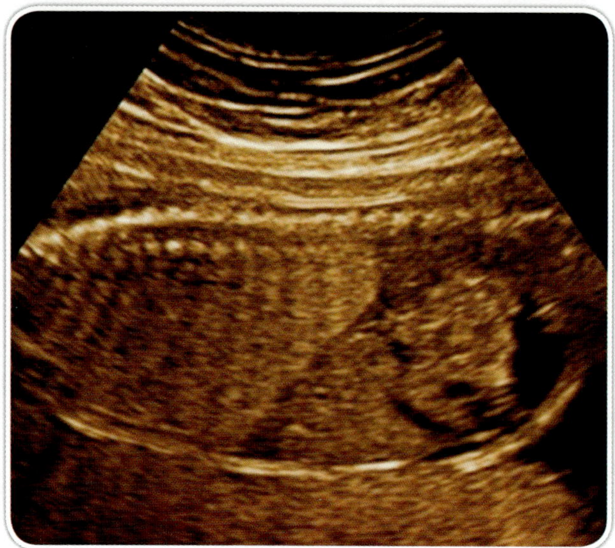

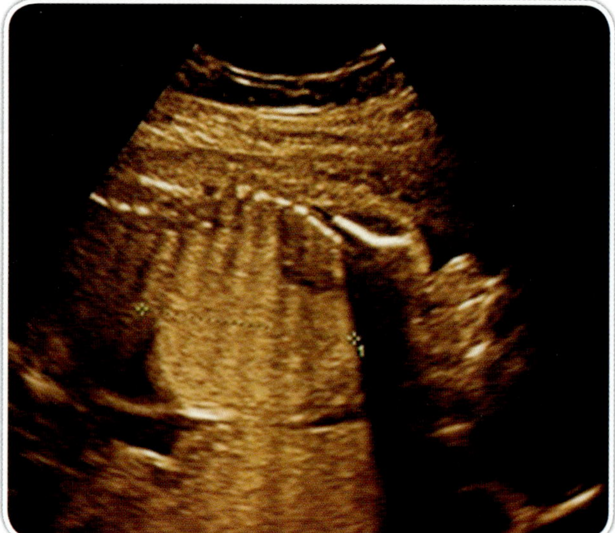

(Lim et al. 2003)

CONGENITAL HIGH AIRWAY OBSTRUCTION (CHAOS): US

- Enlarged hyperechoic lungs
- Flattened/everted diaphragm
- Dilated distal airways
- Mediastinal compression
- Ascites
- Hydrops.

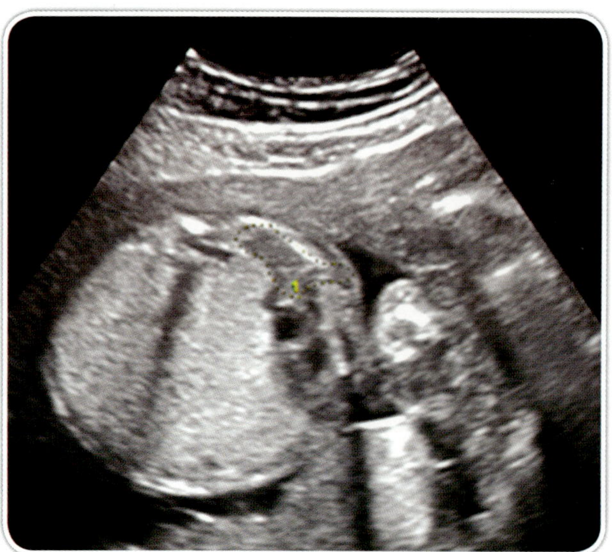

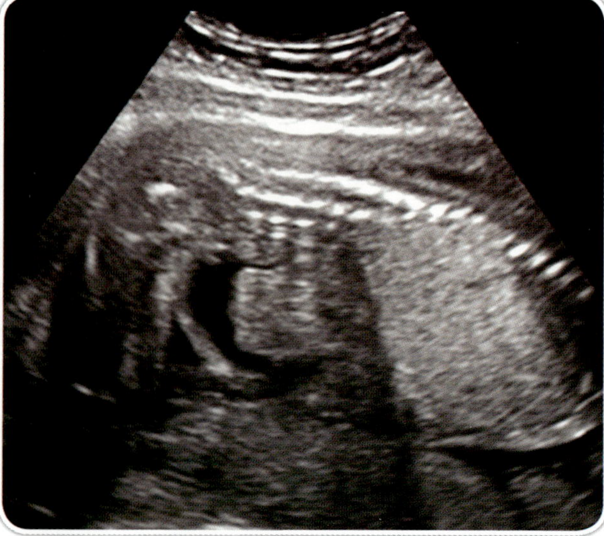

FETAL MRI IN CHAOS

- May confirm features detected on US
- More accurately shows the level of obstruction
- Increased lung signal
- There are only few cases of long-term survival described in literature
- Fetal MRI may lead to fetal tracheo-bronchoscopy, EXIT treatment or more targeted therapy of CHAOS at the time of birth.

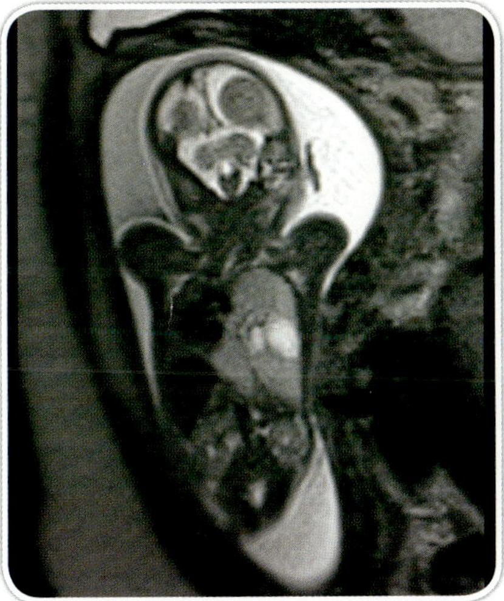

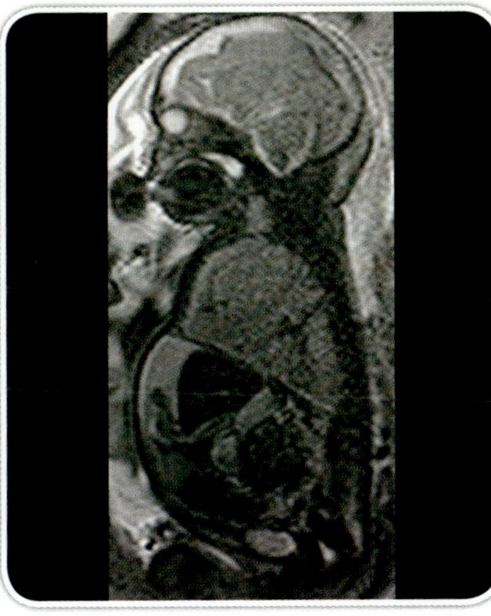

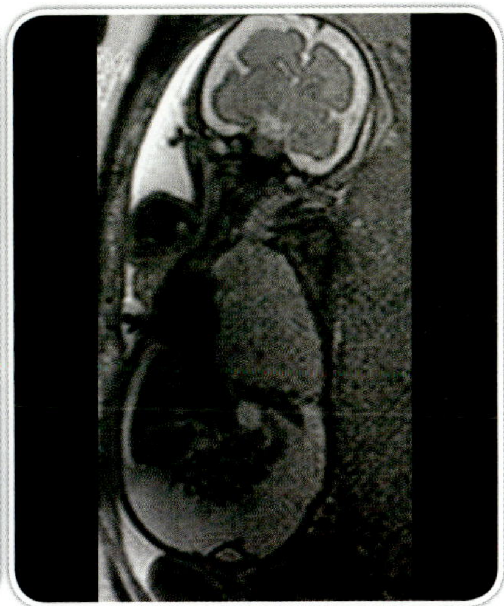

(Guimaraes et al. 2009)

Evaluation of Fetal Intracranial Structures

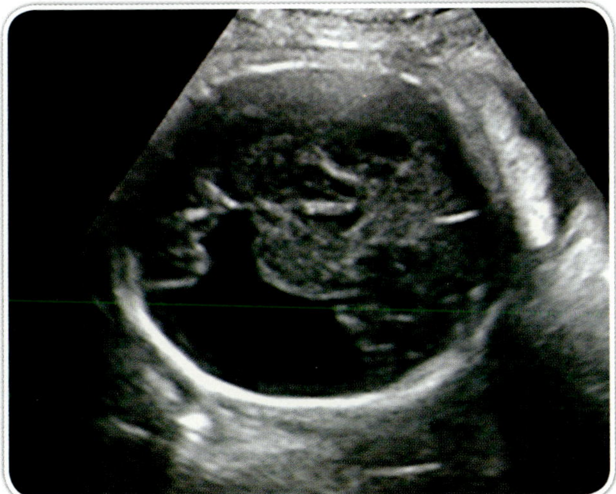

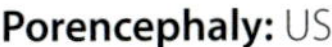

Porencephaly: US

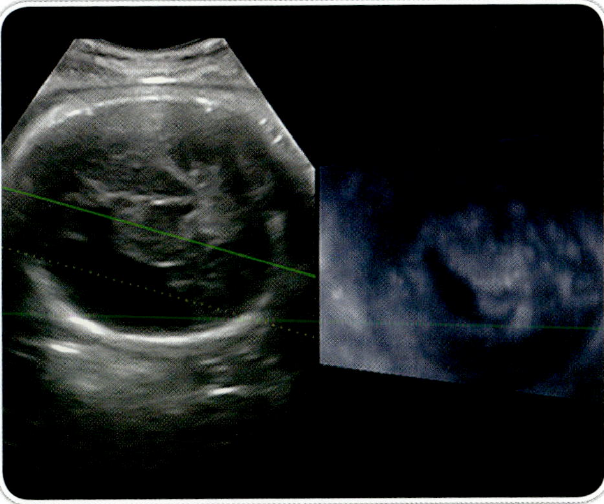

Porencephaly: OmniView™

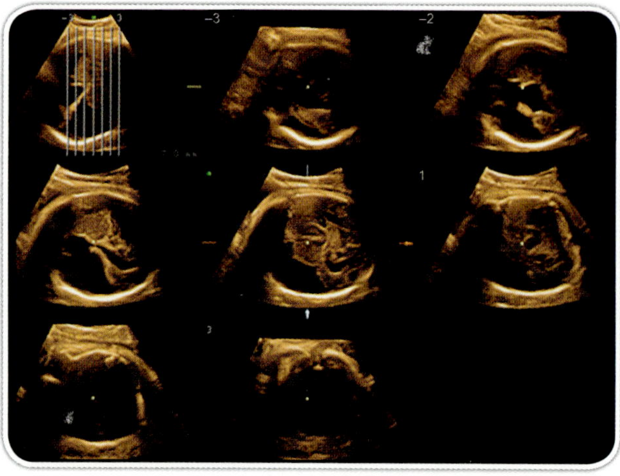

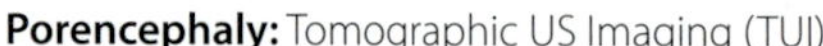

Porencephaly: Tomographic US Imaging (TUI)

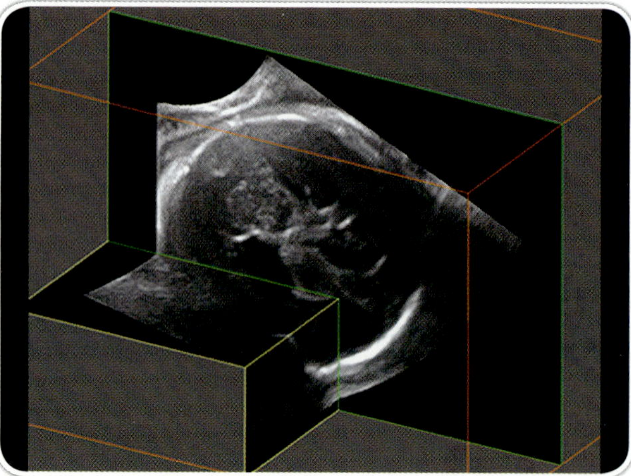

Porencephaly: Niche View™

SEVERE PERINATAL BRAIN DAMAGES

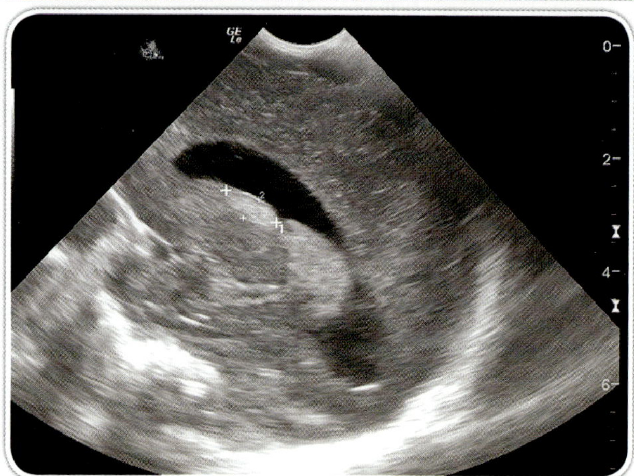

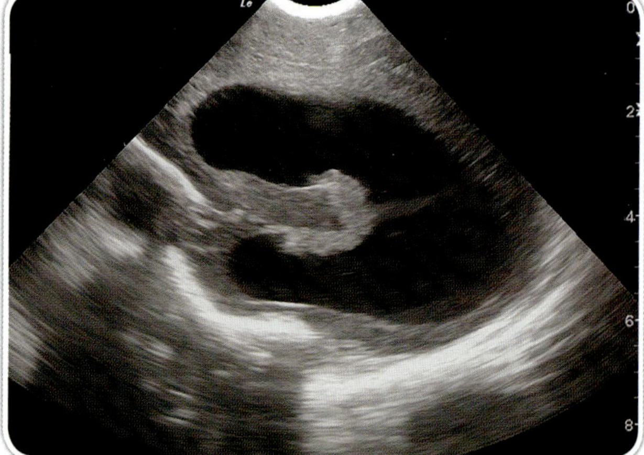

Intraventricular hemorrhage (IVH)

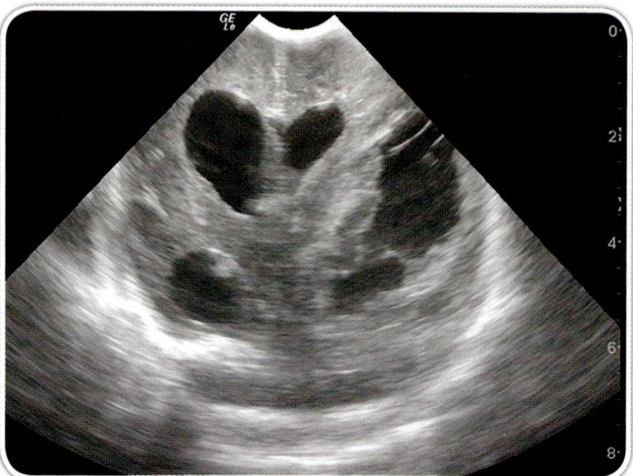

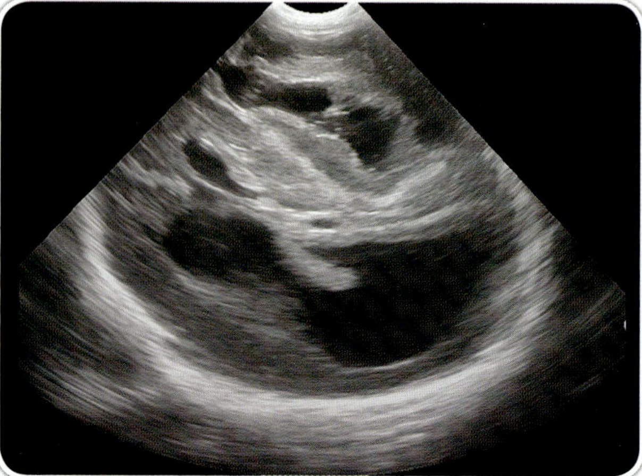

Intraparenchymal hemorrhage

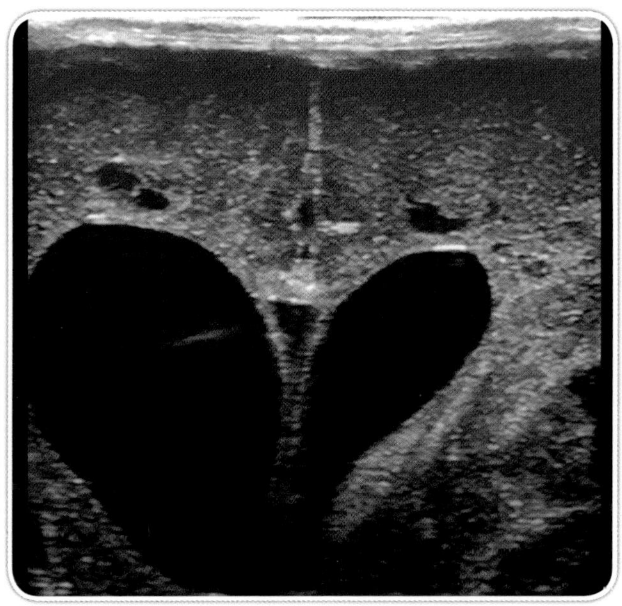

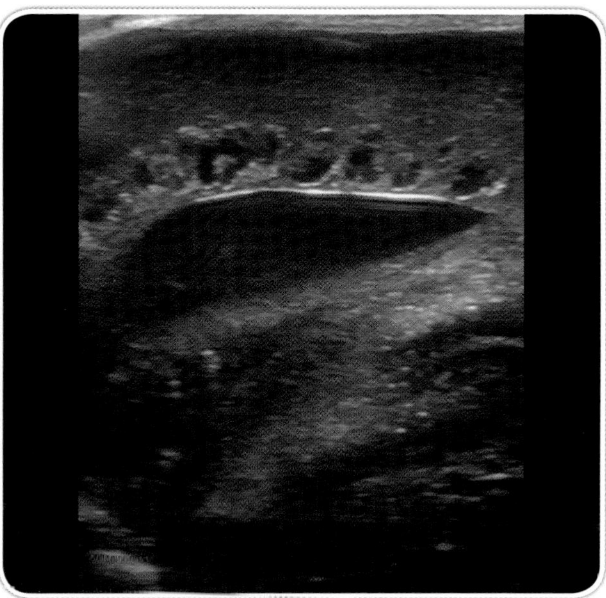

Periventricular leukomalacia

US PREDICTION OF FETAL BRAIN DAMAGE

- High-resolution transabdominal US in non-vertex fetus can detect some intracranial lesions.
- Prognosis of prenatal detection of some conditions, such as aqueductal stenosis or Arnold-Chiari malformations, has been well-documented.

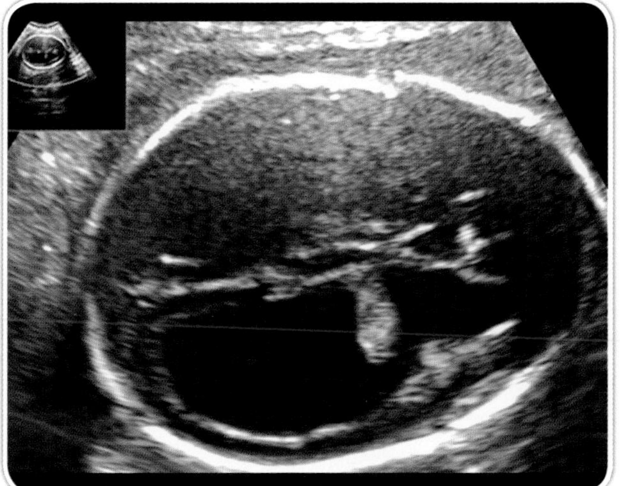

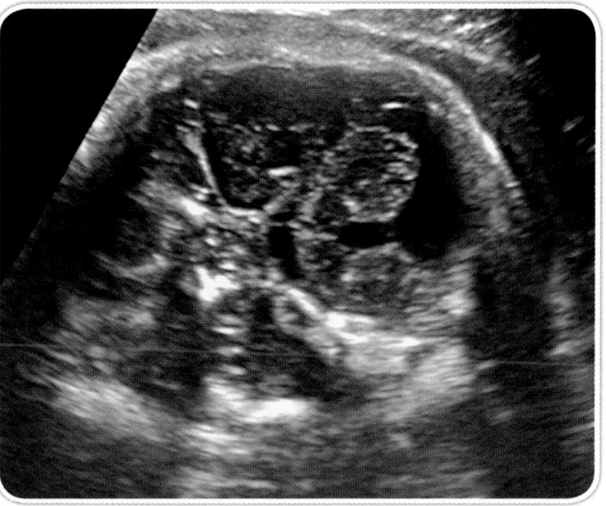

(Yamasaki et al. 2012)

- Transvaginal high-resolution scan is particularly useful when the fetus is in vertex position.

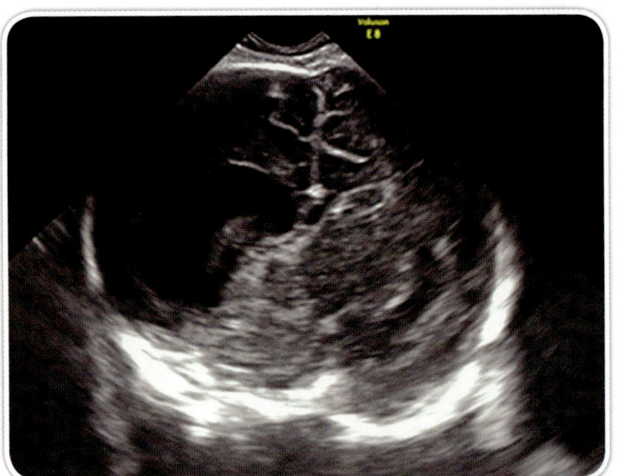

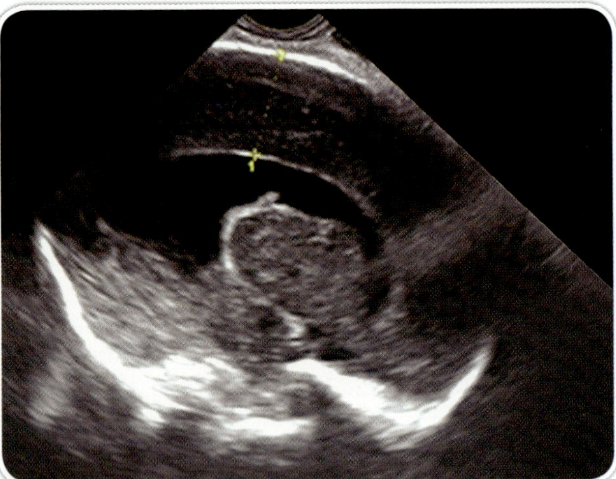

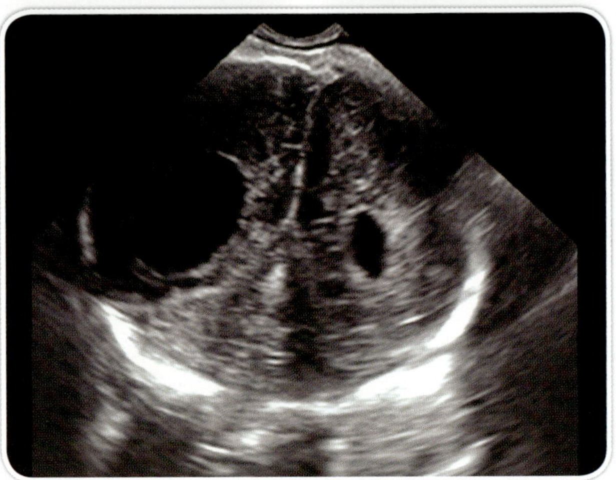

(Pooh et al. 2012)

- Mapping of intracranial vascular anomalies may also predict acquired brain damage in utero.

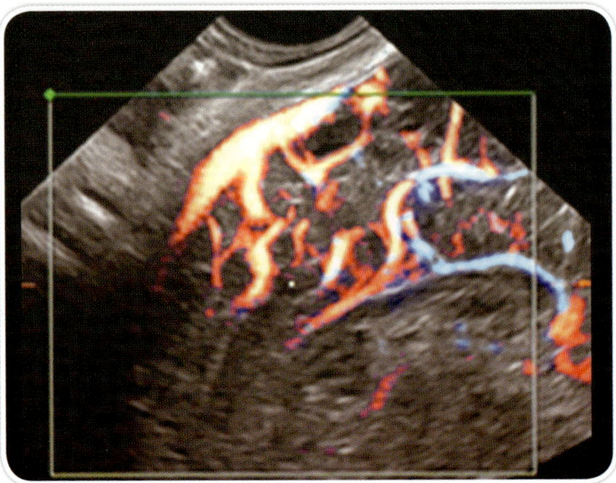

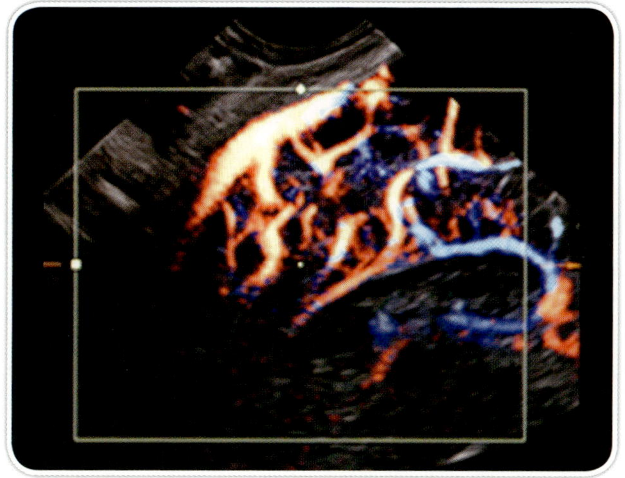

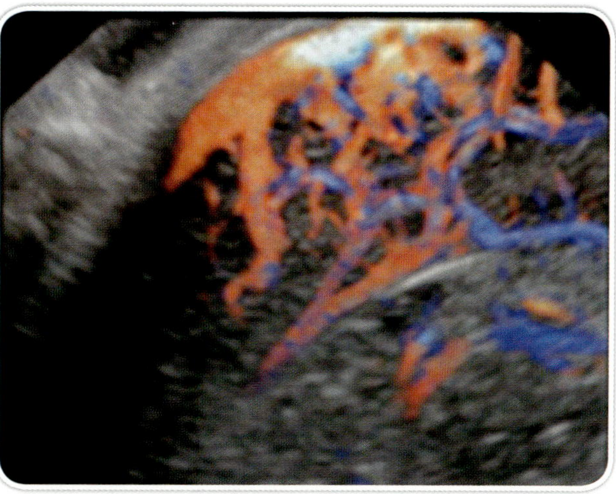

(Pooh et al. 2012)

Indications of MRI Fetal Brain

- Screen 2nd trimester fetus at risk of brain damage
- Borderline US brain anomaly
- Better genetic counseling
- Guide perinatal management.

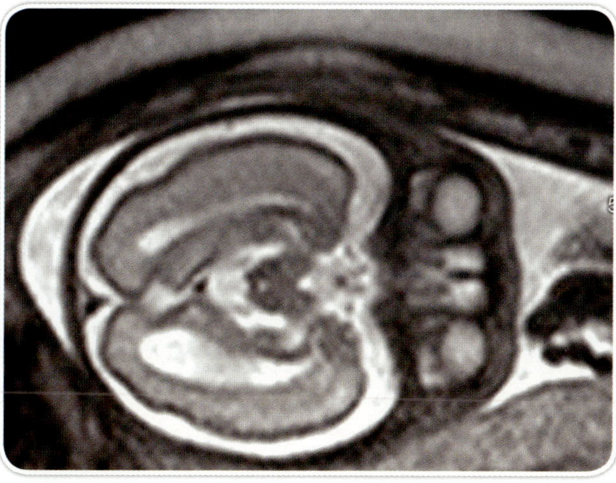

(Saleem, 2013)

UNILATERAL VENTRICULOMEGALY

- Differential diagnoses include atresia of foramen of Monro, toxoplasmosis, brain atrophy, and Weaver syndrome
- If MRI in at 32–34 weeks' show no other abnormality and the cortex is intact, the prognosis is generally good.

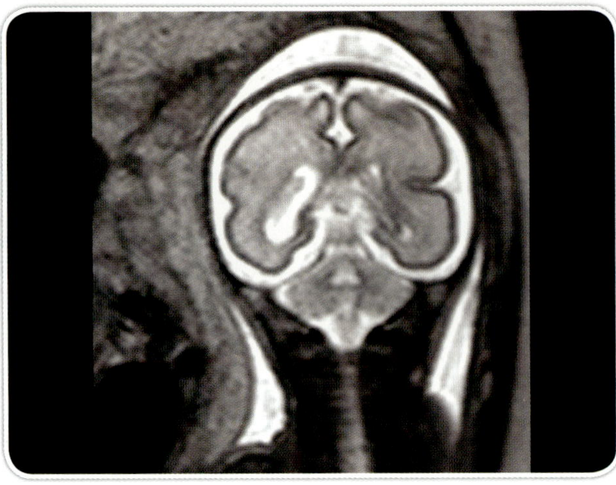

(Senat et al. 1999)

HYDRANENCEPHALY

- Destruction of the cerebral hemispheres
- The brain turns into a sac containing cerebrospinal fluid, with some cerebral remnants
- Termination is usually offered due to its severe neurological handicap

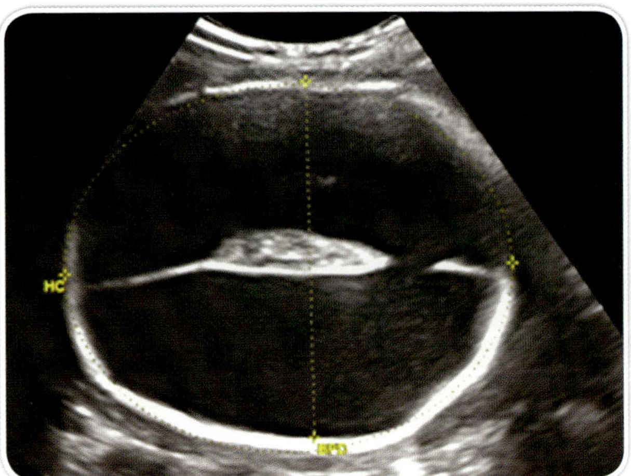

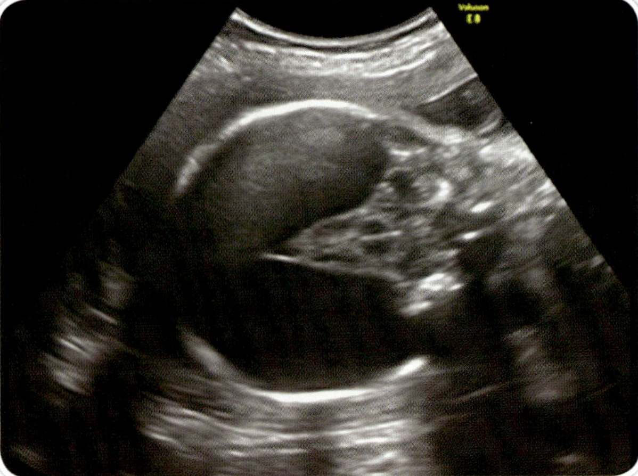

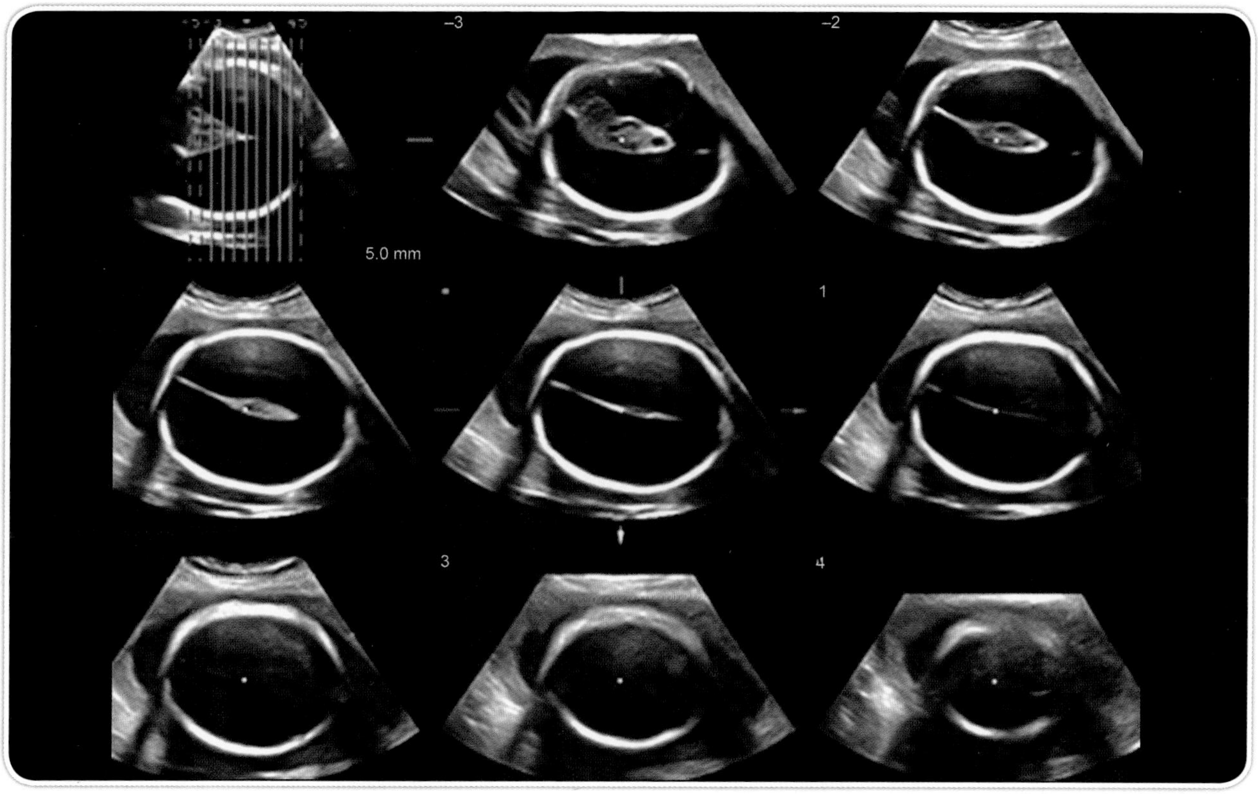

- **Differential diagnosis**
  - Holoprosencephaly: Poor prognosis
  - Schizencephaly: Poor prognosis
  - Obstructive hydrocephalus: Cerebral cortex is still visible, may be by MRI. Postnatal shunt can be offered.

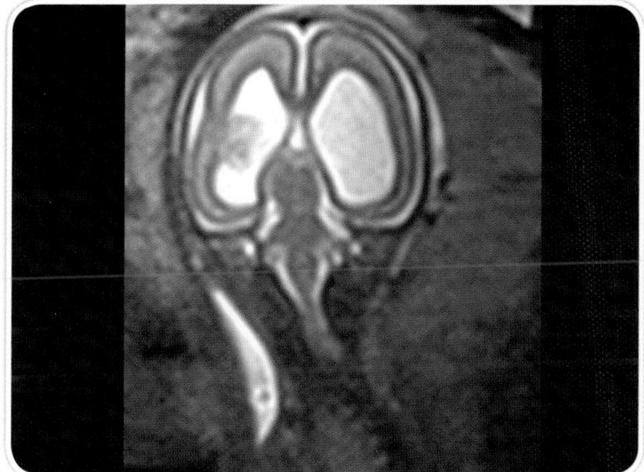

Obstructive hydrocephalous
- Better prognosis
- Postnatal shunt can be offered

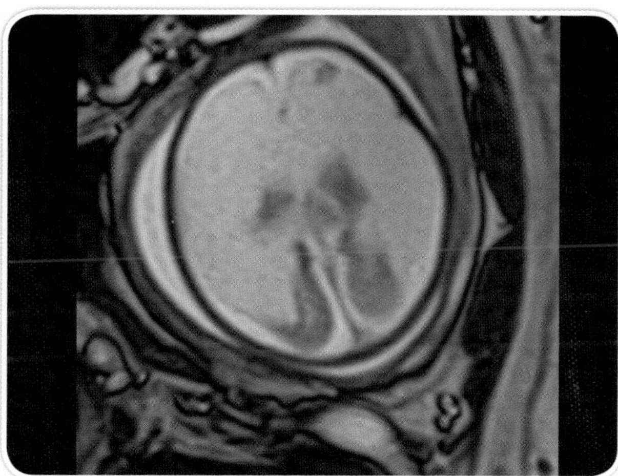

Hydranencephaly
- Grave prognosis
- Termination can be offered

ARACHNOID CYST

- It is lined by arachnoid membranes and filled with cerebrospinal fluid
- Primary maldevelopment of the arachnoid space or secondary to infection or hemorrhage
- It can be associated with other genetic syndrome and delayed developments.

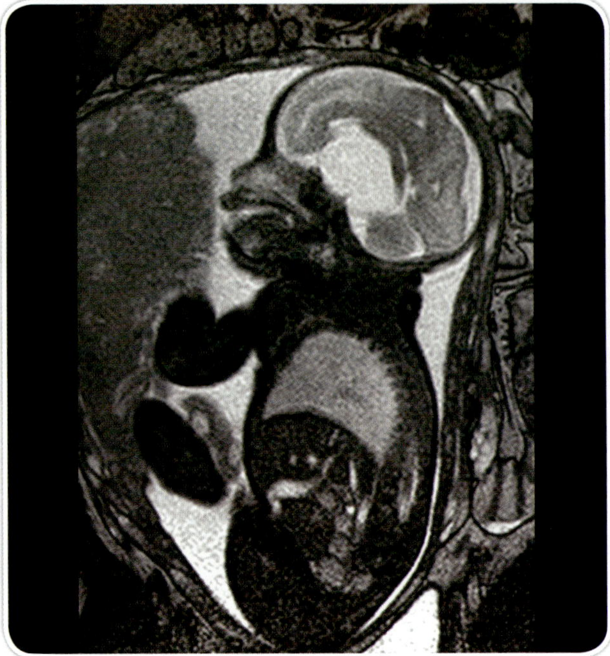

(Bannister et al. 1999)

Fetal MRI and Arachnoid Cyst

- To confirm the diagnosis
- To determine the invasion/compression to adjacent structures
- Aid in counseling by neuropedriatrician

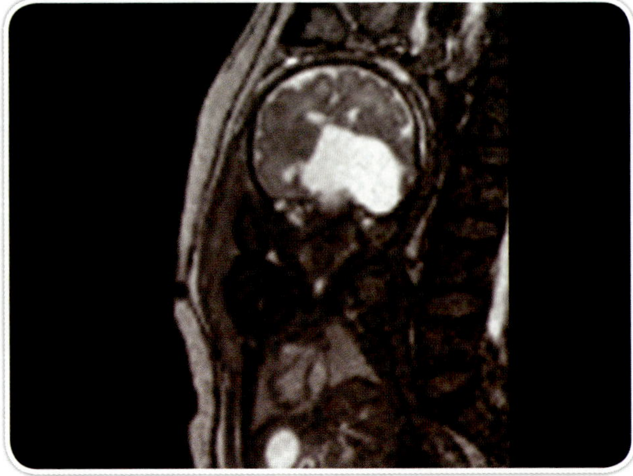

(Garel and Moutard, 2014)

Borderline Ventriculomegaly (11–15 mm)

- Its significance range from normal variation to something more serious
- MRI may be required to determine the real significance
- Associated temporal lobe lesion can be suggestive for cytomegalovirus infection and hearing deficit
- There were 44% ultrasound and 25% MRI examinations disagreement with postnatal diagnosis
- The most commons are migrational abnormalities, callosal dysgenesis/destruction and interval development of hemorrhage.

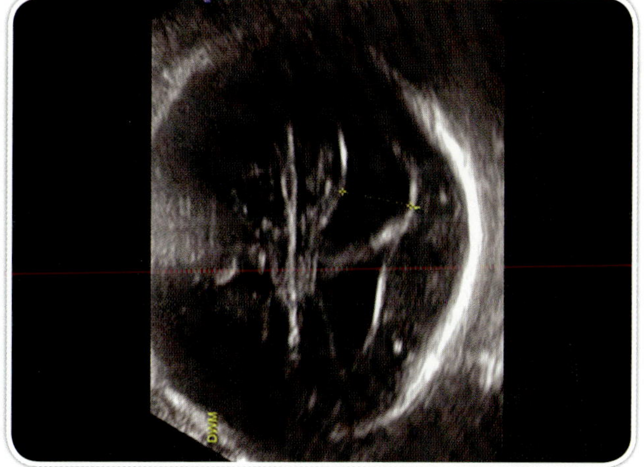

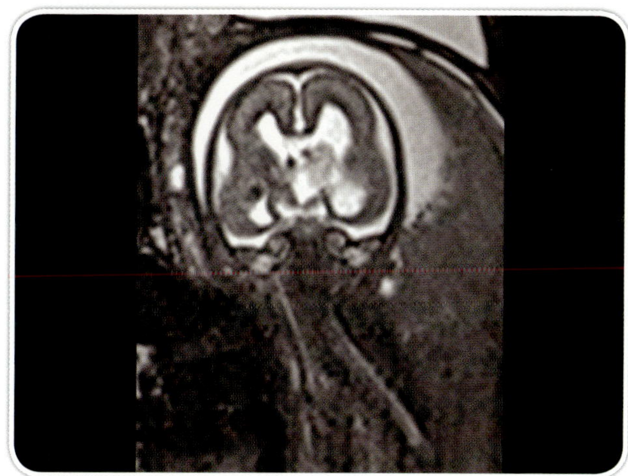

(Senapati et al. 2010)

SIGNIFICANCE OF VENTRICULOMEGALY

- In the era of widespread use of fetal MRI, even in community hospital, the simple diagnosis of 'fetal ventriculomegaly' may no longer satisfy the patients and their family.

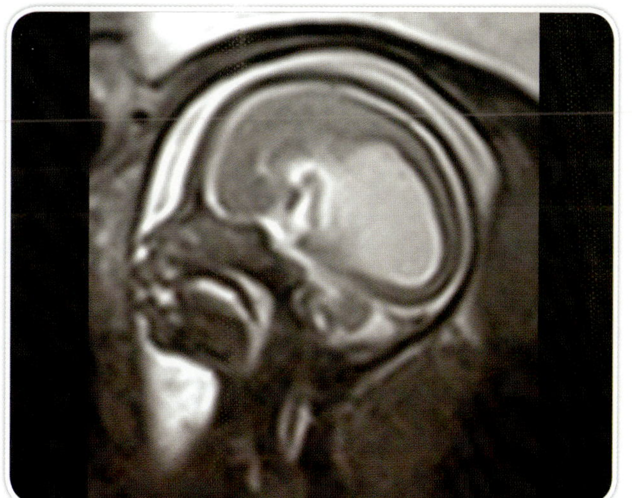

(Ghobrial et al. 2011)

SCHIZENCEPHALY

- Cerebral cortical cleft lined by gray matter
- MRI can show this gray matter lining, which separates it from porencephaly
- Developmental delay, especially in bilateral clefts.

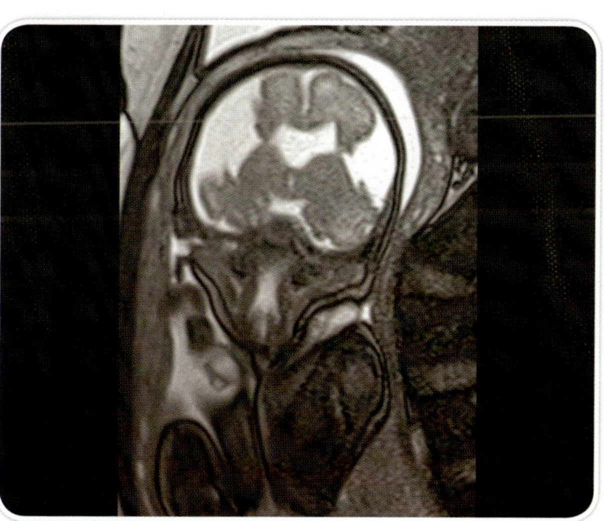

FETAL INFRATENTORIAL STRUCTURES

- Examination of cerebellum using ultrasound is markedly limited after 33 weeks', especially when the fetus is not in vertex position
- Myelomeningocele was associated with tonsillar herniation and a smaller posterior fossa
- MRI can be used to determine the degree of herniation before and after the antenatal surgical repair.

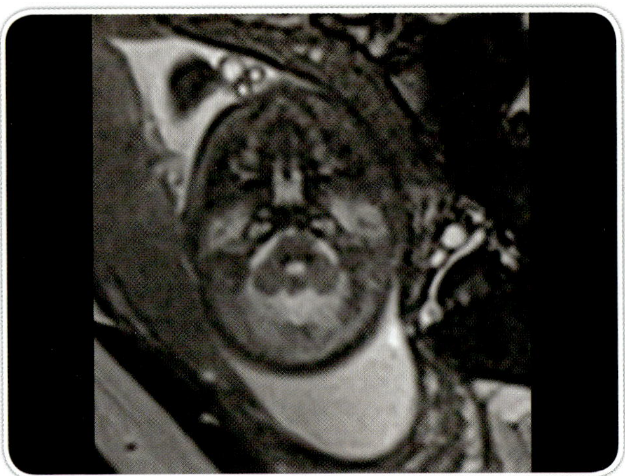

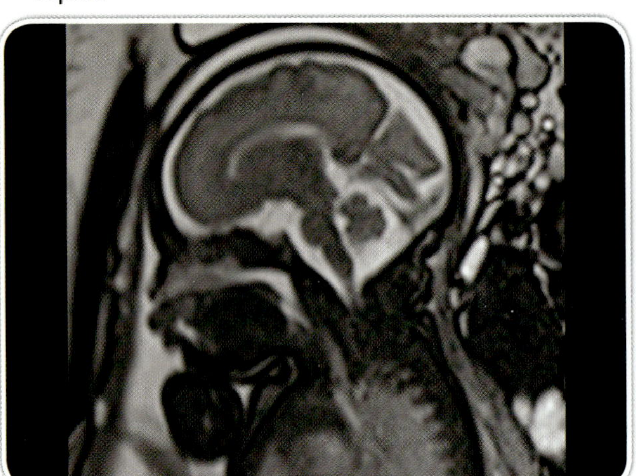

(Grant et al. 2011)

OCCIPITAL MENINGOCELE

- Herniation of meninges through the skull defect, most commonly at the occipital site
- Occipital cephaloceles are associated with genetic syndromes, amniotic band sequence, congenital rubella, and maternal diabetes (as shown in the picture).
- If brain tissue is seen in the sac from MRI (encephalocele), mortality rises to 44%, with 91% delayed development
- MRI may detect associated brain anomalies that may not be seen on the US.

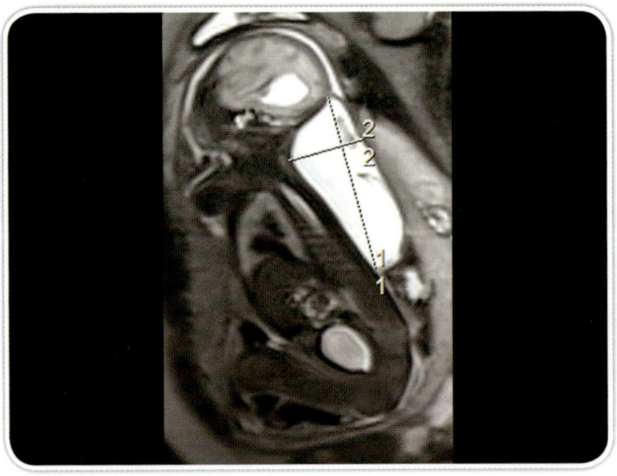

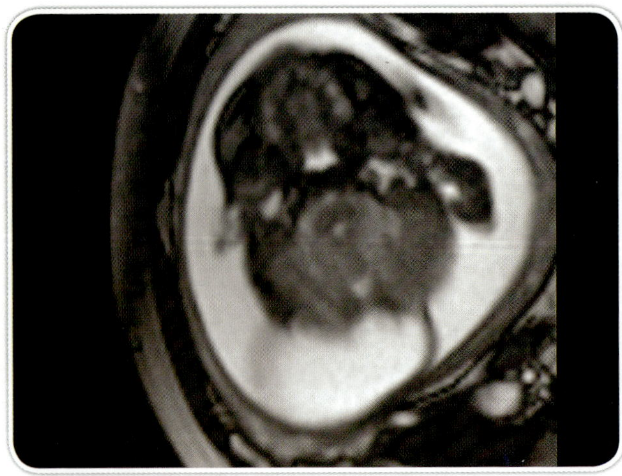

(Budorick et al. 1995)

FETAL MENINGOMYELOCELE

- Defect in the spinal column and skin, exposing the meninges and spinal cord
- Associated herniation of cerebellar vermis (Arnold-Chiari II) and hydrocephalus
- Congenital hip dislocation and clubfeet secondary to inervation deficits.

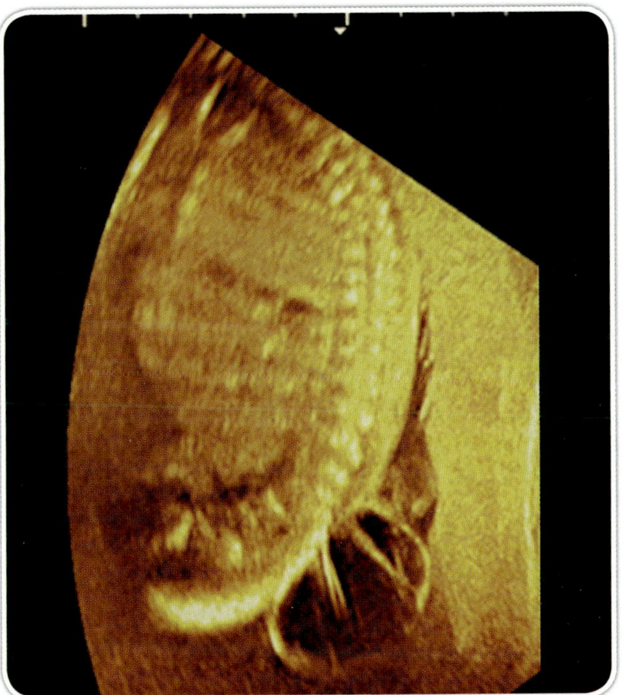

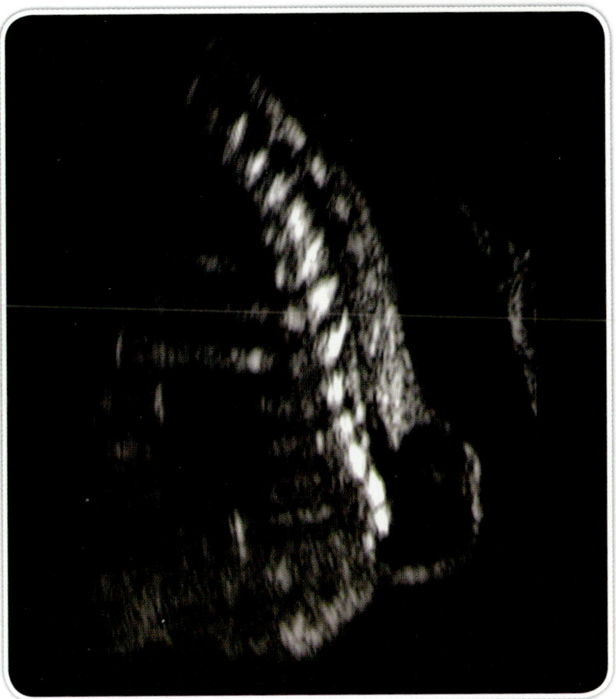

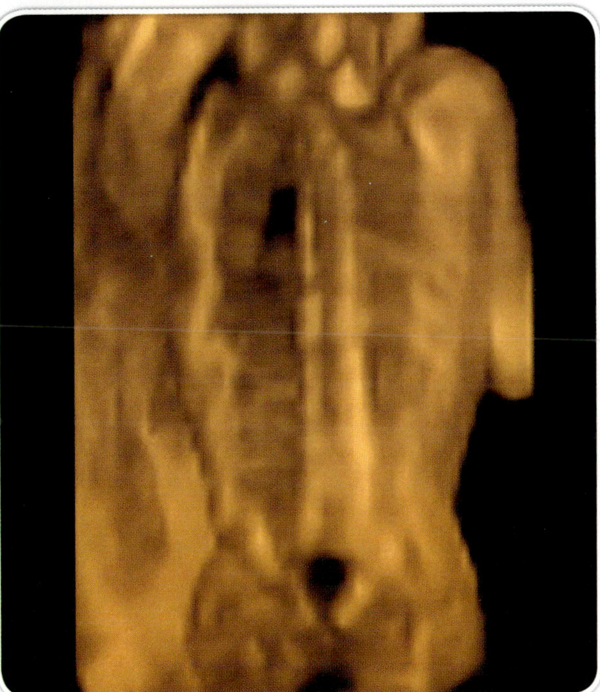

FETAL MENINGOMYELOCELE: INTRACRANIAL SIGNS

- 61% biparietal diameter lower than 5th percentile
- 25% head circumference lower than 5th percentile
- 77% dilated anterior cerebral ventricular horn
- 86% dilated posterior cerebral ventricular horn
- 77% scalloping frontal bone ('Lemon sign')
- 57% curved cerebellum ('banana sign').

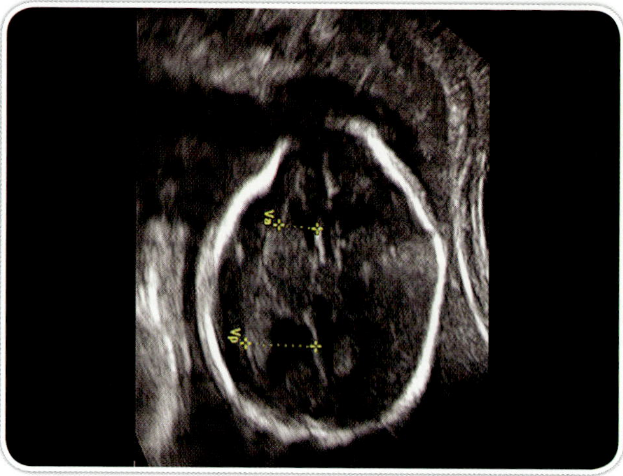

(Nicolaides et al. 1986)

Fetal Meningomyelocele

- Hindbrain herniation is also associated with apnea at birth
- This information is important for neonatal resuscitation.

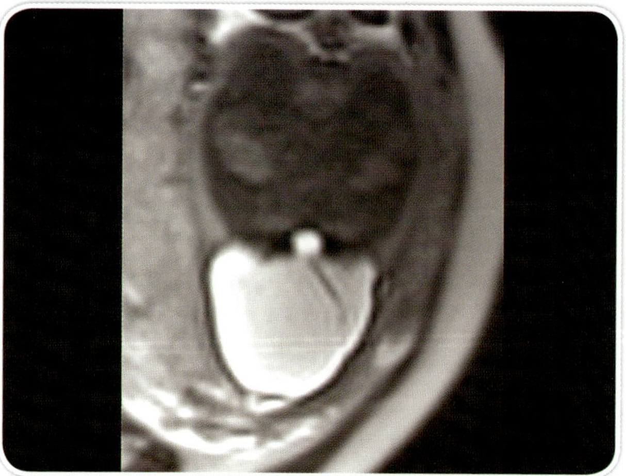

MRI and Antenatal Management

- MRI has been used to show hindbrain herniation in for a proper counseling and candidatation for in-utero repair
- In-utero repair in these selected cases can reduce the neurodeficiency.

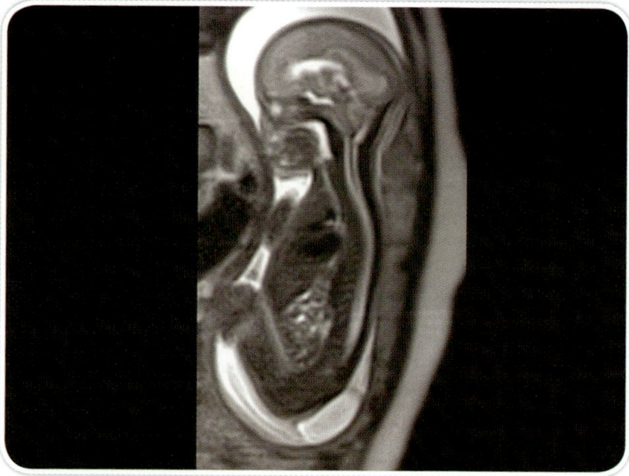

Sacral Defect without Hindbrain Herniation may Perform Well at Birth

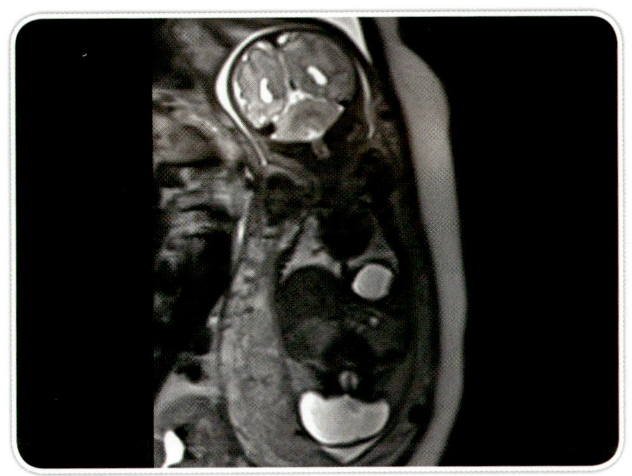

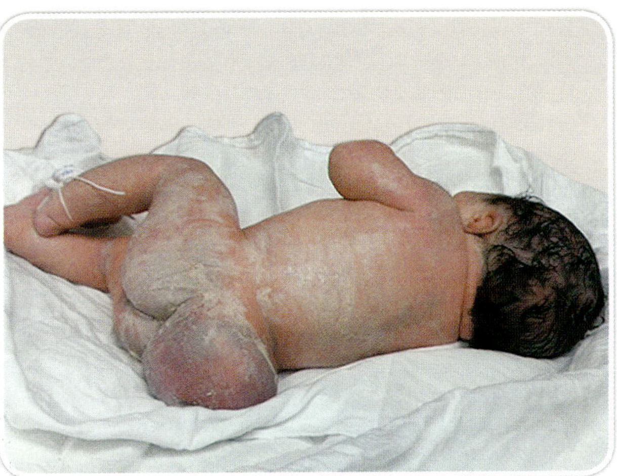

Fetal Soft Tissue/Cystic Tumor

- US may have limitations to determine the
  - Nature
  - Invasion of adjacent structures
  - Compression of adjacent structures.

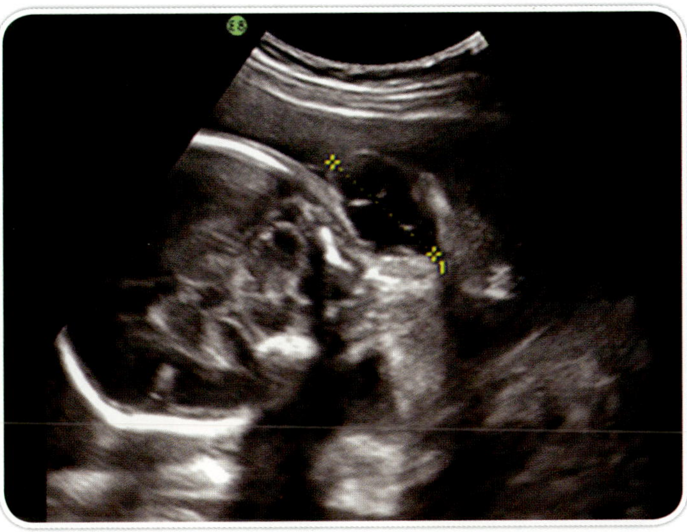

Fetal Lymphangioma

- Lymphangioma frequently develop in the anterior mediastinum or the thymus
- Cystic /multiseptated cyst on US
- Extension to the chest wall, the suprasternal area, or even into the retropharyngeal space.
- Fetal MRI can determine
  - Extent and progression
  - Differential diagnose with other fetal cystic tumors
  - Relationship with the airway: EXIT requirement
  - Mediastinal compression, leading to polyhydramnios and hydrops.
  - Associated pathologies.

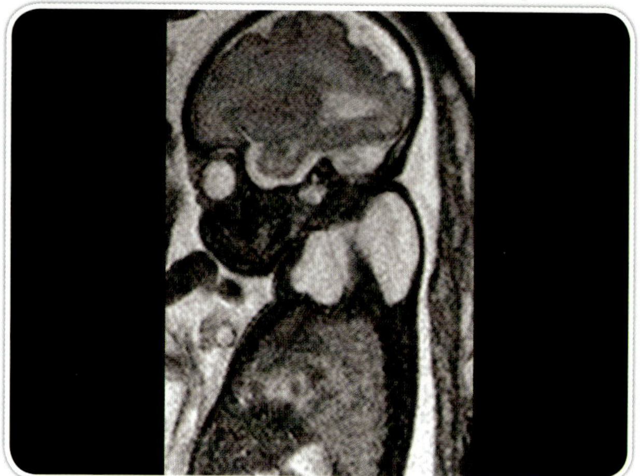

(Avni et al. 2009)

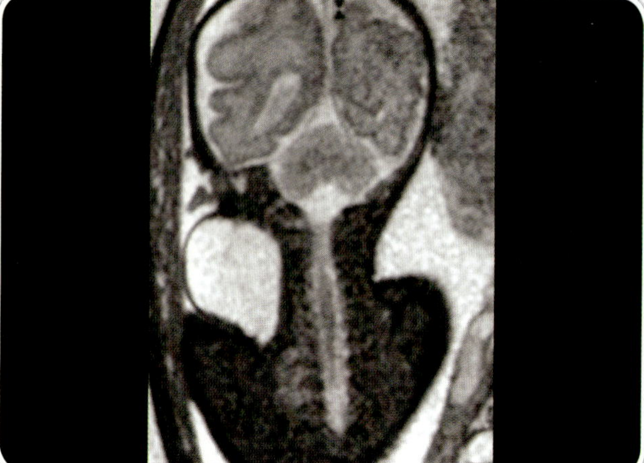

(Comstock et al. 2008)

MRI and Fetal Lymphangioma

- Fetal lymphangiomas display the same MRI features as postnatal lymphangiomas
- Airway management may be altered with respect to the type and location of the tumor.

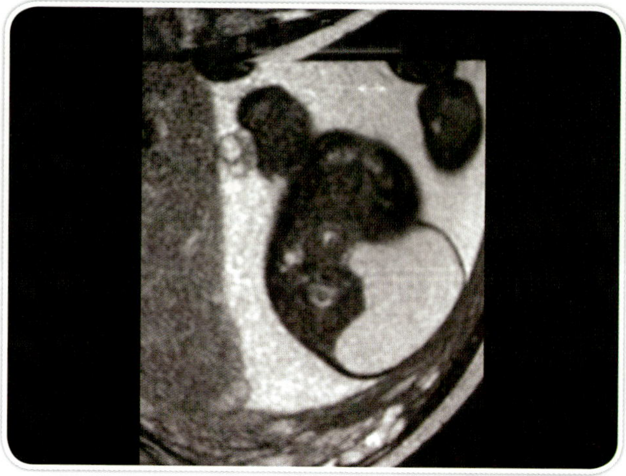

(Koelblinger et al. 2013)

Postnatal Appearance of Lymphangioma

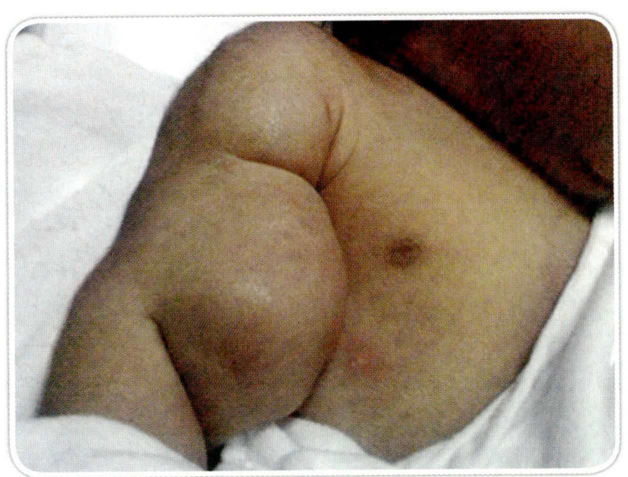

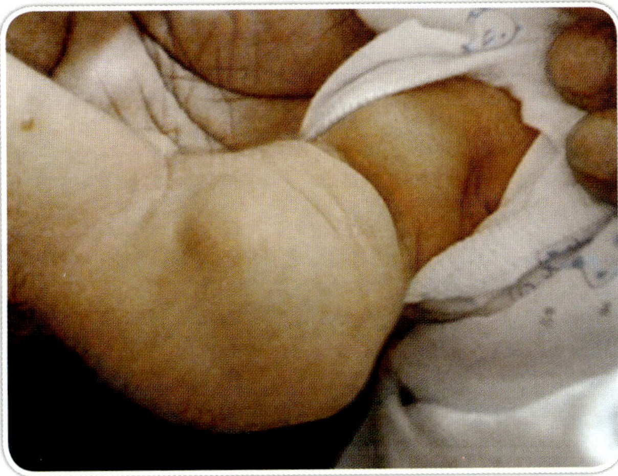

Fetal Solid Tumor

- Solid tumor at the anterior compartment of the fetal neck and chest
- Hyperextended position and polyhydramnios suggested for esophageal and/or airway compromise
- Ex-utero intrapartum treatment was successfully performed in this case.

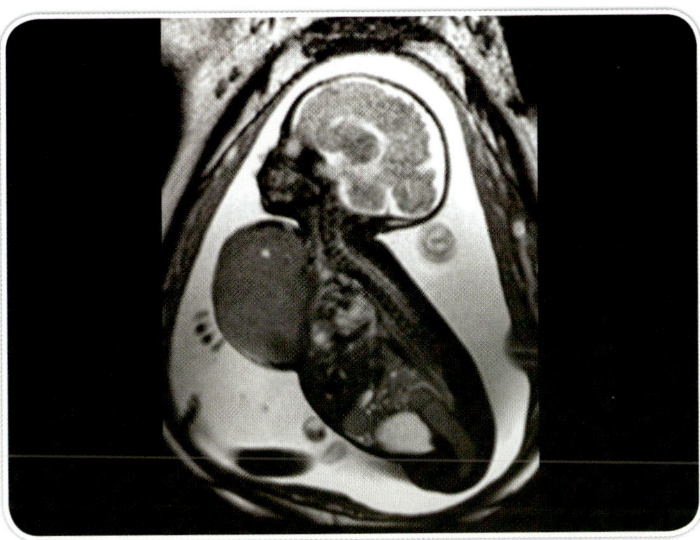

(Wataganara et al. 2007)

Fetal MRI and KUB Anomalies

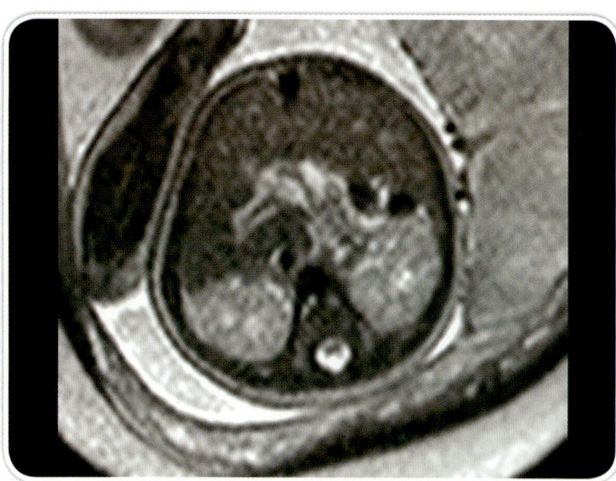

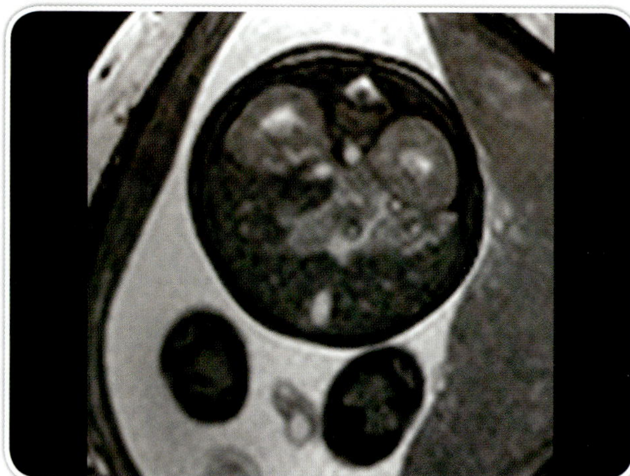

MRI signals of normal fetal kidneys

Fetal Bilateral Renal Agenesis

- Maternal body habitus, fetal position, and anhydramnios can preclude the diagnosis of renal aplasia/agenesis.
- Fetal MRI modified the diagnosis and altered management in 3 to 20% of the cases.

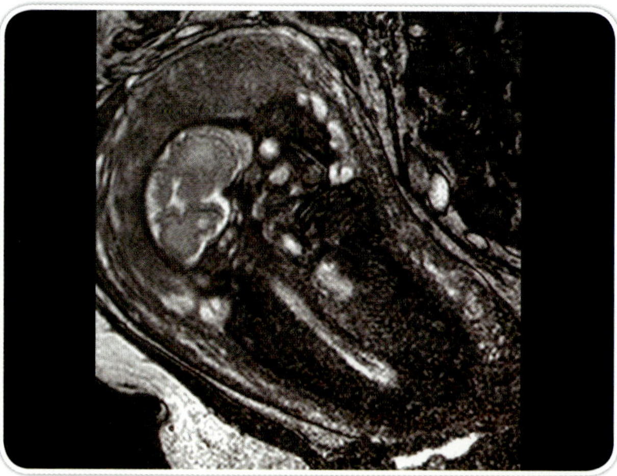

(Barseghyan et al. 2008)

Fetal Bladder Outlet Obstruction

- Posterior urethral valve is the most common cause of bilateral renal obstruction and dysplasia, hydronephrosis, oligohydramnios, and lung hypoplasia.
- US evaluation of non-functioning kidney in the presence of oligohydramnios is a challenge.

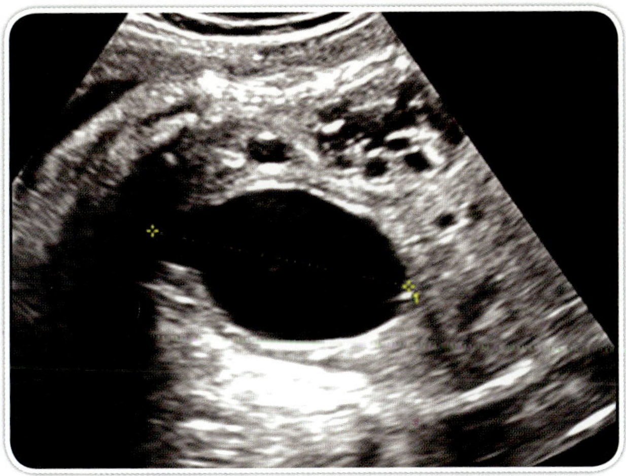

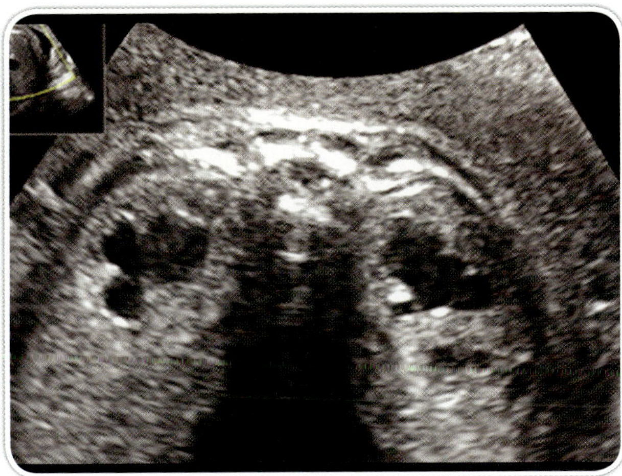

Fetal Posterior Urethral Valve

- Termination of pregnancy may be offered in the presence of bilateral, non-functioning kidneys
- Antenatal vesico-amniotic shunting or laser ablation of posterior urethral valve may be offered in the intact fetal renal parenchyma.

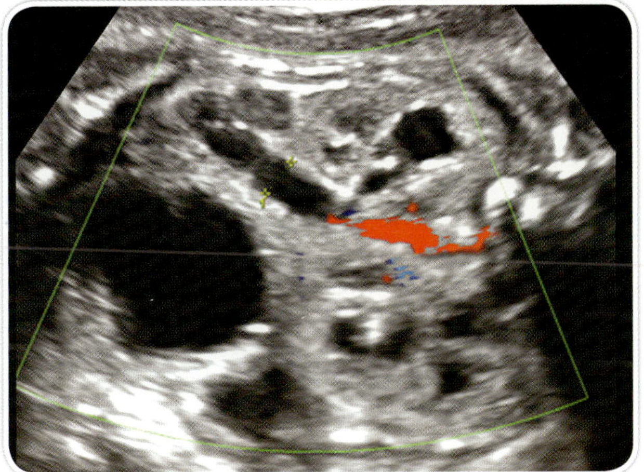

(Salam, 2006)

MRI of Fetal Posterior Urethral Valve

- Male fetus
- Dilatation of the urinary bladder and the proximal urethra
- Thickening of urinary bladder wall
- Reduced liquor volume.

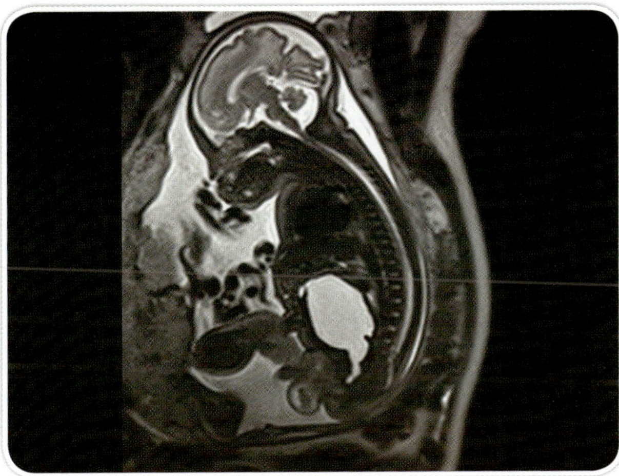

Fetal Kidney Deterioration in Posterior Urethral Valve

- Intact calyces
- Intact cortex
- Normal liquor

- Hydronephrosis
- Clubbed calyceal system
- Cortical thinning
- Reduced liquor

- Cortical scaring
- Anhydramnios

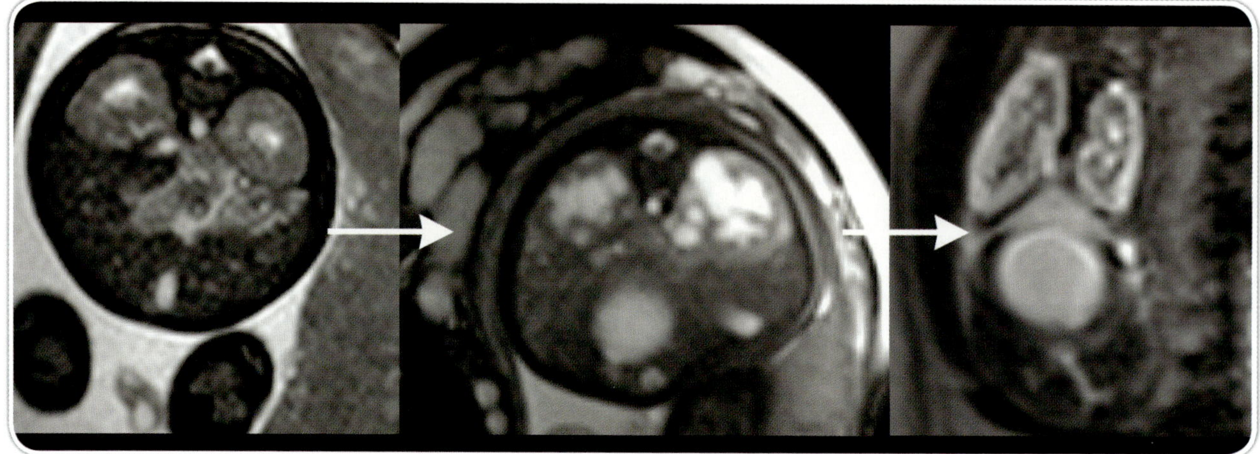

Ureteropelvic Junction (UPJ) Obstruction

- Unilateral/bilateral dilatation of pelvicalyceal system may indicate obstruction, reflux, or other complex KUB anomalies
- MRI can alter the diagnosis, that lead to different prenatal management in some cases.

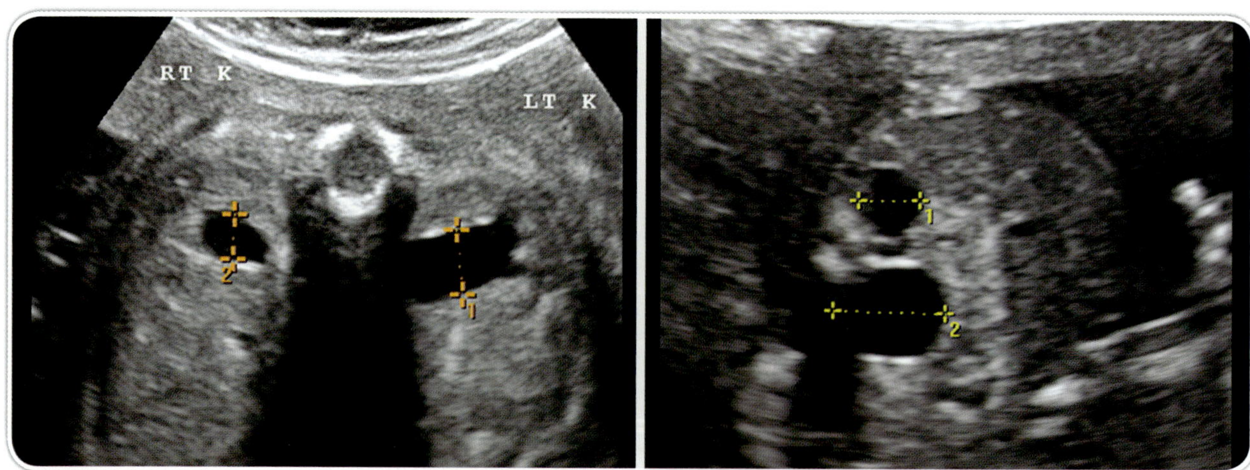

(Cassart et al. 2004)

MRI Feature of Bilateral UPJ Obstruction

- Anhydramnios (preclude accurate US assessment)
- Small bladder
- Dilatated calyces and thin cortex.

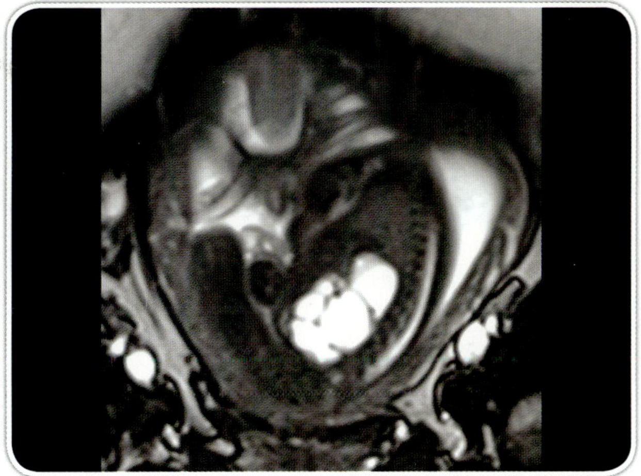

Large MRI Field of View

- Normal colon (exclude megacystis microcolon)
- Normal contralateral kidney (suggest better prognosis)
- Normal amniotic fluid (suggest better prognosis).

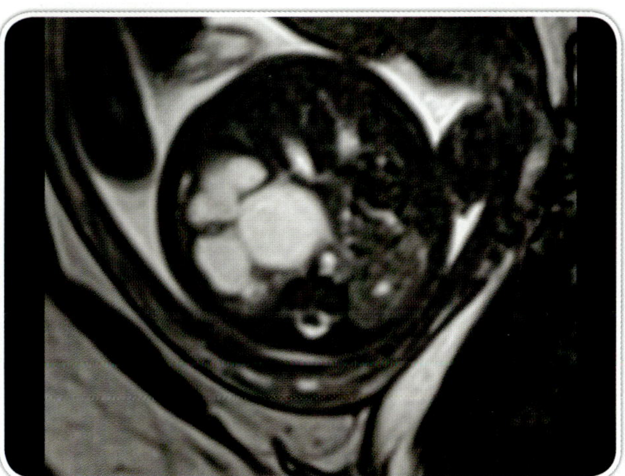

Fetal Sacrococcygeal Teratoma

- Multipotent germ cell tumor arising from Hensen node in the coccyx

(Mintz et al. 1978)

- Mortality 30–50% from heart failure and hydrops

(Flake et al. 1986)

- Pelvic invasion and bleeding.

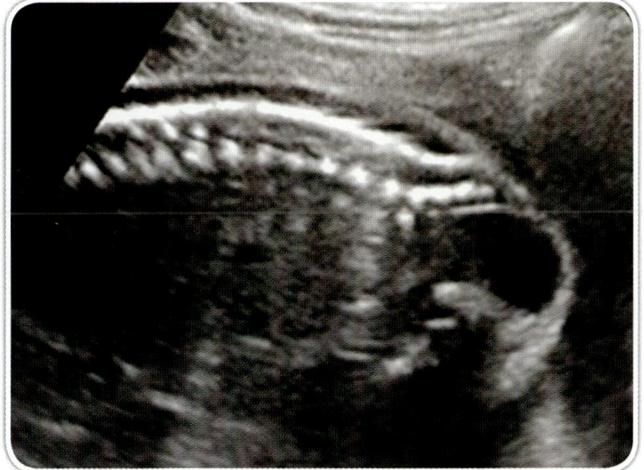

MRI Fetal Sacrococcygeal Teratoma

- Type I: Predominantly external
- Type II: Predominantly external + intrapelvic component
- Type III: Predominantly intrapelvic + intra-abdominal extension
- Type IV: Entirely intrapelvic + intra-abdominal.

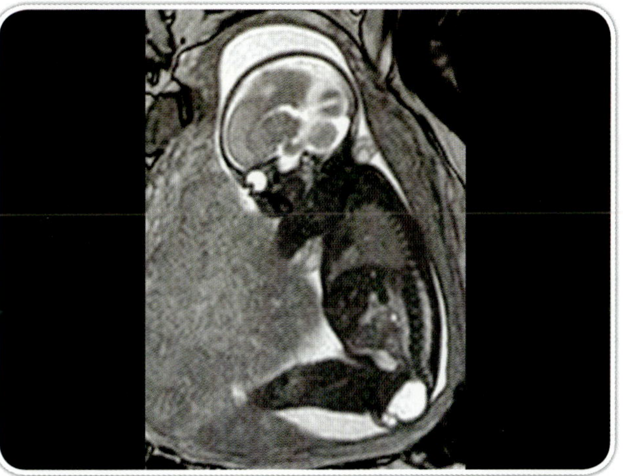

(American Academy of Pediatrics, Surgical Section)

Prediction of Successful Postnatal Resection

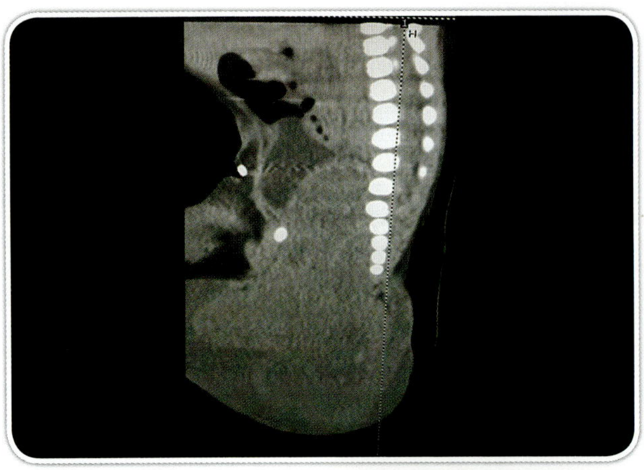

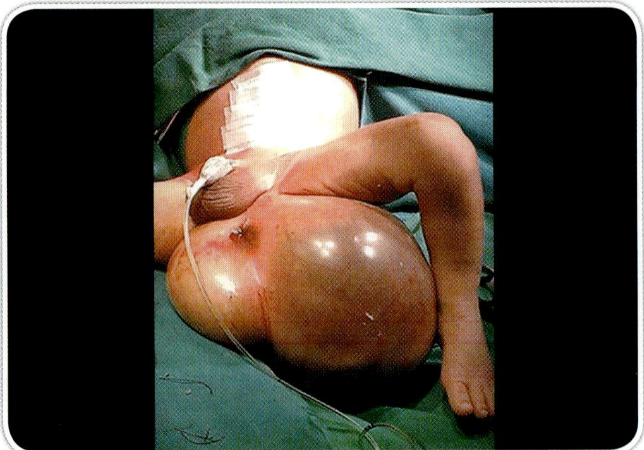

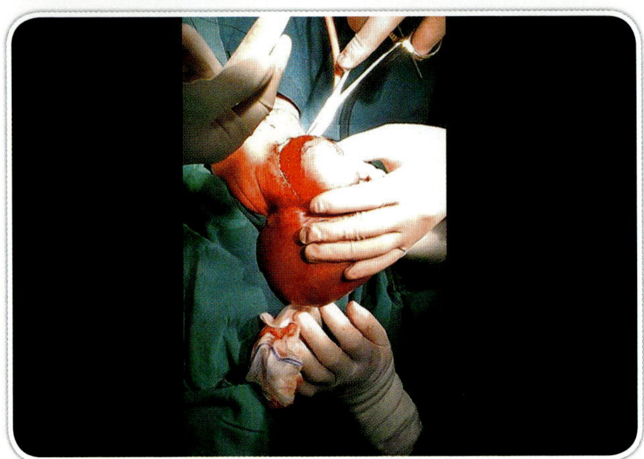

Limitations of Fetal MRI

- Motion artifact
- Maternal claustrophobia
- Maternal pacemaker and ferromagnetic implants.

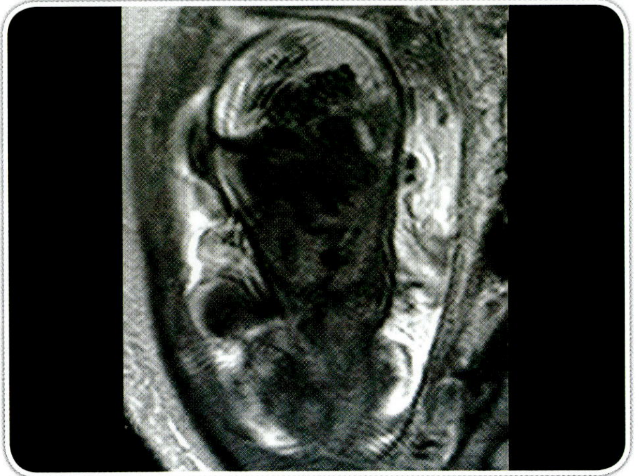

(Glenn et al. 2006)

Potential Pitfalls

Problems	Consequences	How to avoid
Polyhydramnios	Increased motion artifacts	Perform MRI immediately after amnioreduction
Maternal breathing	Increased motion artifacts	Breath-hold sequences (15 sec)

CONCLUSION

- Fetal MRI is unique for its multiplanar with great soft tissue delineation
- Maternal structure assessment; large field of view
- MRI is particularly useful in oligohydramnios and CDH.

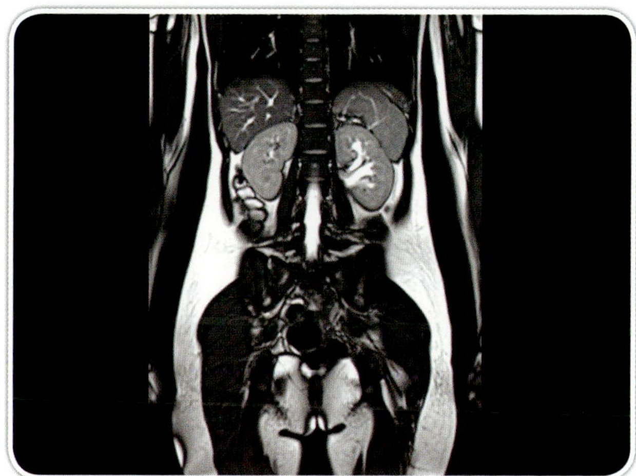

- Developing fetal anatomy and subtle changes can be reviewed by multi-speciality team
- Certain fetal therapy can be guided by MRI
- MRI can support immediate neonatal managements.

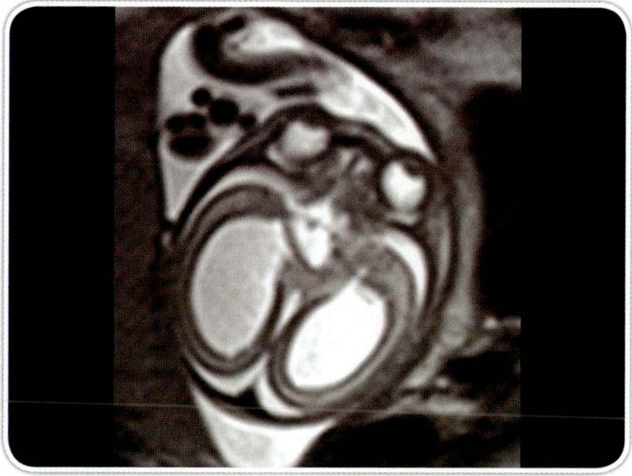

SUGGESTED READING

1. Albanese CT, Lopoo J, Goldstein RB, Filly RA, Feldstein VA, Calen PW, et al. Fetal liver position and perinatal outcome for congenital diaphragmatic hernia. Prenat Diagn.1998;18:1138-42.
2. Alfaraj MA, Shah PS, Bohn D, Pantazi S, O'Brien K, Chiu PP, et al. Congenital diaphragmatic hernia: lung-to-head ratio and lung volume for prediction of outcome. Am J Obstet Gynecol. 2011;205:43:e41-8.
3. Avni FE, Massez A, Cassart M, 2009. Tumours of the fetal body: a review. Pediatric Radiology. 2009;39:147-57.
4. Bannister CM, Russell SA, Rimmer S, Mowle DH. Fetal arachnoid cysts: their site, progress, prognosis and differential diagnosis. Eur J Ped Sur:Official Journal of Austrian Association of Pediatric Surgery. Zeitschrift fur Kinderchirurgie.1999 (Suppl 1); 27-8.
5. Barseghyan K, Jackson KA, Chmait R, De Filippo RE, Miller DA. Complementary roles of sonography and magnetic resonance imaging in the assessment of fetal urinary tract anomalies. J US Med:Official Journal of the American Institute of Ultrasound in Medicine. 2008;27:1563-9.
6. Ben-IshayO, Johnson VM, Wilson JM, Buchmiller TL. Congenital diaphragmatic hernia associated with esophageal atresia: incidence, outcomes, and determinants of mortality. J Am Col Surg. 2013;216: 90-5;e92.
7. Budorick NE, Pretorius DH, McGahan JP, Grafe MR, James HE, Slivka J. Cephalocele detection in utero: sonographic and clinical features. Ultrasound in Obstetrics & Gynecology: The Official Journal of the International Society of Ultrasound in Obstetrics and Gynecology. 1995;5:77-85.
8. Cassart M, Massez A, Metens T, Rypens F, Lambot MA, Hall M, et al. Complementary role of MRI after sonography in assessing bilateral urinary tract anomalies in the fetus. Am J Roentgen.2004;182:689-95.
9. Comstock CH, Lee W, Bronsteen RA, Vettraino I, Wechter D. Fetal mediastinal lymphangiomas. J US Med:Official Journal of the American Institute of Ultrasound in Medicine. 2008;27:145-8.
10. Derman AY, Nikac V, Haberman S, Zelenko N, Opsha O, Flyer M. MRI of placenta accreta: a new imaging perspective. Am J Roentgen. 2011;197:1514-21.
11. Flake AW, Harrison MR, Adzick NS, Laberge JM, Warsof SL. Fetal sacrococcygeal teratoma. J Ped Surg. 1986;21:563-6.
12. Garcia-Bournissen F, Shrim A, Koren G. Safety of gadolinium during pregnancy. Canadian family physician Medecin de famille canadien. 2006;52:309-10.
13. Garel C, Moutard ML. Main Congenital Cerebral Anomalies: How Prenatal Imaging Aids Counseling. Fetal diagnosis and therapy. 2014.
14. Ghobrial PM, Levy RA, O'Connor SC. The fetal magnetic resonance imaging experience in a large community medical center. J Clin Imaging Scien. 2011;1:29.
15. Glenn OA. Fetal central nervous system MR imaging. Neuroimaging clinics of North America. 2006;16:1-17.
16. Grant RA, Heuer GG, Carrion GM, Adzick NS, Schwartz ES, Stein SC, et al. Morphometric analysis of posterior fossa after in utero myelomeningocele repair. J Neur Ped. 2011;7:362-8.
17. Guimaraes CV, Linam LE, Kline-Fath BM, Donnelly LF, Calvo-Garcia MA, Rubio EI, et al. Prenatal MRI findings of fetuses with congenital high airway obstruction sequence. K J Radiol:Official Journal of the Korean Radiological Society. 2009;10:129-34.
18. Harrison MR. Tracheal occlusion works. Fetal diagnosis and therapy. 2011;29:78-9.
19. Kilian AK, Schaible T, Hofmann V, Brade J, Neff KW, Busing KA , et al. Congenital diaphragmatic hernia: predictive value of MRI relative lung-to-head ratio compared with MRI fetal lung volume and sonographic lung-to-head ratio. Am J Roentgen. 2009; 192:153-8.
20. Koelblinger C, Herold C, Nemec S, Berger-Kulemann V, Brugger PC, Koller A, et al. Fetal magnetic resonance imaging of lymphangiomas. J Perin Med. 2013;41:437-43.
21. Lim FY, Crombleholme TM, Hedrick HL, Flake AW, Johnson MP, Howell LJ, et al. Congenital high airway obstruction syndrome: natural history and management. J Ped Surg. 2003;38:940-5.
22. Mintz B, Cronmiller C, Custer RP. Somatic cell origin of teratocarcinomas. Proceedings of the National Academy of Sciences of the United States of America. 1978;75:2834-8.
23. Nicolaides KH, Campbell S, Gabbe SG, Guidetti R. Ultrasound screening for spina bifida: cranial and cerebellar signs. Lancet. 1986;2:72-4.
24. PoohRK. Sonogenetics in fetal neurology. Seminars in fetal and neonatal medicine. 2012;17:353-9.
25. Salam MA. Posterior urethral valve: Outcome of antenatal intervention. Inter J Urol:Official Journal of the Japanese Urological Association. 2006;13:1317-22.
26. Saleem SN. Fetal magnetic resonance imaging (MRI): a tool for a better understanding of normal and abnormal brain development. J Child Neur.2013; 28:890-908.
27. Senapati GM, Levine D, Smith C, Estroff JA, Barnewolt CE, Robertson RL, etal. Frequency and cause of disagreements in imaging diagnosis in children with ventriculomegaly diagnosed prenatally. US Obs & Gynec: The Official Journal of the International Society of Ultrasound in Obstetrics and Gynecology. 2010;36:582-95.
28. Senat MV, Bernard JP, Schwarzler P, Britten J, Ville Y. Prenatal diagnosis and follow-up of 14 cases of unilateral ventriculomegaly. US Obs & Gynec:The Official Journal of the International Society of Ultrasound in Obstetrics and Gynecology. 1999;14:327-32.
29. Shih JC, Palacios Jaraquemada JM, Su YN, Shyu MK, Lin CH, Lin SY, et al. Role of three-dimensional power Doppler in the antenatal diagnosis of placenta accreta: comparison with gray-scale and color Doppler techniques. US Obs & Gynec: The Official Journal of the International Society of Ultrasound in Obstetrics and Gynecology. 2009;33:193-203.

30. Smith FW, Adam AH, Phillips WD. NMR imaging in pregnancy. Lancet. 1983;1:61-2.
31. Stecco A, Saponaro A, Carriero A. Patient safety issues in magnetic resonance imaging: state of the art. La Radiologia medica. 2007; 112:491-508.
32. WataganaraT, Ngerncham S, Kitsommart R, Fuangtharnthip P. Fetal neck myofibroma. J Med Assoc of Thailand (Chotmaihet thangphaet). 2007;90:376-80.
33. Wenstrom KD. Fetal surgery for congrnital diaphragmatic hernia. The New Eng J Med. 2003;349:1887-8.
34. Yamasaki M, Nonaka M, Bamba Y, Teramoto C, Ban C, Pooh RK. Diagnosis, treatment, and long-term outcomes of fetal hydrocephalus. Seminars in fetal and neonatal medicine. 2012;17:330-5.
35. Zhang ZQ, Huang XM, Lu H. Early biomarkers as predictors for bronchopulmonary dysplasia in preterm infants: a systematic review. Eur J Ped. 2014;173:15-23.

Chapter 21

Perfect Baby: Imperfect Expectations

Frank A Chervenak

PERINATAL MEDICINE

Promotes Pursuit of the Perfect Baby

- Imaging
- Genetics
- Fetal treatment
- Consumer Rights Movement
- Termination of pregnancy
- Prematurity and obstetrics
- Prematurity and neonatology

Imaging

- Rapid and dramatic advances in fetal imaging
  - Ultrasound 3D–4D
  - MRI
- Different views
  - Perinatologist sees fetal anatomy and physiology
  - Pregnant woman sees something more arresting and powerful
- The woman's experience of "seeing" the "first baby pictures" can create significant bonding
- Medicine's ability to see what was previously hidden/mysterious, leads to the belief for an ability to control human biology.

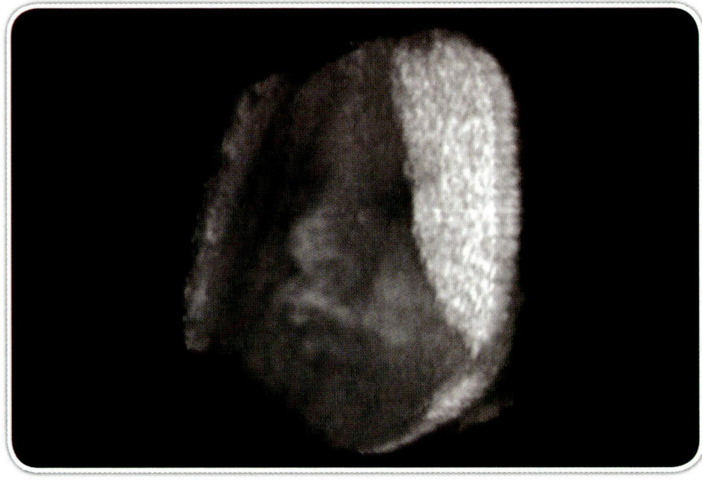

Genetics

- Karyotyping can promote binomial thinking
- Either there is a genomic anomaly or not
- Absence of anomaly results in reassurance
- Microarray analysis simply expands the scope of binomial thinking
- Lay translation: Either something is wrong or everything is fine.

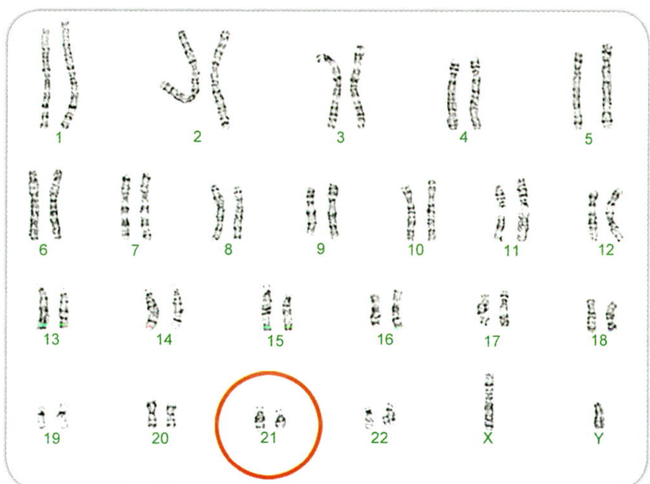

Fetal Treatment

- Fetal imaging and molecular genetics allows for an accurate fetal diagnosis
- "Fetus as a Patient" ethical concept
- Fetal therapy is an expanding option
- Steroid therapy, Rhogam®, and intrauterine blood transfusion: EFFECTIVE
- **Miracles:** Innovative fetal therapy
- Public expectation in the power of perinatal medicine to control human reproductive biology, with few or no limits.

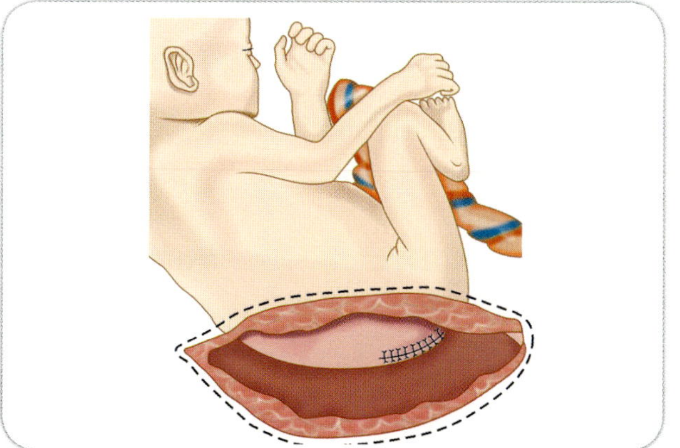

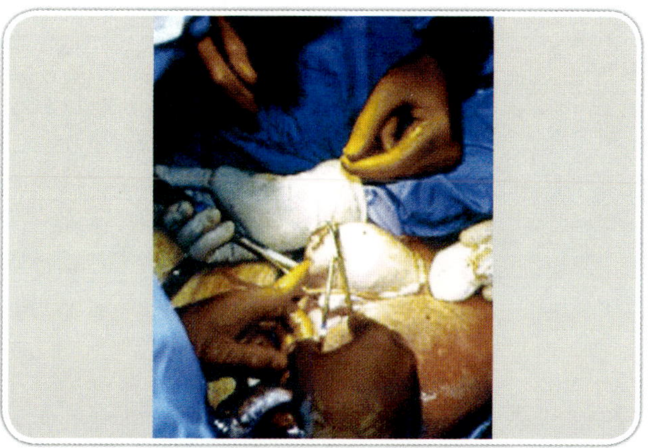

For complete presentation, please refer the accompanying CD-ROM...

SUGGESTED READING

1. Chervenak FA, McCullough LB, Brent RL. The perils of the imperfect expectation of the perfect baby. Am J Obstet Gynecol 2010;203(2):e1-5.

Chapter

22

Ultrasound Diagnosis of Morbidly Adherent Placenta

Giuseppe Cali

MORBIDLY ADHERENT PLACENTA

- Definition
- Pathogenesis
- Epidemiology
- Diagnosis 2nd and 3rd trimester

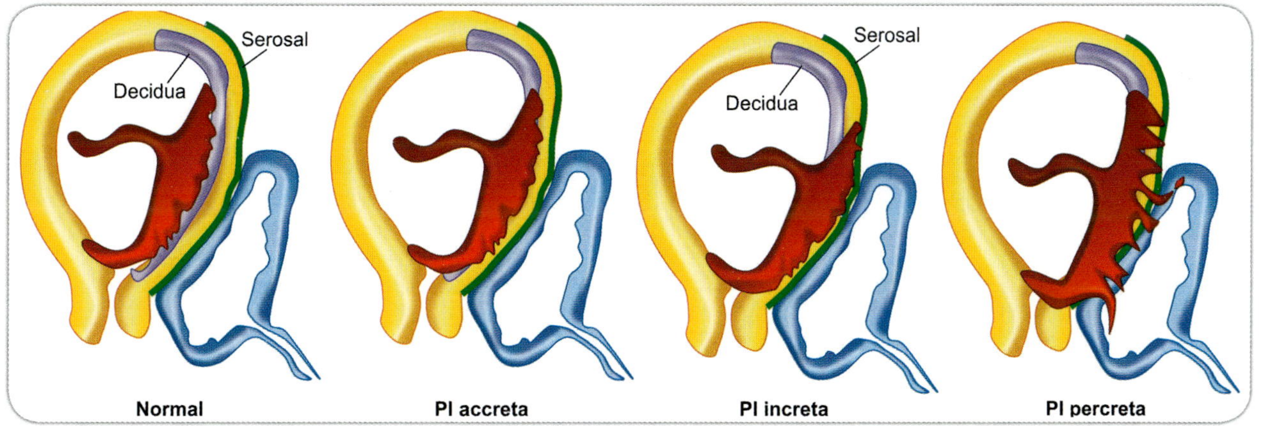

- **Placenta accreta:**
  - A placenta that is abnormally adherent to the uterus
- **Basal decidua** is an ineffective barrier.

Epidemiology

- 1/7,000 deliveries before 1970 — *Breen JL et al. 1977*
- 1/1,851 deliveries between 1996 and 2002
- 1/840 deliveries between 2002 and 2008 — *Eller AG et al. 2009*
- Between 1/540 and 1/2,500 today — *Hull AD et al. 2011*

6 Previous CS!!!

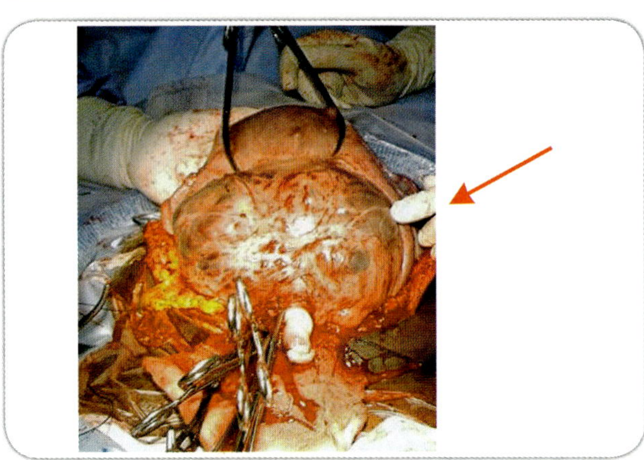

Risk of Placenta Adherent

• Pl previa	5 %
• Pl previa + 1 Previous CS	24 %
• Pl previa + 2 Previous CS	35 %
• Pl previa + 3 Previous CS	51 %
• Pl previa + 4 Previous CS	**67 %**

Clark SL, Koonings PP, Phelan JP. Placenta previa/accreta and prior cesarean section. Obstet Gynecol 1985;66:89–92.

Risk of Placenta Adherent

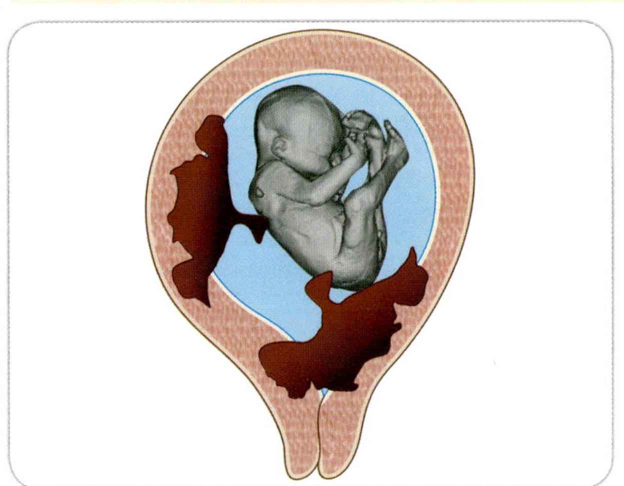

Total 155.670 delivery

- 0.04% in patients without pl previa
- 9.3% in patients with pl previa
- 2% in patients < 35 years/NO CS
- 39% patients ≥ 35 years + 2 CS

Miller DA, Am J Obstet Gyneco 1997

Risk Factors

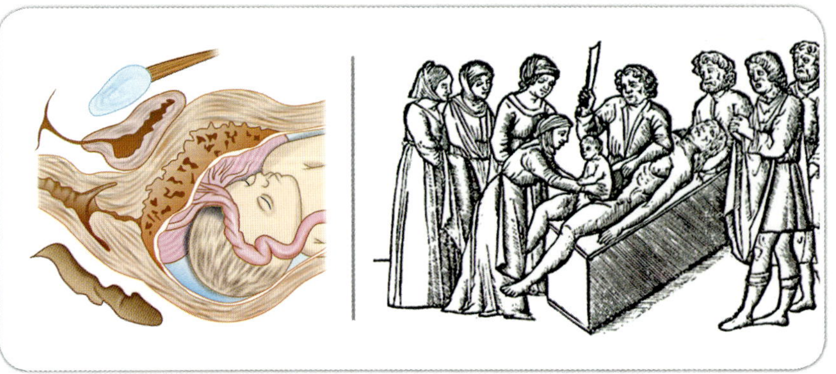

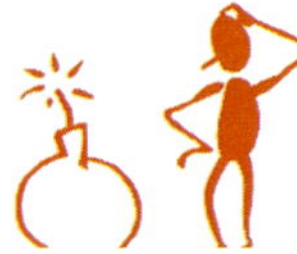

- **Placenta previa**
- **Previous TC**
- Previous uterine surgery
- Advanced maternal age
- Multiparity
- ↑α-fetoprotein

For complete presentation, please refer the accompanying CD-ROM...

SUGGESTED READING

1. Breen JL, Neubecker R, Gregori CA, Franklin JE Jr. Placenta accreta, increta, and percreta. A survey of 40 cases. Obstetrics and gynecology. 1977;49(1):43-7. PubMed PMID: 299782.
2. Cali G, Forlani F. Three-dimensional sonographic virtual cystoscopy in a case of placenta percreta. Ultrasound in obstetrics & gynecology : the official journal of the International Society of Ultrasound in Obstetrics and Gynecology. 2014;43(4):481-2. PubMed PMID: 24481639.
3. Cali G, Giambanco L, Puccio G, Forlani F. Morbidly adherent placenta: evaluation of ultrasound diagnostic criteria and differentiation of placenta accreta from percreta. Ultrasound in obstetrics & gynecology : the official journal of the International Society of Ultrasound in Obstetrics and Gynecology. 2013;41(4):406-12. PubMed PMID: 23288834.
4. Chou MM, Tseng JJ, Ho ES, Hwang JI. Three-dimensional color power Doppler imaging in the assessment of uteroplacental neovascularization in placenta previa increta/percreta. Am J Obstet and Gynecol. 2001;185(5):1257-60. PubMed PMID: 11717667.
5. Chou MM, Tseng JJ, Ho ES. The application of three-dimensional color power Doppler ultrasound in the depiction of abnormal uteroplacental angioarchitecture in placenta previa percreta. Ultrasound in obstetrics & gynecology : the official journal of the International Society of Ultrasound in Obstetrics and Gynecology. 2002;19(6):625-7. PubMed PMID: 12047547.
6. Clark SL, Koonings PP, Phelan JP. Placenta previa/accreta and prior cesarean section. Obstetrics and gynecology. 1985;66(1):89-92. PubMed PMID: 4011075.
7. Comstock CH, Bronsteen RA. The antenatal diagnosis of placenta accreta. BJOG : an international journal of obstetrics and gynaecology. 2014;121(2):171-81;discussion 81-2. PubMed PMID: 24373591.
8. D'Antonio F, Iacovella C, Bhide A. Prenatal identification of invasive placentation using ultrasound: systematic review and meta-analysis. Ultrasound in obstetrics & gynecology: The Official Journal of the International Society of Ultrasound in Obstetrics and Gynecology. 2013;42(5):509-17. PubMed PMID: 23943408.
9. D'Antonio F, Iacovella C, Palacios-Jaraquemada J, Bruno CH, Manzoli L, Bhide A. Prenatal identification of invasive placentation using magnetic resonance imaging: systematic review and meta-analysis. Ultrasound in obstetrics & gynecology : the official journal of the International Society of Ultrasound in Obstetrics and Gynecology. 2014;44(1):8-16. PubMed PMID: 24515654.
10. Eller AG, Bennett MA, Sharshiner M, Masheter C, Soisson AP, Dodson M, et al. Maternal morbidity in cases of placenta accreta managed by a multidisciplinary care team compared with standard obstetric care. Obstetrics and gynecology. 2011;117(2,Pt 1):331-7. PubMed PMID: 21309195.
11. Eller AG, Porter TF, Soisson P, Silver RM. Optimal management strategies for placenta accreta. BJOG : An International Journal of Obstetrics and Gynaecology. 2009;116(5):648-54. PubMed PMID: 19191778.
12. Hull AD, Moore TR. Multiple repeat cesareans and the threat of placenta accreta: incidence, diagnosis, management. Clinics in perinatology. 2011;38(2):285-96. PubMed PMID: 21645796.
13. Hull AD, Salerno CC, Saenz CC, Pretorius DH. Three-dimensional ultrasonography and diagnosis of placenta percreta with bladder involvement. Journal of ultrasound in medicine : official journal of the American Institute of Ultrasound in Medicine. 1999;18(12):853-6. PubMed PMID: 10591451.
14. Miller DA, Chollet JA, Goodwin TM. Clinical risk factors for placenta previa-placenta accreta. American journal of obstetrics and gynecology. 1997;177(1):210-4. PubMed PMID: 9240608.
15. O'Brien JM, Barton JR, Donaldson ES. The management of placenta percreta: conservative and operative strategies. Am J Obstet and Gynecol. 1996;175(6):1632-8. PubMed PMID: 8987952.
16. Shih JC, Palacios Jaraquemada JM, Su YN, Shyu MK, Lin CH, Lin SY, et al. Role of three-dimensional power Doppler in the antenatal diagnosis of placenta accreta: comparison with gray-scale and color Doppler techniques. Ultrasound in obstetrics & gynecology : the official journal of the International Society of Ultrasound in Obstetrics and Gynecology. 2009;33(2):193-203. PubMed PMID: 19173239.
17. Thia EW, Lee SL, Tan HK, Tan LK. Ultrasonographical features of morbidly-adherent placentas. Singapore medical journal. 2007;48(9):799-802;quiz3. PubMed PMID: 17728958.
18. Timor-Tritsch IE, Monteagudo A, Cali G, Palacios-Jaraquemada JM, Maymon R, Arslan AA, et al. Cesarean scar pregnancy and early placenta accreta share common histology. Ultrasound in obstetrics & gynecology : the official journal of the International Society of Ultrasound in Obstetrics and Gynecology. 2014;43(4):383-95. PubMed PMID: 24357257.
19. Timor-Tritsch IE, Monteagudo A, Cali G, Vintzileos A, Viscarello R, Al-Khan A, et al. Cesarean scar pregnancy is a precursor of morbidly adherent placenta. US Obstet and Gynecol: The Official Journal of the International Society of Ultrasound in Obstetrics and Gynecology. 2014;44(3):346-53. PubMed PMID: 24890256.
20. Timor-Tritsch IE, Monteagudo A. Unforeseen consequences of the increasing rate of cesarean deliveries: early placenta accreta and cesarean scar pregnancy. A review. Am J Obstet and Gynecol. 2012;207(1):14-29. PubMed PMID: 22516620.
21. Yang JI, Lim YK, Kim HS, Chang KH, Lee JP, Ryu HS. Sonographic findings of placental lacunae and the prediction of adherent placenta in women with placenta previa totalis and prior Cesarean section. Ultrasound in obstetrics & gynecology : the official journal of the International Society of Ultrasound in Obstetrics and Gynecology. 2006;28(2):178-82. PubMed PMID: 16858740.

Chapter

23

Preeclampsia Screening

Tuangsit Wataganara

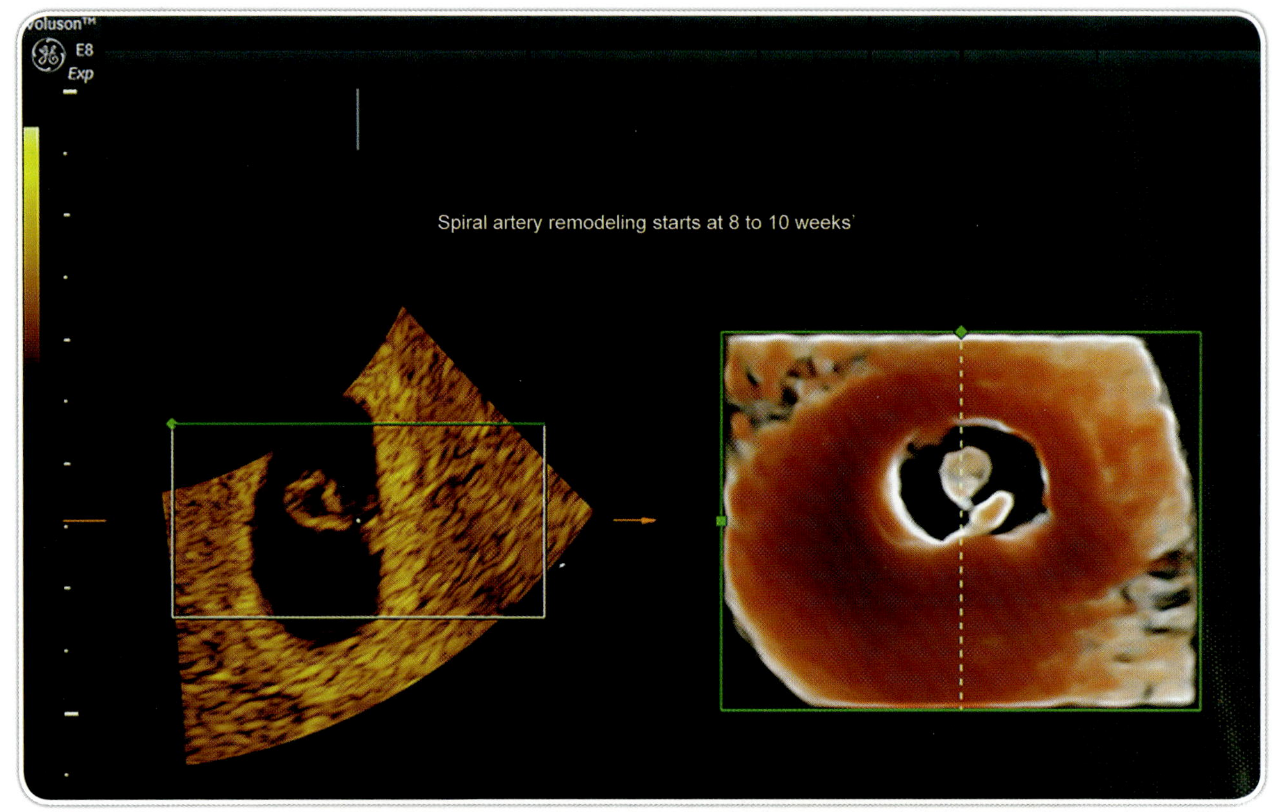

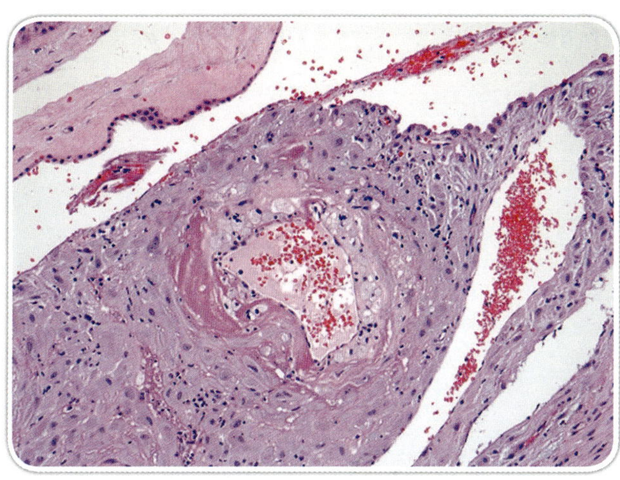

Villous Trophoblast: Cytotrophoblast

PlGF	Fetal DNA/RNA
Flt-1	ADAM12
Endoglin	PAPP-A

Villous Trophoblast: Syncytiotrophoblast

PlGF	Fetal DNA/RNA
sFlt-1	ADAM12
sEndoglin	PAPP-A
PP13	

- Decidual vasculopathy of the spiral artery
- Angiogenic markers released from trophoblasts.

(Modified from Cetin et al. 2011)

Maternal Tissues

P-selectin	Pentraxin-3
PlGF	sFlt-1
sEndoglin	VEGF

Extravillous Trophoblast

PlGF	Fetal DNA/RNA
sFlt-1	ADAM12 (?)
sEndoglin (?)	PAPP-A (?)

Pro-angiogenic factors
- Vascular endothelial growth factor (VEGF)
- Placental growth factor (PlGF)

Anti-angiogenic factors
- Soluble fms-like tyrosine kinase-1 (sFlt-1)
- Soluble endoglin (sEng)

Remodeling of spiral arteries

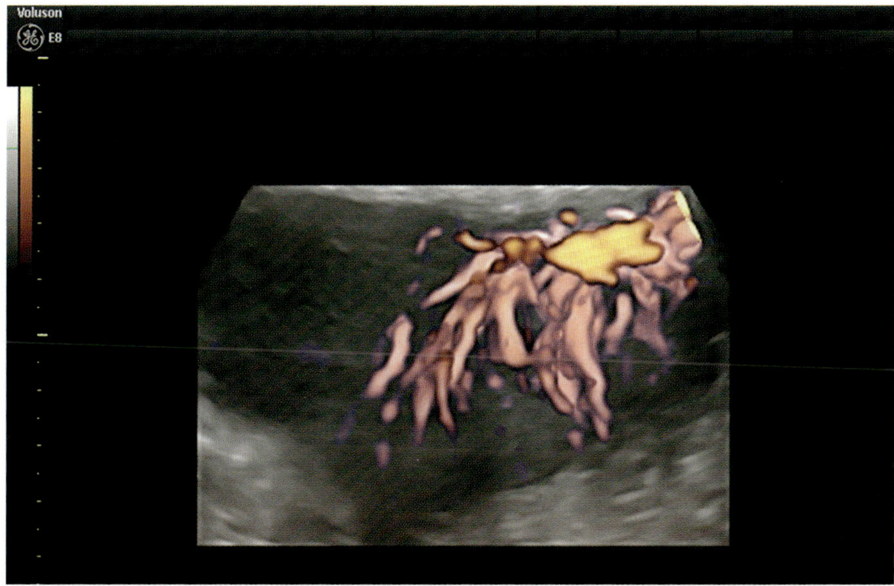

SERUM BIOMARKERS AND PREECLAMPSIA

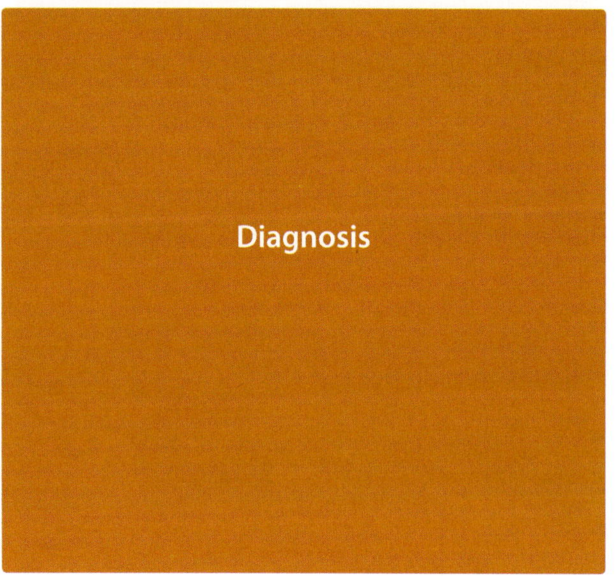

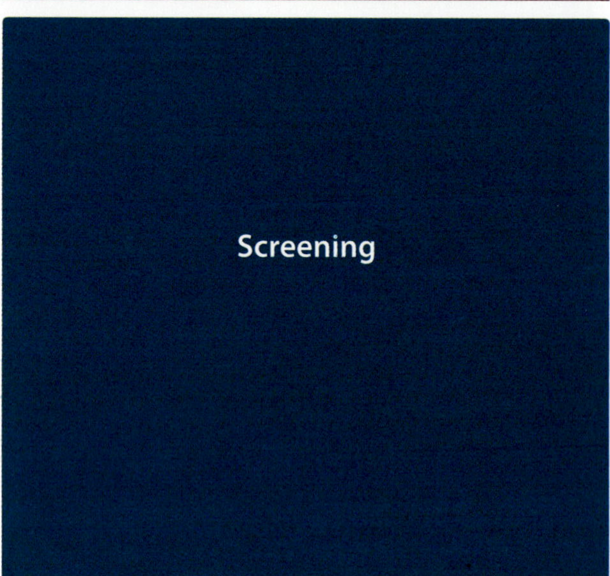

Diagnosis of Preeclampsia: Changing of the landscape

- Preeclampsia is a syndrome before 'eclampsia'
- Edema has been eliminated in 2002. The definition was switched to '**new onset of proteinuric hypertension**'
- Nonproteinuric preeclampsia in 2012. The definition was elusive, yet again. Limitations of the conventional cut-off for 24 hours proteinuria during pregnancy
- **Non-hypertensive preeclampsia?**

What is Preeclampsia, Really?

- Endothelial dysfunction during pregnancy as a result of trophoblast derived vasoactive mediators
- HELLP syndrome, and multiple organ failure
- Recent insights into the pathophysiology of preeclampsia including the role of angiogenic imbalances.

Development of Freshly Dissociated Human Umbilical Vein Endothelial Cell Preparation for Electrophysiological Studies

Wuttinan Theerathananon[1], Wattana B. Wattanapa[1,], Tuangsit Wataganara[2]*
[1]Department of Physiology and [2] Department of Obstetrics and Gynecology, Faculty of Medicine Siriraj Hospital, Mahidol University, Bangkok 10700, Thailand

- Cells isolated from human umbilical vein that has been kept in culture for 48 hours
- Note the abundance and the morphology typical of endothelial cells

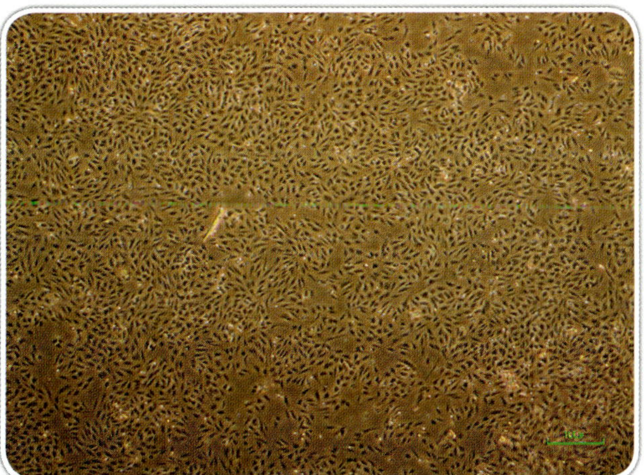

- Immunofluorescent staining
- Isolated cells were stained positive for VEGFR-2 shown in CY3 red.

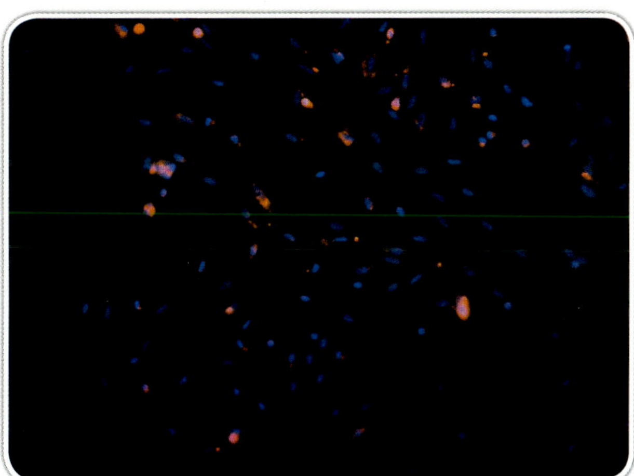

- Immunofluorescent staining
- Isolated cells were stained positive for vWF shown in FITC green.

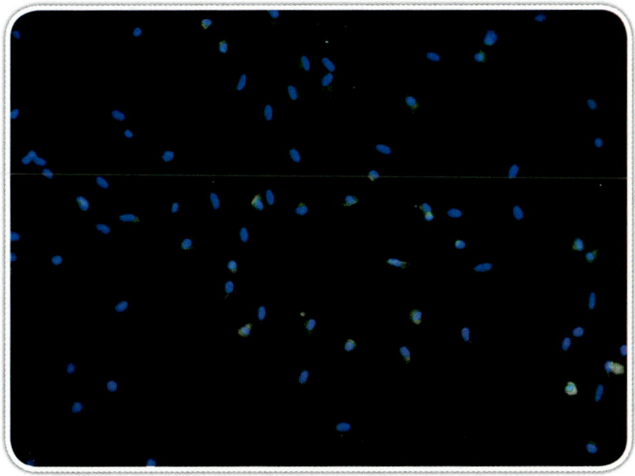

- Immunofluorescent staining
- Isolated cells were stained negative for α-actin shown in CY3 red. Nuclei were stained with DAPI shown in blue.

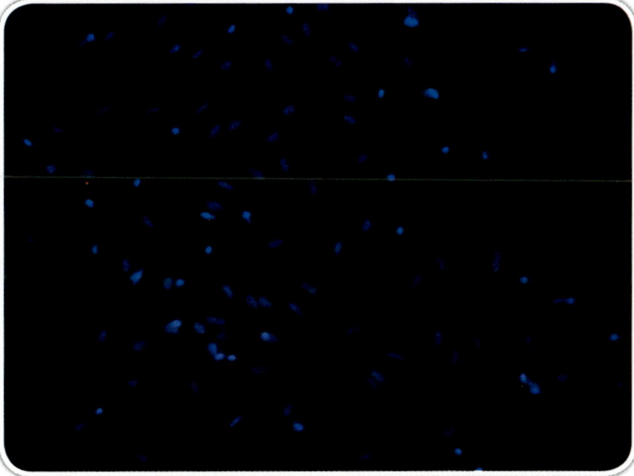

Rationale of Using Angiogenic/Antiangiogenic Proteins in Preeclampsia

Preeclampsia is a two-stage disease: Abnormal implantation

- Predictive claim: presymptomatic identification of pregnant women destined to develop preeclampsia
  - Hypoxic placenta
  - Aberrant angiogenic activity
- Diagnostic claim: exclude preeclampsia mimickers
  - Endothelial cell dysfunction (glomerular endotheliosis)
  - Symptomatic proteinuric hypertension.

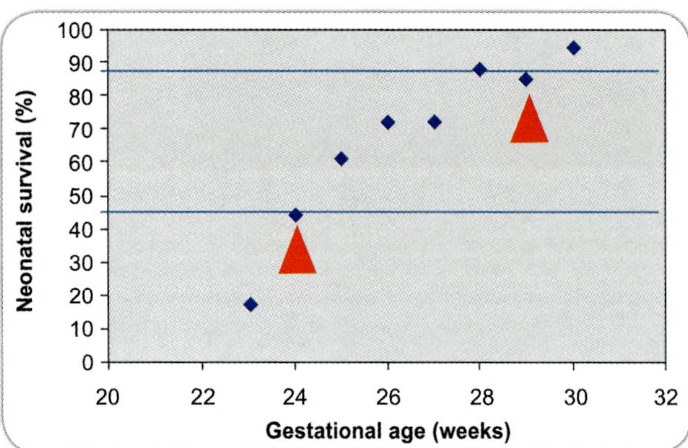

Expectant management in severe preeclampsia remote from term may prolong pregnancy at a median of 5 days (*Bombrys and Sibai, 2009*)

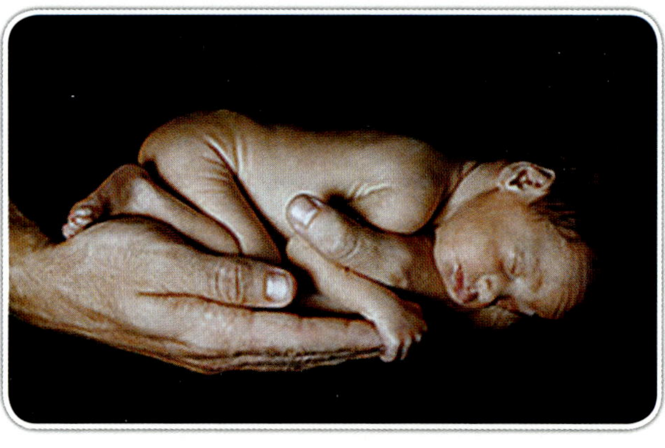

Can the delivery be procrastinated for the benefit of the baby, without jeopardizing the mother's health?

Commercially Available Preeclampsia Biomarker Quantitation Platforms

	Roche Diagnostics	Alere Health	PerkinElmer
Analytes	sFlt-1 PIGF	free PIGF	pp13 PIGF
Analyzer	Cobas, Elecsys 2010	Triage Meter	AutoDELFIA
Comparison has to be made on the same platform.			

Elevation of Serum sFlt-1 and Decrease in PlGF in Preeclamptic Patients

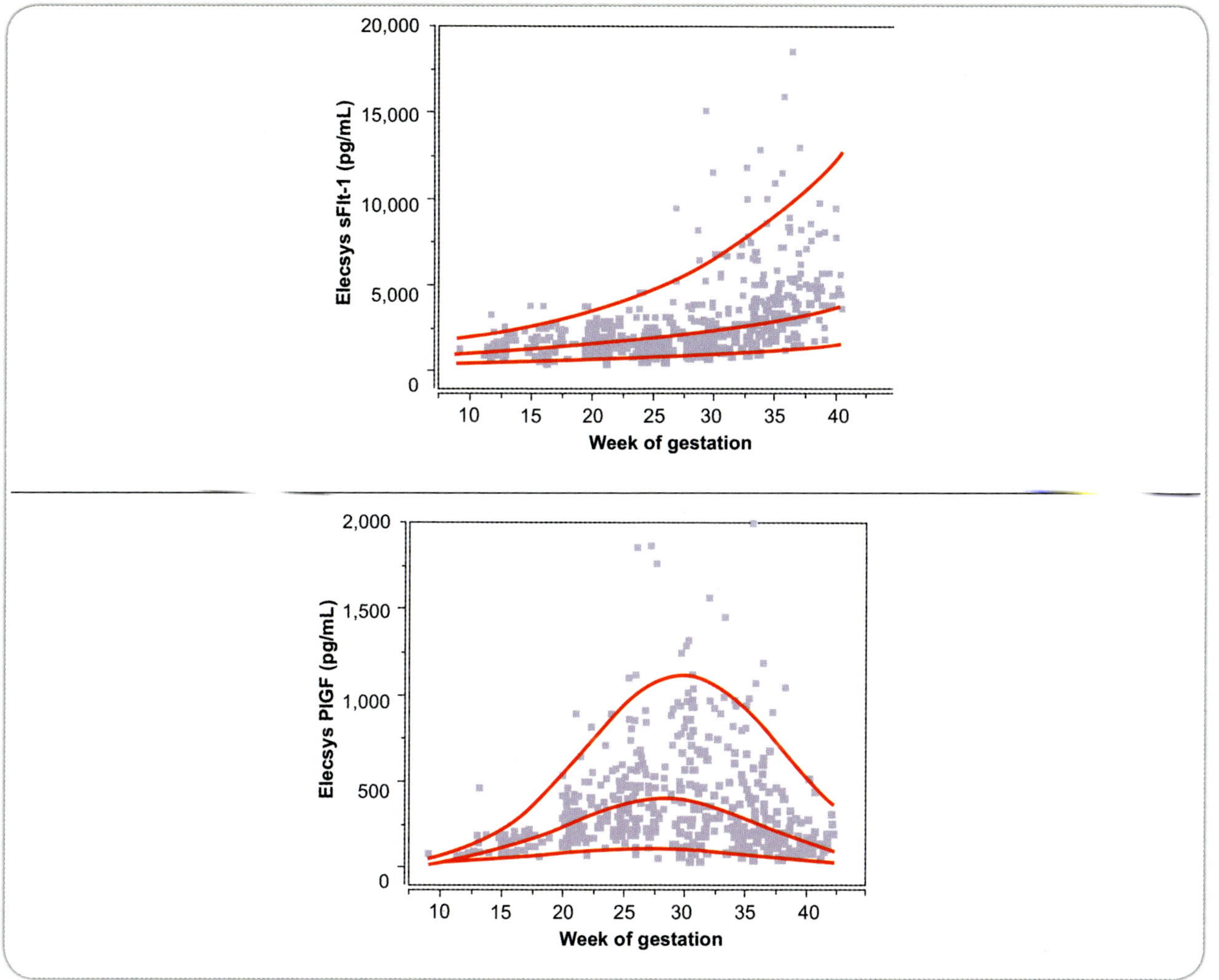

(Verlohren et al. 2010)

Prediction of Disease's Severity

- Markedly elevation of sFlt-1/PlGF has been linked to a shorter time to delivery.

(Verlohren et al. 2012)

	sFlt-1/PlGF ratio
PE/HELLP at < 34 weeks'	506.2 ± 54.3
Normotensive controls < 34 weeks'	9.1 ± 2.1
PE/HELLP ≥ 34 wks'	168.5 ± 17.7
Normotensive controls ≥ 34 weeks'	32.5 ± 4.9

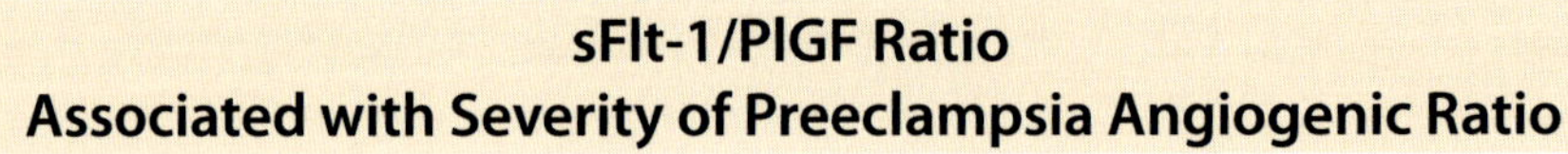

sFlt-1/PlGF Ratio
Associated with Severity of Preeclampsia Angiogenic Ratio

21 to 32 Weeks
Mean concentration (pg/mL)
10,000
9,000
8,000
7,000
6,000
5,000
4,000
3,000
2,000
1,000
0
sFlt-1
PlGF
Angiogenic ratio
P= 0.01
P= 0.02
P= 0.001
P< 0.001
P< 0.001
P< 0.001
P< 0.001
P< 0.001
P< 0.001
Controls
Mild PE
Severe PE
PE < 37 wk
PE+SGA
PE < 34 wk
No. of specimens
102
71
29
26
14
9
33 to 41 Weeks
Angiogenic ratio
Mean concentration (pg/mL)
10,000
9,000
8,000
7,000
6,000
5,000
4,000
3,000
2,000
1,000
0
sFlt-1
PlGF
P< 0.001
P= 0.02
P< 0.001
P< 0.001
P< 0.001
P= 0.02
P< 0.001
P< 0.001
Controls
Mild PE
Severe PE
PE < 37 wk
PE+SGA
No. of specimens
89
55
18
2
7

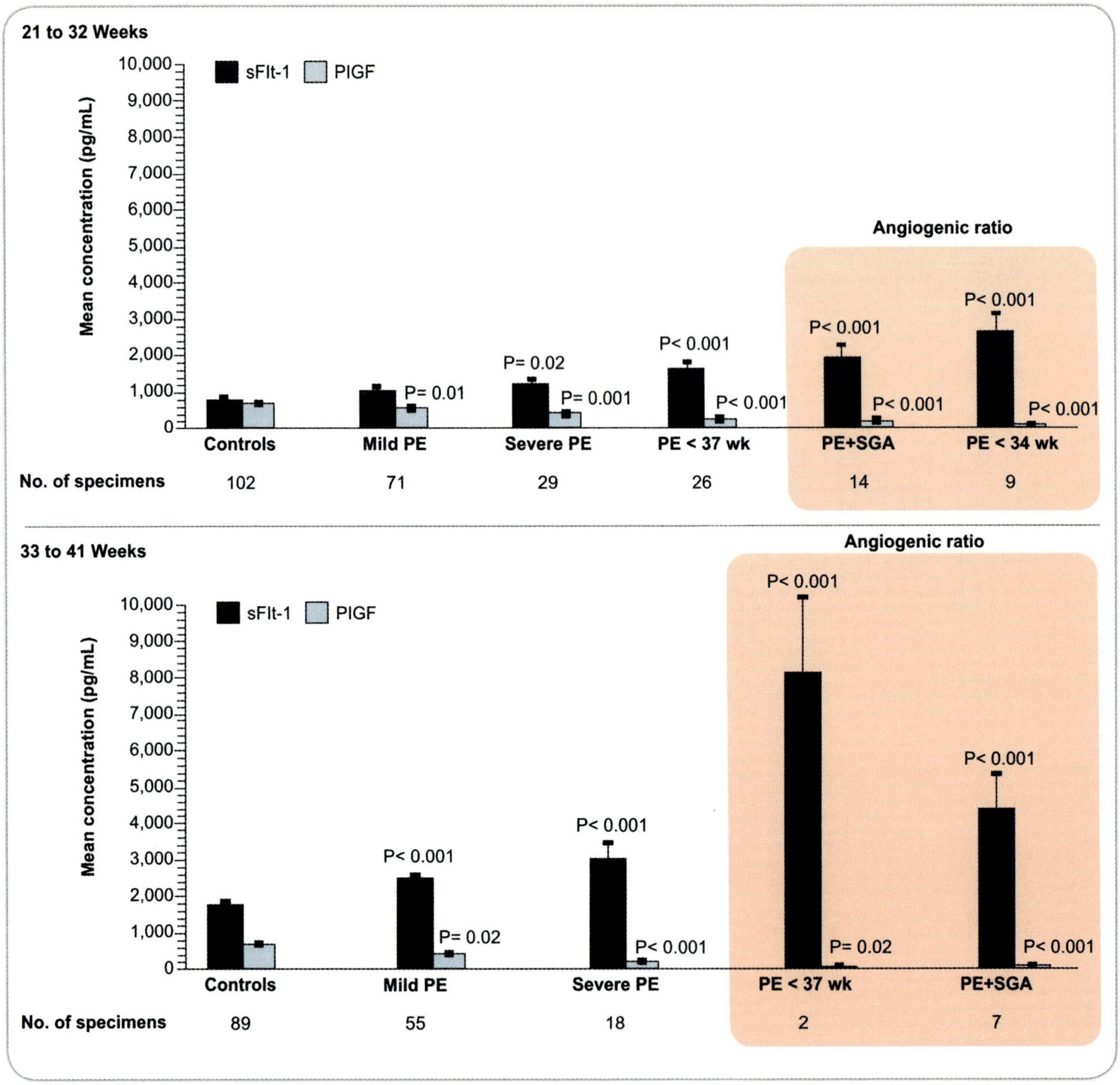

(Levine et al. NEJM 2006)

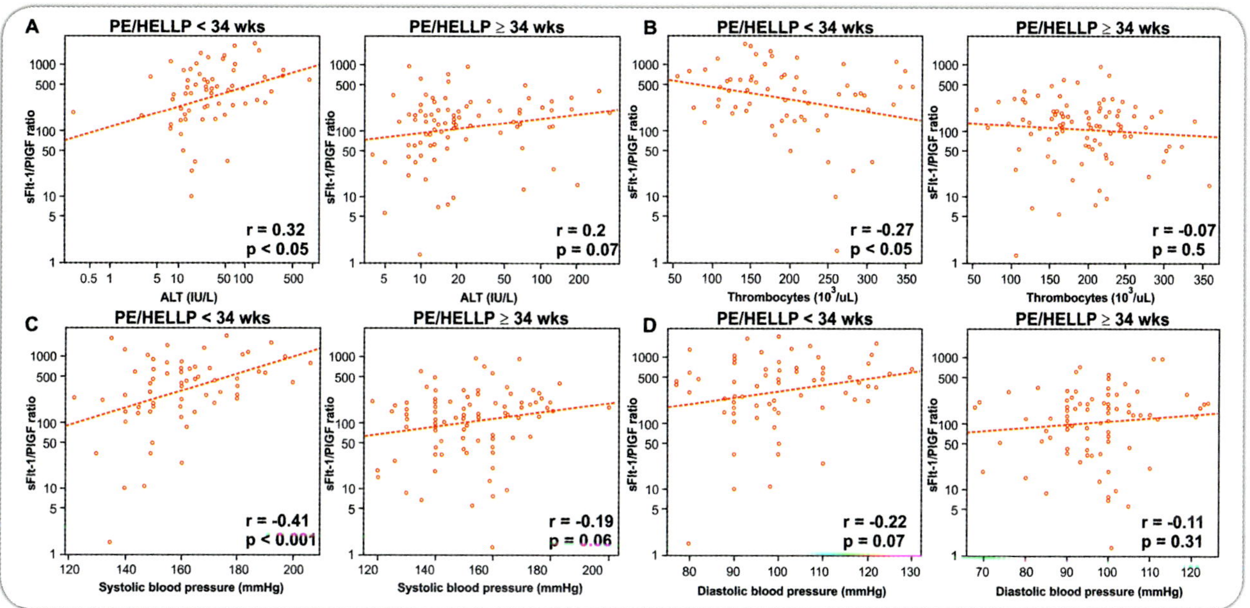

sFlt-1 and PlGF from an automated Elecsys 2010 ratio is slightly related to adverse clinical parameters, i.e. systolic and diastolic BP, AST, ALT, and platelet counts. The correlations are more apparent in early-onset diseases (< 34 weeks'). (*Verlohren et al. 2011*)

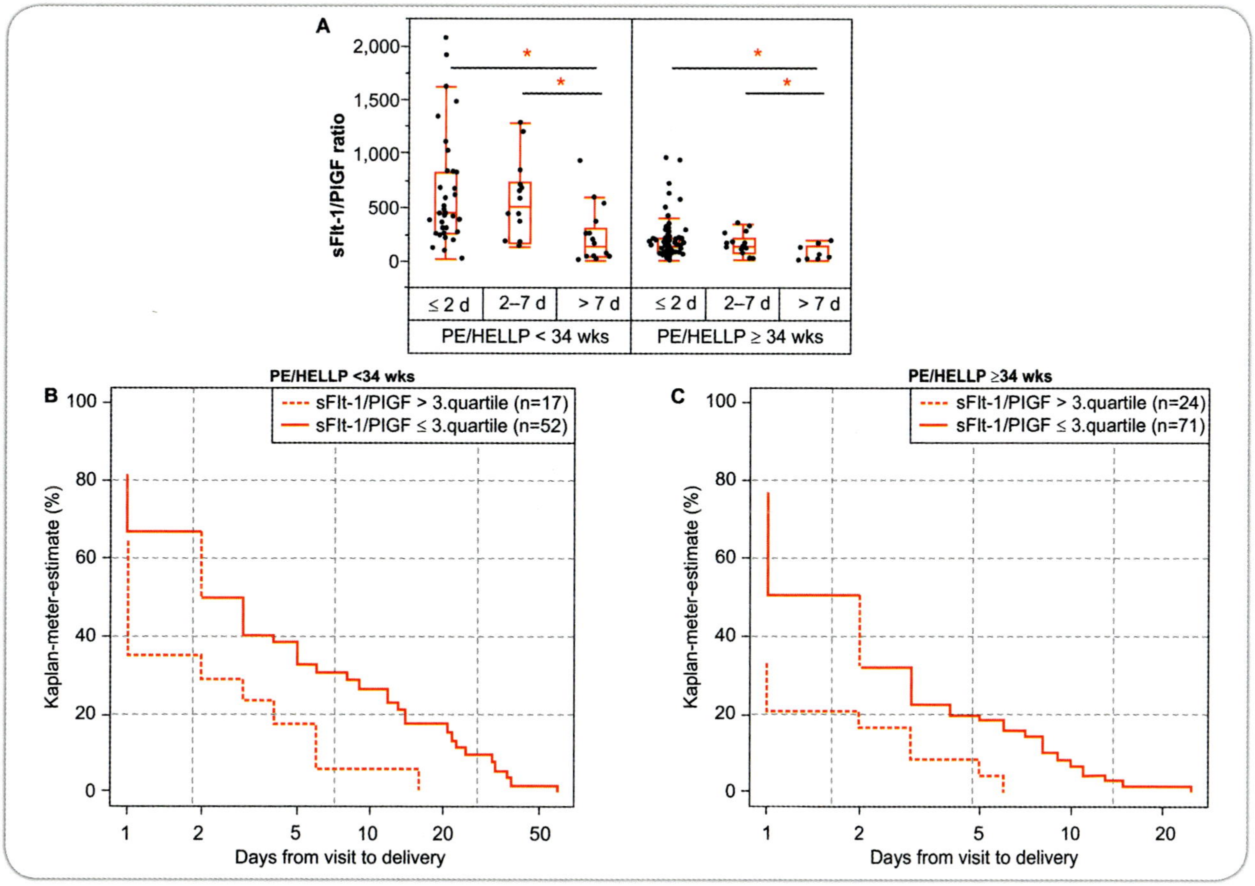

Elevation of sFlt-1 and PlGF ratio is associated with shorter interval to delivery (*Verlohren et al. 2011*)

Extracorporeal Removal of sFlt-1

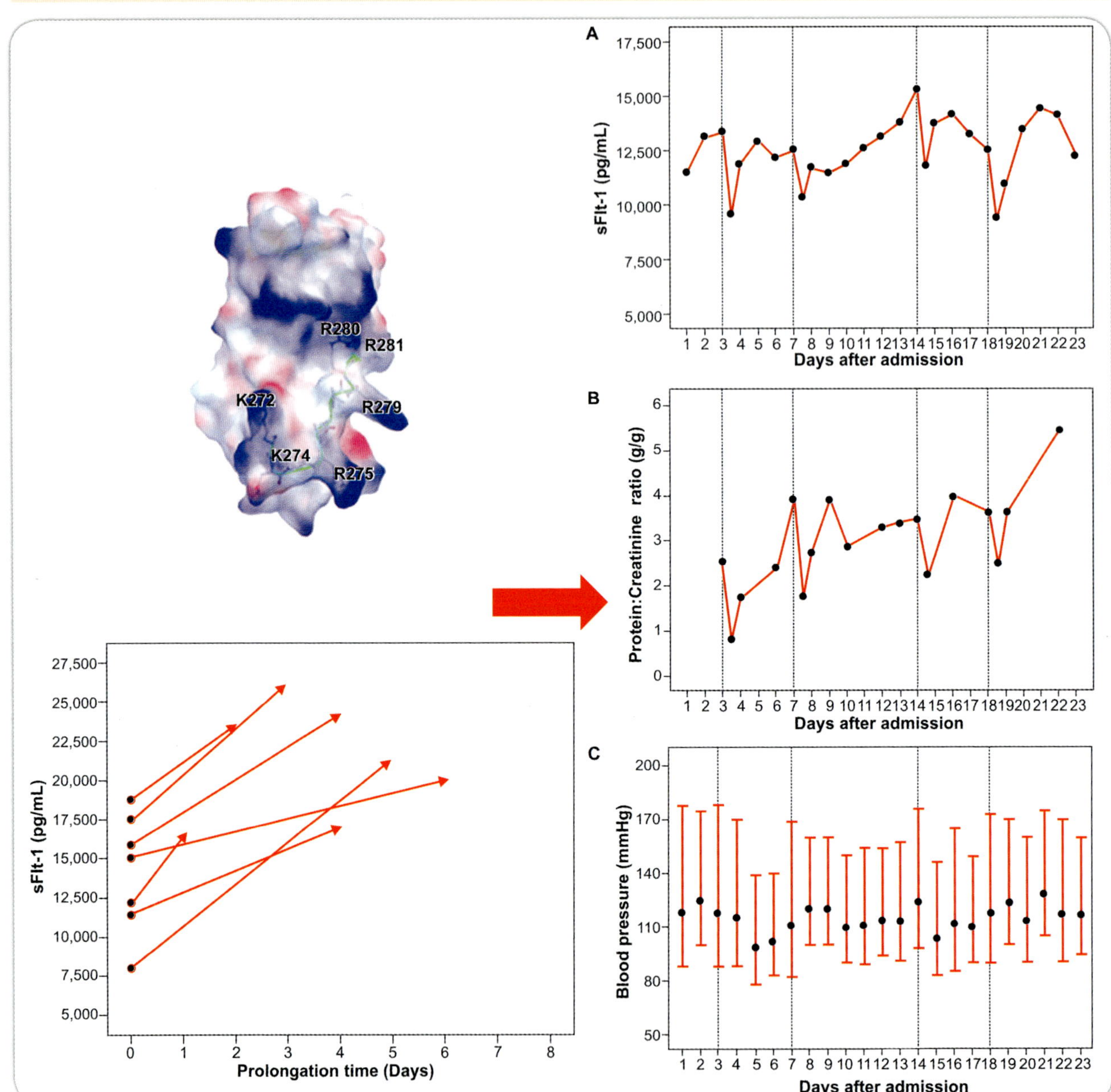

(Thadhani et al. 2011)

SCREENING FOR PREECLAMPSIA

Preeclampsia Screening

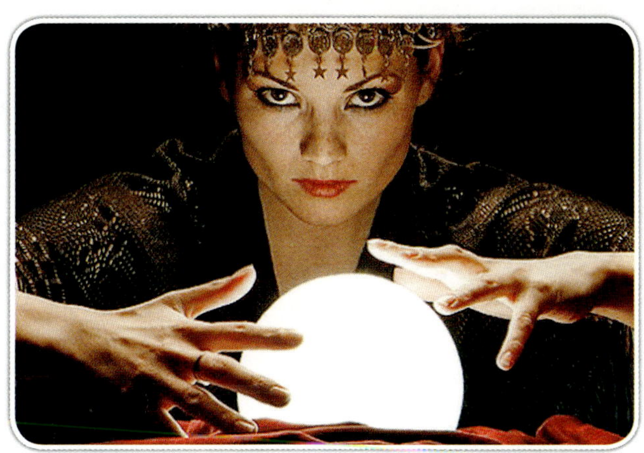

- To identify high-risk population for closer surveillance (resource allocation)
- To initiate prophylactic measures as early as possible (window of opportunity; to modify process of placental development).

Early-onset PE (<34 wks')	Late-onset PE (>34 wks')
• It is commonly associated with IUGR, abnormal uterine, and umbilical artery Doppler waveforms, and adverse maternal as well as neonatal outcomes	• It may be caused by increased maternal vascular susceptibility to the normal inflammatory state of pregnancy or atherosis of a placenta that was initially normally developed
• It is strongly associated with deficient trophoblast invasion and failure of normal spiral artery remodeling.	Is the screening algorithm effective? Does it translate to an improved maternal and perinatal outcomes?

	Early-onset preeclampsia (< 34 wks')	Late-onset preeclampsia (>34 wks')	Recurrent preeclampsia
Course	Minority, rapid progression	Majority, slow progression	Depend on gestational age of onset in first pregnancy
Effective available strategy	Maternal variables + maternal MAP +uterine artery Doppler + PAPP-A and PIGF in First trimester yielded 94.1% sen and 94.3% spec (FPR 5%) (***Poon et al***. 2009)	Poor prediction (35.7%) from Poon's model	By history alone, overall recurrence is 14.7% • < 28 wks': 38.6% • 29–32 wks': 29.1% • 33–36 wks': 21.9% • ≥ 37 wks': 12.9% *(Mostello et al. 2008)*
Reduce maternal and perinatal morbidities	To be proven	Screening may not significantly reduce morbidities	Aspirin 75 mg/D started after 12 wks' *(NICE 2011)*
Pointing to "specific" prevention	To be proven (ASA ?)	To be proven	No
Universally applied	To be proven	To be proven	Yes

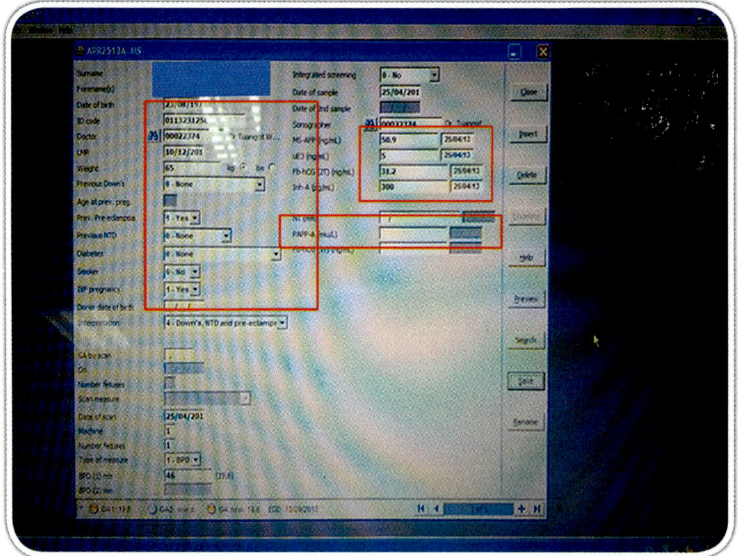

Adding screening for preeclampsia to an existing Down syndrome screening program using the Quadruple test detect over 40% of pregnancies with pre-eclampsia at 6% false-positive rate (about 6%)

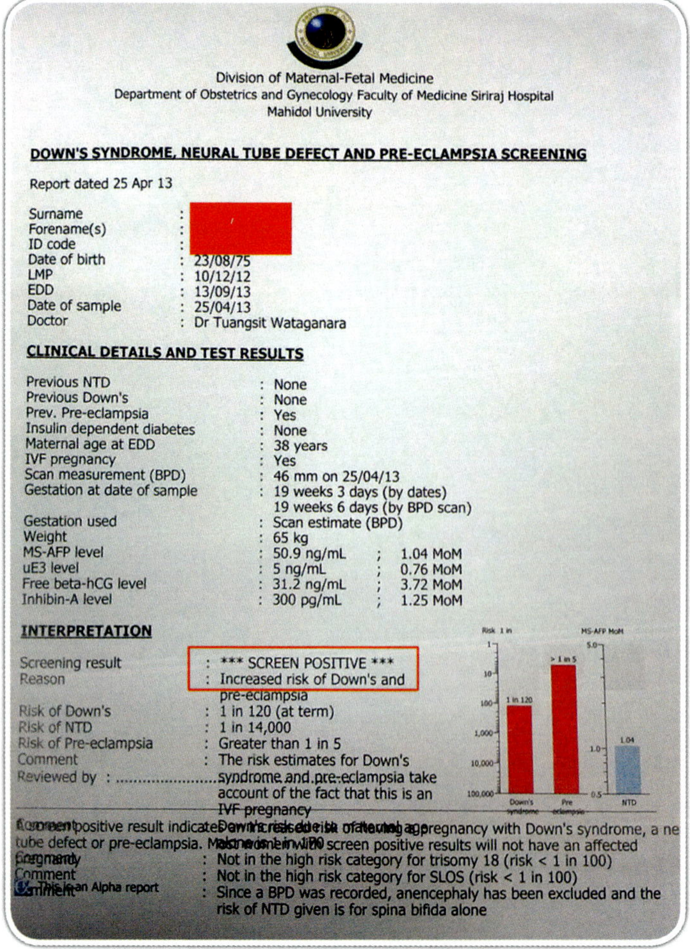

Division of Maternal-Fetal Medicine
Department of Obstetrics and Gynecology Faculty of Medicine Siriraj Hospital
Mahidol University

DOWN'S SYNDROME, NEURAL TUBE DEFECT AND PRE-ECLAMPSIA SCREENING

Report dated 25 Apr 13

Surname	:	
Forename(s)	:	
ID code	:	
Date of birth	:	23/08/75
LMP	:	10/12/12
EDD	:	13/09/13
Date of sample	:	25/04/13
Doctor	:	Dr Tuangsit Wataganara

CLINICAL DETAILS AND TEST RESULTS

Previous NTD	:	None
Previous Down's	:	None
Prev. Pre-eclampsia	:	Yes
Insulin dependent diabetes	:	None
Maternal age at EDD	:	38 years
IVF pregnancy	:	Yes
Scan measurement (BPD)	:	46 mm on 25/04/13
Gestation at date of sample	:	19 weeks 3 days (by dates) 19 weeks 6 days (by BPD scan)
Gestation used	:	Scan estimate (BPD)
Weight	:	65 kg
MS-AFP level	:	50.9 ng/mL ; 1.04 MoM
uE3 level	:	5 ng/mL ; 0.76 MoM
Free beta-hCG level	:	31.2 ng/mL ; 3.72 MoM
Inhibin-A level	:	300 pg/mL ; 1.25 MoM

INTERPRETATION

Screening result	:	*** SCREEN POSITIVE ***
Reason	:	Increased risk of Down's and pre-eclampsia
Risk of Down's	:	1 in 120 (at term)
Risk of NTD	:	1 in 14,000
Risk of Pre-eclampsia	:	Greater than 1 in 5
Comment	:	The risk estimates for Down's syndrome and pre-eclampsia take account of the fact that this is an IVF pregnancy
Reviewed by :		

A screen positive result indicates an increased risk of having a pregnancy with Down's syndrome, a neural tube defect or pre-eclampsia. Most women with screen positive results will not have an affected pregnancy.

Comment	:	Not in the high risk category for trisomy 18 (risk < 1 in 100)
Comment	:	Not in the high risk category for SLOS (risk < 1 in 100)
Comment	:	Since a BPD was recorded, anencephaly has been excluded and the risk of NTD given is for spina bifida alone

This is an Alpha report

Normal uterine artery waveform

Normal uterine artery waveform

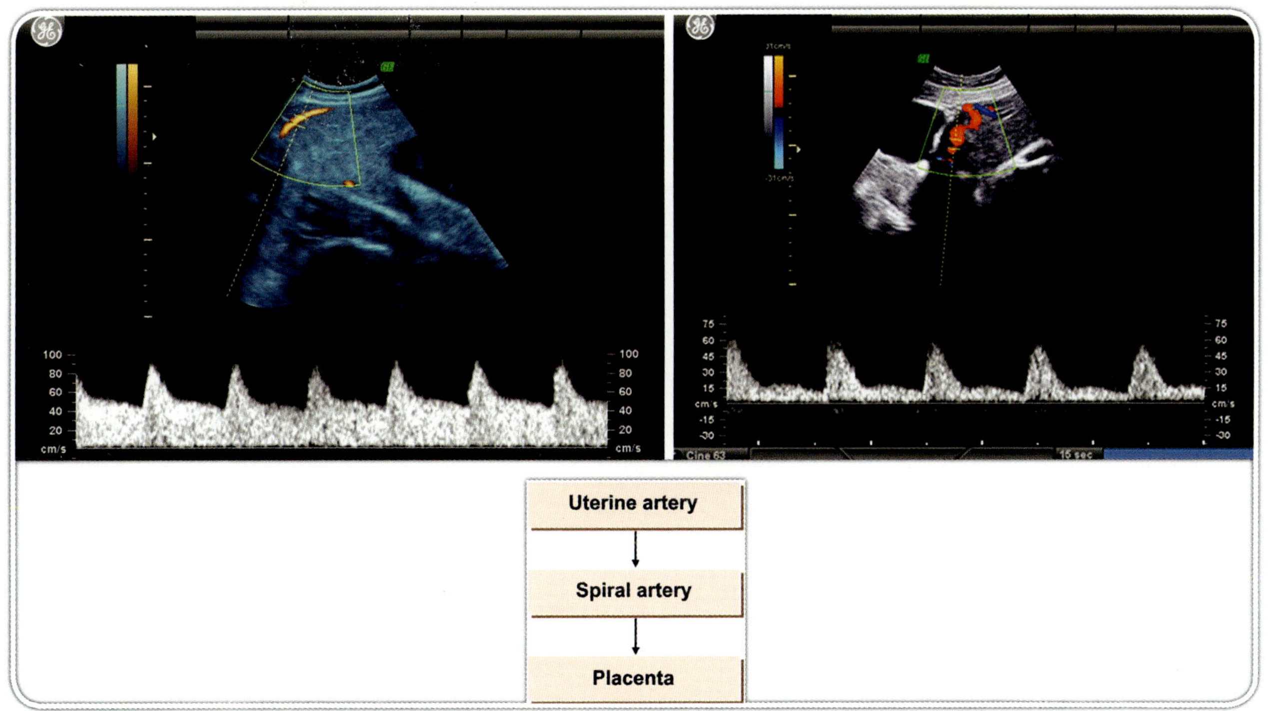

Secondary Prevention of Preeclampsia

Clinical risk factors

- Present → More frequent antenatal visits; Blood pressure monitoring; urine protein monitoring
- Absent → Serum markers; Uterine artery Doppler → More frequent antenatal visits; Blood pressure monitoring; urine protein monitoring

Preeclampsia

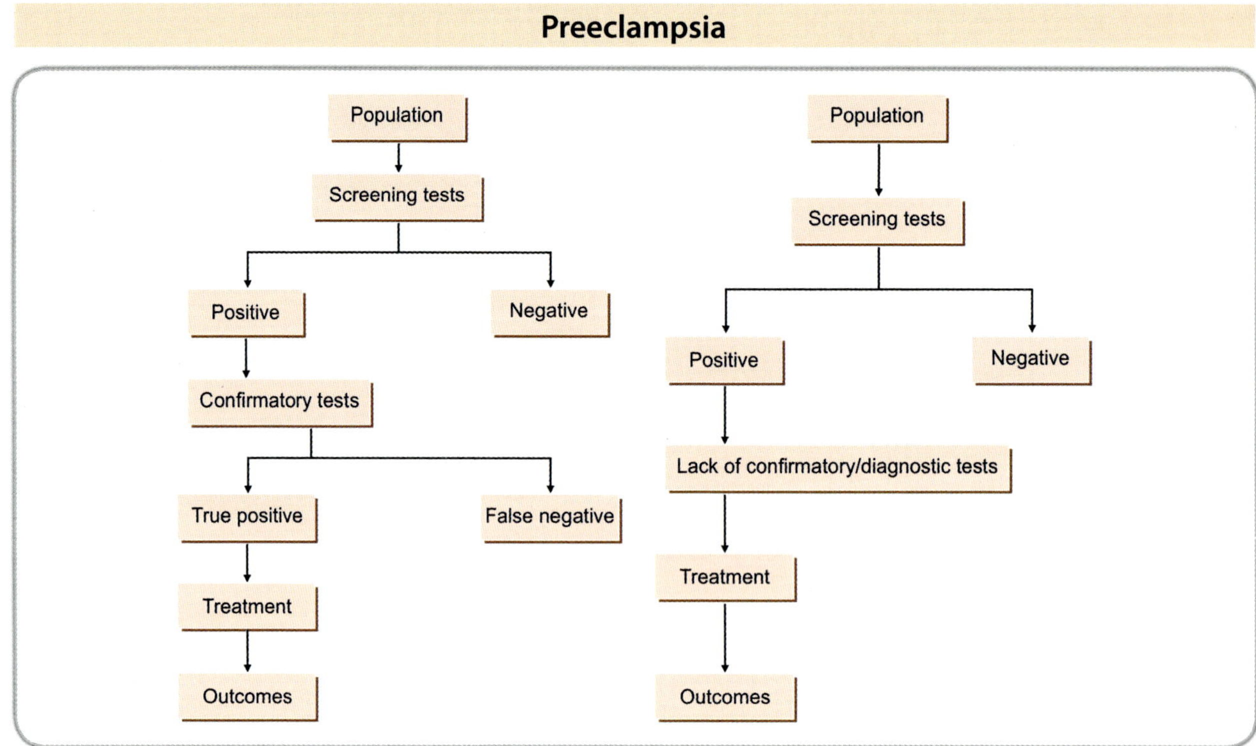

Summary of Potential Serum Biomarkers for Prediction of Preeclampsia

Biomarker	1st trim	2nd trim	Symptomatic	Combination	Also correlated with
PAPP-A	↓	↓	↓		SGA
PP-13	↓	↑	↑	US	IUGR, preterm
fDNA	↑	↑	↑	Inhibin-A	IUGR, polyhydramnios, trisomy 21, 18, preterm
DNA			↑		
sFlt-1		↑	↑	sEng, PlGF, VEGF, US	
PlGF	↓	↓	↓	sEng, sFlt-1	SGA
sEng		↑	↑	sFlt-1, PlGF, US	IUGR, HELLP
P-selectin	↑	↑	↑	Activin A, sFlt-1	
PTX-3	↑	↑	↑		IUGR

Accuracy of Proposed Tests in Predicting Preeclampsia

Tests	RR (95% CI)	Sensitivity (95% CI)	Specificity (95% CI)
Clinical history			
Maternal age > 40 yrs			
Primigravida	1.7 (1.2–2.3)		
Multigravida	2.0 (1.3–3.9)		
Nulliparity	2.9 (1.3–6.6)		
Familial history of PET	2.9 (1.7–4.9)		
Multiple pregnancy			
Twins	2.9 (2.0–4.2)		
Triplets	2.8 (1.3–6.4)		
Preeclampsia in previous pregnancy	7.2 (5.9–8.8)		
History of autoimmune disease	6.9 (4.3–42)		
History of thrombophilia	9.7 (4.3–22)		
Clinical examination			
Body Mass Index (BMI)			
BMI ≥ 25		47% (33–61)	73% (64–83)
BMI ≥ 30		19% (19–20)	90% (88–93)
BMI ≥ 35		21% (12–31)	92% (89–95)
Blood pressure in the first trimester			
Mean arterial pressure ≥ 90 mmHg		62% (35–89)	82% (72–92)
Hemodynamic investigations			
Uterine artery Doppler in second trimester			
High PI and notching in low-risk		23% (14–35)	99% (98–99)
High PI and notching in high-risk		83% (36–100)	96% (90–99)
Unilateral notching		19% (5–42)	99% (97–100)

(Adapted from Thangaratinam et al. 2011)

First Trimester Multiparametric Model Detection Rate for Early-Onset Preeclampsia

DR at 5% FPR	History	MAP	uA-PI	PAPP-A	PlGF	Reference
33	×					*Yu et al.* 2005, *Akolekar et al.* 2011
38			×			*Poon et al.* 2009
47	×			×		*Akolekar et al.* 2011
54	×				×	*Akolekar et al.* 2011
60	×		×	×		*Foidart et al.* 2010
78	×		×		×	*Foidart et al.* 2010
78	×	×	×	×	×	*Akolekar et al.* 2011
84	×	×	×	×		*Poon et al.* 2010
89	×	×	×		×	*Poon et al.* 2010
94	×	×	×	×	×	*Poon et al.* 2009

History: BMI, family history of preeclampsia, previous preeclampsia, ethnicity, and smoking.

(Adapted from Costa Fda S, et al. 2011)

Serum sFlt-1 Elevates Shortly before Onset of the Disease

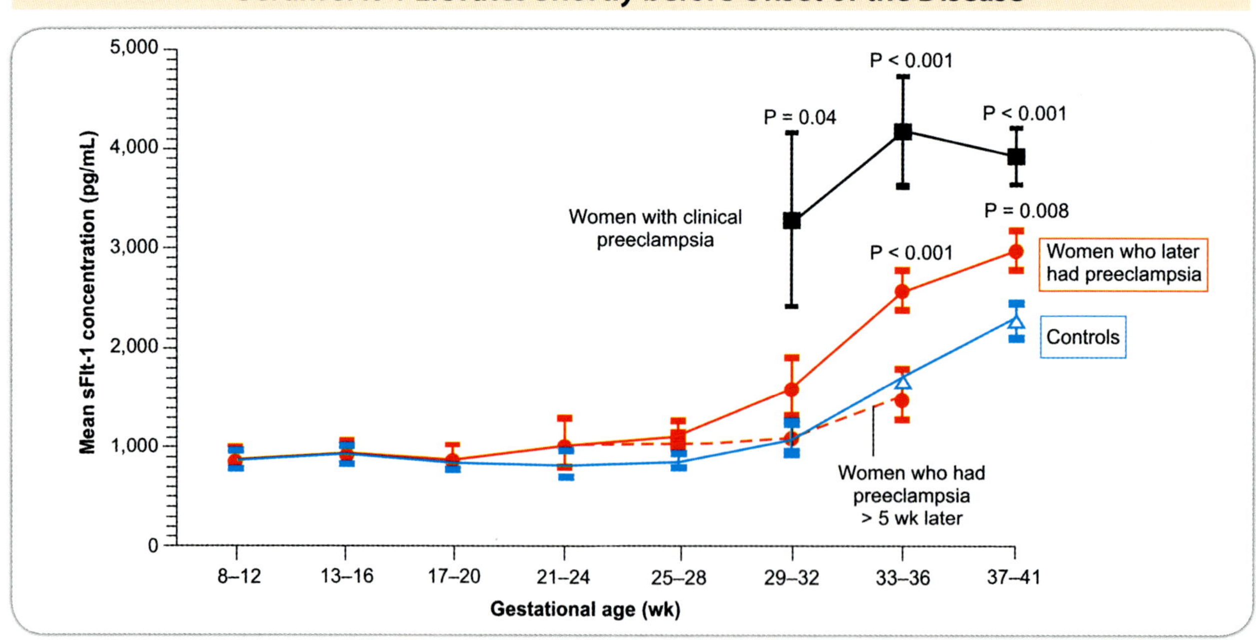

(Levine et al. NEJM 2006)

Two-stage Elevation of Cell-free fetal DNA in Maternal Sera before Onset of Preeclampsia

Richard J. Levine, MD,[a,*] Cong Qian, MS,[b] Erik S. LeShane, BS,[c] Kai F. Yu, PhD,[a] Lucinda J. England, MD,[a] Enreque F. Schisterman, PhD,[a] Tuangsit Wataganara, MD,[c] Roberto Romero, Md,[d] Diana W. Bianchi, MD[c]

Division of Epidemiology, Statistics, and Prevention Research, National Institute of Child Health and Human Development, Department of Health and Human Services, Bethesda, Md[a]; Allied Technology Group, Rockvile, Md[b]; Division of Genetics. Departments of Pediatrics, Obstetrics and Gynecology, Tufts-New England Medical Center and Tufts University School of Medicine, Boston, Mass[c]; Perinatology Research Branch, National Institute of Child Health and Human Development, Department of Health and Human Services, Detroit, Mich[d]

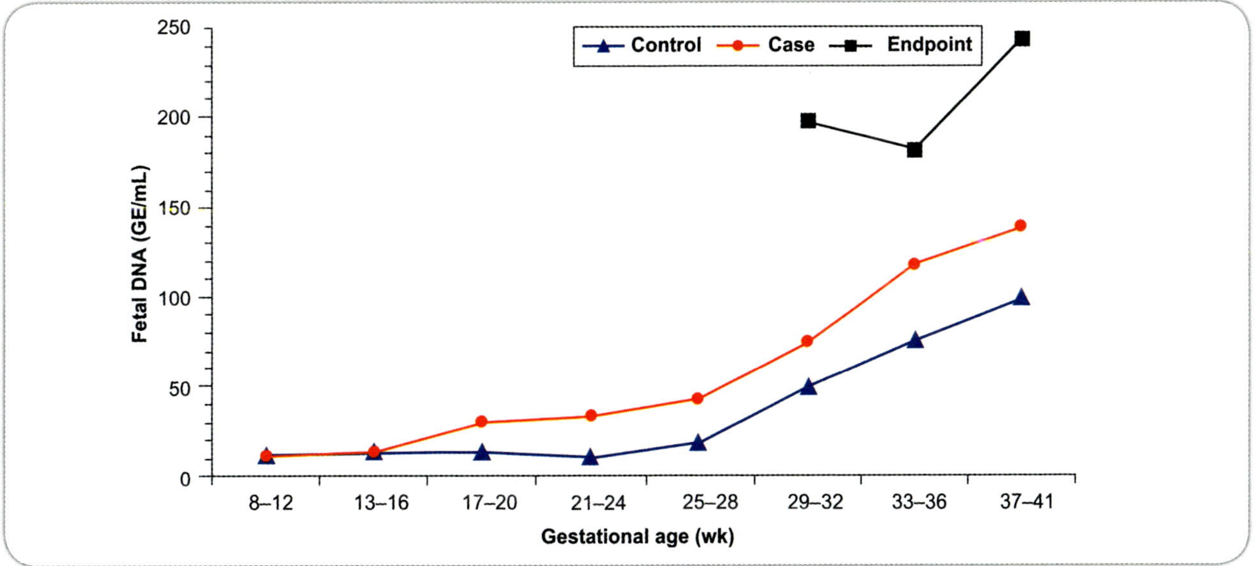

This change mimics the pattern previously found with fetal DNA (surrogate for trophoblastic injuries)

Serum PlGF Decreased Prior to the Onset of the Disease

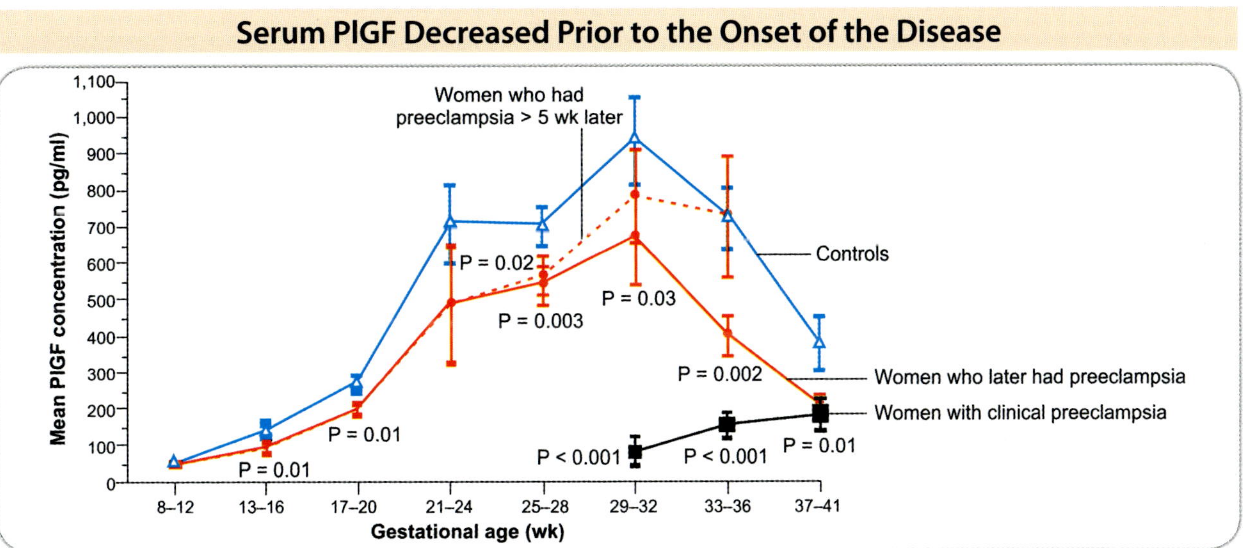

(Levine et al. NEJM 2006)

Issues about Predictive Claim

- Do we need to screen every pregnant women ?
  - In **clinically low risk group**: We need tests that have high negative predictive value.
  - In **clinically high risk group**: We need tests that have high sensitivity and high positive predictive value.
- Therefore, the screening strategy may be different between these two groups ?
- Unlike Down syndrome screening, the disease is not there yet at the time of screening.

Questions to be Addressed ...

- What are the cut-offs? Gestational age specific? sFlt-1/PlGF or PlGF/sFlt-1 ratio?
- When to start the testing, and at what interval ?
- Preeclampsia is a heterogeneous disease. The disease with an earlier onset (<32 weeks') is more homogeneous, and more predictable.
- Incorporation into first or second trimester screening for fetal Down syndrome? Genetic susceptibility must be taken into account.
- Expectant management of severe preeclampsia (prediction of disease progression)?
- Can serum angiogenic peptides help selecting suitable candidate, and predict the perinatal outcomes ?
- Combination with other markers, such as uterine artery Doppler ?
- Multiple markers? Sequential measurements ?

For Screen-positive Individuals...

- **We could offer**...
  - Closer surveillance
  - Timely intervention, e.g. steroids
  - Recruitment for future research studies, e.g. medical treatment of preeclampsia
- **Preventive measures** (?)
  - Aspirin (60–100 mg/D), initiated in the first or second trimester ?
  - Low-dose heparin
  - Calcium, vitamin C and E.

CAN COMBINED SCREENING LEAD TO TARGETED PREVENTATIVE THERAPY ?

Treatments Evaluated for Preeclampsia Prevention

Pharmacological prophylaxis	Nutritional supplement	Lifestyle intervention and diet
• Antiplatelet agents • Nitric oxide agents • Low-molecular weight heparin • Antihypertensives for mild and moderate hypertension • Progesterone • Diuretics	• Calcium • Antioxidant • Folic acid • Magnesium • Marine oil and prostaglandin precursors	• Rest • Exercise • Altered dietary salt • Energy and protein intake • Garlic

(Adapted from Thangaratinam et al. 2011)

Rationale of the Proposed Preventative Measures

Aspirin	Reduce thromboxane and platelet activation, cheap, widely available
Nitric oxide donor	Enhance physiologic vascular adaptation
Low-molecular weight heparin	Reduce ischemic thrombotic lesions in the placenta
Antihypertensives	Commonly used medications
Progesterone	Vascular wall relaxation
Calcium	Moderate parathyroid, calcium, and magnesium channels, resulting in vasodilatation
Antioxidants	Limit endothelial damages from oxidative stress resulting from placental ischemia
Marine oil	Omega-3 fatty acids compete with arachidonic acid (thromboxane A2 precursor)
Exercise	Increase plasma volume, and lower systemic inflammatory response
Garlic	Lower blood pressure, inhibit platelet aggregation

Effectiveness of Proposed Interventions to Prevent Preeclampsia

Intervention	RR (95% CI)
Pharmacologic agents	
Anti-platelets	0.90 (0.84–0.97)
Nitric oxide	0.83 (0.49–1.41)
Low-molecular weight heparin	0.23 (0.08–0.68)
Antihypertensives	0.97 (0.83–1.13)
Progesterone	0.21 (0.03–1.77)
Diuretics	0.68 (0.45–1.03)
Nutritional supplements	
Calcium	0.45 (0.31–0.65)
Anti-oxidants	0.73 (0.51–1.06)
Folic acid	0.46 (0.16–1.31)
Magnesium	0.87 (0.57–1.32)
Marine oil	0.86 (0.59–1.27)
Lifestyle interventions	
Rest	0.05 (0–0.83)
Exercise	0.31 (0.01–7.09)
Altered dietary salt	1.11 (0.46–2.66)
Energy and protein intake	1.2 (0.77–1.89)
Garlic	0.78 (0.31–1.93)

(Adapted from Thangaratinam et al. 2011)

Prevention of Preeclampsia and Intrauterine Growth Restriction with Aspirin Started in Early Pregnancy

A Meta-Analysis

Emmanuel Bujold, MD, MSc, Suphanie Roberge, MSc, Yves Lacasse, MD, MSc, Marc Bureau, MD, Francois Audibert, MD, MSc, Sylvie Marcoux, MD, PhD, Jean-Claude forest, MD, PhD, and Yues Giguere, MD, PhD

1.1 16 or fewer weeks						
August 1994	3	24	5	25	2.5	0.63 (0.17–2.33)
Azar 1990	1	46	4	45	1.1	0.24 (0.03–2.10)
Beaufils 1985	0	48	6	45	0.6	0.07 (0.00–1.25)
Benigni 1989	0	17	0	16		Not estimable
Ebrashy 2005	25	73	40	63	9.3	0.54 (0.37–0.78
Hermida 1997	3	50	7	50	2.6	0.43 (0.12–1.56)
Michael 1992	1	55	5	55	1.1	0.20 (0.02–1.66)
Tulppala 1997	1	33	3	33	1.0	0.33 (0.04–3.04)
Vainio 2002	2	43	10	43	2.2	0.20 (0.05–0.86)
Subtotal (95% CI)		**389**		**375**	**20.5**	**0.47 (0.34–0.65)**
Total events	36		80			
Heterogeneity: Tau^2=0.00; Chi^2=5.45; df=7 (*P*=.61); I^2=0%						
Test for overall effect: Z=4.57 (*P*<.001)						
1.2 More than 16 weeks						
Byaruhanga 1998	17	113	23	117	7.1	0.77 (0.43–1.35)
Caritis 1998	111	663	118	626	10.8	0.89 (0.70–1.12)
CLASP 1994	91	1,259	80	1,233	10.2	1.11 (0.83–1.49)
Davies 1995	5	58	7	60	3.4	0.74 (0.25–2.20)
ECPPA 1996	16	284	22	322	6.6	0.82 (0.44–1.54)
Ferrier 1996	1	23	1	20	0.7	0.87 (0.06–13.02)
Golding 1998	66	1,253	50	1,294	9.4	1.36 (0.95–1.95)
Grab 2000	3	22	2	21	1.7	1.43 (0.27–7.73)
Hauth 1993	5	302	17	302	3.9	0.29 (0.11–0.79)
McParland 1990	1	48	10	52	1.2	0.11 (0.01–0.81)
Morris 1996	4	52	7	50	3.1	0.55 (0.17–1.76)
Rogers 1999	3	118	7	75	2.5	0.27 (0.07–1.02)
Rotchell 1998	10	739	12	746	4.8	0.84 (0.37–1.94)
Schiff 1989	1	34	7	31	1.2	0.13 (0.02–1.00)
Schrocksnadel 1992	0	22	6	19	0.7	0.07 (0.00–1.11)
Wallenburg 1986	0	23	7	23	0.7	0.07 (0.00–1.10)
Yu 2003	49	276	52	278	9.5	0.95 (0.67–1.35)
Zimmerman 1997	4	13	2	13	2	2.00 (0.44–9.08)
Subtotal (95% CI)		**5,302**		**5,282**	**79.5**	**0.81 (0.63–1.03)**
Total events	387		430			
Heterogeneity: Tau^2=0.09; Chi^2=32.49; df =17 (*P*=.01); I^2=48%						
Test for overall effect: Z=1.75 (*P*=.08)						

In high-risk women, low-dose aspirin started before 16 weeks gestation was associated with:

- 53% reduction of developing preeclampsia
- 56% reduction of experiencing IUGR
- 91% reduction of developing severe preeclampsia
- 38% reduction of gestational hypertension
- 78% reduction in preterm birth
- **"High-risk" is usually defined by "clinical" and not by "laboratory" or "sonographic findings".**

(Bujold et al. 2010)

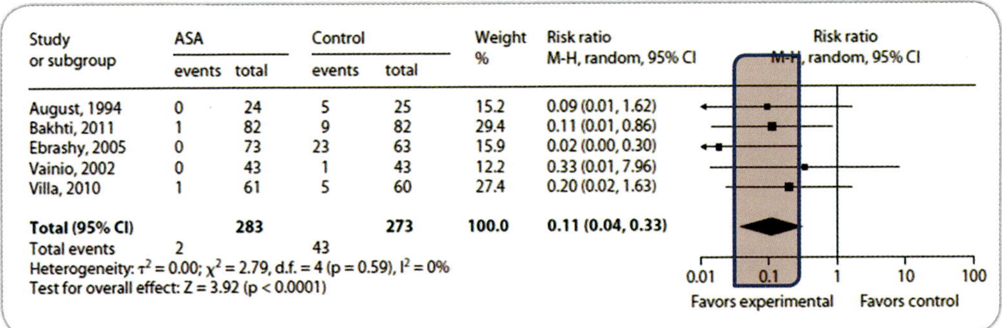

Study or subgroup	ASA events	ASA total	Control events	Control total	Weight %	Risk ratio M-H, random, 95% CI
August, 1994	0	24	5	25	15.2	0.09 (0.01, 1.62)
Bakhti, 2011	1	82	9	82	29.4	0.11 (0.01, 0.86)
Ebrashy, 2005	0	73	23	63	15.9	0.02 (0.00, 0.30)
Vainio, 2002	0	43	1	43	12.2	0.33 (0.01, 7.96)
Villa, 2010	1	61	5	60	27.4	0.20 (0.02, 1.63)
Total (95% CI)		**283**		**273**	**100.0**	**0.11 (0.04, 0.33)**
Total events	2		43			

Heterogeneity: $\tau^2 = 0.00$; $\chi^2 = 2.79$, d.f. = 4 (p = 0.59), $I^2 = 0\%$
Test for overall effect: Z = 3.92 (p < 0.0001)

Forest plot of the effect of low-dose aspirin initiated at or before 16 weeks' gestation on the risk of preterm preeclampsia

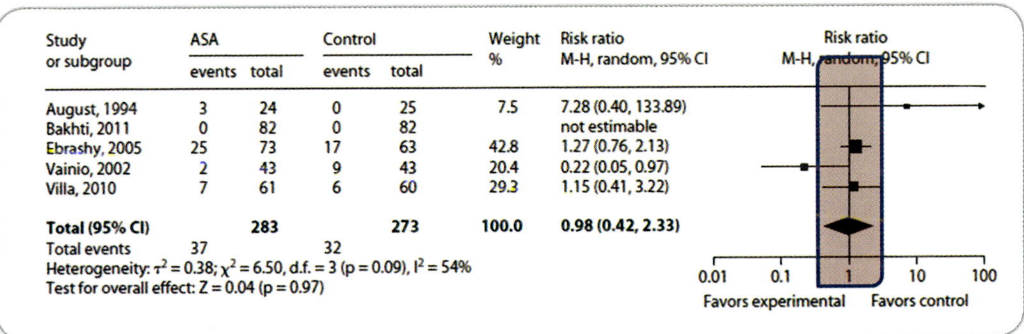

Study or subgroup	ASA events	ASA total	Control events	Control total	Weight %	Risk ratio M-H, random, 95% CI
August, 1994	3	24	0	25	7.5	7.28 (0.40, 133.89)
Bakhti, 2011	0	82	0	82		not estimable
Ebrashy, 2005	25	73	17	63	42.8	1.27 (0.76, 2.13)
Vainio, 2002	2	43	9	43	20.4	0.22 (0.05, 0.97)
Villa, 2010	7	61	6	60	29.3	1.15 (0.41, 3.22)
Total (95% CI)		**283**		**273**	**100.0**	**0.98 (0.42, 2.33)**
Total events	37		32			

Heterogeneity: $\tau^2 = 0.38$; $\chi^2 = 6.50$, d.f. = 3 (p = 0.09), $I^2 = 54\%$
Test for overall effect: Z = 0.04 (p = 0.97)

Forest plot of the effect of low-dose aspirin initiated at or before 16 weeks' gestation on the risk of term preeclampsia

(Roberge et al. 2012)

Severe preeclampsia requiring delivery before 34 weeks' occur in only 0.5% of pregnancies

(Roberge et al. 2012)

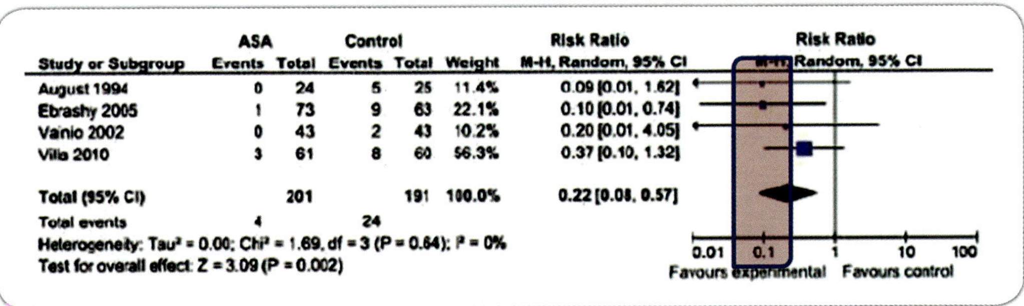

Study or Subgroup	ASA Events	ASA Total	Control Events	Control Total	Weight	Risk Ratio M-H, Random, 95% CI
August 1994	0	24	5	25	11.4%	0.09 [0.01, 1.62]
Ebrashy 2005	1	73	9	63	22.1%	0.10 [0.01, 0.74]
Vainio 2002	0	43	2	43	10.2%	0.20 [0.01, 4.05]
Villa 2010	3	61	8	60	56.3%	0.37 [0.10, 1.32]
Total (95% CI)		**201**		**191**	**100.0%**	**0.22 [0.08, 0.57]**
Total events	4		24			

Heterogeneity: Tau² = 0.00; Chi² = 1.69, df = 3 (P = 0.64); I² = 0%
Test for overall effect: Z = 3.09 (P = 0.002)

Forest plot of the effect of low-dose aspirin initiated at or before 16 weeks' gestation on the prevalence of severe preeclampsia. ASA, acetylsalicylic acid; CI, confidence interval; DPI, dots per inch; M-H, Mantel-Haenszel

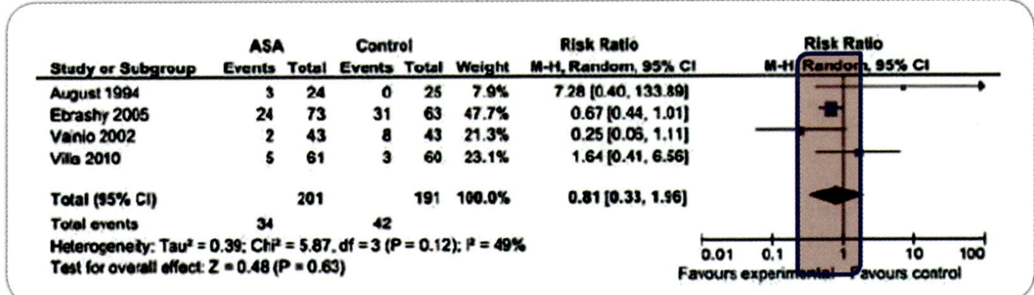

Study or Subgroup	ASA Events	ASA Total	Control Events	Control Total	Weight	Risk Ratio M-H, Random, 95% CI
August 1994	3	24	0	25	7.9%	7.28 [0.40, 133.89]
Ebrashy 2005	24	73	31	63	47.7%	0.67 [0.44, 1.01]
Vainio 2002	2	43	8	43	21.3%	0.25 [0.06, 1.11]
Villa 2010	5	61	3	60	23.1%	1.64 [0.41, 6.56]
Total (95% CI)		**201**		**191**	**100.0%**	**0.81 [0.33, 1.96]**
Total events	34		42			

Heterogeneity: Tau² = 0.39; Chi² = 5.87, df = 3 (P = 0.12); I² = 49%
Test for overall effect: Z = 0.48 (P = 0.63)

Forest plot of the effect of low-dose aspirin initiated at or before 16 weeks' gestation on the prevalence of mild preeclampsia. ASA, acetylsalicylic acid; CI, confidence interval; DPI, dots per inch; M-H, Mantel-Haenszel

(Roberge et al. 2012)

Efficacy of Medications Proposed to Prevent Preeclampsia

Aspirin	Largely ineffective, except in subgroup of "clinically" high-risk women
Nitric oxide donors	Ineffective
Diuretics	Ineffective
Progesterone	Ineffective
Low-molecular weight heparin	Largely ineffective, except in small subgroup of thrombophiliac (investigational)
Recombinant VEGF	Investigational

(National Institute of Clinical Excellence; NICE 2011)

Efficacy of Dietary Supplements Proposed to Prevent Preeclampsia

Calcium	Largely ineffective, except in setting of low dietary calcium intake (< 600 mg/day or corresponding to less than two dairy servings per day)
Magnesium	Ineffective
Folic acid	Ineffective
Antioxidants (vitamin C and E)	Ineffective
Fish oils or algal oils	Ineffective
Garlic	Ineffective

(Adapted from National Institute of Clinical Excellence; NICE 2011)

Health Technology Assessment UK, 2008 Prediction of Preeclampsia

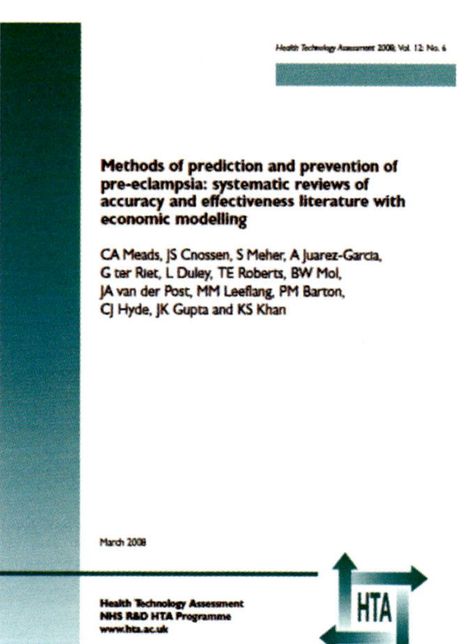

Health Technology Assessment 2008; Vol. 12: No. 6

Methods of prediction and prevention of pre-eclampsia: systematic reviews of accuracy and effectiveness literature with economic modelling

CA Meads, JS Cnossen, S Meher, A Juarez-Garcia, G ter Riet, L Duley, TE Roberts, BW Mol, JA van der Post, MM Leeflang, PM Barton, CJ Hyde, JK Gupta and KS Khan

March 2008

Health Technology Assessment
NHS R&D HTA Programme
www.hta.ac.uk

HTA

Refraining from Testing, but to Initiate Preventative Measure

Recommendations for Practice

Given the generally low sensitivities of the tests evaluated, a practical recommendation for clinicians for prevention of pre-edampsia is to consider refraining from testing, but to initiate preventative treatment.

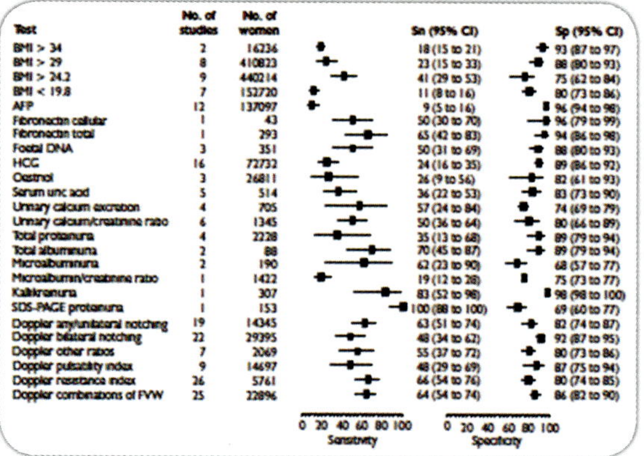

	Treatment	RR	95% CI	Revised RR[a]	95% CI
Group 1[b]	Rest for normotensive women vs unrestricted activity	0.05	0.0 to 0.83	No subgroup analyses	
	Antioxidants vs placebo/no antioxidants	0.61	0.50 to 0.75	0.45[d]	0.31 to 0.66
	Calcium supplement vs placebo	0.48	0.33 to 0.69	0.62[e]	0.32 to 1.20
	Antiplatelets vs placebo/no intervention	0.81	0.75 to 0.88	0.85[f]	0.77 to 0.94
Group 2[c]	Progesterone vs no progesterone	0.21	0.03 to 1.77	NA	
	Diuretics vs placebo/no diuretics	0.68	0.45 to 1.03	NA	
	Garlic vs placebo	0.78	0.31 to 1.93	NA	
	Nitric oxide donors or precursors vs placebo/no intervention	0.83	0.49 to 1.41	NA	
	Marine/fish oils vs placebo/no treatment	0.86	0.59 to 1.27	NA	
	Antihypertensives vs placebo/no treatment	0.99	0.84 to 1.18	NA	
	Advice to reduce dietary salt vs advice to continue normal diet	1.11	0.46 to 2.66	NA	
				Comments	
RRs not used in the models	**Updated review**				
	Antiplatelets vs placebo/no intervention	0.83	0.77 to 0.89	Results virtually identical with older version of review results used in the model	
	Updated review				
	Antihypertensives vs placebo/no treatment	0.97	0.83 to 1.13		
	Exercise	0.31	0.01 to 7.09	Results based on one outcome in 2 small RCTs (n = 16 and 29)	
	Bed rest for hypertension during pregnancy	0.98	0.80 to 1.20	Inappropriate population	
	Nutritional advice during pregnancy	0.89	0.42 to 1.88	Results based on 1 RCT	
	Balanced energy/protein supplementation	1.20	0.77 to 1.89	Risk of harm	
	Isocaloric protein supplementation	1.00	0.57 to 1.75	Results based on 1 RCT	
	Energy/protein restriction	1.13	0.59 to 2.18	Risk of harm	

[a] RRs based on subgroup analyses, defined in detail in the text, and used as parameters in sensitivity analyses.
[b] Group 1 are those treatments with an RR whose upper 95% CI is <1.0.
[c] Group 2 are those treatments with an RR whose 95% CI includes a value compatible with worsened outcome.
[d] Subgroup excluding the single large quasi-randomised trial.
[e] Subgroup of trials carried out in populations with an adequate calcium diet.
[f] Subgroup of trials carried out in populations with mothers at 'moderate risk' of pre-eclampsia rather than both 'moderate' and 'high risk' combined.

Low-dose Aspirin... Calcium Supplement ...Cost-effective Approach...without Prior Testing

Recommendations for Practice

With regard to effectiveness results, low-dose aspirin could be offered to women at risk of preeclampsia and calcium supplementation could be considered for those with low dietary calcium intake. With regard to the economic modelling, the most cost-effective approach to reducing preeclampsia is likely to be the provision of an effective, affordable and safe intervention applied to all mothers without prior testing to assess level of risk. However, we believe that it is probably premature to suggest the implementation of a treat-all intervention strategy such as advice to rest, low-dose aspirin or calcium supplementation on cost-effectiveness grounds at present. Some consideration needs to be given as to whether we should continue to do certain tests reviewed in this report whose main perceived value up to now has been to help identify preeclampsia.

Recommendation from the National Institute of Clinical Excellence (NICE) 2011

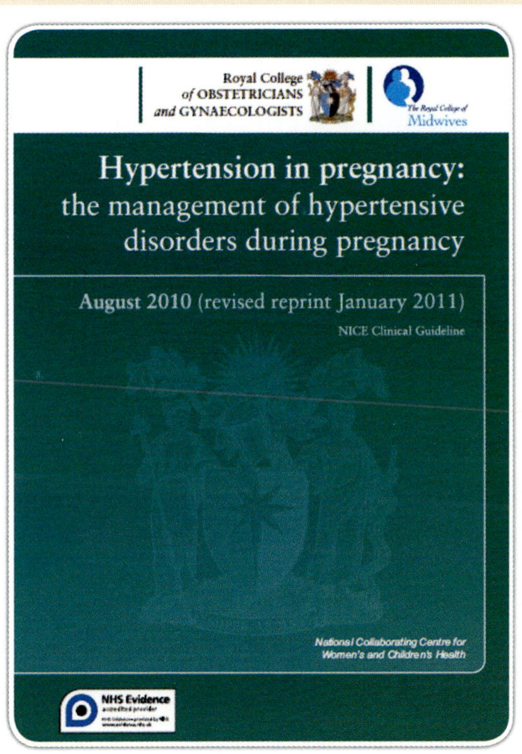

- This screening strategy based on maternal history and characteristics (and not by sonographic or laboratory)

High-risk (1)	Moderate Risk (≥2)
• Hypertensive disease during previous pregnancy	• First pregnancy
• Chronic hypertension	• Age ≥ 40 years
• Chronic kidney disease	• Pregnancy interval > 10 years
• Autoimmune disease (i.e. SLE, Antiphospholipid syndrome)	• BMI ≥ 35 kg/m^2 on 1st visit
• Type 1 or 2 diabetes	• Family history of preeclampsia
	• Multiple pregnancies

Aspirin 75 mg/D from 12 weeks' until delivery

CONCLUSION

Remaining challenges for screening, prediction, and therapy for preeclampsia

- Serum biomarkers aids in diagnosis in controversial cases
- Serum biomarkers are a part of effective multivariate algorithm for prediction of preeclampsia
- Prophylaxis and novel therapy for preeclampsia may eventually based on serum bioinformatics
- These biomarkers may have an additional role in other placental related diseases, i.e. preterm delivery and placental growth restriction.

SUGGESTED READING

1. Bombrys AE, Barton JR, Habli M, Sibai BM. Expectant management of severe preeclampsia at 27(0/7) to 33(6/7) weeks' gestation: maternal and perinatal outcomes according to gestational age by weeks at onset of expectant management. Am J Perinatol. 2009;26:441-6.
2. Bujold E, Roberge S, Lacasse Y, et al. Prevention of preeclampsia and intrauterine growth restriction with aspirin started in early pregnancy: a meta-analysis. Obstetrics and gynecology. 2010;116:402-14.
3. Levine RJ, Qian C, Leshane ES, et al. Two-stage elevation of cell-free fetal DNA in maternal sera before onset of preeclampsia. Am J Obstet and Gynecol. 2004;190:707-13.
4. Levine RJ, Qian C, Maynard SE, Yu KF, Epstein FH, Karumanchi SA. Serum sFlt1 concentration during preeclampsia and mid trimester blood pressure in healthy nulliparous women. Am J Obstet and Gynecol. 2006;194:1034-41.
5. Ozkan H, Cetinkaya M, Koksal N, Ozmen A, Yildiz M. Maternal preeclampsia is associated with an increased risk of retinopathy of prematurity. Journal of perinatal medicine. 2011;39:523-7.
6. Roberge S, Giguere Y, Villa P, et al. Early administration of low-dose aspirin for the prevention of severe and mild preeclampsia: a systematic review and meta-analysis. Am J Perinat. 2012;29:551-6.
7. Thangaratinam S, Langenveld J, Mol BW, Khan KS. Prediction and primary prevention of pre-eclampsia. Best practice and research in clinical obstetrics and gynaecology. 2011;25:419-33.
8. Verlohren S, Galindo A, Schlembach D, et al. An automated method for the determination of the sFlt-1/PlGF ratio in the assessment of preeclampsia. Am J Obstet and Gynecol. 2010;202:161;e1- e11.
9. Verlohren S, Herraiz I, Lapaire O, et al. The sFlt-1/PlGF ratio in different types of hypertensive pregnancy disorders and its prognostic potential in preeclamptic patients. Am J Obstet and Gynecol. 2012;206:58;e1-8.

Chapter

24

Fetal Urinary Tract Anomalies

Mandy Abushama, Badreldeen Ahmed

Urinary Tract Anomalies

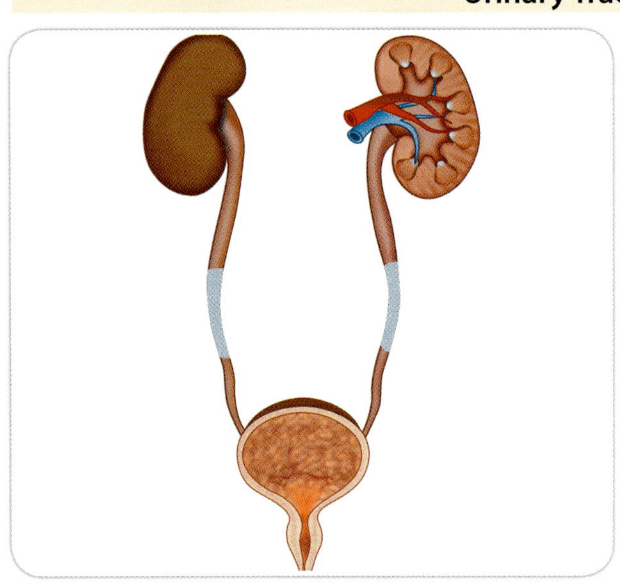

- Fetal kidneys and urinary bladder (KUB) should be sonographically visible at 20 wks'
- Severe KUB anomalies can be visible as early as 12 wks'
- But some KUB anomalies may not be visible until 3rd trimester.

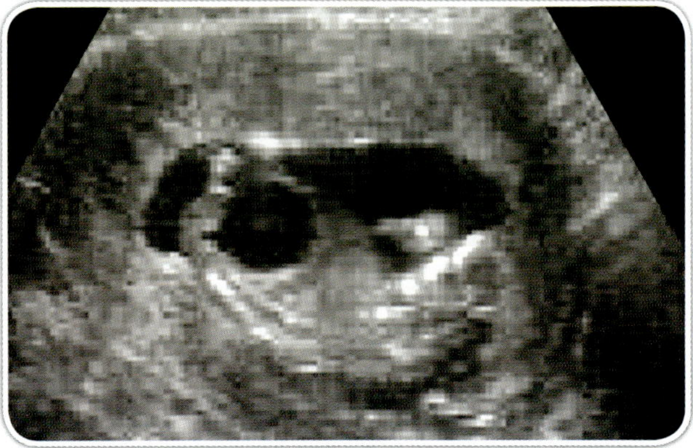

- Common fetal anomalies (34%) of all anomalies)
- Usually occurs in low-risk women
- 32% = Isolated
- 20% = Associated with other nephro-urological diseases
- 48% = Syndrome/Chromosome.

(Stoll C et al. 2014, Mishrat et al. 2010)

Embryology

- Fetal kidneys develop from the intermediate mesoderm in the form of pro-, meso-, and metanephros starting at age 5 wks'
- Mesonephric duct is the origin of the ureteric bud from which collecting ducts including the renal pelvis develop
- The bladder is formed from the distal part of the mesonephric duct (the trigone) and part of the cloaca
- Production of fetal urine begins by 10th wks'.

(Potter EL. 1972)

Normal Anatomy: Kidneys

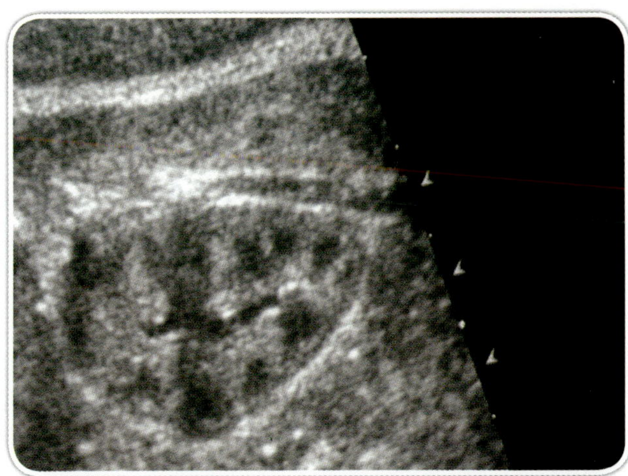

- Circumference of normal fetal kidneys: Circumference of fetal abdomen remains constant at **0.27–0.30**
- The normal length of the kidney also remains at the height of 4–5 vertebrae.

(Chitty et al. 2003, Zoltan et al. 2011)

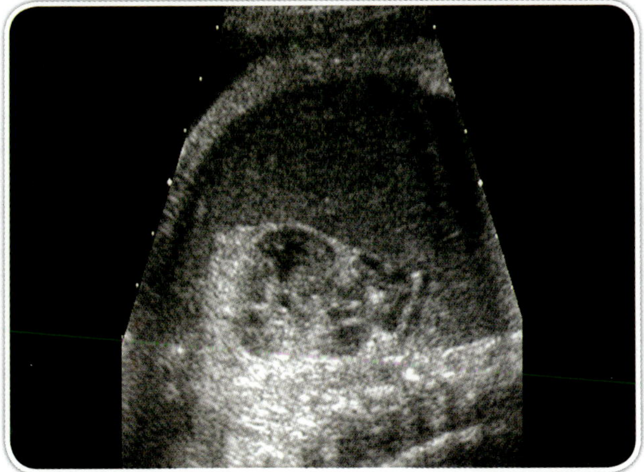

- May be visible at 11–12 wks'
- Consistently seen in mid-trimester and thereafter.

(Chitty et al. 2003, Zoltan et al. 2011)

For complete presentation, please refer the accompanying CD-ROM...

REFERENCES

1. Adra AM, Mejides AA, Dennaoui MS, Beydoun SN. Fetal pyelectasis: is it always "physiologic"? Am J Obstet Gynecol 1995; 173:1263-6.
2. Avni F E, Garel L, Cassart M, Massez A, Eurin D, Didier F, etal. Perinatal assessment of hereditary cystic renal diseases: the contribution of sonography. Pediat Radiol. 2006; 36(5): 405-14.
3. Bromley B, Lieberman E, Shipp TD, et al. The genetic sonogram, a method for risk assessment for Down syndrome in the mid trimester. J Ultrasound Med 2002; 21:1087.
4. Chitty LS. Charts of fetal size: kidney and pelvis measurements. Prenat Diagn 2003; 23(11):891-7.
5. Corteville JE, Gray DL, Crane JP. Congenital hydronephrosis: correlation of fetal ultrasound findings with infant outcome. Am J Obstet Gynecol. 1991; 165(2): 384-8.
6. Dremsek PA, Gindl K, Voitl P, Strobl R, Hafner E, Geissler W, etal . Renal pyelectasis in fetuses and neonates: diagnostic value of renal pelvis diameter in pre- and postnatal sonographic screening. AJR Am J Roentgenol. 1997; 168(4):1017-9.
7. Droste S, Fitzsimmons J, Pascoe-Mason J, Shepard TH, Mack LA. Size of the fetal adrenal in bilateral renal agenesis. Obstet Gynecol.1990;76(2):206-9.
8. Dubbins PA, Kurtz AB, Wapner RJ, Goldberg BB. Renal agenesis: spectrum of in utero findings. J Clin Ultrasound.1981; 9(4):189-93.
9. Feldman DM, DeCambre M, Kong E, Borgida A, Jamil M, McKenna P, Egan JF. Evaluation and follow-up of fetal hydronephrosis. J Ultrasound Med. 2001; 20(10):1065–9.
10. Helin I, Persson PH. Prenatal diagnosis of urinary tract abnormalities by ultrasound. Pediatrics .1986;78 (5) : 879 -83.
11. Hobbins J C, Romero R, Grannum P, Berkowitz RL, Cullen M, Mahoney M. Antenatal diagnosis of renal anomalies with ultrasound : I. Obstructive uropathy. Am J Obstet Gynecol.1984; 148(7): 868-77.
12. Lee RS, Cendron M, Kinnamon DD, Nguyen HT. Antenatal hydronephrosis as a predictor of postnatal outcome: a meta analysis. Pediatrics 2006; 118:586-93.
13. Mishra OP, Pandey N, Shukla RC, Agarwal NR, Prasad R. Antenatal detection of urinary tract abnormalities by ultrasonography. Int J Nephrol Urol. 2010; 2(2): 373-8.
14. Moore KL, Persaud TVN. The Developing Human: Clinically Oriented Embryology, 8th ed. Philadelphia: Saunders, 2003; chapter 12, pp. 243-283. Edition: 9th
15. Nyberg DA, Souter VL, El-Bastawissi A, et al. Isolated sonographic markers for detection of fetal Down syndrome in the second trimester of pregnancy. J Ultrasound Med 2001; 20(10):1053-63.
16. Odibo AO, Raab E, Elovitz M, Merrill JD, Macones GA.Prenatal mild pyelectasis: evaluating the thresholds of RPD associated with normal postnatal renal function. J Ultrasound Med. 2004; 23(4): 513-7.
17. Ouzounian JG, Castro MA, Fresquez M, Al Sulyman OM, Kovacs BW. Prognostic significance of antenatally detected fetal pyelectasis. Ultrasound Obstet Gynecol .1996; 7(6):424-8.
18. Parkhouse HF, Barratt TM. Investigation of the dilated urinary tract. Pediatr Nephrol. 1988;2(1):43-7.
19. Potter EL: Normal and abnormal development of the kidney, Chicago, 1972, Year Book Medical Publishers .
20. Promsonthi P. Viseshsindh W. Case report and review: prenatal diagnosis of congenital megalourethra. Fetal Diagn Ther .2010;28(2):123-8.
21. Rinat C, Farkas A, Frishberg Y. Familial inheritance of crossed fused renal ectopia. Pediatr Nephrol . 2001; 16(3):269-270.
22. Roberto R, Cullen M, Peter Grannum, Jeanty P, Reece EA, Venus I, etal. Antenatal diagnosis of renal anomalies with ultrasound III. Bilateral renal agenesis.Am J Obstet Gynecol.1985;151(1); 38-43.
23. Roodhooft AM, Birnholz JC, Holmes LB. Familial nature of congenital absence and severe dysgenesis of both kidneys. N Engl J Med.1984; 310(21):1341.
24. Sabbagha R, Tamura R, et al, Glob. libr. women's med., Ultrasound Diagnosis of Fetal Anomalies (ISSN: 1756-2228) 2008; DOI 10.3843/GLOWM.10205.
25. Sanders RC, James AE (Eds).The principles and practice of ultrasonography in obstetrics and gynaecology, 3rd edition, Norwalk, Connecticut :Appleton Century Crofts:1985.pp.195-209. CT (USA); ISBN 0-8385-7956-6.
26. Sanders RC. Blackman LR, Hogge WA, Wulfsberg EA, Spevak PJ. Structural fetal abnormalities . Mosby 2002 second edition.
27. Schreuder MF, Rik Westland R,Joanna AE, van Wijk2. Unilateral multicystic dysplastic kidney: a meta-analysis of observational studies on the incidence, associated urinary tract malformations and the contralateral kidney. Nephrol DialTransplant. 2009; 24 (6): 1810-8.
28. Stoll C, Dott B, Alembik Y, Roth MP. Associated nonurinary congenital anomalies among infants with congenital anomalies of kidney and urinary tract (CAKUT). Eur J Med Genet. 2014;57(7):322-8.
29. Thornburg LL, Pressman EK, Chelamkuri S, etal. Third trimester ultrasound of fetal pyelectasis: predictor for postnatal surgery. J Pediatr Urol. 2008; 4:51-4.
30. Woodward M, Frank D . Postnatal management of antenatal hydronephrosis. BJU Int. 2002; 89:149-56.
31. Yamamura Y, Swartout JP, Anderson EA, et al. Management of mild pyelectasis: a comparison analysis. J Ultrasound Med. 2007 ; 26(11):1539-43.
32. Zoltan et al. Diagnostic sonography of Fetal urinary tract anomalis. Donald school textbook Ultrasound in Obstetrics and Gynecology. Asim Kurjak, Frank Chervenak. Jaypee Brothers Medical Publishers, 2011.

Chapter 25

Fetal Skeletal Dysplasia and Malformations

Ritsuko Kimata Pooh

DEVELOPMENT OF BONE IN THE EARLY STAGE

- Endochondral ossification
  - Bone tissue replaces hyaline cartilage
  - Forming all bones below the skull except for the clavicles
- Osteoblasts secrete osteoid, creating a bone collar around the diaphysis of the hyaline cartilage model
- Cartilage in the center of the diaphysis calcifies and deteriorates, forming cavities
- Periosteal bud invades the internal cavities
- Spongy bone forms around the remaining fragments of hyaline cartilage
- The diaphysis elongates as the cartilage in the epiphyses continues to lengthen
- Medullary cavity forms through the action of osteoclasts within the center of the diaphysis
- Epiphyses ossify shortly after birth through the development of secondary ossification centers.

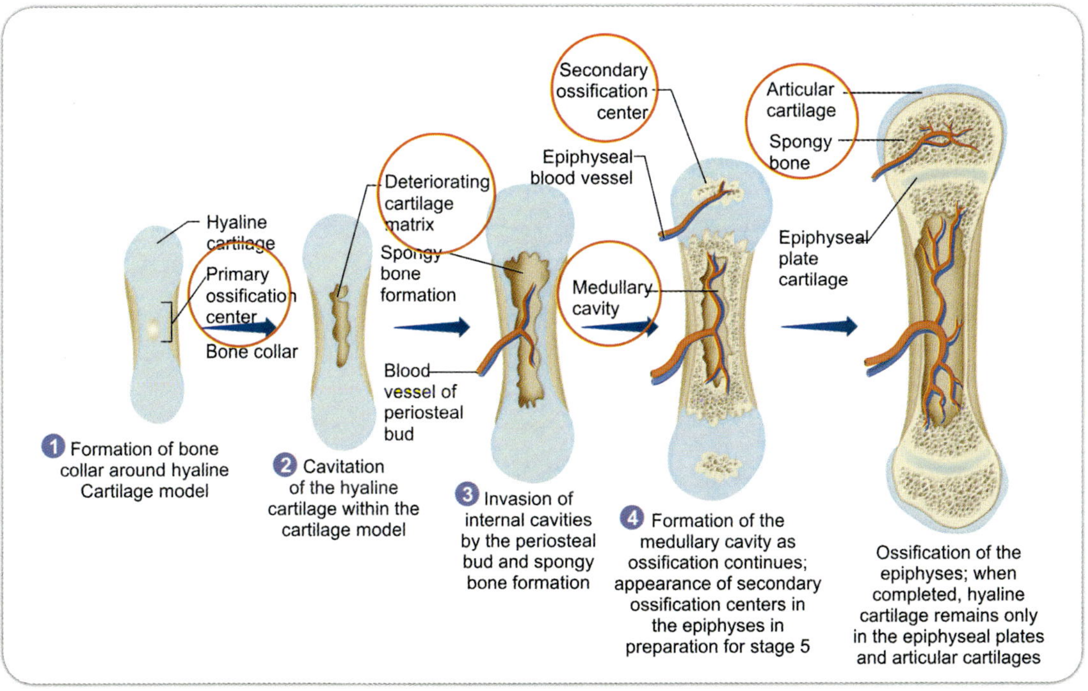

Classes.midlandstech.edu. Chapter 6: Bones And Skeletal Tissues. http://classes.midlandstech.edu/carterp/Courses/bio210/chap06/lecture1.html

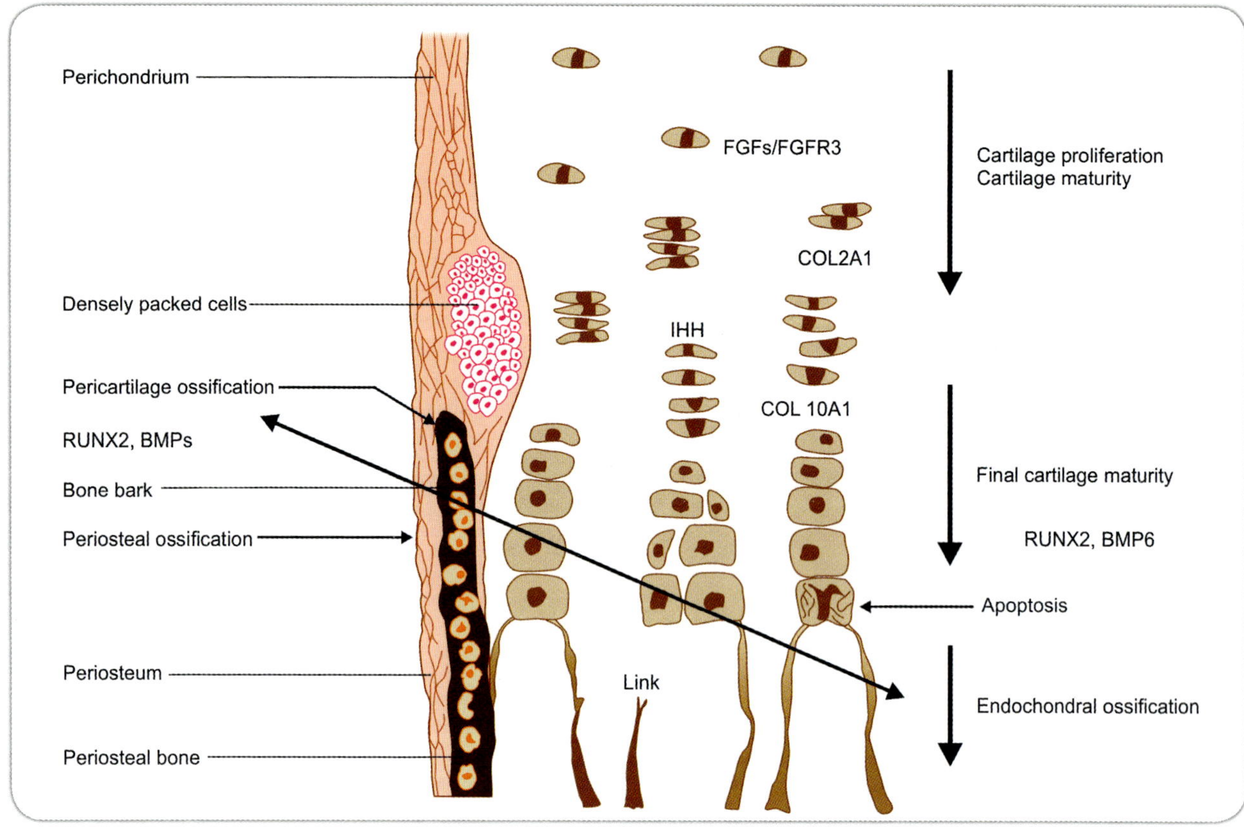

RUNX2 ; Runt-related transcription factor 2, BMP; bone morphogenetic protein, FGF; fibroblast growth factor, FGFR; FGF receptor, COL2A1; collagen, type II, alpha 1

PATTERN RECOGNITION OF SKELETAL DYSPLASIAS

- FGFR3 (Thanatophoric dysplasia/Achondroplasia)
- Short rib (polydactyly) group
- Type 2 collagenopathies:
  - ACGII/HCG/SEDC; Stickler/Kniest dysplasia
- Disorders with dumbbell deformity:
  - Dyssegmental dysplasia/FCG/Schneckenbecken dysplasia/Metatropic dysplasia
- ACG 1A
- DTDST disorders:
  - ACG 1 B, AO2, Diastrophic dysplasia
- Filaminopathy B:
  - Larsen dysplasia/Boomerang dysplasia/AO 1/3
- Bent and fragile bone groups
  - OI/campomelic dysplasia/hypophosphatasia/I-cell disease
- Chondrodysplasia punctata.

For complete presentation, please refer the accompanying CD-ROM…

SUGGESTED READING

1. Classes.midlandstech.edu. Chapter 6: Bones and skeletal tissues. http://classes.midlandstech.edu/carterp/Courses/bio210/chap06/lecture1.html
2. Spranger JW, Brill PW, Nishimura G, Superti-Furga A, Unger S. Bone dysplasia. An atlas of genetic disorders of skeletal development. 3rd Edition. Oxford University Press. New York. 2012

Chapter
26

Sonogenetics

Ritsuko Kimata Pooh

EUPLOID

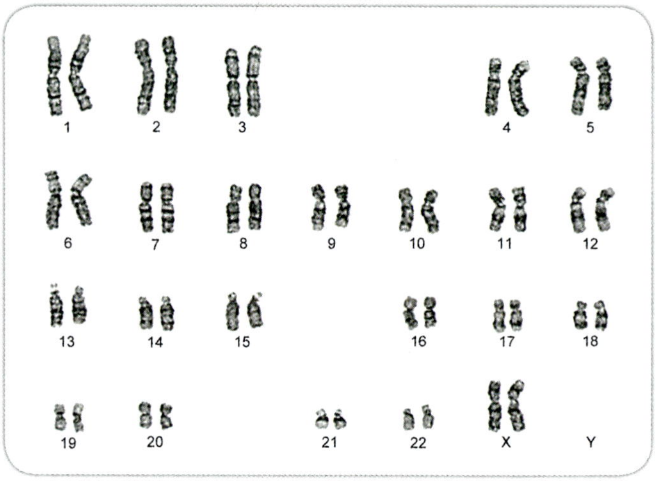

1 2 3 4 5
6 7 8 9 10 11 12
13 14 15 16 17 18
19 20 21 22 X Y

TRISOMY

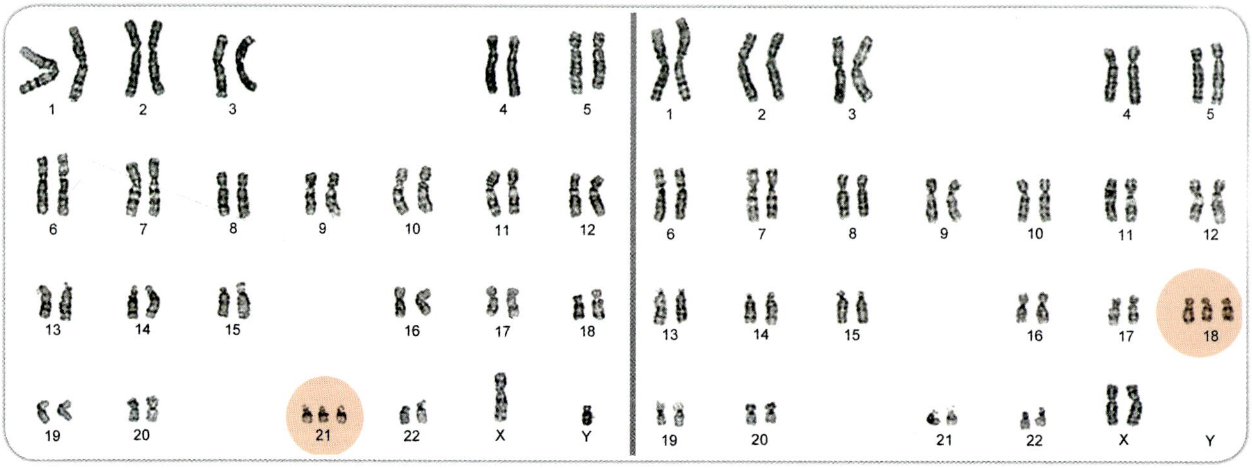

1 2 3 4 5
6 7 8 9 10 11 12
13 14 15 16 17 18
19 20 21 22 X Y

1 2 3 4 5
6 7 8 9 10 11 12
13 14 15 16 17 18
19 20 21 22 X Y

MONOSOMY

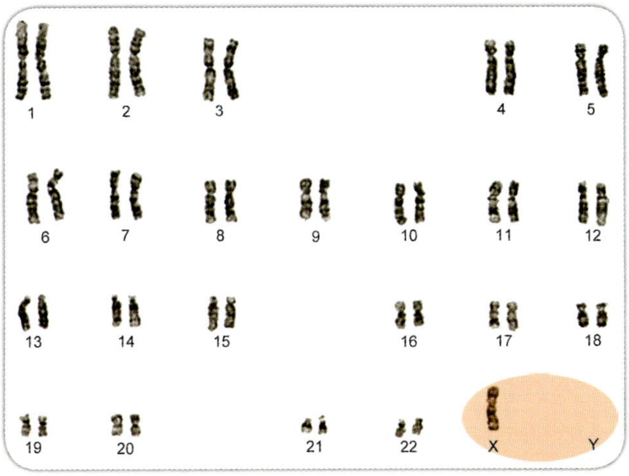

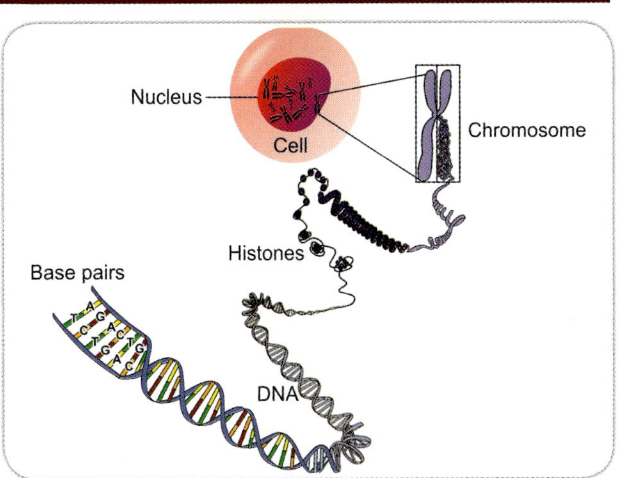

CHROMOSOME PROFILE

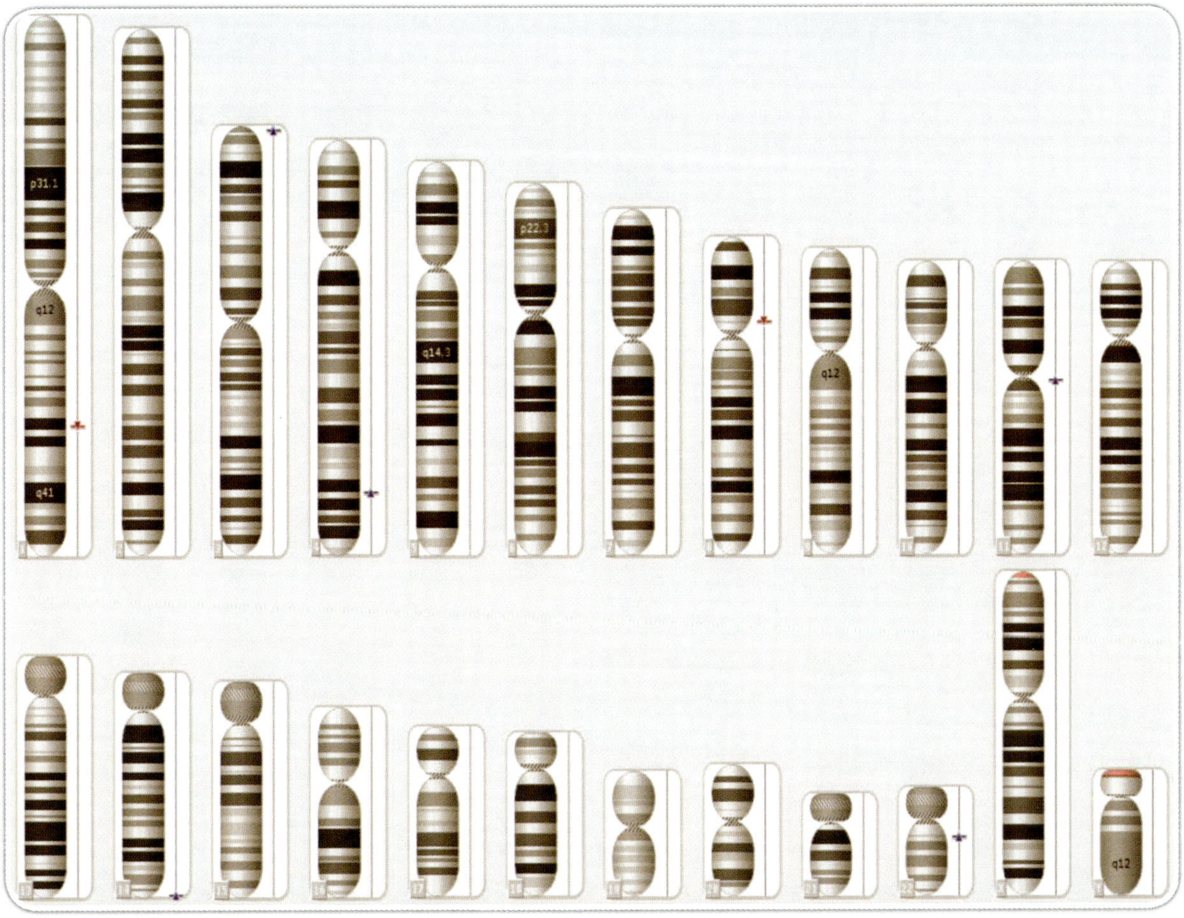

For complete presentation, please refer the accompanying CD-ROM…

SUGGESTED READING

1. Brunetti-Pierri N, Berg JS, Scaglia F, et al. Recurrent reciprocal 1q21.1 deletions and duplications associated with microcephaly or macrocephaly and developmental and behavioral abnormalities. Nat Genet. 2008; 40(12):1466-71.
2. Bruno DL, Ganesamoorthy D, Schoumans J, et al. Detection of cryptic pathogenic copy number variations and constitutional loss of heterozygosity using high resolution SNP microarray analysis in 117 patients referred for cytogenetic analysis and impact on clinical practice. J Med. Genet. 2009;46:123-31.
3. Campeau PM, Ah Mew N, Cartier L, Mackay KL, Shaffer LG, Der Kaloustian VM, etal. Prenatal diagnosis of monosomy 1p36: a focus on brain abnormalities and a review of the literature. Am J Med Genet A. 2008;146 A(23):3062-9.
4. Choy KW, Setlur SR, Lee C, Lau TK. The impact of human copy number variation on a new era of genetic testing. BJOG. 2010;117(4):391-8.
5. Faas BH, van der Burgt I, Kooper AJ, Pfundt R, Hehir-Kwa JY, Smits AP, et al. Identification of clinically significant, submicroscopic chromosome alterations and UPD in fetuses with ultrasound anomalies using genome-wide 250k SNP array analysis. J Med Genet. 2010; 47:586-94.
6. Hillman SC, Pretlove S, Coomarasamy A, McMullan DJ, Davison EV, Maher ER , et al. Additional information from array comparative genomic hybridization technology over conventional karyotyping in prenatal diagnosis: a systematic review and meta-analysis. Ultrasound Obstet Gynecol. 2011;37:6-14.
7. Law LW, Lau TK, Fung TY, Leung TY, Wang CC, Choy KW. De novo 16p13.11 microdeletion identified by high-resolution array CGH in a fetus with increased nuchal translucency. BJOG. 2009; 116(2):339-43.
8. Leung TY, Pooh RK, Wang CC, Lau TK, Choy KW. Classification of pathogenic or benign status of CNVs detected by microarray analysis. Expert Rev Mol Diagn. 2010; 10(6):717-21.
9. Pooh RK, Choy KW, Leung TY, Lau TK. Sonogenetics –a breakthrough in prenatal diagnosis. Donald School J Ultrasound Obstet Gynecol. 201; 5(1)75-9.
10. Pooh RK. Sonogenetics in fetal neurology. Semin Fetal Neonatal Med. 2012; 17(6):353-9.
11. Shinawi M, Cheung SW. The array CGH and its clinical applications. Drug Discov Today. 2008; 13:760-70.
12. Soong YK, Wang TH, Lee YS, Chen CP, Chang CL, Ho SY, et al. Genome-wide detection of uniparental disomy in a fetus with intrauterine growth restriction using genotyping microarrays. Taiwan J Obstet Gynecol. 2009; 48:152-8.
13. Srebniak MI, Boter M, Oudesluijs GO, Cohen-Overbeek T, Govaerts LC, Diderich KE, et al. Genomic SNP array as a gold standard for prenatal diagnosis of foetal ultrasound abnormalities. Mol Cytogenet. 2012; 5:14.

Chapter 27

Fetal Thorax: Anatomy and Defects

Cihat Şen

THORAX
Normal Anatomy

- Conotruncal shape
- Upper borders by the clavicles and the neck
- Inferior by the diaphragm
- Laterally by the ribs
- Anteriorly by the sternum
- Posteriorly by the shoulder

- Lungs
- Heart
- Mediastinum with the great vessels
- The thymus (larger in the fetus than in the neonate).

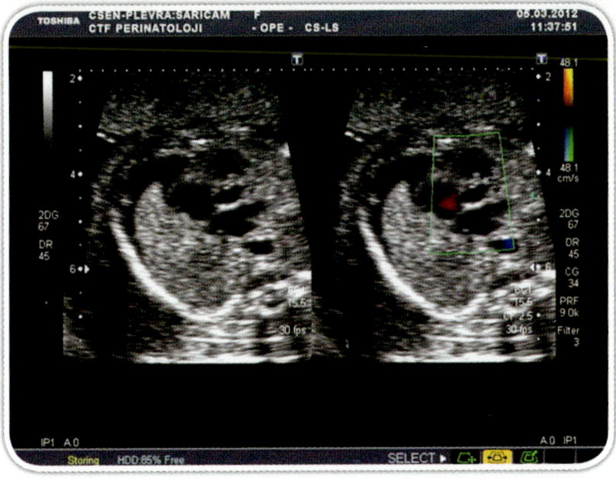

Thorax Anomalies

- May appear only in the 3rd trimester
- F/U late 3rd trimester scan
- May regress before birth
- Initial assessment of the thorax and the heart: 12–14 wks'.

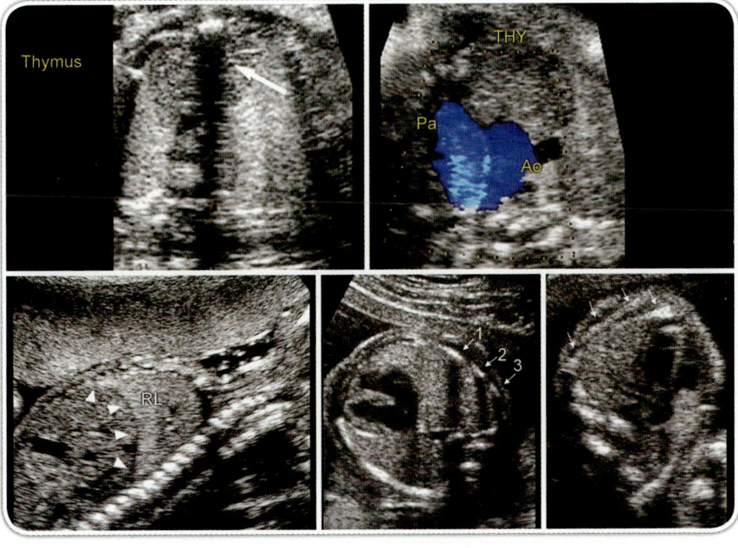

NORMAL THORAX

- Classic **4-chamber view**
- Also examine ribs, sternum, and the cutaneous outline
- The diaphragm shows a curved outline, convex towards the thorax

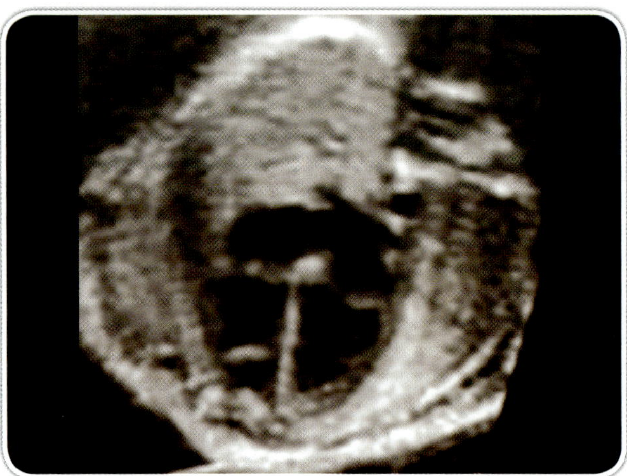

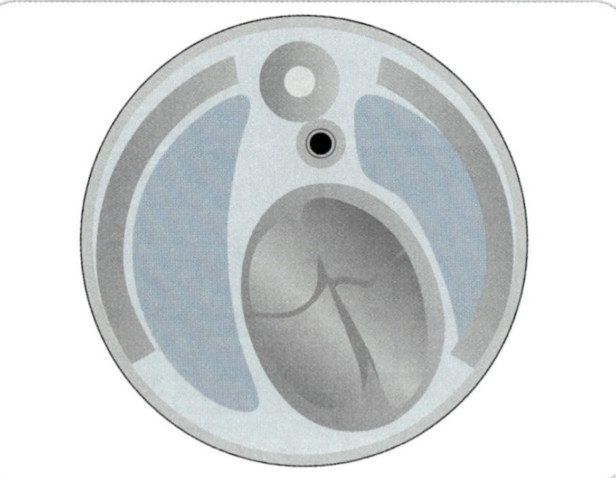

- Axial plane: Lungs appear as solid, homogeneous, weakly hyperechoic structures that almost completely surround the heart
- Heart is mainly located in the left hemithorax
- Therefore, right lung will appear larger than the left one
- **Pleural cavity** is virtual, and does not show up
- **Pericardial cavity**, on the contrary, often contain a film of fluid, especially insonated with high-frequency transducers.

AXIAL VIEW OF THE MEDIASTINUM (3-VESSEL VIEW)

- Parallel to the 4-chamber view, but more cranial
- To demonstrate the aortic and pulmonary arches and the corresponding flows on color Doppler for the detection of ductus dependence
  - The thymus and its relationship with the great vessels
  - Easier to recognize from the late 2nd trimester onwards when it starts to undergo significant hypertrophy.

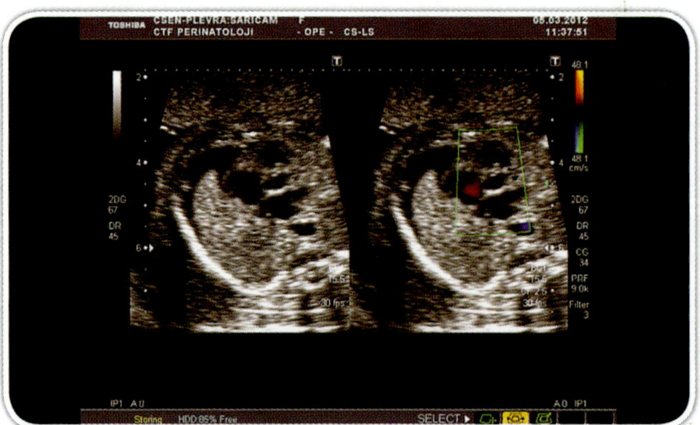

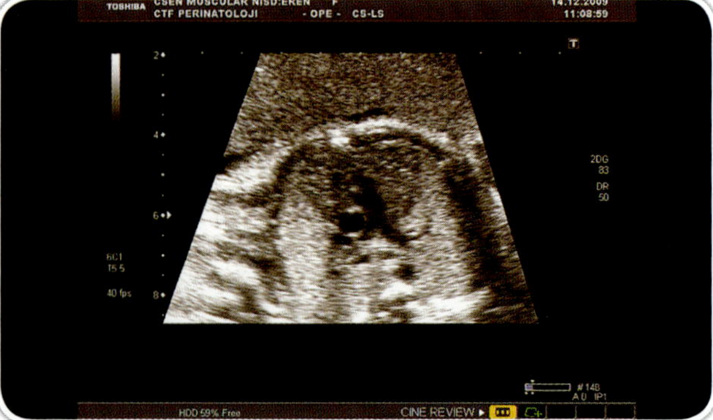

For complete presentation, please refer the accompanying CD-ROM...

SUGGESTED READING

1. Stevens TP, Chess PR, McConnochie KM, SinkinRA, Guillet R, Maniscalco WM,et al. Survival in early- and late-term infants with congenital diaphragmatic hernia treated with extracorporeal membrane oxygenation. Pediatrics. 2002;110:590-6.
2. Witlox RS, Lopriore E, Oepkes D. Prenatal interventions for fetal lung lesions. Prenatal Diagn. 2011; 31:628-36.
3. YinonY, Grisaru-Granovsky S, Chaddha V, Windrim R, Seaward PG, Kelly EN,et al. Perinatal outcome following fetal chest shunt insertion for pleural effusion. Ultrasound Obstet Gynecol : the official Journal of the International Society of Ultrasound in Obstetrics and Gynecology. 2010; 36:58-64.

Chapter

28

Ultrasound in Fetal and Neonatal Alloimmune Thrombocytopenia

Simona Vladareanu, Vlad Zamfirescu, Radu Vladareanu

INTRODUCTION

- Fetal and neonatal alloimmune thrombocytopenia (FNAIT) is the most common cause of severe neonatal thrombocytopenia
- FNAIT is analogous to the fetal/neonatal anemia caused by hemolytic disease of the fetus and newborn (HDFN)
- Fetal platelet antigens are normally expressed on platelets as early as the 16th week of pregnancy
- Feto-maternal incompatibility for human platelet alloantigens (HPAs) may cause maternal alloimmunization
- Fetal and neonatal thrombocytopenia may result from placental transfer of IgG antibodies.

(Kaplan, 2007, Murphy et al. 2007)

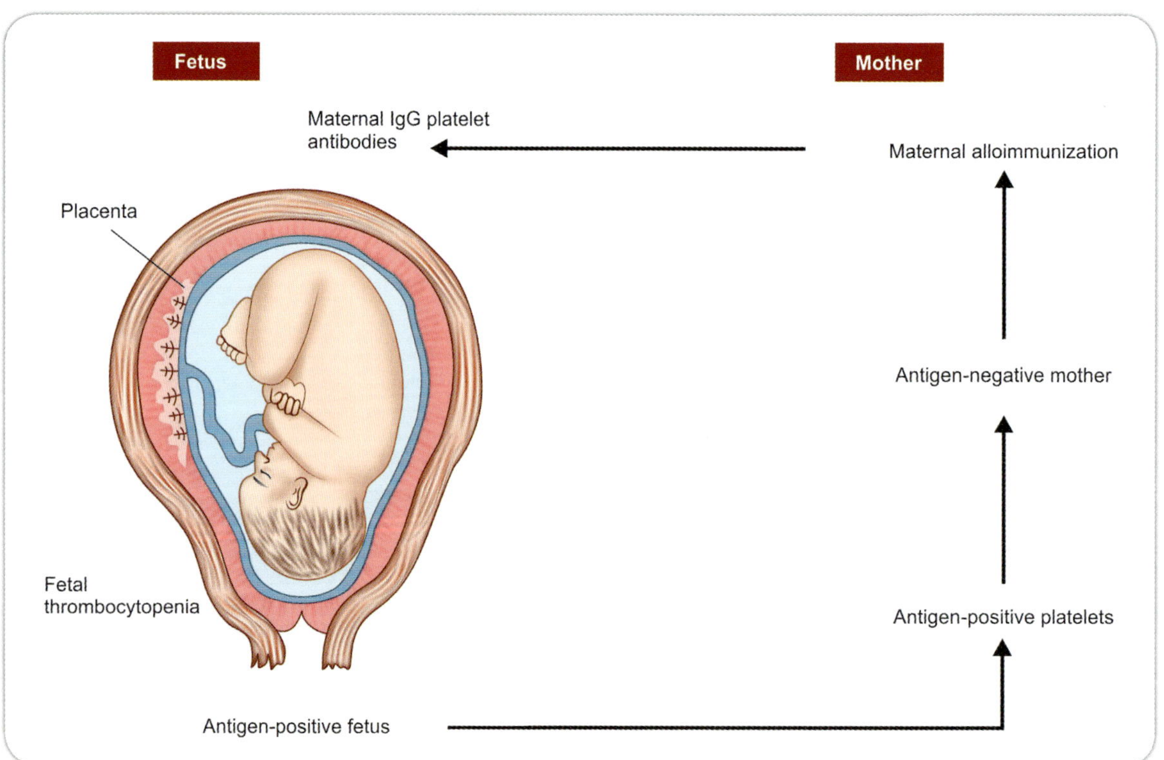

FNAIT mechanism

- The fetal opsonized platelets are then cleared in the reticulo-endothelial system
- The resulting thrombocytopenia is not only due to increased platelet destruction but also to impaired platelet production
- The majority of HPA antigens such as HPA-1a are located on the β3 subunit of the αIIbβ3 integrin (GPIIb/IIIa, CD41/CD61), which is present at high density on the platelet membrane
- Others such as HPA- 5b are on α2β1 (GPIa/IIa, CD49b)
- Antigenic incompatibility HPA-1a is found in 80% of cases of FNAIT in Caucasians
- In contrast to HDFN, FNAIT frequently occurs in first pregnancies
- Considerable progress has been made in the laboratory investigation of FNAIT since it was first recognized in the 1950s
- There have also been improvements in its management, particularly in the antenatal management of women with a history of one or more pregnancies affected by FNAIT
- Better understanding of severe hemorrhage and advances in fetal and transfusion medicine.

(Ouwehand et al. 2006)

Epidemiology

- The normal platelet count in the fetus and the neonate is the same as in adults
- Neonatal thrombocytopenia has many causes, and is the commonest hematological problem in the newborn infant
- A platelet count of <150 ×10⁹/l occurs in about 1% of unselected neonates, and is <50 × 10⁹/l in about 0.2%
- FNAIT is the most important cause of severe fetal and neonatal thrombocytopenia (frequency and bleeding severity)
- For example, FNAIT is associated with more severe fetal/neonatal bleeding than with maternal autoimmune thrombocytopenic purpura (associated platelet and/or endothelial dysfunction)
- A fetal or neonatal platelet count of <20 × 10⁹/l is usually caused by FNAIT due to anti-HPA-1a as approximately half of the cases in which the neonatal platelet count is <50 × 10⁹/l.

Incidence

- The frequency of HPAs varies across the world
- The HPA-1a that predominates in the Caucasian population is rare in the Asian population, where HPA-5b incompatibility is the most common cause of feto-maternal alloimmune thrombocytopenia
- Prospective studies in Caucasian populations for FNAIT due to anti-HPA-1a indicate that about 2% of women are HPA-1a-negative, and that about 10% of HPA-1a-negative women develop anti-HPA-1a.
- Alloimmunization to HPA-1a is HLA class II restricted. There is a strong association with HLADRB3*0101 (HLADRw52a), which is present in 1 in 3 of Caucasian women, and HPA-1a alloimmunization is rare in HPA-1a-negative women who lack this antigen
- Incidence of FNAIT due to anti-HPA-1a is 1 in 1163 live births (86 per 100,000)
- Incidence of severe thrombocytopenia (platelet count 50 ×10⁹/l) to be 1 in 1695 (or 59 per 100,000)
- FNAIT is under-diagnosed in routine clinical practice. Only 7–23% of cases of FNAIT, and only 37% of severe cases, are detected clinically
- The incidence of an intracranial hemorrhage (ICH) as a result of alloimmunization to the HPA-1a antigen is approximately 20%

For complete presentation, please refer the accompanying CD-ROM...

SUGGESTED READING

1. Donal B et al., 2000; Benacerraf BR et al., 2005; Baba K et al., 2000; Desser TS et al., 2001; Mercé LT et al., 2006; Kupesic S et al., 2003; Hill ML, 1992; Soares SR et al., 2000; Salle B et al., 1999; De Kroon CD et al., 2003; Oliveira FG et al., 2004; Kurjak A et al., 1992; Grimbizis GF et al., 2001; Acien P, 1997; Salim Daya, 1994; Heinonen PK, 2006; Troiano RN et al., 2004; Stassart JP et al. 1992; Kurjak A et al., 1991; Bourne TH et al., 1996; Ilan Timor - Trisch educational ppt
2. Kaplan, 2007; Murphy et al., 2007; Ouwehand et al., 2006; Rayment et al., 2005; Turner et al., 2005; Spencer et al., 2001; Dreyfus et al., 1997; Blanchette et al., 2000; Rader et al., 2003; Murphy et al., 2002; Kjeldsen-Kragh et al., 2007; Tiller et al., 2009; Kanhai et al., 2007; Fretheim, 2008; Killie et al., 2007; Birchall et al., 2003; Silver et al., 2000; Berkowitz et al., 2006; Paidas et al., 1995; Simon et al., 2003; Rayment et al., 2005; Berkowitz et al., 2007; Bussel et al., 1996; Berkowitz et al., 2006; Radder et al., 2001; Bussel et al., 2008; Ouwehand et al., 2000; Mueller-Eckhardt et al., 1989; Bassler et al., 2008; Kiefel et al., 2006; Allen et al., 2007; Bakchoul et al., 2008; Derycke et al., 1985; Sidiropoulus et al., 1984; Suarez et al., 1987; Ballin et al., 1988; Linder et al., 1990; Bussel et al., 2005; Kanhai et al., 2007.

Chapter

29

Management of Prenatally Diagnosed Congenital Anomalies in Africa

Aliyu Labaran Dayyabu

OUTLINE

- Definition/Epidemiology
- Why prenatal diagnosis in Africa
- Problems of prenatal diagnosis in Africa
- Spectrum of congenital anomalies in Africa
- Our approach and experience
- Cases of prenatally diagnosed anomalies
- The future of prenatal diagnosis in Africa
- Prevention of congenital anomalies in Africa
- Conclusion

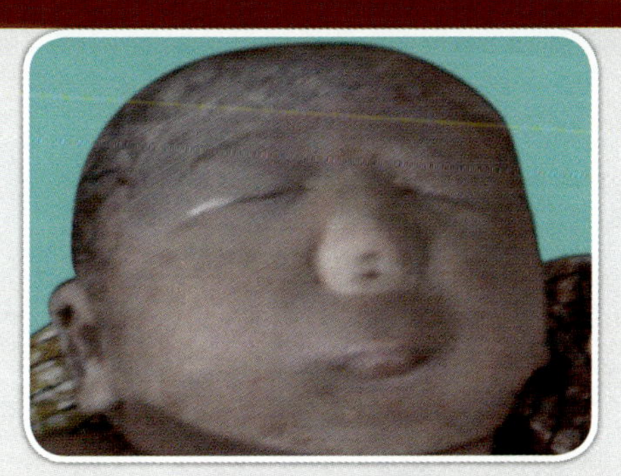

Definition and Epidemiology

Definition

- Prenatal diagnosis is testing for disease or conditions in a fetus before it is born[WHO]
- Aim is to detect birth defects which can be morphological, genetic, or biochemical
- Ultrasound is meant to detect morphological aberrations such as spina bifida or serve as a means of getting access to fetal tissues for further analysis
- "Congenital/fetal anomalies" = structural, functional and/or biochemical-molecular defects present at birth whether detected at that time or not [WHO]
- Prevalence in developing countries especially in Africa is underestimated because of deficiencies in diagnostic capabilities
- Lack of reliable medical records and statistics (*Victor et al. 2002*)
- Incidence 2–3% of newborns (*ICBDM 1991*)
- 94% of severe birth defects are seen in low- resource countries particularly in Africa
- 71% of births go unrecorded in sub-Saharan Africa (UNICEF 2001)
- It follows that the number anomalies recorded is far below the actual number.

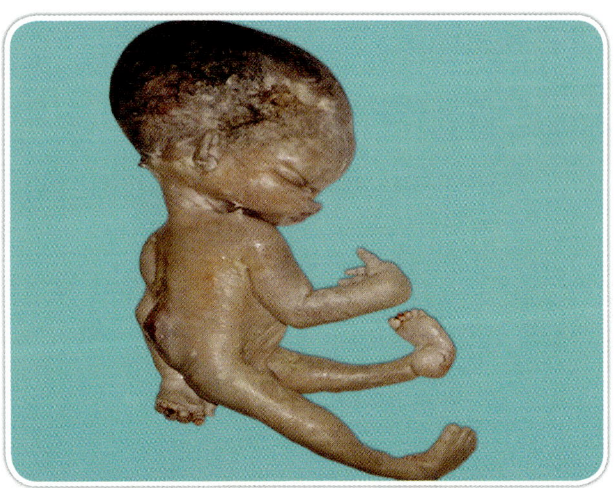

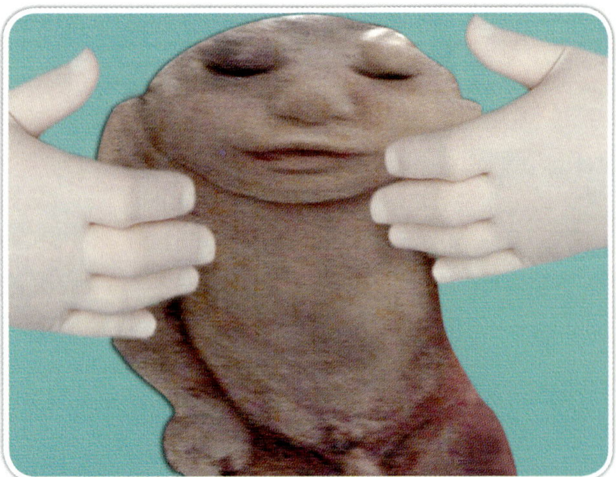

CONGENITAL ANOMALIES SEEN IN AFRICA

Particular environmental conditions/diseases

- Iodine/Folate deficiencies
- Diseases such Diabetes
- Infections
  - Rubella: 25% of infants born to mothers who had the disease in the first trimester have CRS
  - Syphilis: In Sub-Saharan Africa 6–16% of pregnant women have active Syphilis (*Murray et al. 1998*)

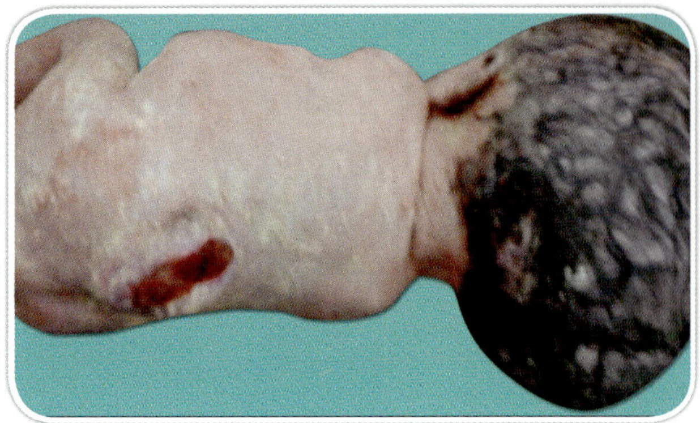

Usually, the presentation is of multiple anomalies

- Neural tube defects
- Hydrocephalus
- Limb deformities
- Sacrococcygeal teratoma
- Cystic hygroma
- Cleft lip/Palate
- Others.

Causes

- 50% are idiopathic (*Cutts et al. 1997*)
- Most are multifactorial in nature

Other causes include:

- Chromosomal anomalies, e.g. Down syndrome
- Environmental factors
  - Intrauterine infections, e.g. Rubella, Syphilis
  - Drugs, e.g. Thalidomide, Phenytoin
  - Alcohol
  - Deficiencies, e.g. Folic acid, Iodine
  - Ionizing radiation.

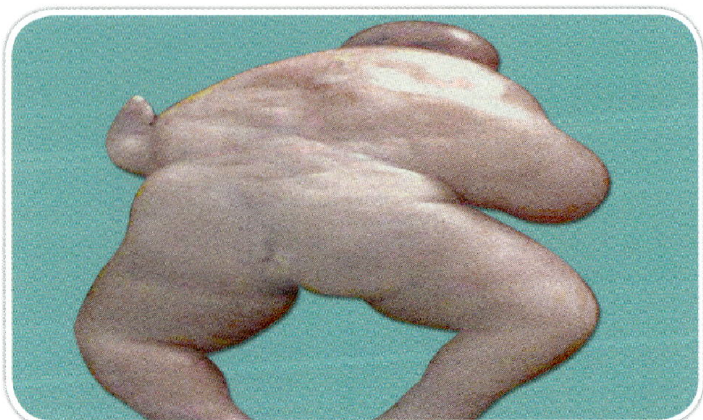

For complete presentation, please refer the accompanying CD-ROM...

SUGGESTED READING

1. Adeleye AO, Dairo MD, Olowookere KG. Central nervous system congenital malformations in a developing country: Issues and their challenges against their prevention. Child Nerv Syst. 2010;26(7):914-24.
2. Adetiloye VA, Dare FO, Oyelami OA. A ten-year review of Encephalocele in a teaching hospital. Int J Gynecol Obstet. 1993;41(3):241-9.
3. Berry RJ, Zhu I, Erickson JD, Song I, et al. Prevention of neural tube defects with folic acid in China. N Eng J Med. 1999;341: 1485-90.
4. Controlling Birth Defects: Reducing the Hidden Toll of Dying and Disabled Children in Low-Income Countries [Disease Control Priority Project].
5. Cutts FT, Wynnyck E. Modelling the incidence of congenital rubella syndrome in developing countries. Int J Epidemiol. 1997;28:1176-84.
6. Fact sheet N°370 [Updated January 2014.
7. ICBDM, 1991.
8. Jose M Carrera. Obstetric Ultrasound in Africa is it necessary to promote their appropriate use? DSJOG. 2011;289-96.
9. Lakhoo K, et al. Best clinical practice: surgical conditions of the fetus and newborn. Early Human Dev. 2006;82:281-324.
10. Mourali M, Fkih C, Essoussi-Chikhaoui J, Ben Haj Hassine A, Binousi N, Ben Zineb N, Boussed H. Gestational Trophoblastic disease in Tunisia. Tunis Med. 2008;86(7):665-9.
11. MRC Vitamin Study Research Group. Prevention of neural tube defects: Results of the Medical Research Council Vitamin Study. Lancet. 1991;338:131-7.
12. Murray CJL, Lopez AD. Health Dimensions of Sex and Reproduction: The Global Burden of Sexually Transmitted Diseases, HIV, Maternal Conditions, Perinatal Disorders and Congenital Anomalies,1998. Boston: Harvard School of Public Health.
13. Pan American Health Organization. Report on Vaccines and Immunization. 128th Session of the Executive Committee, 25-29 June 2001. CE128/10, Washington DC, USA.2001; pp. 10-11.
14. Pharoah PO. Iodine supplementation trials. Am J Clin Nutr. 1993;57(suppl): 276S-279S.
15. Robertson SE, Cutts FT, Samuel R, et al. Control of rubella and congenital rubella syndrome (CRS) in developing countries. Part 2: Vaccination against rubella. Bull World Health Organ. 1997;75:55-68.
16. Todd C, Haw T, Kromberg J, Christianson A. Genetic Counselling in a South African Community. Jounal of Genetic Counselling. 2010:19(3):247-54.
17. UNFPA 1998. The state of the world population. New York. United Nations Fund for population activities.
18. UNICEF. Report about world infancy health. Report Geneve, 2001.
19. Victor B Penchaszadeh. Preventing congenital anomalies in developing countries. Community Genet. 2002;5:61-9.
20. WHO
21. WHO 2000. Primary health care approaches for the prevention and control of congenital and genetic disorders. Geneva, WHO/HGN/WG/001.

Chapter

30

Ultrasound in Labor

Dominic Iliescu, Panos Antsaklis, Asim Kurjak

ULTRASOUND IN LABOR: INTRODUCTION

1. Clinical assessment of labor progress is one of the basic skills that is taught during training (residency).
2. Abdominal palpation, digital examination, cervical dilatation, head position, head station, head rotation etc.
3. Use of PARTOGRAM for more than 50 years in Obstetrics.

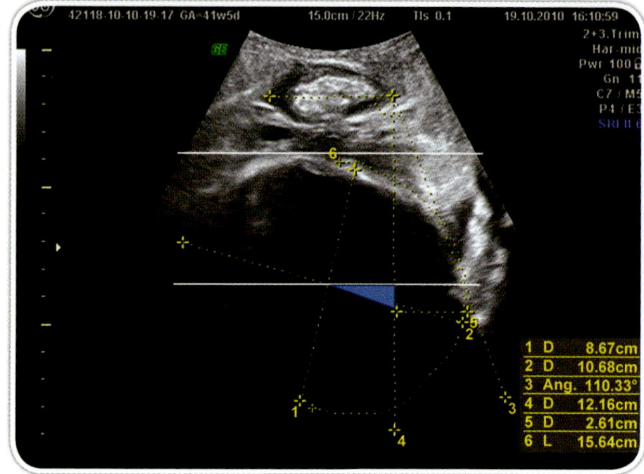

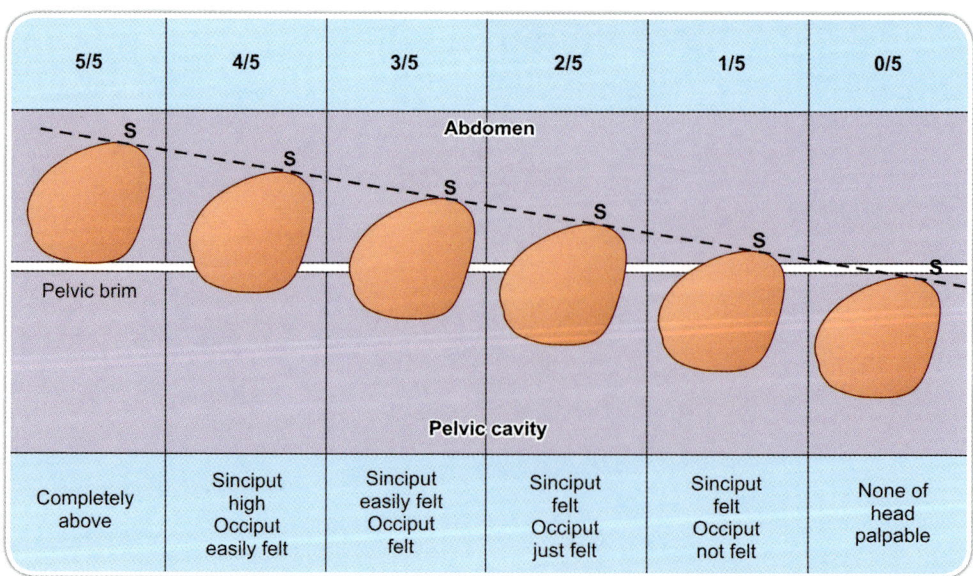

Clinical estimation of descent of head in fifths palpable above the pelvic brim

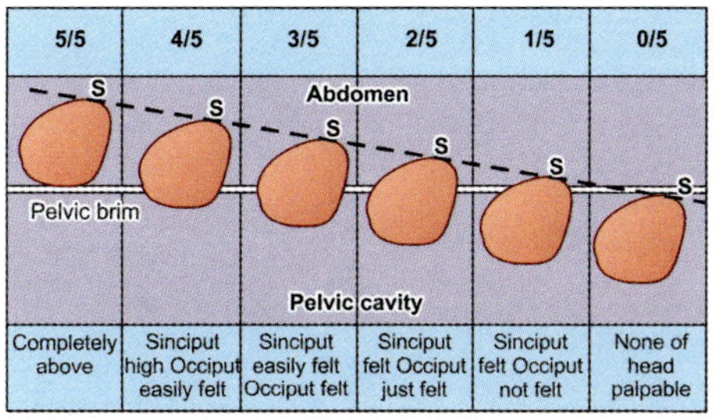

5/5	4/5	3/5	2/5	1/5	0/5
Completely above	Sinciput high Occiput easily felt	Sinciput easily felt Occiput felt	Sinciput felt Occiput just felt	Sinciput felt Occiput not felt	None of head palpable

Abdomen
Pelvic brim
Pelvic cavity
S

Clinical estimation of descent of head in fifths palpable above the pelvic brim

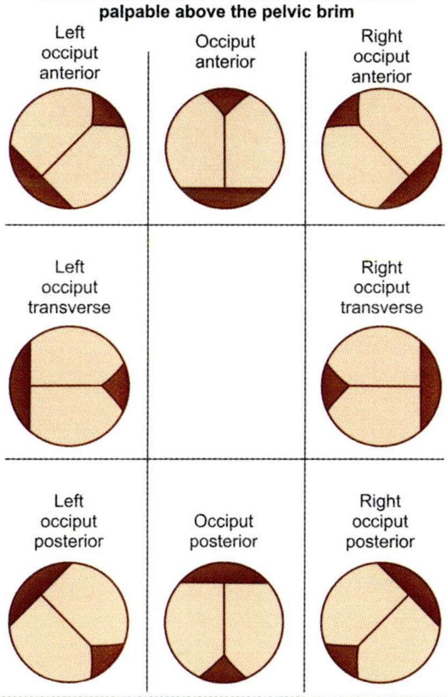

Left occiput anterior — Occiput anterior — Right occiput anterior

Left occiput transverse — Right occiput transverse

Left occiput posterior — Occiput posterior — Right occiput posterior

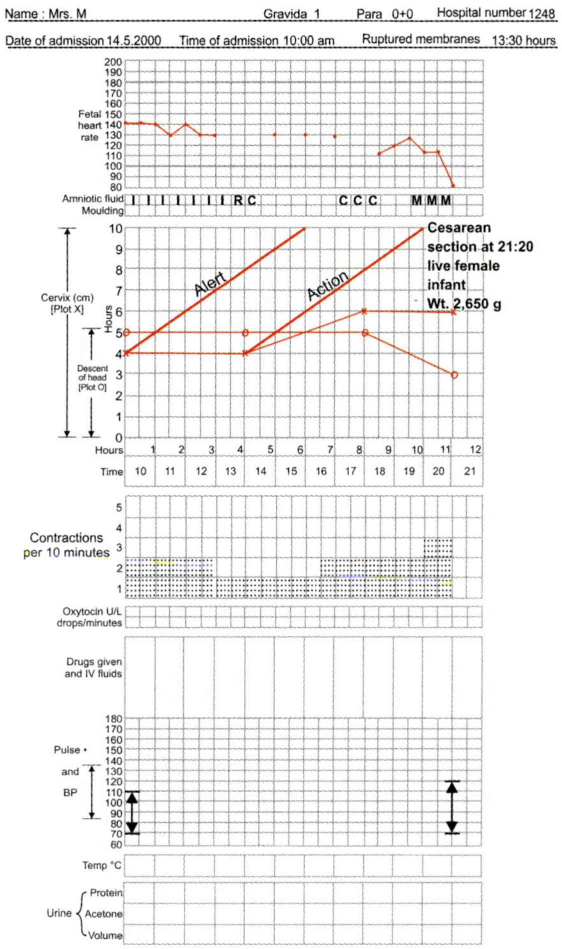

Name : Mrs. M Gravida 1 Para 0+0 Hospital number 1248

Date of admission 14.5.2000 Time of admission 10:00 am Ruptured membranes 13:30 hours

Fetal heart rate (80–200)

Amniotic fluid / Moulding: I I I I I I I R C C C C M M M

Cervix (cm) [Plot X]

Descent of head [Plot O]

Alert

Action

Cesarean section at 21:20 live female infant Wt. 2,650 g

Hours: 1 2 3 4 5 6 7 8 9 10 11 12

Time: 10 11 12 13 14 15 16 17 18 19 20 21

Contractions per 10 minutes

Oxytocin U/L drops/minutes

Drugs given and IV fluids

Pulse • and BP

Temp °C

Urine: Protein, Acetone, Volume

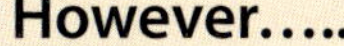

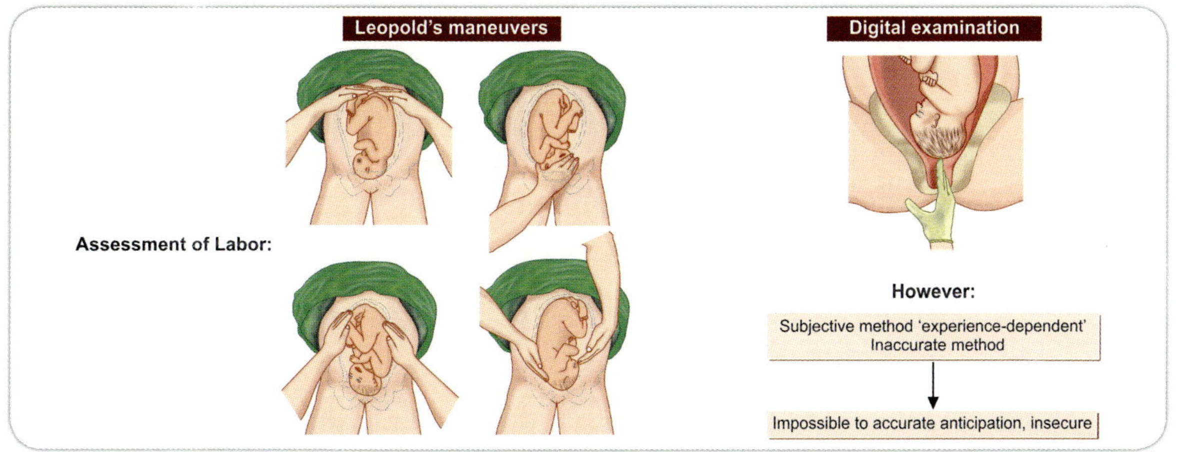

For complete presentation, please refer the accompanying CD-ROM...

SUGGESTD READING

1. ACOG, Practice Bulletin #107, "Induction of Labor," published in the August 2009 issue of Obstetrics & Gynecology.
2. Akmal S, Kametas N, Tsoi E, Hargreaves C, Nicolaides KH. Comparison of transvaginal digital examination with intrapartum sonography to determine fetal head position before instrumental delivery. Ultrasound Obstet Gynecol. 2003;21:437-40.
3. Akmal S, Tsoi E, Howard R, Osei E, Nicolaides KH. Investigation of occiput posterior delivery by intrapartum sonography. Ultrasound Obstet Gynecol. 2004;24:425-8.
4. Akmal S, Tsoi E, Kametas N, Howard R, Nicolaides KH. Intrapartum sonography to determine fetal head position. J Matern Fetal Neonatal Med. 2002;12:172-7.
5. Barbera AF, Imani F, Becker T, Lezotte DC, Hobbins JC. Anatomic relationship between the pubic symphysis and ischial spines and its clinical significance in the assessment of fetal head engagement and station during labor. Ultrasound Obstet Gynecol. 2009;33:320-5.
6. Barbera AF, Pombar X, Perugino G, Lezotte DC, Hobbins JC. A new method to assess fetal head descent in labor with transperineal ultrasound. Ultrasound Obstet Gynecol. 2009;33:313-9.
7. Björklund K, Lindgren PG, Bergström S, Ulmsten U. Sonographic assessment of symphyseal joint distension intrapartum. Acta Obstet Gynecol Scand. 1997;76:227–32.
8. Crane JM. Factors predicting labor induction success: a critical analysis. Clin Obstet Gynecol 2006;49:573-84.
9. Crowley P. Interventions for preventing or improving the outcome of delivery at or beyond term. Cochrane Database Syst Rev. 2000;2:CD000170.
10. Dietz H, Moore KH. Pelvic organ mobility is associated with delivery mode. Aust NZJ Obstet Gynaecol. 2003;43:70-4.
11. Dietz HP, Bennett MJ. The effect of childbirth on pelvic organ mobility. Obstet Gynecol. 2003; 102:223-8.
12. Dietz HP, Lanzarone V, Simpson JM. Predicting operative delivery. Ultrasound Obstet Gynecol. 2006;27:409-15.
13. Dietz HP, Lanzarone V. Measuring engagement of the fetal head: validity and reproducibility of a new ultrasound technique. Ultrasound Obstet Gynecol 2005; 25: 165–168.
14. Dietz HP, Wilson PD. Anatomical assessment of the bladder outlet and proximal urethra using ultrasound and videocystourethrography. Int Urogynecol J Pelvic Floor Dysfunct. 1998;9:365-9.
15. Dietz HP. Ultrasound imaging of the pelvic floor. Part I: two-dimensional aspects. Ultrasound Obstet Gynecol. 2004;23:80-92.
16. Dupuis O, Ruimark S, Corinne D, Simone T, André D, René-Charles R. Fetal head position during the second stage of labor: comparison of digital vaginal examination and transabdominal ultrasonographic examination. Eur J Obstet Gynecol Reprod Biol. 2005;123(2):193-7. Epub 2005 May 31.
17. Dupuis O, Silveira R, Zentner A, Dittmar A, Gaucherand P, Cucherat M, Redarce T, Rudigoz RC. Birth simulator: reliability of transvaginal assessment of fetal head station as defined by the American College of Obstetricians and Gynecologists classification. Am J Obstet Gynecol. 2005; 192:868-74.
18. Dückelmann AM, Bamberg C, Michaelis SA, Lange J, Nonnenmacher A, Dudenhausen JW, Kalache KD. Measurement of fetal head descent using the 'angle of progression' on transperineal ultrasound imaging is reliable regardless of fetal head station or ultrasound expertise. Ultrasound Obstet Gynecol. 2010;35:216-22.
19. Ecker J, Chen K, Cohen A, Riley L, Lieberman E. Increased risk of cesarean delivery with advancing maternal age: Indications and associated factors in nulliparous women. Am J Obstet Gynecol. 2001;185:883-7.
20. Eggebø TM, Gjessing LK, Heien C, Smedvig E, Økland I, Romundstad P, Salvesen KA. Prediction of labor and delivery by transperineal ultrasound in pregnancies with prelabor rupture of membranes at term. Ultrasound Obstet Gynecol. 2006;27:387-91.
21. Eggebø TM, Heien C, Økland I, Gjessing LK, Romundstad P, Salvesen KA. Ultrasound assessment of fetal head-perineum distance before induction of labor. Ultrasound Obstet Gynecol. 2008; 32:199-204.
22. Fitzpatrick M, McQuillan K, O'Herlihy C. Influence of persistent occiput posterior position on delivery outcome. Obstet Gynecol. 2001;98:1027-31.
23. Fuchs I, Tutschek B, Henrich W. Visualization of the fetal fontanels and skull sutures by three-dimensional translabial ultrasound during the second stage of labor. Ultrasound Obstet Gynecol. 2008;31(4):484-6.
24. Ghi T, Farina A, Pedrazzi A, Rizzo N, Pelusi G, Pilu G. Diagnosis of station and rotation of the fetal head in the second stage of labor with intrapartum translabial ultrasound. Ultrasound Obstet Gynecol. 2009;33:331-6.
25. Gonen R, Degani S, Ron A. Prediction of successful induction of labor: comparison of transvaginal ultrasonography and the Bishop score. Eur J Ultrasound. 1998;7:183-7.
26. Government Statistical Service. NHS Maternity Statistics, England: 2003–04. Bulletin 2005/10: March 2005; http://www.dh.gov.uk/assetRoot/04/10/70/61/04107061.pdf [Accessed 1 September 2007].
27. Grau T, Leipold RW, Horter J, Conradi R, Martin EO, Motsch J. Paramedian access to the epidural space: the optimum window for ultrasound imaging. J Clin Anesth. 2001;13:213-7.
28. Grylack L. Prenatal sonographic diagnosis of cephalhematoma due to pre-labor trauma. Pediatr Radiol. 1982;12:145-7.
29. Henrich W, Dudenhausen J, Fuchs I, Kamena A, Tutschek B. Intrapartum translabial ultrasound (ITU): sonographic landmarks and correlation with successful vacuum extraction. Ultrasound Obstet Gynecol. 2006;28:753-60.

30. Kalache KD, Dükelmann AM, Michaelis SAM, Lange J, Cichon G, Dudenhausen JW. Transperineal ultrasound imaging in prolonged second stage of labor with occipitoanterior presenting fetuses: how well does the 'angle of progression' predict the mode of delivery? Ultrasound Obstet Gynecol. 2009;33:326-30.
31. Knight D, Newnham JP, McKenna M, Evans S. A comparison of abdominal and vaginal examinations for the diagnosis of engagement of the fetal head. Aust NZJ Obstet Gynacol. 1993;33:154-8.
32. Kreiser D, Schiff E, Lipitz S, Kayam Z, Avraham A, Achiron R. Determination of fetal occiput position by ultrasound during the second stage of labor. J Matern Fetal Med. 2001;10:283-6.
33. Lieberman E, Davidson K, Lee-Paritz A, Shearer E. Changes in fetal position during labor and their association with epidural anesthesia. Obstet Gynecol. 2005;105:974-82.
34. Maesel A, Lingman G, Marsal K. Cerebral blood flow during labor in the human fetus. Acta Obstet Gynecol Scand. 1990;69:493-5.
35. Molina F, Nicolaides K. Ultrasound in Labor and Delivery. Fetal Diagn Ther. 2010;27:61-7.
36. Molina FS, Terra R, Carrillo MP, Puertas A, Nicolaides KH. What is the most reliable ultrasound parameter for assessment of fetal head descent? Ultrasound Obstet Gynecol. 2010;36:493-9.
37. Pandis GK, Papageorghiou AT, Ramanathan VG, Thompson MO, Nicolaides KH. Preinduction sonographic measurement of cervical length in the prediction of successful induction of labor. Ultrasound Obstet Gynecol. 2001;18:623-8.
38. Pearl ML, Roberts JM, Laros RK, Hurd WW. Vaginal delivery from the persistent occiput posterior position. Influence on maternal and neonatal morbidity. J Reprod Med. 1993;38:955-61.
39. Peregrine E, O'Brien P, Omar R, Jauniaux E. Clinical and ultrasound parameters to predict the risk of cesarean delivery after induction of labor. Obstet Gynecol. 2006;107:227-33.
40. Petrikovsky BM, Schneiner E, Smith-Levitin MM, Gross B. Cephalhematoma and caput succedaneum: do they always occur in labor? Am J Obstet Gynecol. 1998;179:906-8.
41. Rane SM, Guirgis RR, Higgins B, Nicolaides KH. Models for the prediction of successful induction of labor based on pre-induction sonographic measurement of cervical length. J Matern Fetal Neonatal Med. 2005;17:315-22.
42. RCOG: Induction of labor; in Evidence-Based Clinical Guideline Number 9. London, RCOG Clinical Support Unit, 2001.
43. Rozenberg P, Chevret S, Ville Y. Comparison of pre-induction ultrasonographic cervical length and Bishop score in predicting risk of cesarean section after labor induction with prostaglandins. Gynecol Obstet Fertil. 2005;33:17-22.
44. Schiwmer SR, Lebovic J. In utero sonographic demonstration of a caput succedaneum. J Ultrasound Med. 1986;5:711.
45. Shapiro JL, Sherer DM, Hurley JT, Metlay LA, Amstey MS. Postpartum ultrasonographic findings associated with placenta accreta. Am J Obstet Gynecol. 1992;167:601-2.
46. Sherer DM, Abulafia O. Intrapartum assessment of fetal head engagement: comparison between transvaginal digital and transabdominal ultrasound determinations. Ultrasound Obstet Gynecol. 2003;21:430-6.
47. Sherer DM, Allen TA, Ghezzi F, Goncalves LF. Enhanced transvaginal sonographic depiction of caput succedaneum prior to labor. J Ultrasound Med. 1994;13:1005-8.
48. Sherer DM, Miodovnik M, Bradley KS, Langer O. Intrapartum fetal head position II: comparison between transvaginal digital examination and transabdominal ultrasound assessment during the second stage of labor. Ultrasound Obstet Gynecol. 2002;19:264-8.
49. Sherer DM, Schwartz BM, Mahon TR. Intrapartum ultrasonographic depiction of fetal malpositioning and mild parietal bone compression in association with uterine leiomyoma. J Matern Fetal Med. 1999;8:28-31.
50. Sherer DM. Intrapartum ultrasound. Ultrasound Obstet Gynecol. 2007;30:123-39.
51. Souka AP, Haritos T, Basayiannis K, Noikokyri N, Antsaklis A. Intrapartum ultrasound for the examination of the fetal head position in normal and obstructed labor. J Matern Fetal Neonatal Med. 2003;13:59-63.
52. To WW, Li IC. Occipital posterior and occipital transverse positions: reappraisal of the obstetric risks. Aust NZJ Obstet Gynaecol 2000;40: 275-9.
53. Williams KP, Galemeav F, Wilson S. Effect of labor on maternal cerebral blood flow. Am J Obstet Gynecol. 1998;178:59-61.
54. Williams KP, Wilson S. Evaluation of cerebral perfusion changes in laboring women: effects of epidural anesthesia. Ultrasound Obstet Gynecol. 1999;14:393-6.
55. Yagel S, Anteby E, Lavy Y, Ben Chetrit A, Palti Z, Hochner-Celnikier D, Ron M. Fetal middle cerebral artery blood flow during normal active labour and in labour with variable decelerations. Br J Obstet Gynaecol. 1992;99:483-5.
56. Yeo ST, French R. Combined spinal-epidural in the obstetric patient with Harrington rods assisted by ultrasonography. Br J Anaesth. 1999;83:670-2.
57. Zhang J, Troendle JF, Yancey MK. Reassessing the Labor Curve in Nulliparous Women. American Journal of Obstetrics and Gynecology. 2002;187(4):824-8.
58. Zilianti M, Azuaga A, Calderon F, Pages G, Mendoza G. Monitoring of the effacement of the uterine cervix by transperineal ultrasonography. J Ultrasound Med. 1995;14:719-24.

Chapter 31

Ultrasound Screening in Perinatal Medicine

Aris Antsaklis

Ultrasound Proved to be the Most Important Diagnostic Breakthrough in the Practice of Obstetrics and Gynecology in this Century

Indications for ultrasound:

- Diagnosis
- Assessment of fetal well-being
- Invasive procedures by ultrasound guidance for fetal diagnosis and therapy

- Ultrasonography is widely accepted by parents and their families
- Women consider the use of ultrasound as a barometer for the adequacy of the maternal care.

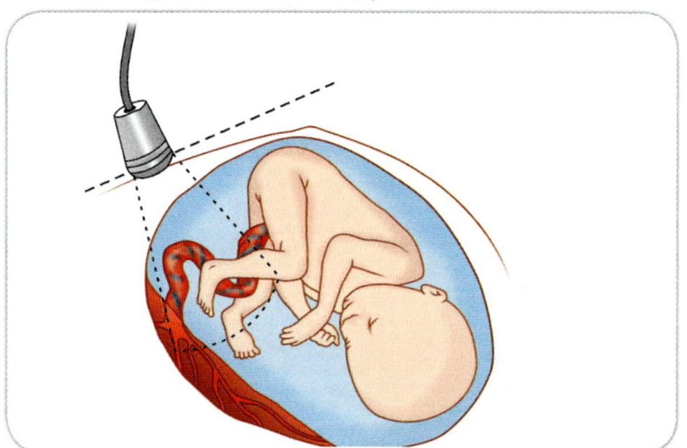

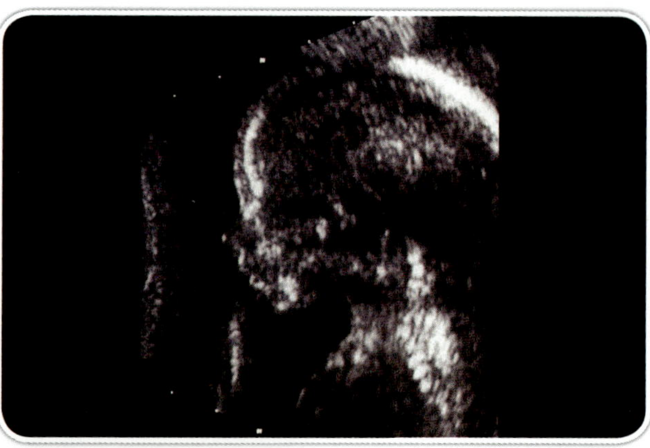

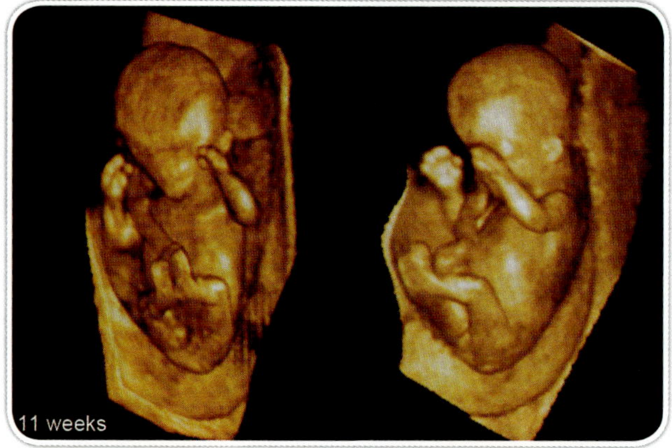

Ultrasound Screening in Perinatal Medicine

The question

Does routine ultrasound improves the overall perinatal mortality and morbidity?

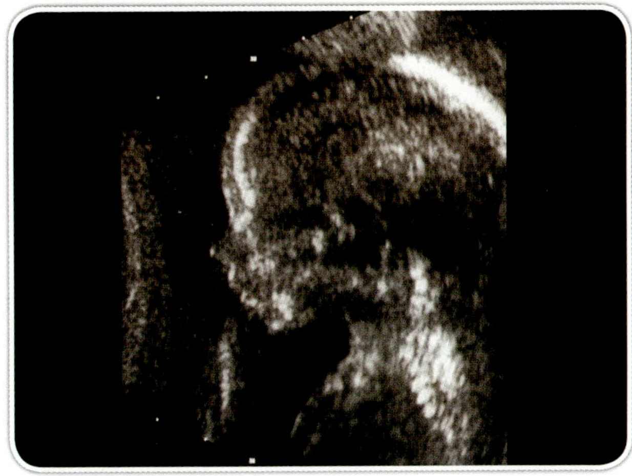

WHAT IS ULTRASOUND SCREENING?

Technical improvements in ultrasonic instrumentation opened up new ways in the visualization and evaluation of normal fetal anatomy and normal and pathological conditions of the female pelvis

To understand and to use

The high technology you need knowledge and experience

Ultrasound Dating

- Reduces the number of births considered to be post term, and reduces the number of inductions

Hyberg, Act Obst Gynecol 76: 907-912, 1997

- Reliable dating is important when interpreting Down's syndrome serum screening results

Wald et al, Prenat Diagn 16: 143-153, 1996

Ultrasound measurement of BPD and CRL gives a better estimation of estimated date of delivery (EDD) than the date of the last menstural period (LMP) even for IVF pregnancies

Gardosi et al 1997, Br J Obst Gynecol 104: 792-797, 1997
Mul et al 1996, Ultras Obst Gynecol 8: 397-402, 1996

More than 60–70% of pregnant women undergo ultrasound at various times on gestation.

For complete presentation, please refer the accompanying CD-ROM...

SUGGESTED READING

1. Benacerraf BR, Neuberg D, Bromley B, Frigoletto FD, Jr. Sonographic scoring index for prenatal detection of chromosomal abnormalities. Journal of Ultrasound in Medicine: official journal of the American Institute of Ultrasound in Medicine. 1992;11:449-58.
2. Carvalho JS, Senat MV, Schwarzler P, Ville Y. Increased nuchal translucency and ventricular septal defect in the fetus. Circulation. 1999;99:E10.
3. Gardosi J. Dating of pregnancy: time to forget the last menstrual period. Ultrasound Obstet Gynecol: the official journal of the International Society of Ultrasound in Obstetrics and Gynecology. 1997;9:367-8.
4. Mul T, Mongelli M, Gardosi J. A comparative analysis of second-trimester ultrasound dating formulae in pregnancies conceived with artificial reproductive techniques. Ultrasound in Obstet Gynecol: the official journal of the International Society of Ultrasound in Obstetrics and Gynecology. 1996;8:397-402.
5. Pilalis A, Souka AP, Antsaklis P, et al. Screening for pre-eclampsia and fetal growth restriction by uterine artery Doppler and PAPP-A at 11-14 weeks' gestation. Ultrasound Obstet Gynecol: the official journal of the International Society of Ultrasound in Obstetrics and Gynecology. 2007;29:135-40.
6. Souka AP, Pilalis A, Kavalakis Y, Kosmas Y, Antsaklis P, Antsaklis A. Assessment of fetal anatomy at the 11-14-week ultrasound examination. Ultrasound Obstet Gynecol: the official journal of the International Society of Ultrasound in Obstetrics and Gynecology. 2004;24:730-4.
7. Wald NJ, Watt HC. Serum markers for Down's syndrome in relation to number of previous births and maternal age. Prenatal diagnosis. 1996;16:699-703.
8. Whitlow BJ, Chatzipapas IK, Lazanakis ML, Kadir RA, Economides DL. The value of sonography in early pregnancy for the detection of fetal abnormalities in an unselected population. British Journal of Obstetrics and Gynaecology. 1999;106:929-36.

Chapter 32

Ultrasound Safety in Obstetrics

Kazuo Maeda

PRINCIPLE OF DIAGNOSTIC ULTRASOUND SAFETY

- The ultrasound (US) user is responsible to the diagnostic ultrasound safety
  - Knowledge of output intensity of US device
  - Possible US bio-effects
  - ALARA (As Low As Reasonably Achievable) principle.
  - US machine function
  - Prudent use of US

Frequent Questions on the Safety of US

- Biological effect in the diagnostic US?
- Tissue heated by US exposure?
- Avoiding US thermal effect in US diagnosis?
- Mechanical bioeffects of US?
- Avoiding mechanical bioeffects?
- Nonmedical use of US permitted?
- Who is responsible to diagnostic US safety?

Pulse-wave and Continuous-wave US

	Pulse-wave (PW)	Continuous-wave (CW)
Average	Low	Low
Peak	High	Low

Pulse-Wave (PW)

- PW; Imaging: Real-time B-mode, transvaginal scan, 3D and 4D ultrasound, pulsed Doppler, color/ power flow mapping

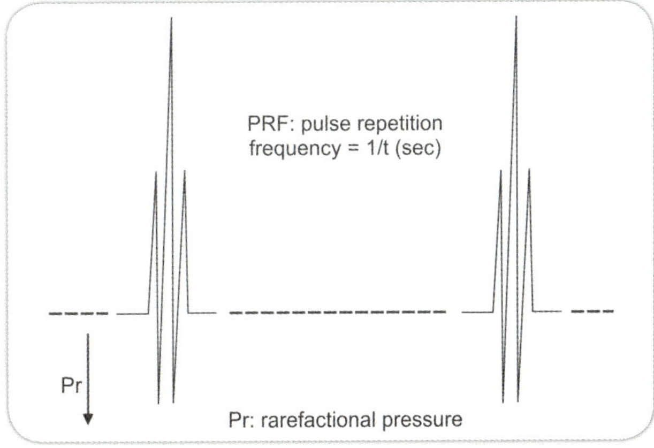

Continuous-Wave (W)

- CW; Functional study: Fetal heart detector, Fetal heart rate monitor [cardiotocogram (CTG), actocardiogram (ACG)]

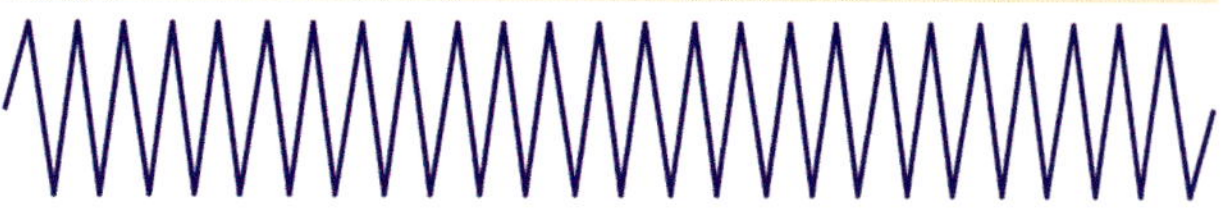

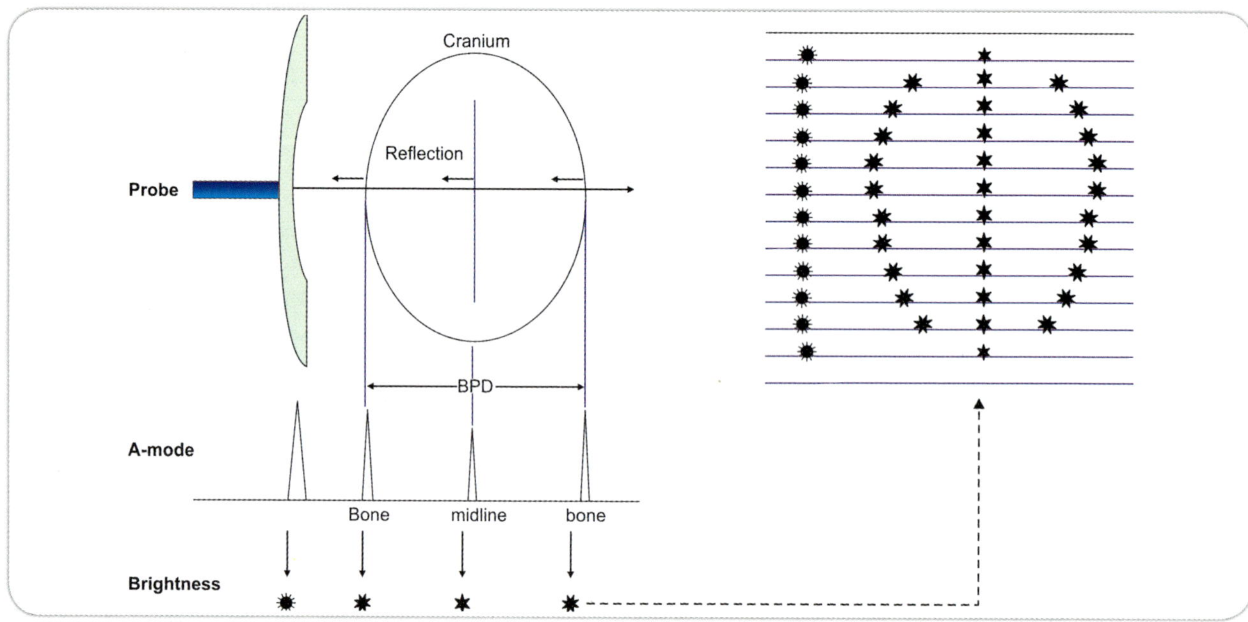

Formation of A- and B-mode images, e.g. fetal cranium

Focusing in the Real-time Electronic Scan B-mode

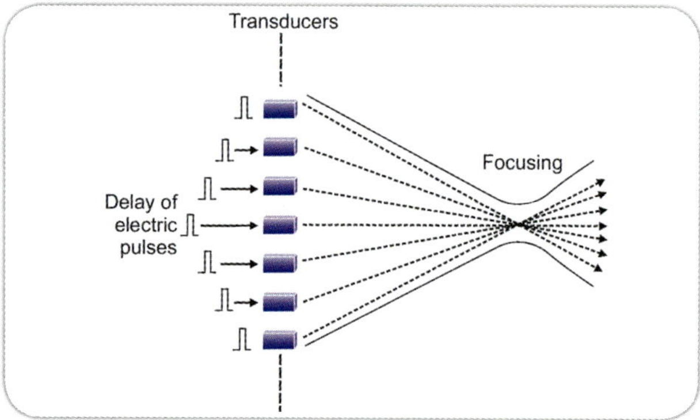

Image sharpness and **ultrasound intensity** increase at the focus

Physical US Effect

- Temperature elevation (heating) by US absorption
- Positive and negative (rarefactional) pressure
- Cavitation: heating, pressure, free radical were developed
- Streaming
- Red blood cell stasis by standing wave.

Reported Biological US Effect (bioeffect)

- Anomaly of fetal animal developed by heated transducer attached maternal abdomen
- **This is not directly developed by ultrasound, when** the transducer was separated from animal by temperature stabilized water
- Sister chromatid exchange was caused by toxic substance produced by cell container, **not by US**
- Small for gestational age neonate would originally be growth restricted fetus
- Left handedness **was statistically insignificant difference**
- Disturbed neuronal migration in mice fetuses that exposed to diagnostic B-mode US for > 30 minutes
- **US probe would be separated from animal by temperature stabilized water**
- Transient hepatic cell apoptosis by diagnostic pulsed Doppler US in rat fetus
- **Neonatal state** would be reported
- Repeated animal experiment with reduced TI and MI is hoped.

For complete presentation, please refer the accompanying CD-ROM...

SUGGESTED READING

1. American Institute of Ultrasound in Medicine/ National Electrical Manufacturers Association; Standard for Real Time Display of Thermal and Mechanical Acoustic Output Indices on Diagnostic Ultrasound Equipment. 1992.
2. Ang Jr ESBC, Glucic V, Duque A, et al. Prenatal exposure to ultrasound waves impacts neuronal migration in mice. Doi/10.1073/pnas06052934103.
3. Bioeffects and Safety Committee, ISUOG, Opinion, Safe use of Doppler ultrasound during the 11 to13+6-week scan: is it possible? Ultrasound Obstet Gynecol. 2011;37:625-8; DOI: 10.1002/uog.9025.
4. Florianski J, Fuchs T, Zimmer M, et al. The role of ductus venosus Doppler flow in the diagnosis of chromosomal abnormalities during the first trimester of pregnancy. Adv Clin Exp Med. 2013;22:295-401.
5. Maeda K, Ide M. The limitation of the ultrasound intensity for diagnostic devices in the Japanese Industrial standards. IEEE Trans Ultrasonics, Ferroelectrics and Frequency Control, 1986; UFFC-33: 241-4.
6. Maeda K, Murao F, Yoshiga T, Yamauchi C, Tsuzaki T. Experimental studies on the suppression of cultured cell growth curves after irradiation with CW and pulsed ultrasound. IEEE Trans Ultrasonics, Ferroelectrics and Frequency Control, 1986; UFFC-33: 186-93.
7. National Council on Radiation Protection and Measurements (NCRP). Exposure Criteria for Medical Diagnostic Ultrasound: I. Criteria based on Thermal Mechanisms. NCRP Report No. 113, 1992.
8. Pellicer B, Herraiz S, Taboas E, et al. Ultrasound bioeffects in rats: quantification of cellular damage in the fetal liver after pulsed Doppler imaging. Ultrasound in Obstet Gynecol. 2011;37:643-648.
9. Sande RK, Mate K, Elde GE, Kiserud T. The effects of reducing the thermal index from 1.0 to 0.5 and 0.1 on common obstetric pulsed wave Doppler measurements in the second half of pregnancy. Acta Obstet Gynecol Scand. 2013;92:790-796.
10. Sande RK, Matre K, Eld GE, Kisserad T. Ultrasound safety in early pregnancy: reduced energy setting does not compromise obstetric Doppler measurements. Ultrasound Obstet Gynecol. 2012;39:438-443.
11. Sande RK, Matre K, Elde GE, Kiserud T. The effect of ultrasound output level on obstetric biometric measurements. Ultrasound Med Biol. 2013;39:37-43.

Chapter

33

Basic Use of Ultrasound in Neonatology

Milan Stanojevic

NEONATAL IMAGING

- Radiogram
- CT scan
- Ultrasound (US)
- Magnetic resonance imaging (MRI)
- 3- or 4-dimensional US

Which Imaging Method Should be Used in Neonates?

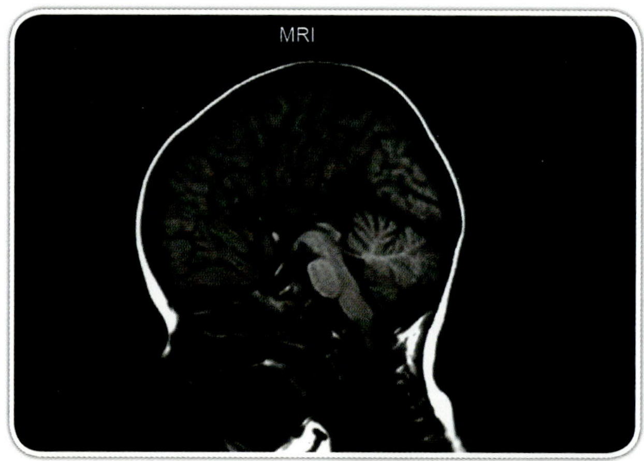

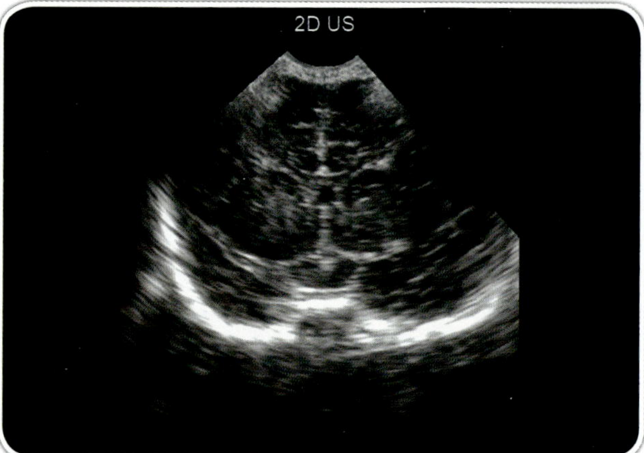

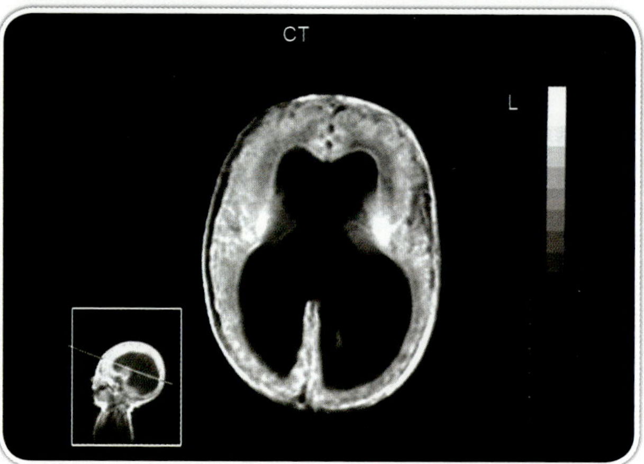

- MRI spectroscopy
- Single photon emission CT (SPECT)
- Positron emission tomography (PET)
- fNMR

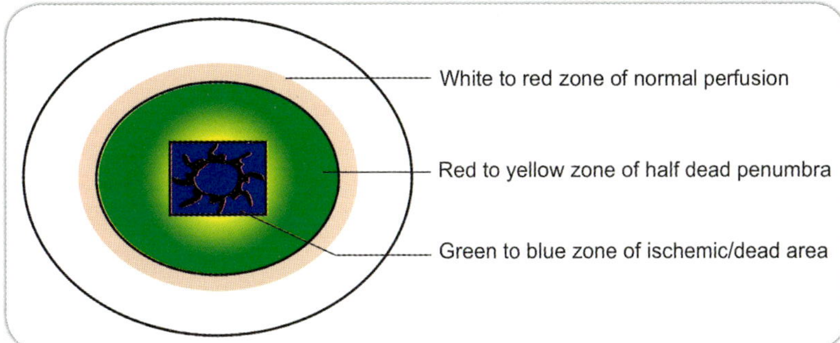

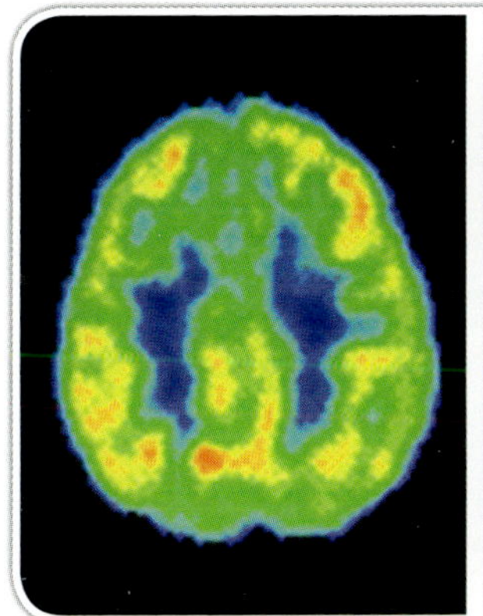
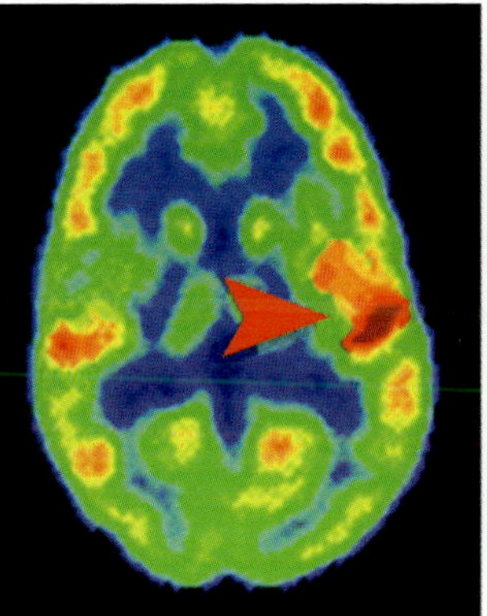
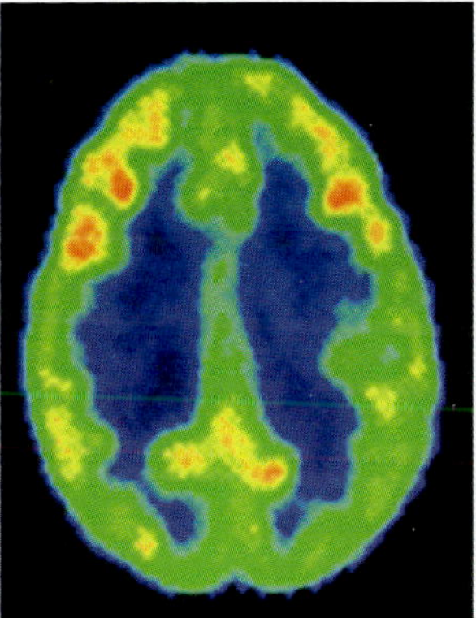
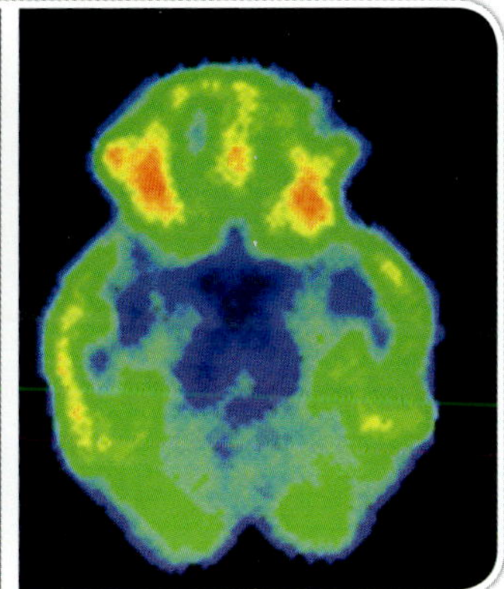

History of US Diagnostics

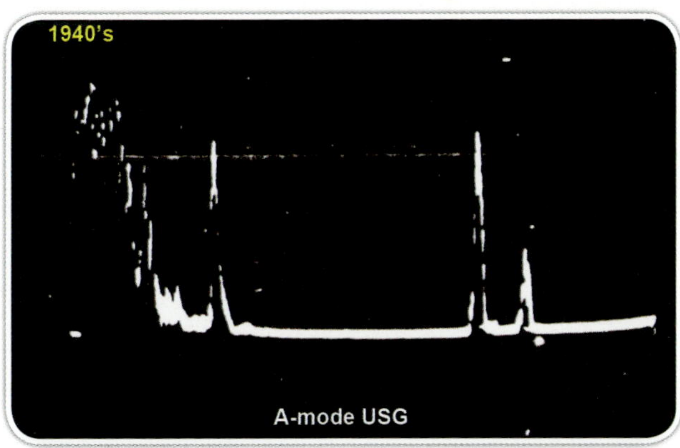

A-mode USG

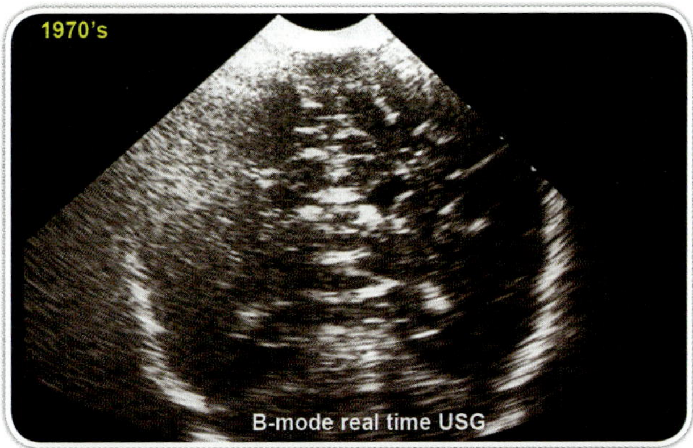

B-mode real time USG

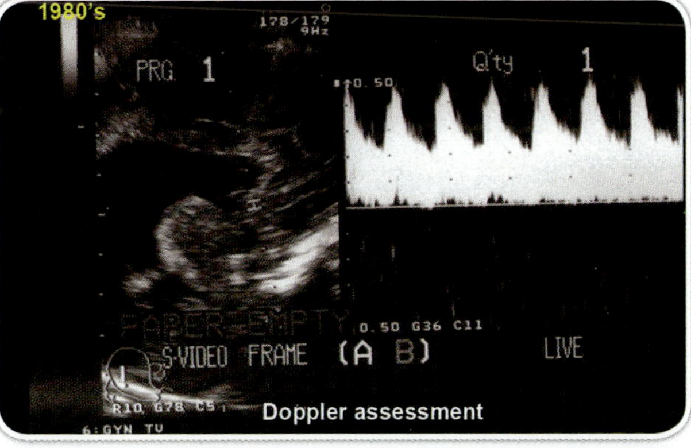

Doppler assessment

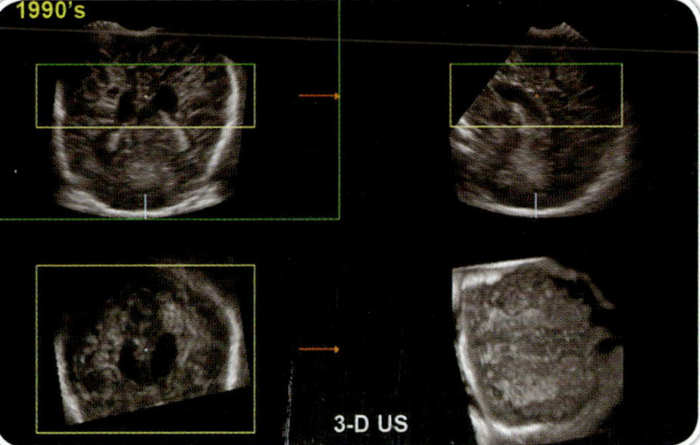

3-D US

For complete presentation, please refer the accompanying CD-ROM...

SUGGESTED READING

1. Abdool Z, Shek KL, Dietz HP. The effect of levator avulsion on hiatal dimension and function. Am J Obstet Gynecol. 2009;201(1):89.e1-e5.
2. Bader W, Degenhardt F, Kauffels W, Nehls K, Schneider J. Ultrasound morphologic parameters of female stress incontinence. Ultraschall Med. 1995;16(4):180-5.
3. Deindl FM, Vodusek DB, Hesse U, Schüssler B. Activity patterns of pubococcygeal muscles in nulliparous continent women. Br J Urol. 1993;72(1):46-51.
4. DeLancy JOL. Stress urinary incontinence: Where are we now, where should we go? Am J Obstet Gynecol. 1996;175:311-9.
5. DeLancy JOL. Structural support of the urethra as it relates to stress urinary incontinence: the hammock hypothesis. Am J Obstet Gynecol. 1994; 170: 1713-20
6. Dietz HP, Clarke B. The urethral pressure profile and ultrasound imaging of the lower urinary tract. Int Urogynecol J Pelvic Floor Dysfunct. 2001;12(1):38-41.
7. Dietz HP, Shek C, Clarke B. Biometry of the pubovisceral muscle and levator hiatus by three-dimensional pelvic floor ultrasound. Ultrasound Obstet Gynecol. 2005;25(6):580-5.
8. Dietz HP, Wilson PD, Clarke B. The use of perineal ultrasound to quantify levator activity and teach pelvic floor muscle exercises. Int Urogynecol J Pelvic Floor Dysfunct. 2001;12(3):166-168
9. Dietz HP, Wilson PD. The influence of bladder volume on the position and mobility of the urethrovesical junction. Int Urogynecol J Pelvic Floor Dysfunct. 1999;10(1):3-6.
10. Dietz HP, Wilson PD. The 'iris effect': how two-dimensional and three-dimensional ultrasound can help us understand anti-incontinence procedures. Ultrasound Obstet Gynecol. 2004; 23(3): 267-71.
11. Gordon D, Pearce M, Norton P, Stanton SL. Comparison of ultrasound and lateral chain urethrocystography in the determination of bladder neck descent. Am J Obstet Gynecol. 1989;160(1):182-5.
12. Gosling JA. The structure of the bladder neck, urethra and pelvic floor in relation to female urinary continence. Int Urogynecol J. 1996;7(4):177-8.
13. Howard D, Delancey JO, Tunn R, Ashton-Miller JA. Racial differences in the structure and function of the stress urinary continence mechanism. Obstet Gynecol. 2000; 95(5):713-7.
14. Jung SA, Pretorius DH, Padda BS, Weinstein MM, Nager CW, den Boer DJ, Mittal RK. Vaginal high-pressure zone assessed by dynamic 3-dimensional ultrasound images of the pelvic floor. Am J Obstet Gynecol. 2007;197(1):52.e1-e7.
15. Khullar V, Cardozo LD, Salvatore S, Hill S. Ultrasound: a noninvasive screening test for detrusor instability. Br J Obstet Gynaecol. 1996;103(9):904-8.
16. Khullar V, Salvatore S, Cardozo L, Bourne TH, Abbott D, Kelleher C. A novel technique for measuring bladder wall thickness in women using transvaginal ultrasound. Ultrasound Obstet Gynecol. 1994;4(3):220-3.
17. King JK, Freeman RM. Is antenatal bladder neck mobility a risk factor for postpartum stress incontinence? Br J Obstet Gynaecol. 1998;105 (12):1300-7.
18. Koelbl H, Bernaschek G, Wolf G. A comparative study of perineal ultrasound scanning and urethrocystography in patients with genuine stress incontinence. Arch Obstet Gynecol. 1988;244:39-45.
19. Kohorn EI, Scioscia AL, Jeanty P, Hobbins JC. Ultrasound cystourethrography by perineal scanning for the assessment of female stress urinary incontinence. Obstet Gynecol. 1986;68(2):269-72.
20. Kruger JA, Heap SW, Murphy BA, Dietz HP. Pelvic floor function in nulliparous women using three-dimensional ultrasound and magnetic resonance imaging. Obstet Gynecol. 2008;111(3) 631-8.
21. Martan A, Masata M, Halaska M, Voigt R. Ultrasound imaging of the urethral sphincter. Ceska Gynekol. 1997;62(6):330-2.
22. Martan A, Massata J, Halaska M, Otcenasek M, Svabik K. Ultrasound Imaging of paravaginal defects in women with stress incontinence before and after paravaginal defect repair. Ultrasound Obstet Gynecol 2002;19:496-500.
23. Miller JM, Perucchini D, Carchidi LT, DeLancey JO, Ashton-Miller J. Pelvic floor muscle contraction during a cough and decreased vesical neck mobility. Obstet Gynecol. 2001;97(2):255-60.
24. Monga A. Fascia--defects and repair. Curr Opin Obstet Gynecol. 1996; 8(5): 366-371.
25. Mouritsen L, Strandberg C. Vaginal ultrasonography versus colpo-cysto-urethrography in the evaluation of female urinary incontinence. Acta Obstet Gynecol Scand. 1994;73(4):338-42.
26. Pantazis K, Freeman RM. Investigation and treatment of urinary incontinence. Current Obstetrics and Gynecology 2006;16(6):344-52.
27. Peschers U, Schaer G, Anthuber C, Delancey JO, Schuessler B. Changes in vesical neck mobility following vaginal delivery. Obstet Gynecol. 1996; 88(6): 1001-6.
28. Peschers UM, Vodusek DB, Fanger G, Schaer GN, DeLancey JO, Schuessler B. Pelvic muscle activity in nulliparous volunteers. Neurourol Urodyn. 2001;20(3):269-75.
29. Peschers UM, Vodušek DB, Fanger G, Schaer GN, DeLancey JO, Schuessler B. Pelvic muscle activity in nulliparous volunteers. Neurourol Urodyn. 2001;20(3):269-75.
30. Petri E, Koelbl H, Schaer G. What is the place of ultrasound in urogynecology? A written panel. Int Urogynecol J Pelvic Floor Dysfunct. 1999;10(4):262-73.

31. Poon CI, Zimmern PE. Role of three-dimensional ultrasound in assessment of women undergoing urethral bulking agent therapy. Curr Opin Obstet Gynecol. 2004;16(5):411-7.
32. Reddy AP, DeLancey JO, Zwica OM, Ashton-Miller JA. On-screen vector-based ultrasound assessment of vesical neck movement. Am J Obstet Gynecol. 2001; 185(1): 65-70.
33. Sapsford RR, Hodges PW, Richardson CA, Cooper DH, Markwell SJ, Jull GA. Co-activation of the abdominal and pelvic floor muscles during voluntary exercises. Neurourol Urodyn. 2001;20(1):31-42.
34. Schaer G, Koelbl H, Voigt R, Merz E, Anthuber C, Niemeyer R, et al.. Recommendations of the German Association of Urogynecology on functional sonography of the lower female urinary tract. Int Urogynecol J Pelvic Floor Dysfunct. 1996;7(2):105-8.
35. Schaer GN, Koechli OR, Schuessler B, Haller U. Improvement of perineal sonographic bladder neck imaging with ultrasound contrast medium. Obstet Gynecol. 1995; 86(6): 950-4.
36. Schaer GN, Koechli OR, Schuessler B, Haller U. Perineal ultrasound: determination of reliable examination procedures. Ultrasound Obstet Gynecol 1996;7(5): 347-52.
37. Schaer GN, Koechli OR, Schuessler B, Haller U. Perineal ultrasound for evaluating the bladder neck in urinary stress incontinence. Obstet Gynecol. 1995;85(2):220-4.
38. Schaer GN, Perucchini D, Munz E, Peschers U, Koechli OR, Delancey JO. Sonographic evaluation of the bladder neck in continent and stress-incontinent women. Obstet Gynecol. 1999;93(3):412-6.
39. Tunn R, Perucchini D. Morphologic assessment for diagnosing urogynaecologic disorders. Zentralbl Gynakol. 2001;123(12):672-9.
40. Tunn R, Petri E. Introital and transvaginal ultrasound as the main tool in the assessment of urogenital and pelvic floor dysfunction: an imaging panel and practical approach. Ultrasound Obstet Gynecol. 2003;22(2):205-13.
41. Umek WH, Laml T, Stutterecker D, Obermair A, Leodolter S, Hanzal E. The urethra during pelvic floor contraction: observations on three-dimensional ultrasound. Obstet Gynecol. 2002;100(4):796-800.
42. Unger CA, Weinstein MM, Pretorius DH. Pelvic Floor Imaging. Ultrasound Clinics. 2010;5(2):313-30.
43. Viereck V, Bader W, Skala C, Gauruder-Burmester A, Emons G, Hilgers R, Krauss T. Determination of bladder neck position by intraoperative introital ultrasound in colposuspension: outcome at 6-month follow-up. Ultrasound Obstet Gynecol. 2004;24(2):186-91.
44. Weber AM, Abrams P, Brubaker L, Cundiff G, Davis G, Dmochowski RR, et al. The standardization of terminology for researchers in female pelvic floor disorders. Int Urogynecol J Pelvic Floor Dysfunct. 2001;12(3): 78-86.
45. Weinstein MM, Jung SA, Pretorius DH, Nager CW, den Boer DJ, Mittal RK. The reliability of puborectalis muscle measurements with 3-dimensional ultrasound imaging. Am J Obstet Gynecol. 2007; 197(1): 68.e1-e6.
46. White RD, McQuown D, McCarthy TA, Ostergard DR. Real-time ultrasonography in the evaluation of urinary stress incontinence. Am J Obstet Gynecol. 1980; 138(2): 235-7.
47. Wijma J, Weis Potters AE, de Wolf BT, Tinga DJ, Aarnoudse JG. Anatomical and functional changes in the lower urinary tract during pregnancy. BJOG. 2001;108(7):726-32.
48. Yang JM, Huang WC. Discrimination of bladder disorders in female lower urinary tract symptoms on ultrasonographic cystourethrography. J Ultrasound Med. 2002;21(11):1249-55.
49. Yang JM, Yang SH, Huang WC. Biometry of the pubovisceral muscle and levator hiatus in nulliparous Chinese women. Ultrasound Obstet Gynecol. 2006; 28(5): 710-6.
50. Yang JM, Yang SH, Huang WC. Dynamic morphological changes in the anterior vaginal wall before and after laparoscopic Burch colposuspension in primary urodynamic stress incontinence. Ultrasound Obstet Gynecol. 2005; 25(3): 289-95.

Chapter 34

Normal Pelvic Anatomy on Ultrasound: Uterus and Endometrium

Sonal Panchal

INTRODUCTION

- Examination of pelvic organs was previously done only by digital vaginal examination
- This is a blind examination and only gives information of consistency and position of the uterus
- Uterine or ovarian masses can be suspected only when they are large
- Digital vaginal examination has a clear disadvantage of not being able to see the internal anatomy of uterus and ovaries
- To study the internal anatomy of pelvic organs, various imaging modalities have been explored:
  - X-rays
  - Ultrasound (US)
  - MRI (Magnetic Resonance Imaging).

X-RAYS FOR THE UTERUS

- X-rays alone cannot show anatomy of the uterus an ovaries (soft tissues).
- Hysterosalpingography (HSG) = Instillation of uterine cavity with iodinated contrast prior to X-ray.
- HSG can show the shape of the endometrial cavity and can outline the tubes.

HSG

- Advantages
  - Simple
  - Not expensive
  - Prolonged history of usage.
- Disadvantages
  - Damage of the ovaries by repeated X-rays
  - Adverse effects from iodinated contrast, i.e. allergic reaction.

HSG: Limitations

- Can be painful
- Invasive
- Shows only the cavity, and no details of either the myometrium or junctional zone
- Not informative for ovarian pathologies or tubo-ovarian relationship (for fertility treatment).

US AND MRI
Less Invasive, More Informative

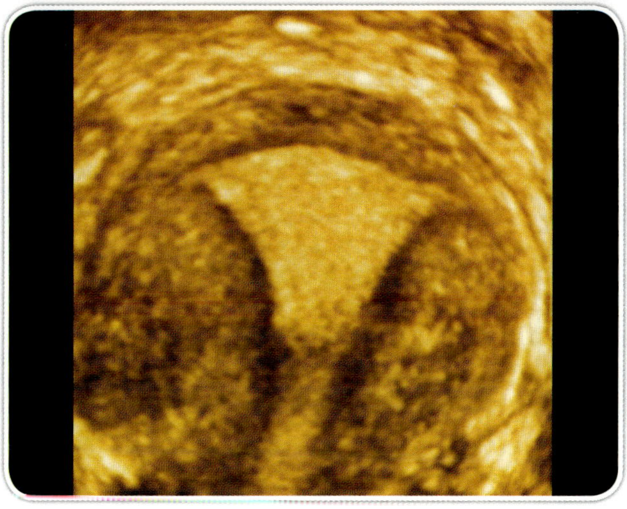

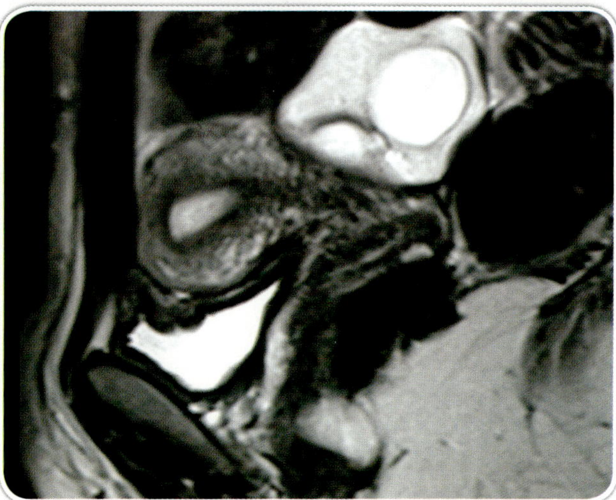

Advantages of US

- Widely available
- Cheaper
- Patient friendly
- Reproducible
- Real-time assessment
- Easy to repeat for follow up.

MRI

- Advantages
  - More detailed anatomy
  - Tissue differentiation.
- Disadvantages
  - Expensive
  - Difficult to repeat for follow up.

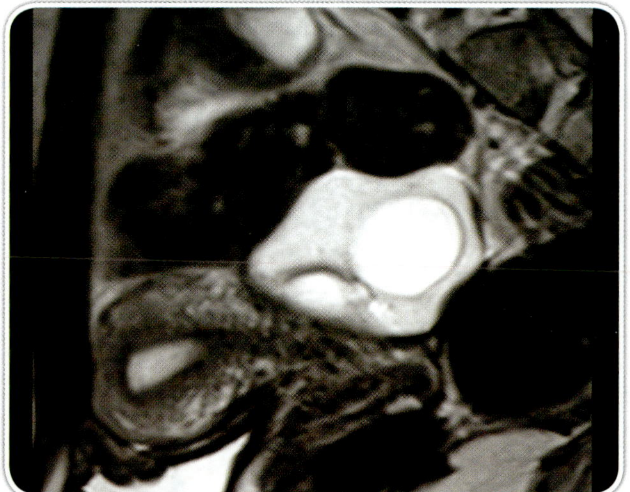

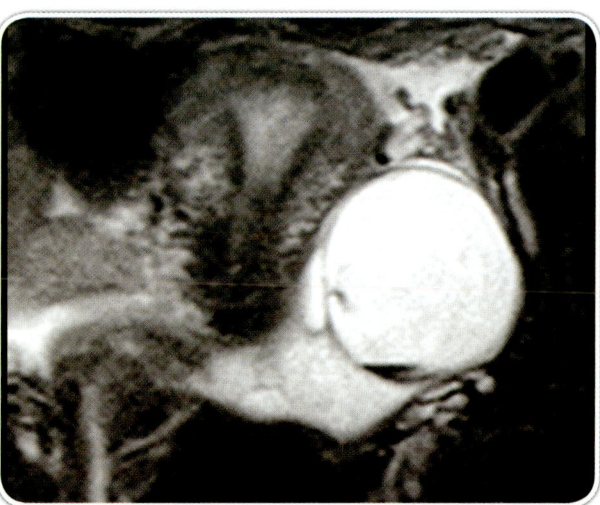

For complete presentation, please refer the accompanying CD-ROM...

SUGGESTED READING

1. Abdalla HI, Brooks AA, Johnson MR, et al. Endometrial thickness: a predictor of implantation in ovum recepients. Hum Reprod. 1994;9(2):363-5.
2. Applebaum M. The 'steel' or 'teflon' endometrium—ultrasound visualization of endometrial vascularity in IVF patients and outcome. Presented at The Third World Congress of Ultrasound in Obstetrics and Gynecology. Ultrasound Obstet Gynecol. 1993;3(Suppl 2):10.
3. Bald R, Hackeloer BJ. Ultraschall-darstellung verschiedener Endometriumformen. In: Otto R, Jan FX (Eds). Ultraschalldiagnostik 1982. Stuttgart:Thieme. 1983;187.
4. Honemeyer U, Kurjak A, Monni G. Normal and abnormal early pregnancy in Donald School Textbook of Ultrasound in Obstetrics and Gynecology, 2nd Edition, Published by Jaypee Brothers Medical Publishers; 2011. pp. 106-29.
5. Hull MGR. Polycystic ovarian disease: clinical aspects and prevalence. Res Clin Forums. 1989;11:21-34.
6. Kurjak A, Kupesic S. Ovarian senescence and its significance on uterine and ovarian perfusion. Fertil Steril. 1995;64:532-8.
7. Smith B, Porter R, Ahuja K, Craft I. Ultrasonic assessment of endometrial changes in stimulated cycles in an in vitro fertilization and embryo transfer program. J In Vitro Fertil Embryo Transf. 1984;1:233-8.
8. Wikland M, Granberg S. Endometrial changes as imaged by transvaginal sonography in fertile and infertile women. In: Fleischer A, Kurjak A, Granberg S (Eds). Ultrasound and endometrium. New York. Parthenon Publishing, London; 1996:17-23.
9. Zaidi J, Campbell S, Pitroff R, Tan SL. Endometrial thickness, morphology, vascular penetration and velocimetry in predicting implantation in an in vitro fertilization program. Ultrasound Obstet Gynecol. 1995;6:191-8.

Chapter

35

Normal Pelvic Anatomy on Ultrasound: Fallopian Tubes and Ovaries

Sonal Panchal

- Anatomical location of ovaries and fallopian tubes is not amenable to any direct inspection
- Modality of choice for assessment of these pelvic organs is transvaginal ultrasound.

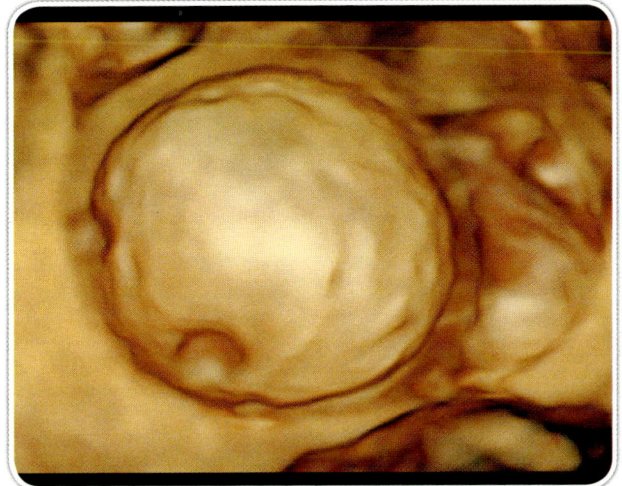

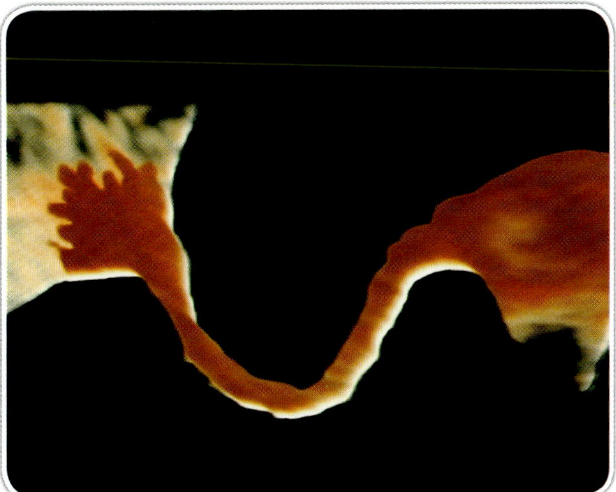

Transvaginal Scan

- It is the primary examination after clinical assessment as it gives more information than any other single test and is noninvasive.

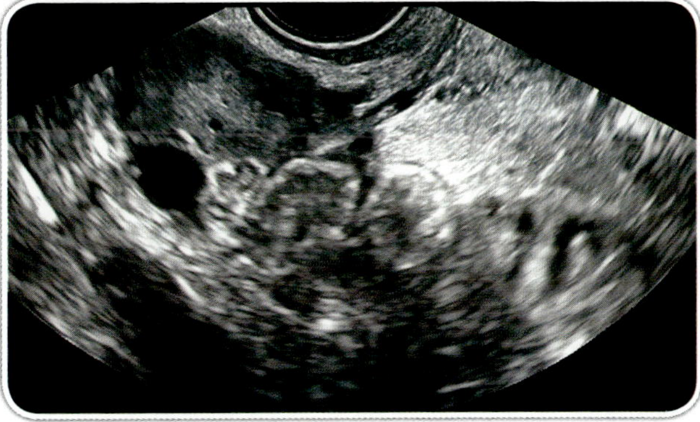

Advantage of Transvaginal Route

- Probe closest to pelvic organs
- High resolution due to high frequency probe
- No bowel preparation
- No bladder distention
- But transvaginal scans cannot be done…
  - When patient is virgin
  - When patient is not cooperative
  - When there is severe vaginismus or vaginal disease
  - Rarely when vagina is absent.

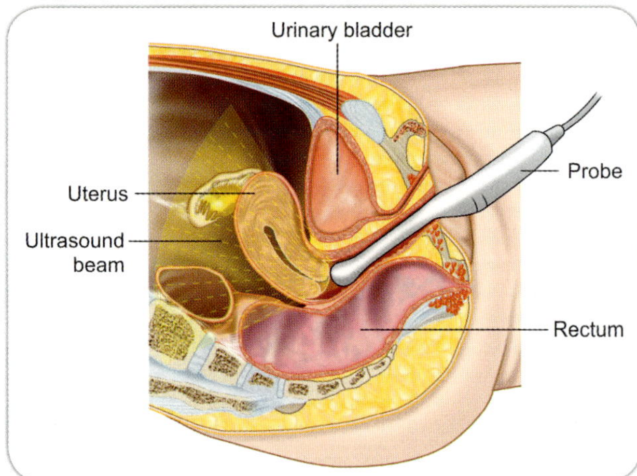

- In these cases transabdominal or transrectal scan may be done
- But transabdominal scan gives little details about the anatomy of the ovaries

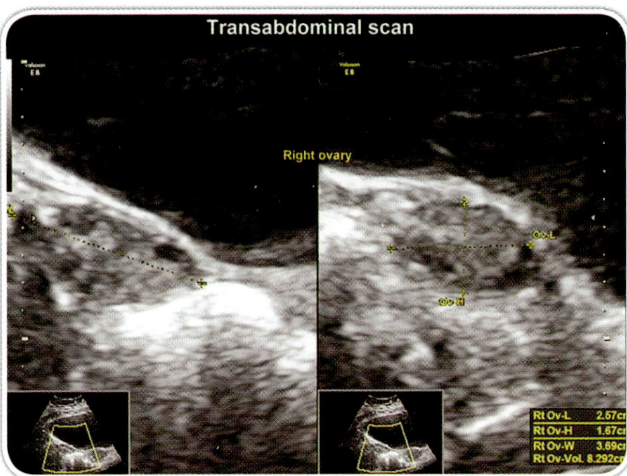

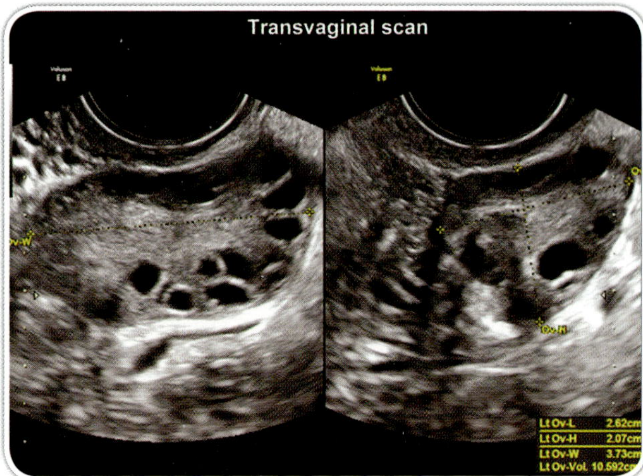

- Transrectal scan has disadvantages of discomfort, but still gives thee resolution comparable with the transvaginal scan as it uses a high frequency endocavitary probe
- B-mode ultrasound and Doppler are satisfactorily sufficient for assessment of ovarian pathologies but 3D and 3D power Doppler is of help for understanding and interpreting the ovarian physiology by ultrasound.

For complete presentation, please refer the accompanying CD-ROM…

SUGGESTED READING

1. Ardaens Y, Robert Y, Lemaitre L, Fossati P, Dewailly D. Polycystic ovarian disease: contribution of transvaginal endosonography and reassessment of ultrsonographic diagnosis. Fertil Steril. 1991;55:1062-8.
2. Bourne T, Jurkovic D, Waterstone J, Campbell S, Collins WP. Intrafollicular blood flow during human ovulation. Ultrasound Obstet Gynecol. 1991;1:53-9.
3. Bridges NA, Cooke A, Healy MJR, et al. Standards for ovarian volume in childhood and puberty. Fertil Steril. 1993;60(3):456-60.
4. Chan CC, Ng EH, Tang OS, et al. Comparison of three-dimensional hysteron-contrast-sonography and diagnostic laparoscopy with chromopertubation in the assessment of tubal patency for the investigation of subfertility. Acta Obstet Gynecol Scand. 2005;84(9):909-13.
5. Cohen HL, Shapiro MA, Mundel FS, et al. Normal ovaries in neonates and infants: a sonographic study of 77 patients 1 day to 24 months old. Am J Roentgenol. 1993;160:583-6.
6. Dewailly D, Gronier H, Poncelet E, Robin G, Leroy M, Pigny P, et al. Diagnosis of polycystic ovarian syndrome (PCOS): revisiting the threshold values of follicle count on ultrasound and of the serum AMH level for the definition of polycystic ovaries. Hum Reprod. 2011;26(11):3123-29.
7. Dewailly D, Robert Y, Helin I, et al. Ovarian stromal hypertrophy in hyperandrogenic women. Clin Endocrinol(oxf). 1994;41:557-62.
8. Faddy MJ, Gosden RG, Gougeon A, et al. Accelerated disappearance of ovarian follicles in mid-life: implications for forecasting menopause. Hum Reprod. 1992;7(10):1342-6.
9. Falghesu M, Ciampelli M, Belosi C, Apa R, Pavone V, Lanzone A. A new ultrasound criterion for the diagnosis of polycystic ovary syndrome: the ovarian stroma: total area ratio. Fertil Steril. 2001;76:326-31.
10. Glock JL, Brumsted JR. Color flow pulsed Doppler ultrasound in diagnosing luteal phase defect. Fertil Steril. 1995;64:500-4.
11. Haadsma MLA, Bukman H, Groen EMA, Roeloffzen FR, Groenewoud MJ. The number of small antral follicles (2–6 mm) determines the outcome of endocrine ovarian reserve tests in a subfertile population. Hum Reprod. 2007;22:1925-31.
12. Hamilton CJ, Evers JL, Tan FE, et al. The reliability of ovulation prediction by single ultrasonic follicle measurement. Hum Reprod. 1987;2(2):103-7.
13. Higgins RV, Van Nagell JR, Woods CH, et al. Interobserver variation in ovarian measurements using transvaginal sonography. Gynecol Oncol. 1990;39(1):69-71.
14. Jokubkeine L, Sladkevicius P, Rovas L, Valentine L. Assessment of changes in volume and vascularity of ovaries during the normal menstrual cycle using three-dimensional power Doppler ultrasound. Hum Reprod. 2006;21(10):2661-8.
15. Kalogirou D, Antoniou G, Botsis D, et al. Is colour Doppler necessary in the evaluation of tubal patency by hysterosalpingo-contrast sonography. Clin Exp Obstet Gynecol. 1997;24(2):101-3.
16. Kiyokawa K, Masuda H, Fuyuki T, Koseki M, Uchida N, Fukuda T, et al. Three-dimensional hysterosalpingo-contrast sonography (3D-HyCoSy) as an outpatient procedure to assess infertile women: a pilot study. Ultrasound Obstet Gynecol. 2000;16(7):648-54.
17. Kupesic S, Kurjak A. The assessment of normal and abnormal luteal function by transvaginal colour Doppler sonography. Eur J Obstet Gynecol. 1997;72:83-7.
18. Kupesic S, Kurjak A. Uterine and ovarian perfusion during the periovulatory period assessed by transvaginal colour Doppler. Fertil Steril. 1993;3:439-43.
19. Lam PM, Jhonson IR, Rainne-Fenning NJ. Three-dimensional ultrasound features of the polycystic ovary and the effect of different phenotypic expressions on these parameters. Hum Reprod. 2007;22:3116-23.
20. Legro RS, Gnatuk CL, Kunselman AR, Dunaif A. Changes in glucose tolerance over time in women with polycystic ovary syndrome: a controlled study. J Clin Endocrinol Metab. 2005;90:3236-42.
21. Lucaino DE, Exacoustos C, Johns DA, et al. Transabdominal saline contrast sonohysterography: Can it replace Hysterosalpingography in low resource countries? Am J Obstet Gynecol. 2011;204(1):79.
22. Lujan ME, Jarrett BY Brooks ED, Reines JK, Peppin AK, Muhn N, et al. Updated ultrasound criteria for polycystic ovary syndrome: reliable thresholds for elevated follicle population and ovarian volume. Hum Reprod. 2013;28(5):1361-68.
23. Nagori CB, Panchal SY, Assessing correlation between ovarian and stromal volumes and fasting and postprandial insulin levels in PCOS patients. Presented at ISUOG 2008, Chicago.
24. Nugent D, Smith J, Balen AH. Ultrasound and the ovary. In: Kupesic S, de Ziegler D (Eds). Ultrasound in Infertility London: Parthenon Publishing; 2000. pp. 23-43.
25. Robert Y, Dubrulle F, Gailandre L, et al. Ultrasound assessment of ovarian stroma hypertrophy in hyperandrogenism and ovulation disorders: visual analysis versus computerized quantification. Fertil Steril. 1995;64:307-12.
26. Rotterdam ESHRE/ASRM-Sponsored PCOS Consensus Workshop Group. Revised 2003 consensus on diagnostic criteria and long-term health risks related to polycystic ovary syndrome. Fertil Steril. 2004;81(1):19-25.
27. Seal SL, Ghosh D, Saha D. Comaparative evaluation of sonosalpingography, hysterosalpingography and laparoscopy for determination of tubal patency. J Obstet and Gynecol India. 2007;57(2):158-61.
28. Tanawattanachaeron S, Suwajanakorn S, Uerpairojkit B, Boonkasemsamti W, Virutamasen P. Transvaginal hystero-contrast sonography (HyCoSy) compared with chromolaparoscopy. J Obstet Gynecol Resear. 2000;26(1):71-5.
29. Tan SL, Zaidi J, Campbell S, Doyle P, Collins W. Blood flow changes in the ovarian and uterine arteries during the normal menstrual cycle. Am J Obstet Gynecol. 1996;175:625-31.
30. Wu M-H, Tang H-H, Hsu C-C, Wang S-T, Huang KE. The role of three-dimensional ultrasonographic images in ovarian measurement. Fertil Steril. 1998;69:1152-55.

Chapter

36

Color Doppler in Gynecology

Ashok Khurana

COLOR DOPPLER IN GYNECOLOGY

Overview of Current Applications

- To assess the presence or absence of flow in a "cystic' space
- As a landmark to confirm the ovary
- To identify isoechoic lesions
- To study cyclical changes
- To assess ovarian torsion
- Differential diagnosis of endometrial lesions
- Tumor neovascularity
- Pelvic congestion.

FLOW IN A "CYSTIC SPACE"

Confirmation of Nature of Fluid

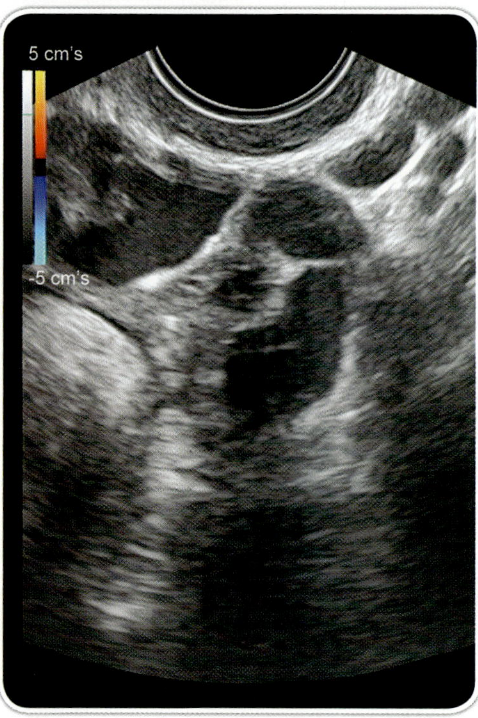

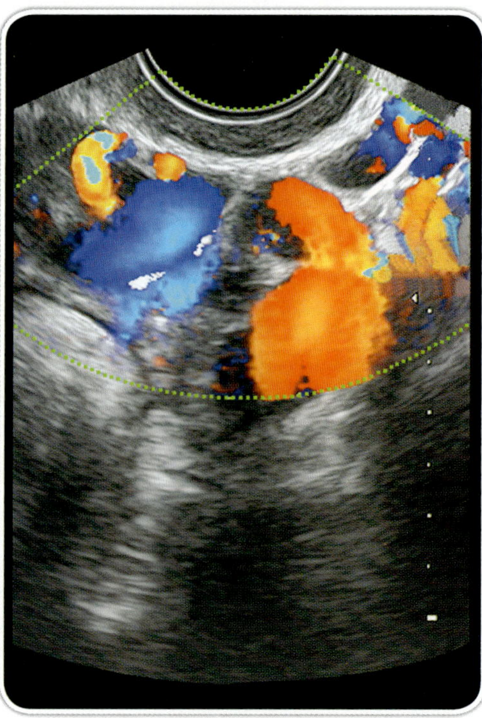

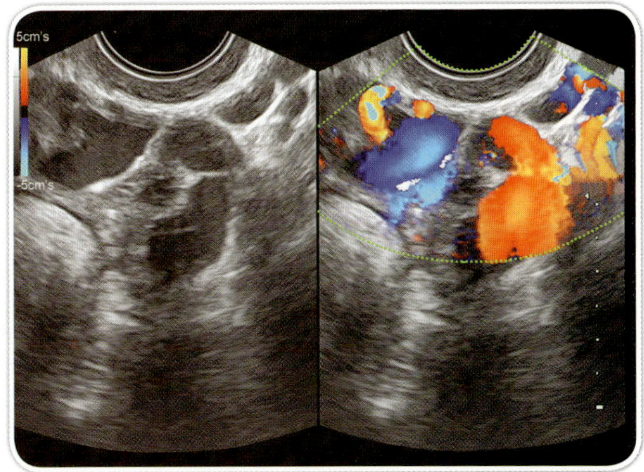

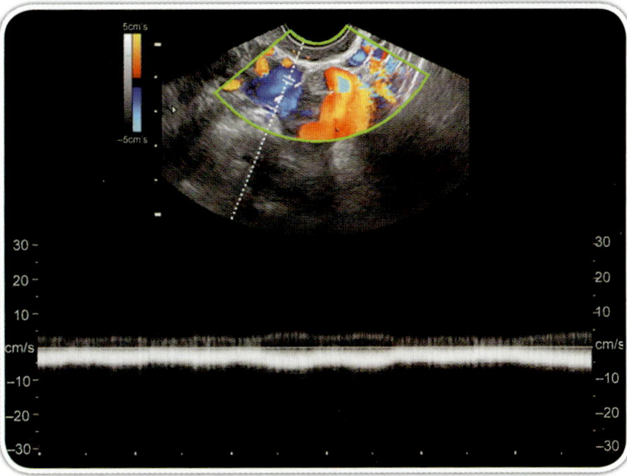

AS A LANDMARK FOR THE OVARY

Iliac Artery and Vein

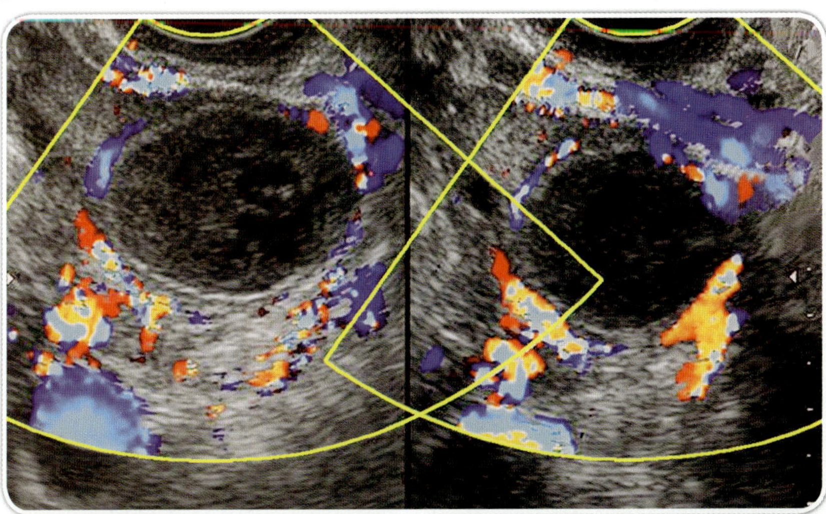

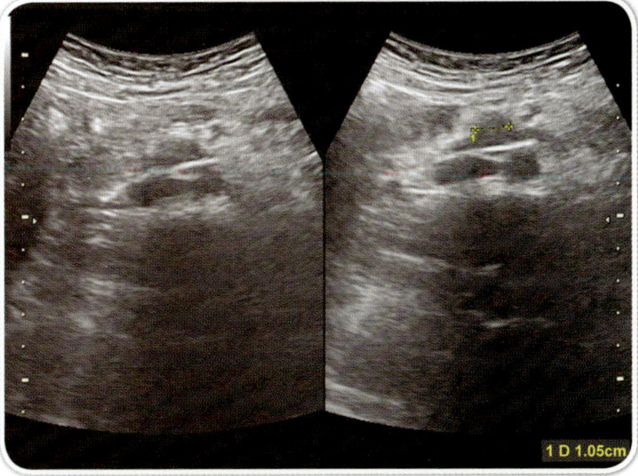

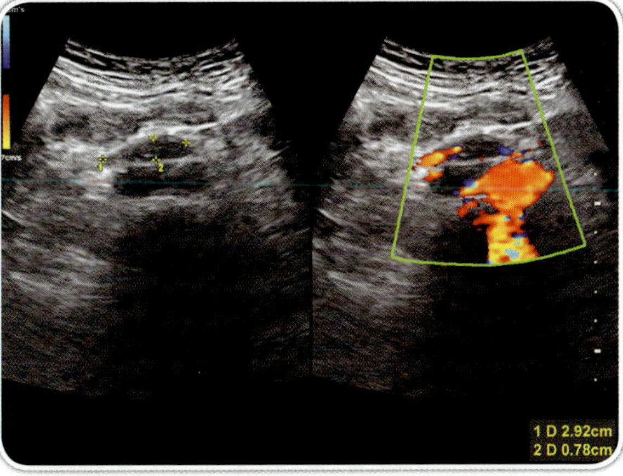

For complete presentation, please refer the accompanying CD-ROM...

SUGGESTED READING

1. Ardaens Y, Gougeon A, Lefebvre C, Thomas P, Lerov M, Lerov JL, et al. Contribution of ovarian and uterine color Doppler in medically assisted reproduction techniques (ART). Gynecol Obstet Fertil. 2002;30(9):663-72.
2. Ashton D, Amin HK, Richart RM, Neuwirth RS. The incidence of asymptomatic uterine anomalies in women undergoing transcervical tubal sterilization. Obstet Gynecol. 1988;72:28-30.
3. Balen FG, Allen CM, Gardener JE, Siddle NC, Lees WR. Three-dimensional reconstruction of ultrasound images of the uterine cavity. Br J Radiol. 1993;66(787):588-91.
4. Baruffi RL, Contart P, Mauri AL, Peterson C, Felipe V, Garbellini E, et al. A uterine ultrasonographic scoring system as a method for the prognosis of embryo implantation. J Assist Reprod Genet. 2002;19(3):99-102.
5. Bega G, Lev-Toaff AS, O'Kane P, Becker E Jr, Kurtz AB. Three-dimensional ultrasonography in gynecology: Technical aspects and clinical applications. J Ultrasound Med. 2003;22(11):1249-69.
6. Bourgain C. Devroey P. The endometrium in stimulated cycles for IVF. Hum Reprod. Update 2003;9(6):515-22.
7. Buckett WM, Chian RC, Tan SL. Human chorionic gonadotropin for in vitro oocytes maturation: does it improve the endometrium or implantation? J Reprod Med. 2004;49(2):93-98.
8. Buyuk E, Durmusoglu F, Erenus M, Karakoc B. Endometrial disease diagnosed by transvaginal ultrasound and dilatation and curettage. Acta Obstet Gynecol. 1999;79:419-22.
9. Cararach M, Penella J, Ubeda J, Iabastida R. Hysteroscopic incision of the septate uterus: scissors versus resectoscope. Hum Reprod. 1994;9:87-9.
10. Carbillon L, Perrot N, Uzan M, Uzan S. Doppler ultrasonography and implantation: a critical review. Fetal Diagn Ther. 2001;16(6):327-32.
11. Carrington BM, Hricak M, Naruddin RN. Mullerian duct anomalies: MR evaluation. Radiology. 1990;170:715-20.
12. Chien LW, Lee WS, Au HK, Tzeng CR. Assessment of changes in utero-ovarian arterial impedance during the peri-implantation period by Doppler sonography in women undergoing assisted reproduction. Ultrasound Obstet Gynecol. 2004;23(5):496-500.
13. Dabrashrafi H, Bahadori M, Mohammad K, Alavi M, Moghadami-Tabrizi N, Zandinejad R. Septate uterus: New idea on the histologic features of the septum in this abnormal uterus. Am J Obstet Gynecol. 1995;172:105-7.
14. Delisle M-F, Villeneuve M, Boulvain M. Measurement of endometrial thickness with transvaginal ultrasonography: is it reproducible? J Ultrasound Med. 1998;17:481-4.
15. Dietz HP, Wilson PD. The 'iris effect': how two-dimensional and three-dimensional ultrasound can help us understand anti-incontinence procedures. Ultrasound Obstet Gynecol. 2004;23(3):267-71.
16. Epstein E, Valentin L. Rebleeding and endometrial growth in women with postmenopausal bleeding and endometrial thickness <5 mm managed by dilatation and curettage or ultrasound follow-up: a randomized controlled study. Ultrasound Obstet Gynecol. 2001;18(5):499-504.
17. Fedele L, Arcaini L, Parazzini F, Vercellini P, Nola GD. Metroplastic hysteroscopy and fertility. Fertil Steril. 1993;59:768-70.
18. Fedele L, Bianchi S, Marchini M, Franchi D, Tozzi L, Dorta M. Ultrastructural aspects of endometrium in infertile women with septate uterus. Fertil Steril. 1996;65:750-2.
19. Goldenberg M, Sivan E, Sharabi Z. Reproductive outcome following hysteroscopic management of intrauterine septum and adhesions. Hum Reprod. 1995;10:2663-5.
20. Goldstein RB, Bree RL, Benson CB, Benacerraf BR, Bloss JD, Carlos R, et al. Evaluation of the woman with postmenopausal bleeding: Society of Radiologists in Ultrasound-Sponsored Consensus Conference statement. J Ultrasound Med. 2001;20(10):1025-36.
21. Heinonen PK, Saarikoski S, Pystynen P. Reproductive performance of women with uterine anomalies. An evaluation of 182 cases. Acta Obstet Gynecol Scand. 1982;61:157-62.
22. Homer HA, Li TC, Cooke ID. The septate uterus: a review of management and reproductive outcome. Fertil Steril. 2000;73:1-4.
23. Jorizzo JR, Riccio GJ, Chen MYM, Carr JJ. Sonohysterography: the next step in the evaluation of the abnormal endometrium. Radiographics. 1999;119:S117-30.
24. Jurkovic D, Giepel A, Gurboeck K, Jauniaux E, Natucci M, Campbell S. Three-dimensional ultrasound for the assessment of uterine anatomy and detection of congenital anomalies: a comparison with hysterosalpingography and two-dimensional sonography. Ultrasound Obstet Gynecol. 1995;5:233-7.
25. Kupesic S, Bekavac I, Bjelos D, Kurjak A. Assessment of endometrial receptivity by transvaginal color Doppler and three-dimensional power Doppler ultrasonography in patients undergoing in vitro fertilization procedures. J Ultrasound Med. 2001;20(2):125-34.
26. Kupesic S, Kurjak A, Bjelos D. Sonographic imaging in infertility. In: Kurjak A, Chervenak FA (Eds). Donald School Textbook of Ultrasound in Obstetrics and Gynecology, 1st edn. New Delhi: Jaypee Brothers Medical Publishers; 2003 pp. 658-90.
27. Kupesic S, Kurjak A, Skenderovic S, Bjelos D. Screening for uterine abnormalities by three-dimensional ultrasound improves perinatal outcome. J Perinat Med. 2002;30:9-17.
28. Kupesic S, Kurjak A. Septate uterus: detection and prediction of obstetrical complications by different forms of ultrasonography. J Ultrasound Med. 1998;17:631-6.
29. Kupesic S, Kurjak A. Three-dimensional ultrasound and power Doppler assessment of the septate uterus. In: Kurjak A (Ed). Three-dimensional power Doppler in Obstetrics and Gynecology, 1st edn. New York: Parthenon Publishing; 2000 pp. 85-91.

30. Kupesic S. Three-dimensional ultrasonographic uterine vascularization and embryo implantation. J Gynecol Obstet Biol Reprod (Paris). 2004;33(1 Pt 2):S18-20.
31. La Torre R, Prosperi Porta R, Franco C, Sansone M, Mazzocco M, Pergolini I, et al. Three-dimensional sonography and hysterosalpingosonography in the diagnosis of uterine anomalies. Clin Exp Obstet Gynecol. 2003;30(4):190-2.
32. Marshall C, Mintz DI, Thickman D, Gussman H, Kressel Y. MR evaluation of uterine anomalies. Radiology. 1987;148:287-9.
33. Ng EHY, Chan CCW, Tang OS, Yeung WSB, Ho PC. Comparison of endometrial and subendometrial blood flow measured by three-dimensional power Doppler ultrasound between stimulated and natural cycles in the same patients. Hum Reprod. 2004;19(10):2385-90.
34. Nicolini U, Belloti M, Bonazzi B, Zamberletti D, Candiani GB. Can ultrasound be used screen uterine malformations? Fertil Steril. 1987;47:89-93.
35. Pierson RA. Imaging the endometrium: are there predictors of uterine receptivity? J Obstet Gynaecol Can. 2003;25(5):360-8.
36. Poon CI, Zimmern PE. Role of three-dimensional ultrasound in assessment of women undergoing urethral bulking agent therapy. Curr Opin Obstet Gynecol. 2004;16(5):411-7.
37. Raga F, Bonilla-Musoles F, Blanes J, Osborne NG. Congenital Mullerian anomalies: diagnostic accuracy of three-dimensional ultrasound. Fertil Steril. 1996;65(3):523-8.
38. Raine-Fenning NJ, Campbell BK, Kendall NR, Clewes JS, Johnxon IR. Quantifying the changes in endometrial vascularity throughout the normal menstrual cycle with three-dimensional power Doppler angiography. Hum Reprod. 2004;19(2):330-8.
39. Randelzhofer B, Prompeler HJ, Sauerbrei W, Madjar H, Emons G. Value of sonomorphological criteria of the endometrium in women with postmenopausal bleeding: a multivariate analysis. Ultrasound Obstet Gynecol. 2002;19(1):62-8.
40. Randolph J, Ying Y, Maier D, Schmidt C, Riddick D. Comparison of real-time ultrasonography, and laparoscopy/hysteroscopy in the evaluation of uterine abnormalities and tubal patency. Fertil Steril. 1986;5:828-32.
41. Reuter KL, Daly DC, Cohen SM. Septate versus bicornuate uteri: errors in imaging diagnosis. Radiology. 1989;172:749-52.
42. Richman TS, Viscomi GN, Cherney AD, Polan A. Fallopian tubal patency assessment by ultrasound following fluid injection. Radiology. 1984;152:507-10.
43. Salim R, Regan L, Woelfer B, Backos M, Jurkovic D. A comparative study of the morphology of congenital uterine anomalies in women with and without a history of recurrent first trimester miscarriage. Hum Reproduct. 2003;18(1):162-6.
44. Salim R, Woelfer B, Backos M, Regan L, Jurkovic D. Reproducibility of three-dimensional ultrasound diagnosis of congenital uterine anomalies. Ultrasound Obstet Gynecol. 2003;21(6):578-82.
45. Salle B, Sergeant P, Galcherand P, Guimont I, De Saint Hilaire P, Rudigoz RC. Transvaginal hysterosonographic evaluation of septate uteri: a preliminary report. Hum Reprod. 1996;11:1004-7.
46. Schild RL, Knobloch C, Dorn C, Fimmers R, van der Ven H, Hansmann M. Endometrial receptivity in an in vitro fertilization program as assessed by spiral artery blood flow, endometrial thickness, endometrial volume, and uterine artery blood flow. Fertil Steril. 2001;75(2):361-6.
47. Sheikh M, Sawhney S, Khurana A, Al-Yatama M. Alteration of sonographic texture of the endometrium in postmenopausal bleeding: A guide to further management. Acta Obstet Gynecol Scand 2000; 79: 1006-1010.
48. Sorenson S. Estimated prevalence of mulerian anomalies. Acta Obstet Gynecol Scand 1988; 67: 441-445.
49. Sousa R, Silvestre M, Almeida e Sousa L, Falcao F, Dias I, Silva T, De Oliveira C, Oliveira HM. Transvaginal ultrasonography and hysteroscopy in postmenopausal bleeding: a prospective study. Acta Obstet Gynecol Scan 2001 Sep; 80(9): 856-862.
50. The American Fertility Society. The American Fertility Society classifications of adnexal adhesions, distal tubal occlusion, tubal occlusion secondary to tubal ligation, tubal pregnancies, mullerian anomalies and intrauterine adhesions. Fertil Steril 1988; 49(6): 944-955.
51. Valdes C, Malini S, Malinak LR. Ultrasound evaluation of female genital tract anomalies: a review of 64 cases. Am J Obstet Gynecol 1984; 149: 285-290.
52. Weigel M, Friese K, Strittmatter HJ, Melchert F. Measuring the thickness – is that all we have to do for sonographic assessment of endometrium in postmenopausal women. Ultrasound Obstet Gynecol 1995; 6(2): 97-102.
53. Weinraub Z, Maymon R, Shulman A, Bukovsky J, Kratochwil A, Lee A, Herman A. Three-dimensional saline contrast rendering of uterine cavity pathology. Ultrasound Obstet Gynecol 1996; 8(4): 277-282.
54. Wu MH, Hsu CC, Huang KE, Detection of congenital mullerian duct anomalies using three-dimensional ultrasound. J Clin Ultrasound 1997; 25: 487-492.
55. Yokota A, Nakai A, Oya A, Koshino T, Araki T. Changes in uterine and ovarian arterial impedance during the periovulatory period in conception and nonconception cycles. J Obstet Gynaecol Res. 2000; 26(6): 435-440.

Chapter

37

Three- and Four-Dimensional Ultrasound in Gynecology

Sonal Panchal, CB Nagori, Narendra Malhotra

Benefits of 3DUS in Gynecology

- 3DUS provides information of the structure and morphology of the whole volume, instead of a plane
- It explains the anatomy better
- 3D power Doppler assesses global vascularity
- Can calculate volumes more accurately
- Combination with transvaginal scan.

3DUS = three-dimensional ultrasound

Volume Ultrasound and 3D Power Doppler on the Followings

- Uterus
- Tubal status
- Ovarian lesions
- Infertility evaluation.

Uterus

- Shape of uterine (endometrial) cavity
- Health of the uterus
  - Endometrial lesions
  - Myometrial lesions
- Receptivity of endometrium

Shape of the Endometrial Cavity

Potential (Empty) Cavity

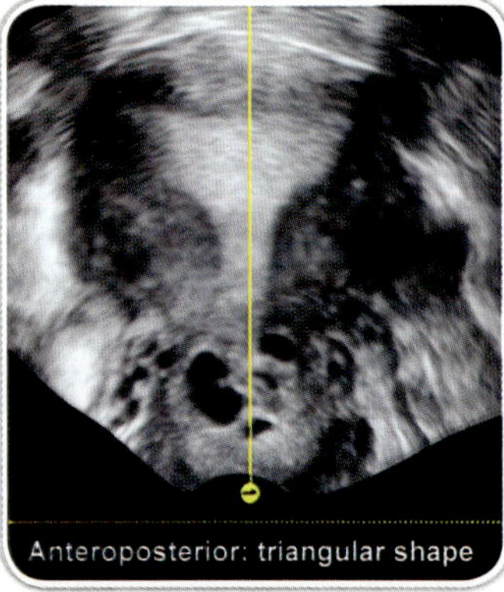
Anteroposterior: triangular shape

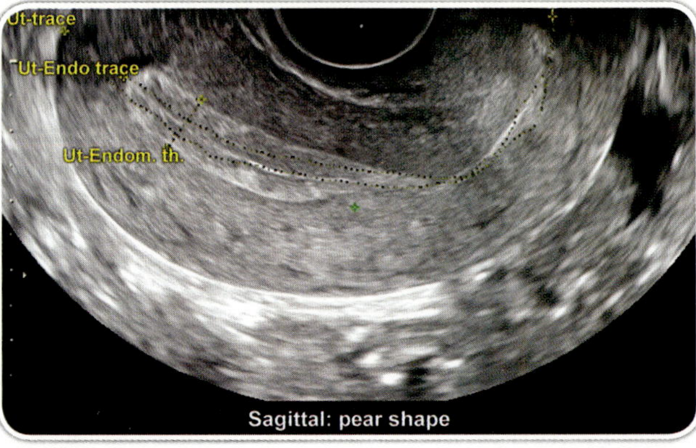

Sagittal: pear shape

Distortion of the Endometrial Cavity

- Congenital uterine abnormalities:
  - These can diagnosed based on external fundal contour and endometrial contour.
- Acquired lesions distorting or invading endometrium.

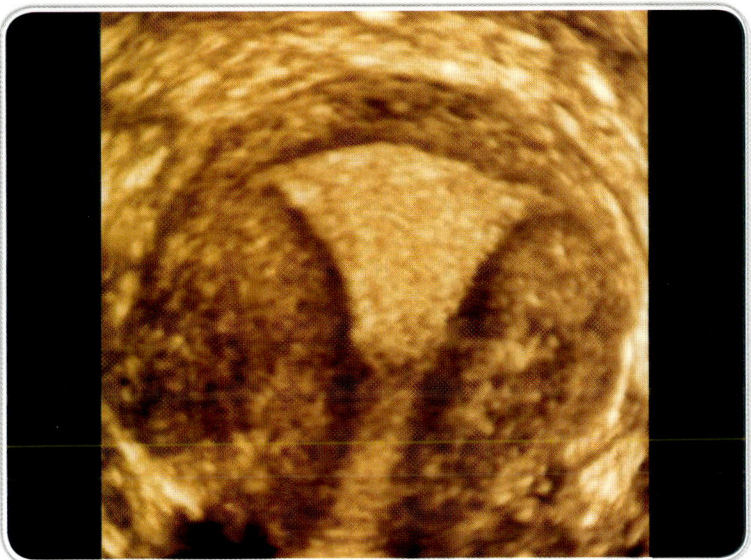

- Greatest advantage of 3D is reconstruction of the coronal plane

Unicornuate Uterus: Diagnosed with 3DUS

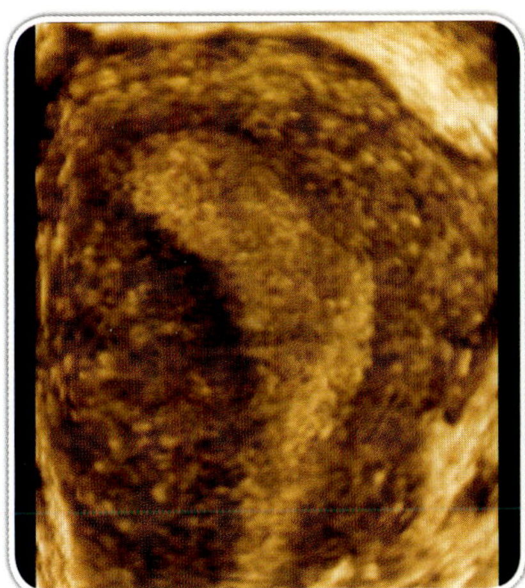

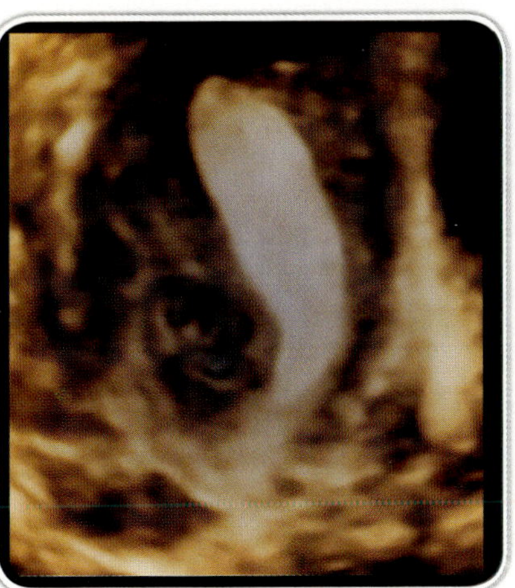

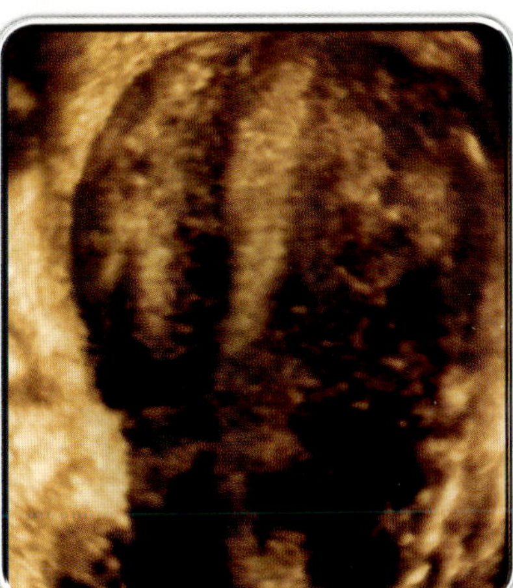

For complete presentation, please refer the accompanying CD-ROM...

SUGGESTED READING

1. Barbot J. Hysteroscopy and Hysterography. Obstet Gynecol Clin North Am. 1995;22:591-603.
2. Bonilla-Musoles F, Raga F, Osborne NG. Three-dimensional ultrasound evaluation of ovarian masses. Gynecol Oncol. 1995;59:129-35.
3. Chan CC, Ng EH, Tang OS, et al. Comparison of three-dimensional hysteron-contrast-sonography and diagnostic laparoscopy with chromopertubation in the assessment of tubal patency for the investigation of subfertility. Acta Obstet Gynecol Scand. 2005;84(9):909-13.
4. Crade M. Tissue block ultrasound and ovarian cancer—a pictorial presentation of findings. Donald School Journal of Ultrasound in Obstetrics and Gynecology. 2009;3(1):41-7.
5. Deb S, Campbell BK, J.S.Clewes, Rainne-Fenning NJ. Quantitative analysis of AFC and size: a comparison of 2D & automated three-dimensional ultrasound techniques. Ultrasound Obstet Gynecol. 2010;35:354-60.
6. Kupesic S, et al, Assessment of endometrial receptivity by transvaginal colour Doppler and three-dimensional power Doppler ultrasonography in patients undergoing in vitro fertilization procedures. J Ultrasound Med. 2001;20:125-34.
7. Kupesic S, Kurjak A. Contrast enhanced three-dimensional power Doppler sonography for the differentiation of adnexal masses. Obstet Gynecol. 2000;96(3):452-8.
8. Kupesic S, Plavsic MB. 2D and 3D hysterosalpingocontrast-sonography in the assessment of uterine cavity and tubal patency. Eur J Obstet Gynecol Reprod Biol. 2007;133(1):64-9.
9. Kurjak A, Kupesic S, Sparac V, et al. Preoprative evauation of pelvic tumours by Doppler and three-dimensional sonography. J Ultrasound Med. 2001;20(8):829-40.
10. Kurjak A, Kupesic S, Sparac V, Prka M, Bekavac I. The detection of stage 1 ovarian cancer by three-dimensional sonography and power Doppler. Gynecol Oncol. 2003;90:258-64.
11. Kyei-Mensah A, Zaidi J, Pittrof R, Shaker A, Campbell S, Tan SL. Transvaginal three-dimensional ultrasound reproducibility of ovarian and endometrial volume measurements. Fertil Steril. 1996;66:718-22.
12. Lam PM, Jhonson IR, Rainne-Fenning NJ. Three dimensional ultrasound features of the polycystic ovary and the effect of different phenotypic expressions on these parameters. J Hum Reprod. 2007;22:3116-23.
13. Lee CN, Cheng WF, Chen CA, et al. Angiogenesis of endometrial carcinomas assessed by measurement of intratumoral blood flow, microvessel density and vascular endothelial growth factor levels. Obstet Gynecol. 2000;96(4):615-21.
14. Legro RS, Chiu P, Kunselman AR, Bentley CM, Dodson WC, Dunaif A. Polycystic ovaries are common in women with hyperandrogenic chronic anovulation but do not predict metabolic or reproductive genotype. JCEM. 2005;90(5):2571-79.
15. Merce LT, Barco MJ, Kurjak A. Ultrasound Markers of implantation. Donald School Journal of Ultrasound in Obstetrics and Gynecology. 2012;6(1):14-26.
16. Oyesanya OA, Parsons JH, Collins WP, Campbell S. Total ovarin volume before human chorionic gonadotrophins administration for ovulation induction may predict the hyperstimulation syndrome. Hum Reprod. 1995;10:3211-2.
17. Panchal SY, Nagori CB. Can 3D PD be a better tool for assessing the pre- HCG follicle and endometrium? A randomized study of 500 cases. Presented at 16th World Congress on Ultrasound in Obstetrics and Gynecology, London. J Ultrasound Obstet Gynecol. 2006;28(4):504.
18. Raine-Fenning N, Jayaprakasan K, Deb S. Three-dimensional ultrasonographic characteristics of endometriomata. Ultrasound Obstet Gynecol 2008;31:718-24.
19. Rempen A. The shape of endometrium evaluated with three-dimensional ultrasound: an additional predictor of extrauterine pregnancy. Hum Reprod. 1998;13(2):450-4.
20. Richman TS, Viscomi GN, Cherney AD, Polan A. Fallopian tubal patency assessment by ultrasound following fluid injection. Radiology. 1984;152:507-10.
21. Sladkevicius P, Jokubkiene L, Valentin L. Vascular morphology and ovarian masses. Ultrasound Obstet and Gynecol. 2007;30(6):874-82.
22. Valentin L. Ultrasound and endoscopic surgery in obstetrics and gynaecology. In: Timmerman D, et al (Eds). Springer-Verlag:London; 2002 pp. 153-64.
23. Wu MH, Tsai SJ, Pan HA, Hsiao KY, Chang FM. Three-dimensional power Doppler imaging of ovarian stromal blood flow in women with endometriosis undergoing in vitro fertilization. Ultrasound Obstet Gynecol. 2003;21:480-5.

Chapter

38

Additional Benefits of 3-Dimensional Sonogram in Gynecology

Tuangsit Wataganara

PELVIC ORGAN EXAMINATIONS

- **Uterus**
  - Position: Anteflexed, axial, retroflexed
  - Myometrium: Fibroids, adenomyosis
  - Endometrial cavity: Appearance, shape, content
  - Serosal surface.
- **Ovaries**
  - Shape and contour
  - Follicles and function.
- **Miscellaneous**
  - Urinary bladder
  - Free fluid.
  - Rectum

UTERUS

3D US can Create Unconventional View of the Uterus

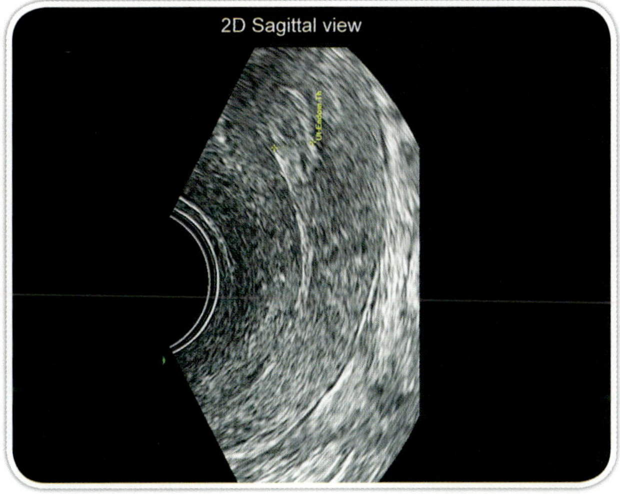
2D Sagittal view

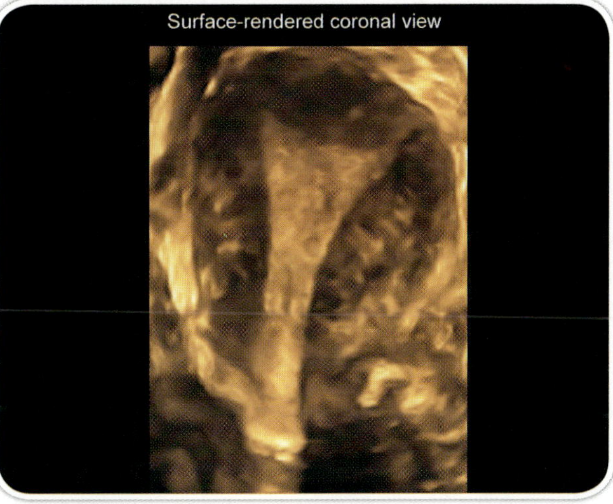
Surface-rendered coronal view

Endometrial Cavity Contour

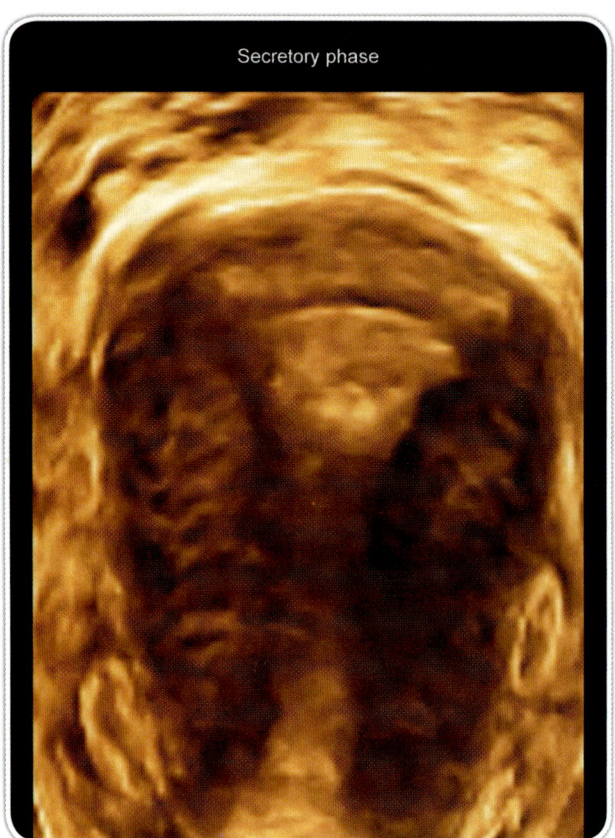

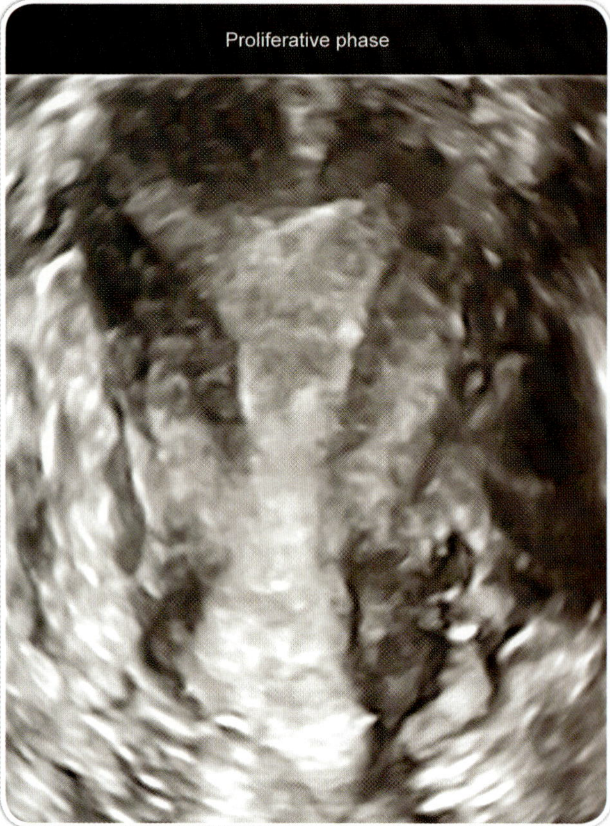

Endometrial Cavity Appearance

'Triple Layer' Late Proliferative Phase

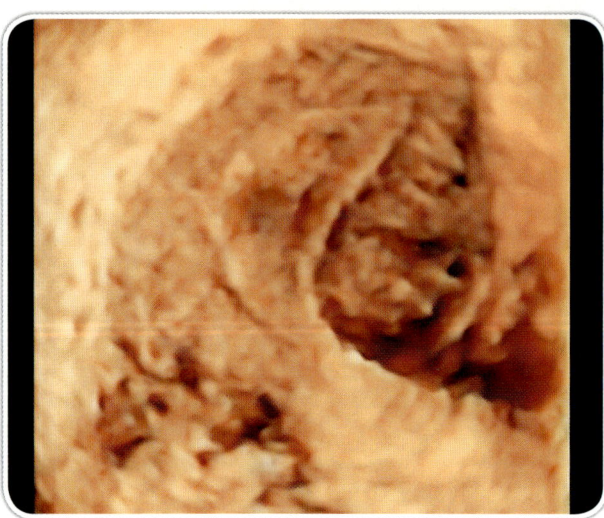

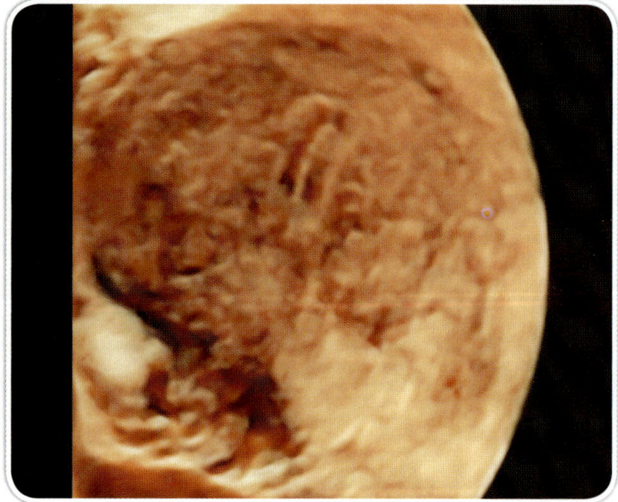

ABNORMAL UTERINE CAVITY

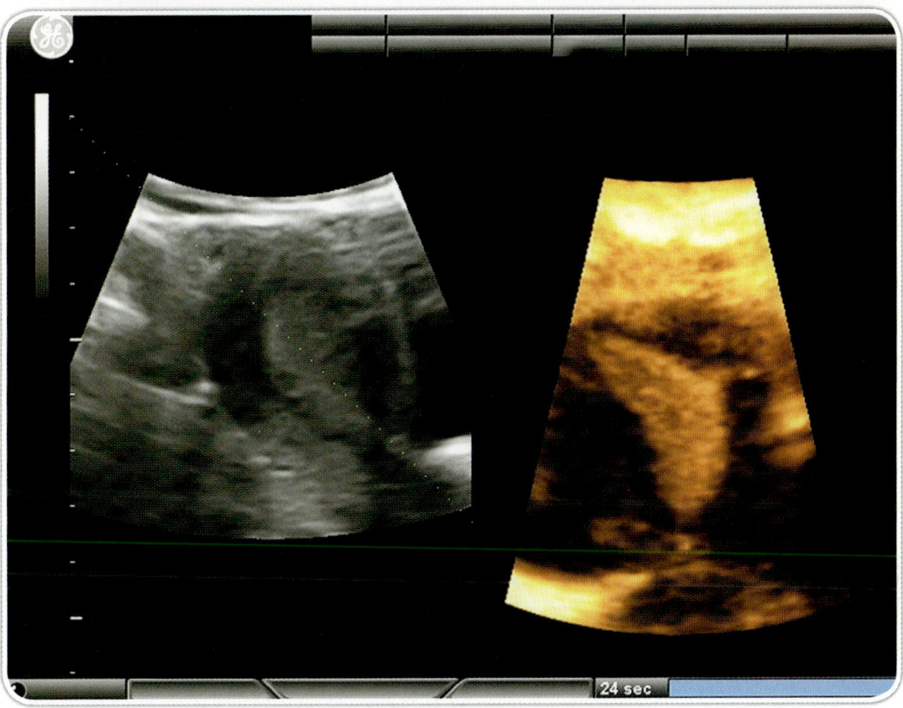

Endometrial assessment should be performed with transabdominal or transrectal, but not transabdominal approach

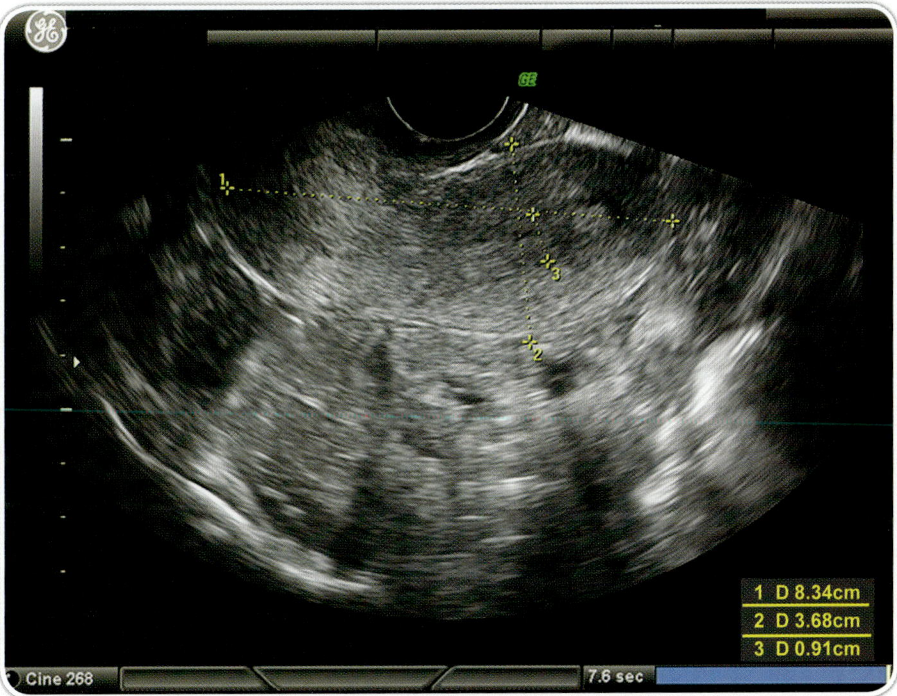

Endometrial cavity looks almost normal on the conventional 2D sagittal view

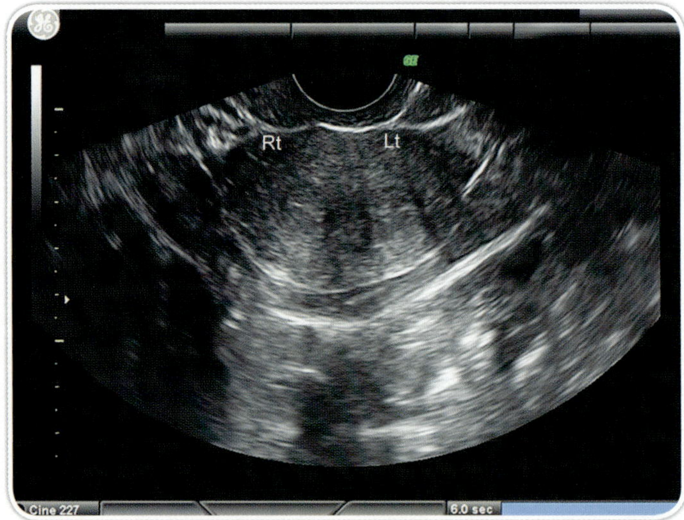

Axial view shows 2 endometrial cavities

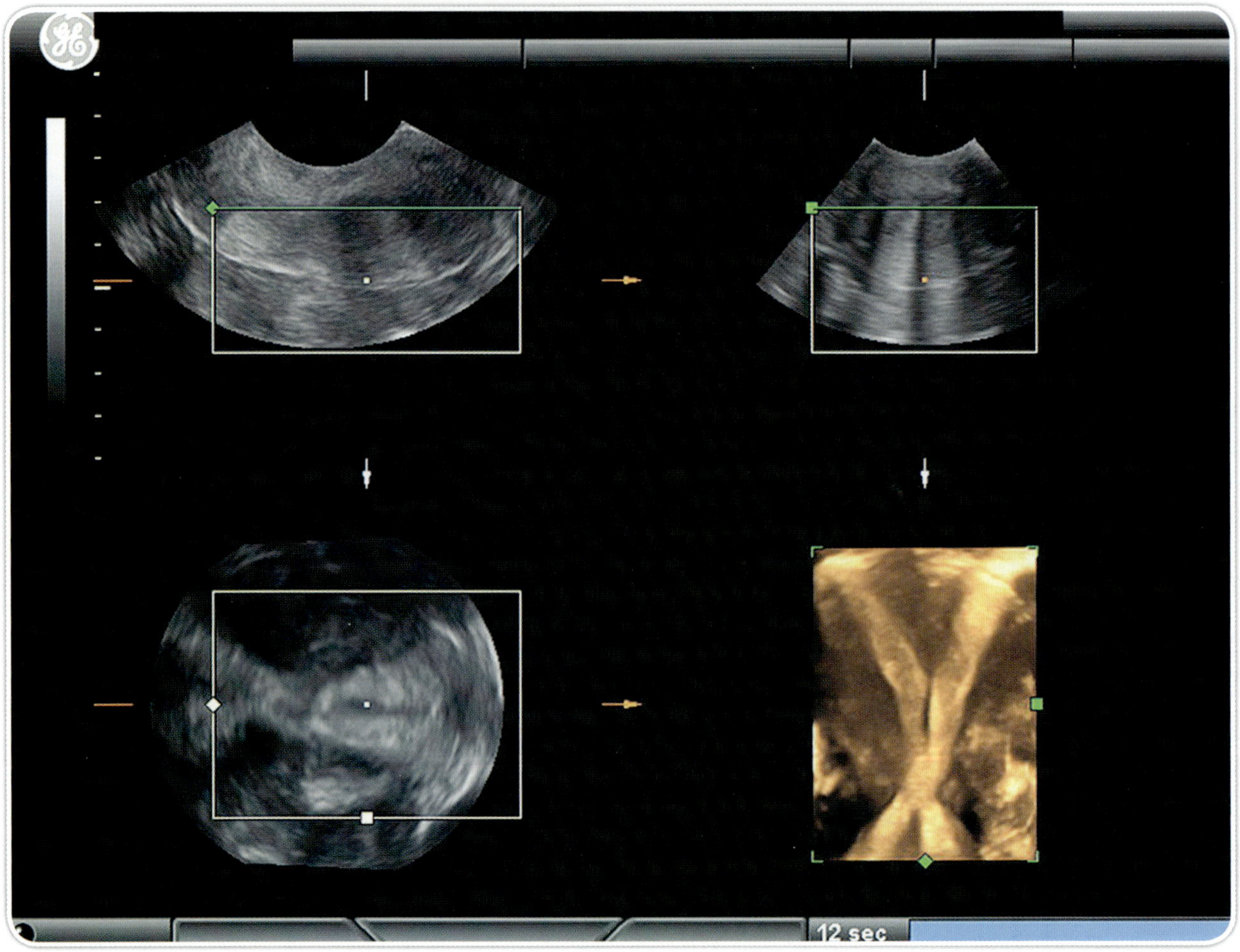

3D surface rendered

Septate Uterus

- In septate uterus, there is a wedge of fibrous tissue that divide the uterine cavity
- Uterine fundus is preserved
- The differential diagnosis can be bicornuate uterus, which has 2 uterine fundi.

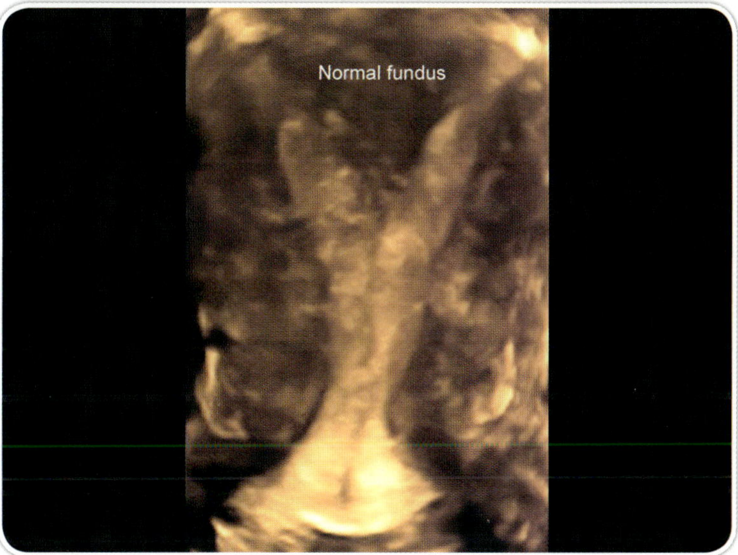

Arcuate Uterus

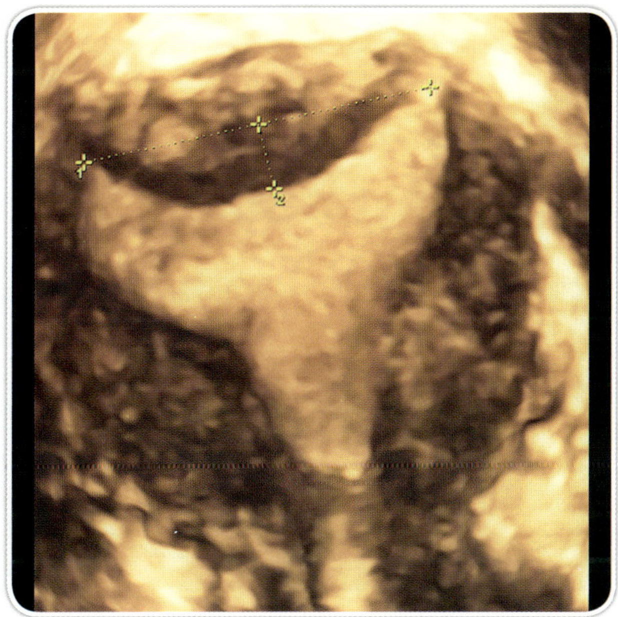

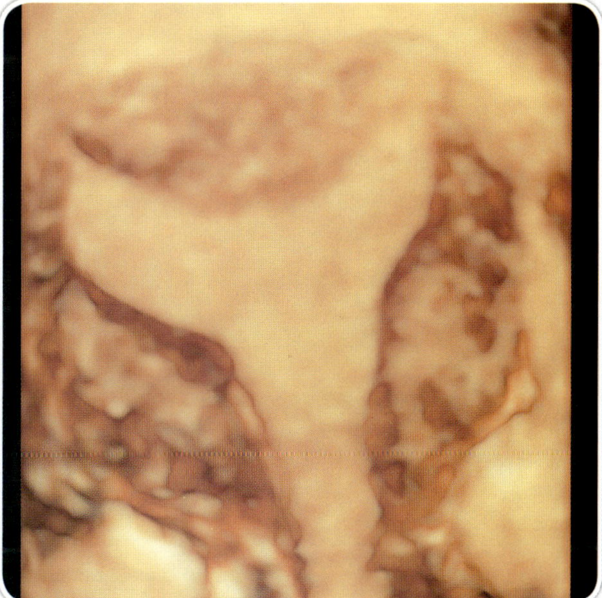

- Mullerian anomaly
- Concave contour of fundal part of the uterine cavity
- May have a higher risk for miscarriage, premature birth, and malpresentation.

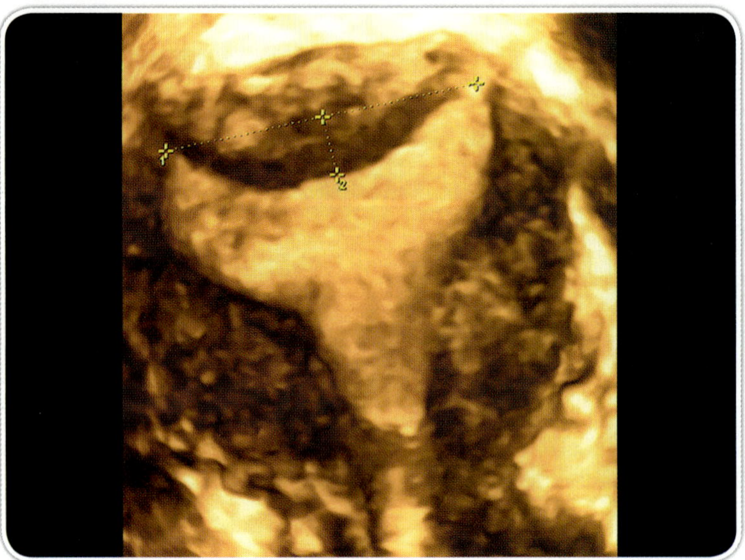

Hematometra in Cervical Stenosis

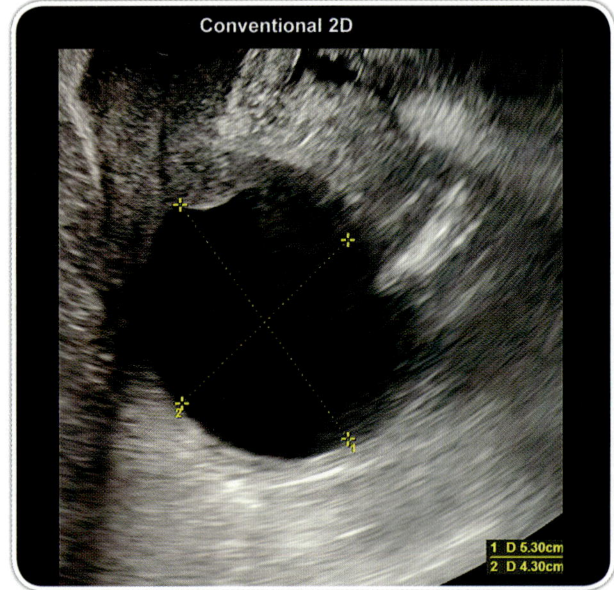

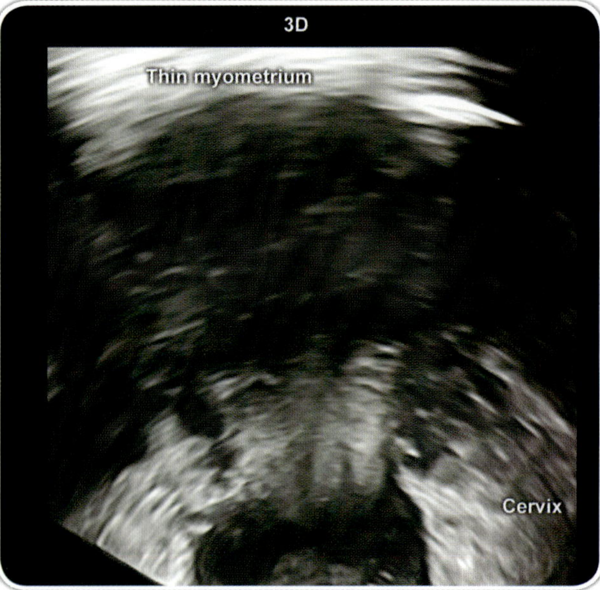

ENDOMETRIAL LESIONS

Focal Endometrial Lesion; Polyp

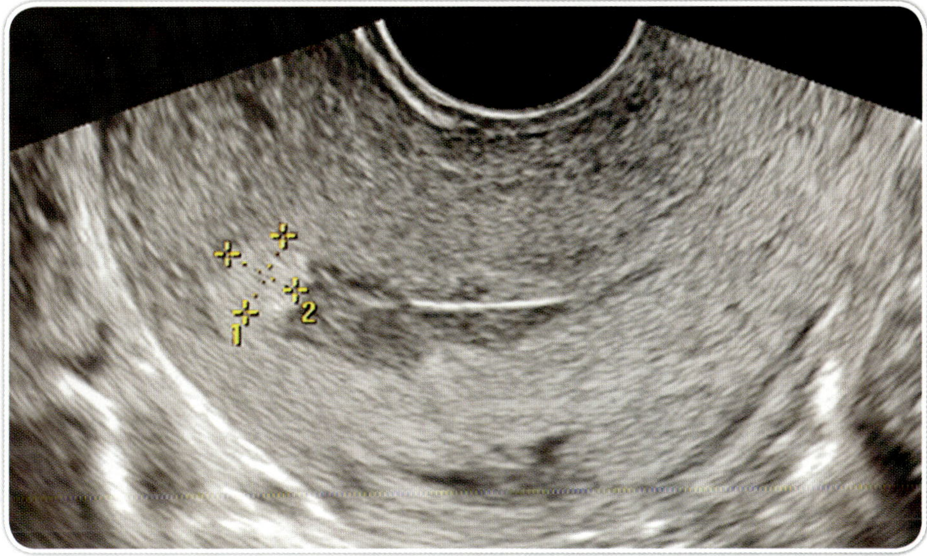

Focal endometrial lesions are best visualized during proliferative phase (sonolucent endometrial layers)

Endometrial Polyp

- May be sessile (wide-base) or pedunculated
- Vaginal spotting
- Should be removed, especially when symptomatic, to exclude endometrial hyperplasia.

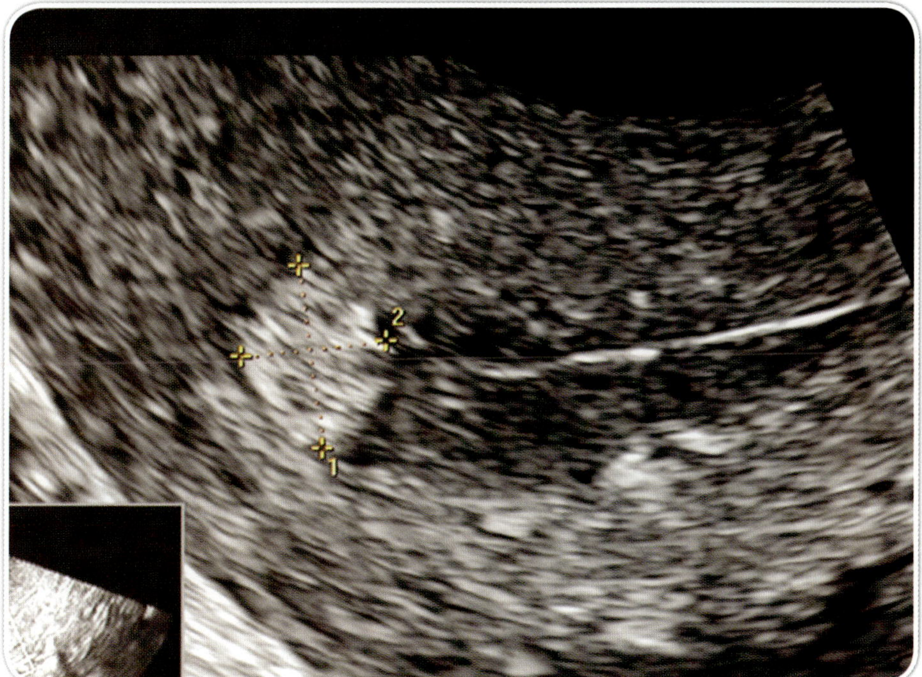

Endometrial Polyp: Removal

- Uterine curettage
- Hysteroscopic resection
- Hysterectomy (in association with the other diseases)

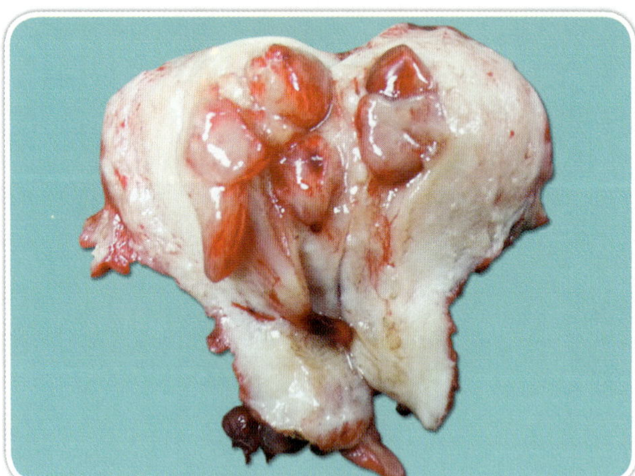

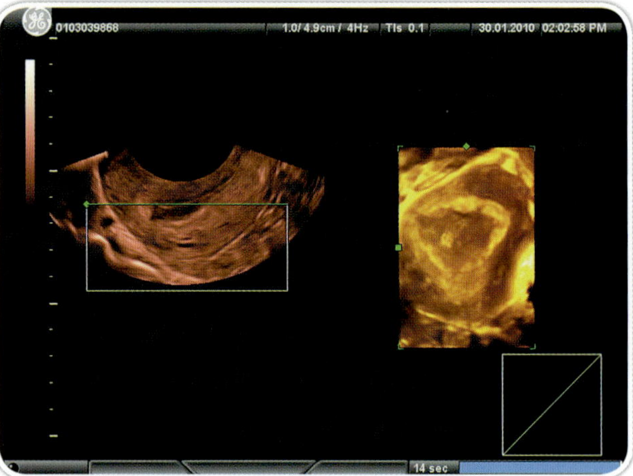

Echogenic endometrium during secretory phase can impair visualization of small focal endometrial lesions

Visualization of Small Focal Endometrial Lesions

Small amount of fluid can enhance the visualization of endometrial lesions, particularly in the secretory phase.

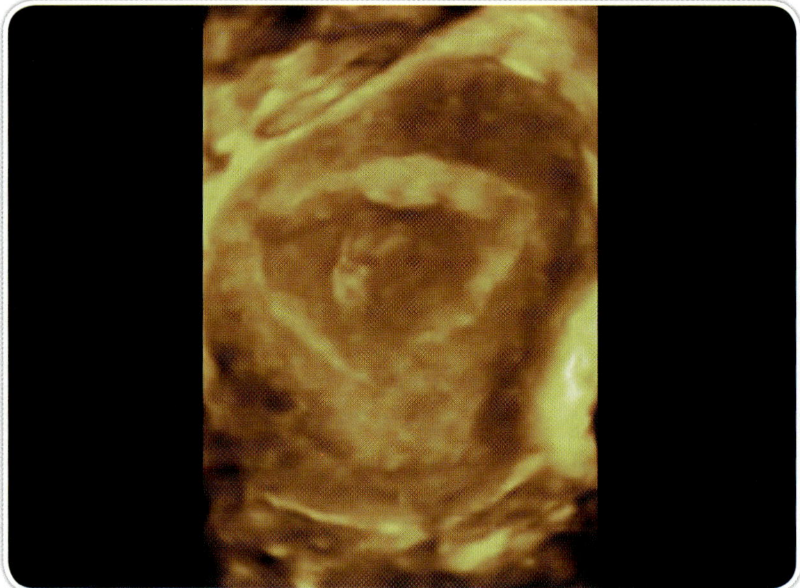

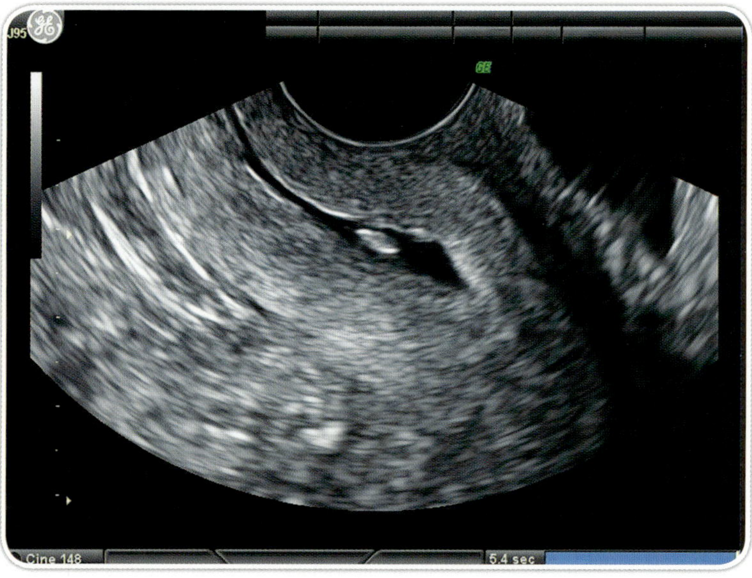

Endometrial fluid facilitates the rendering

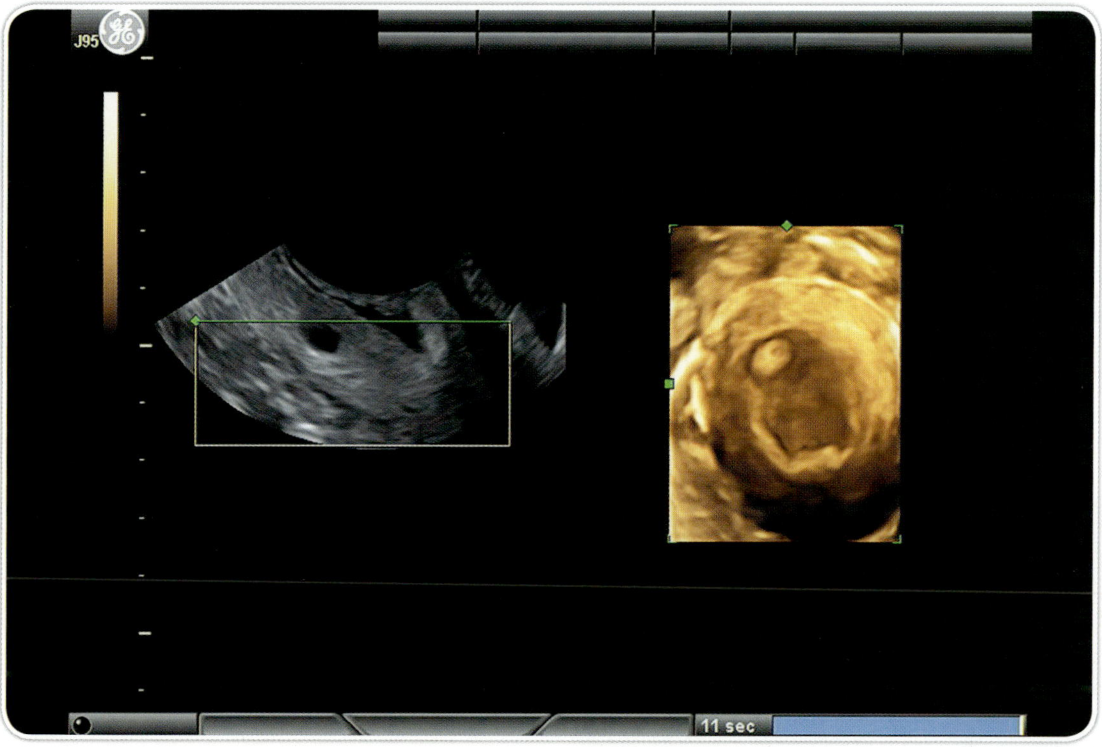

Endometrial polyp seen after saline infusion sonohysterography (SIS)

Saline Infusion Sonohysterography (SIS)

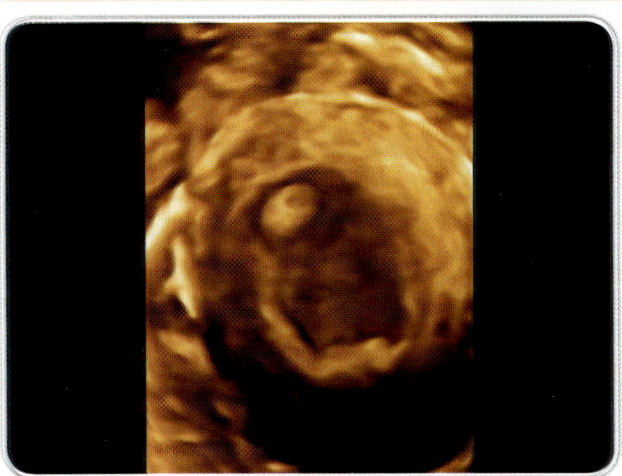

- Instillation of a small amount of saline solution into the uterine cavity
- Enhancement of small focal lesions
  - Endometrial polyp
  - Uterine synechiae (Asherman's syndrome).

Submucous Myoma

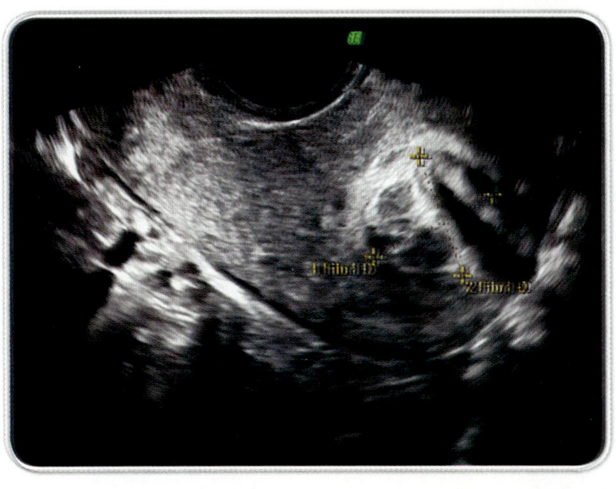

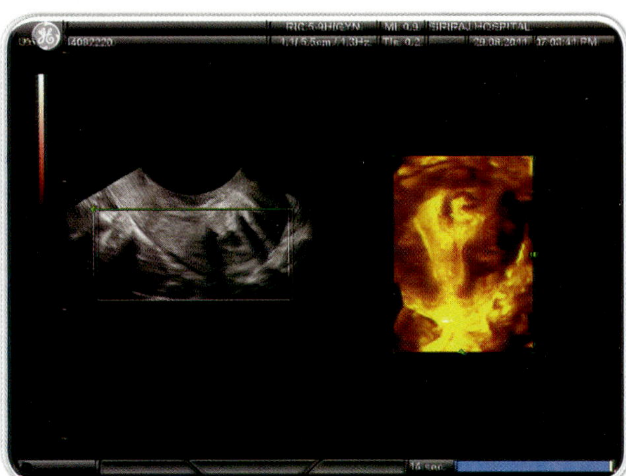

Submucous Myoma and Fertility

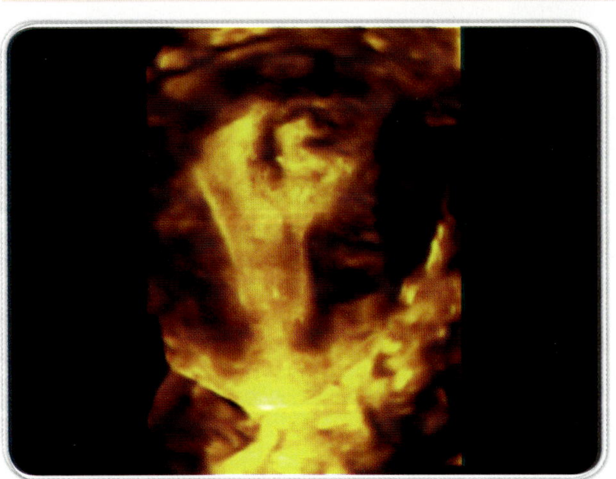

(Jayakrishnan et al. 2013)

- Size and location of submucous myoma
- Hysteroscopic resection can improve the pregnancy outcomes
- Location and depth of myometrial/intracavitary involvement may be better visualized with 3DUS.

INTRAUTERINE DEVICES (IUD)

Pyometra with IUD (uncertain history)

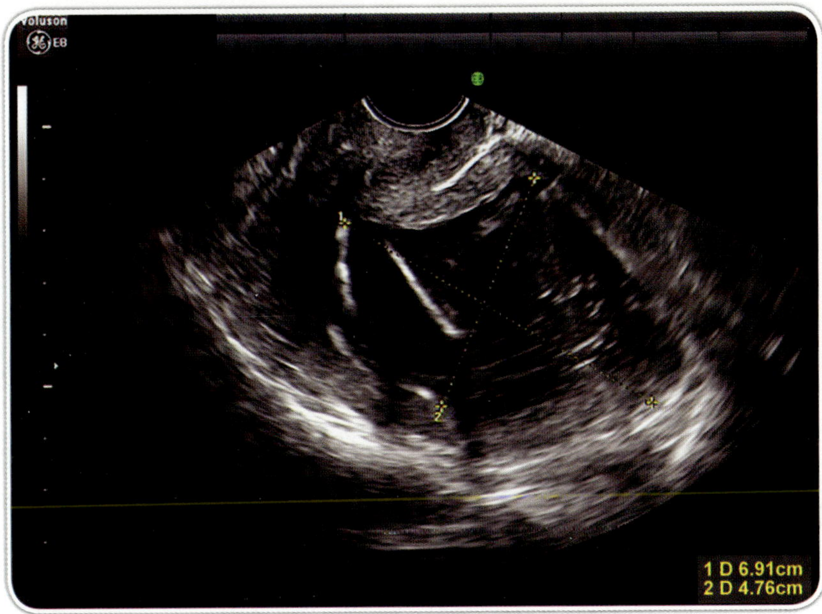

Lippes Loop

2D is informative enough for IUDs with unique shapes.

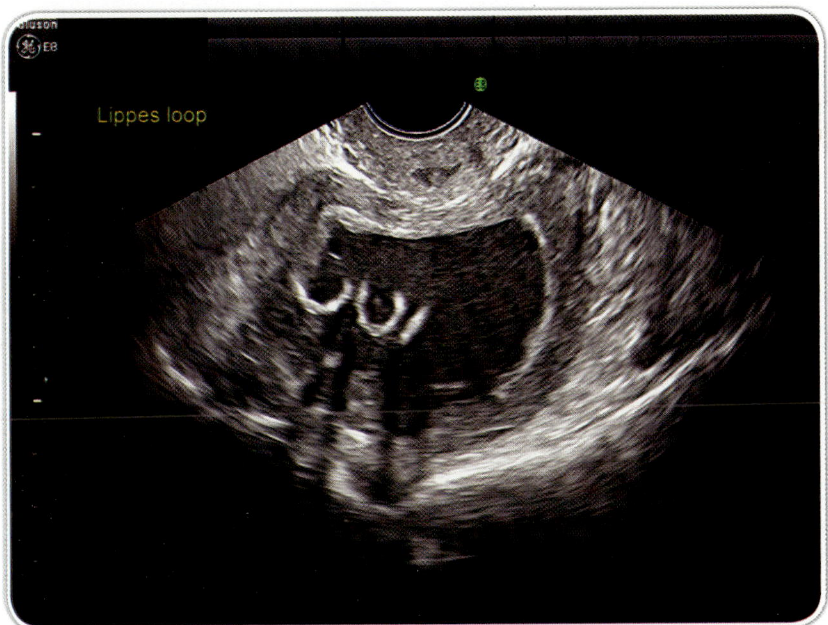

For other Types of IUDs

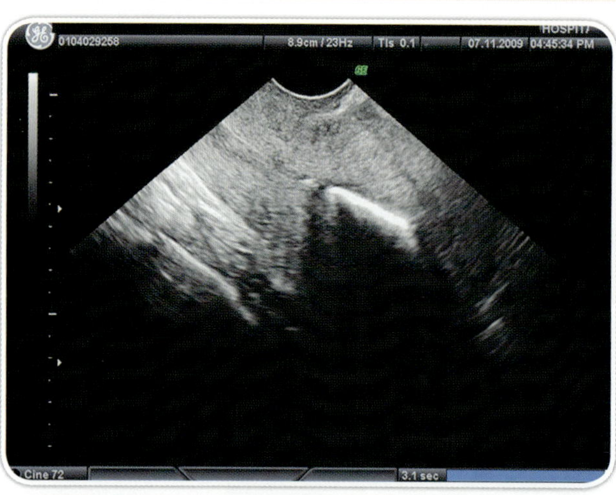

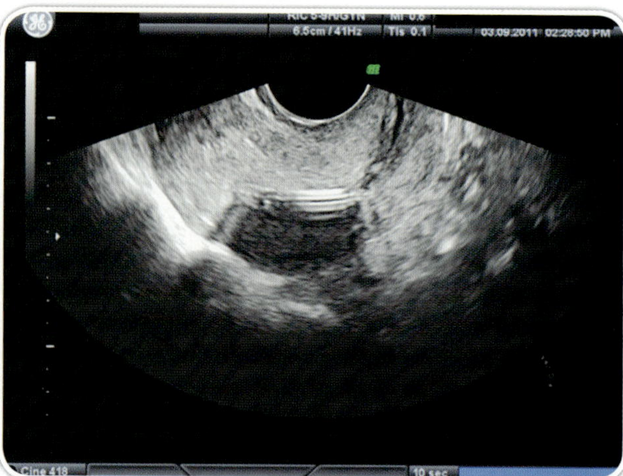

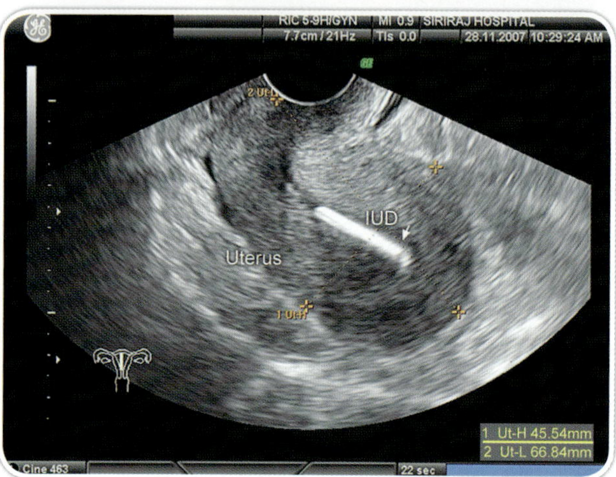

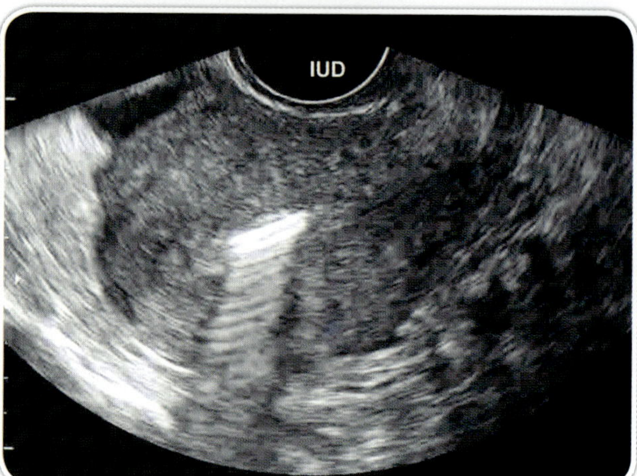

They have similar appearances on the conventional 2D

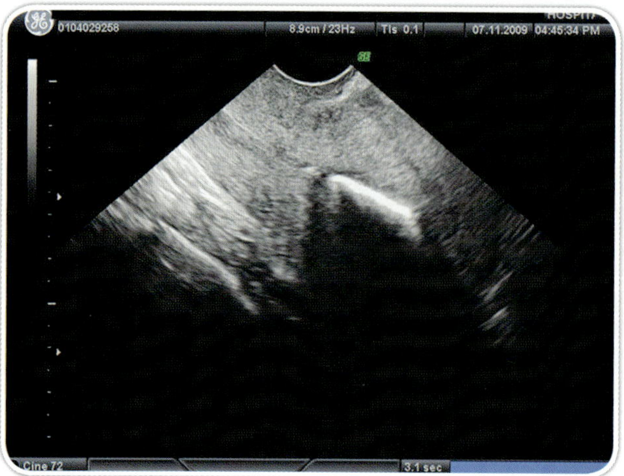

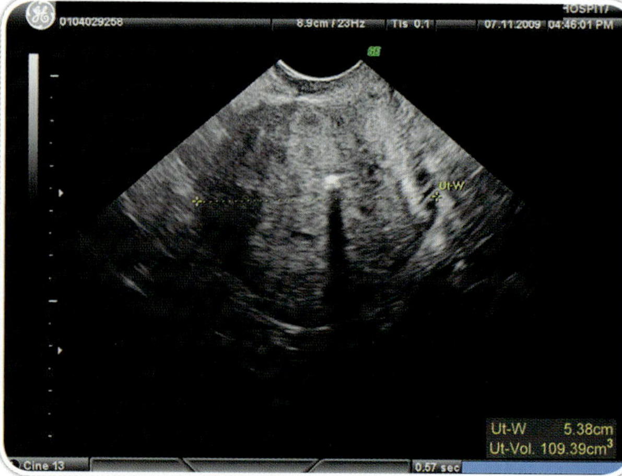

Single metallic rod without metallic components on the wings

Single Metallic Rod without Metallic Components on the Wings

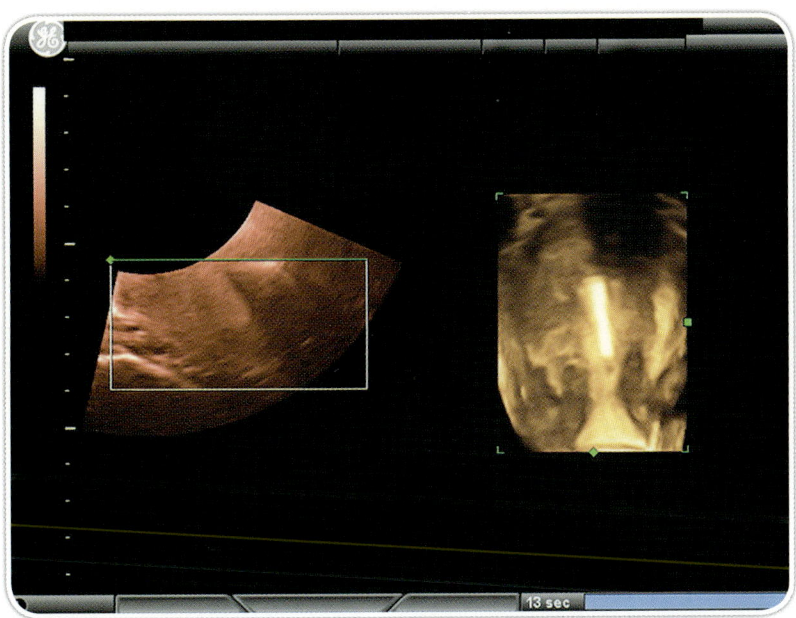

Single Metallic Rod without Metallic Components on the Wings: Multiload IUD

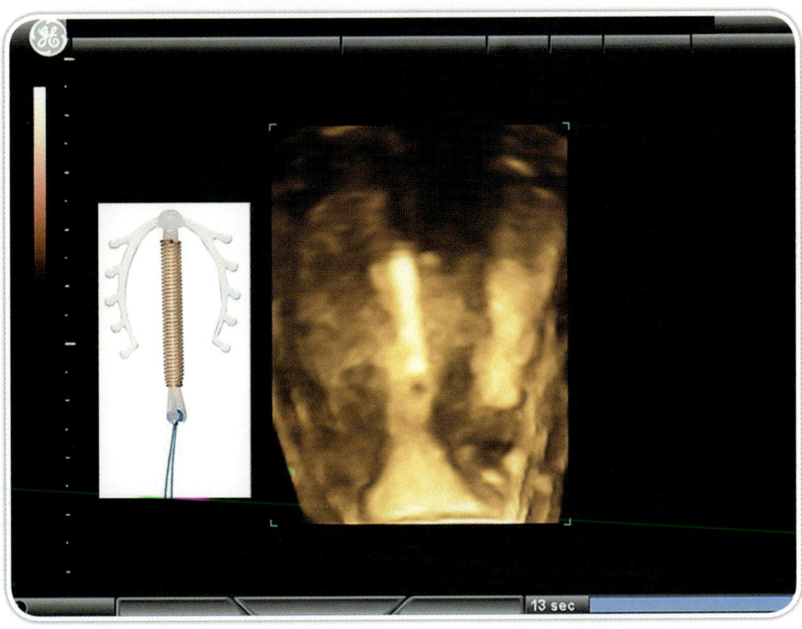

Multiload IUD

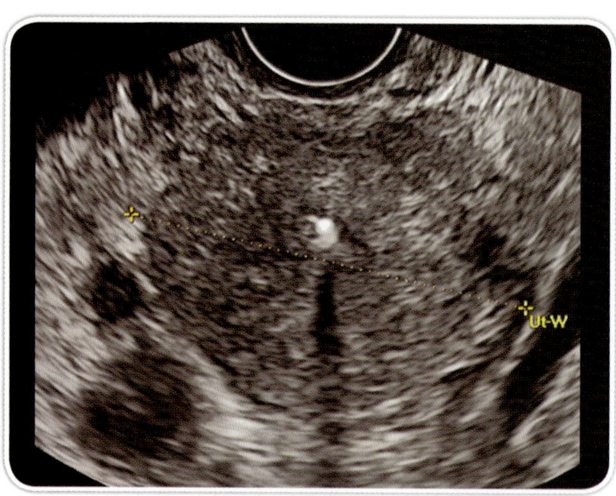

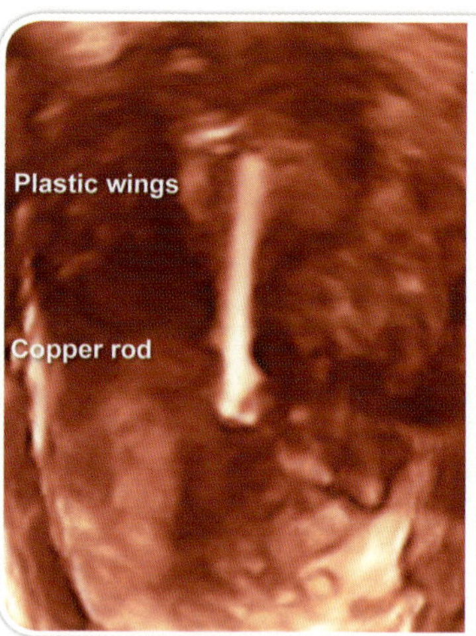

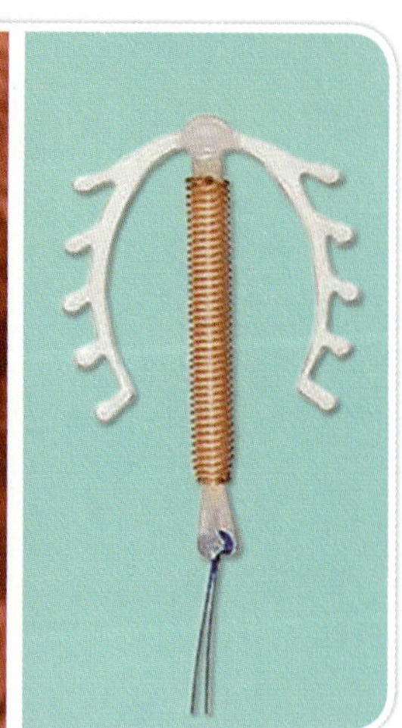

Multiload IUD: Various 3DUS demonstrations

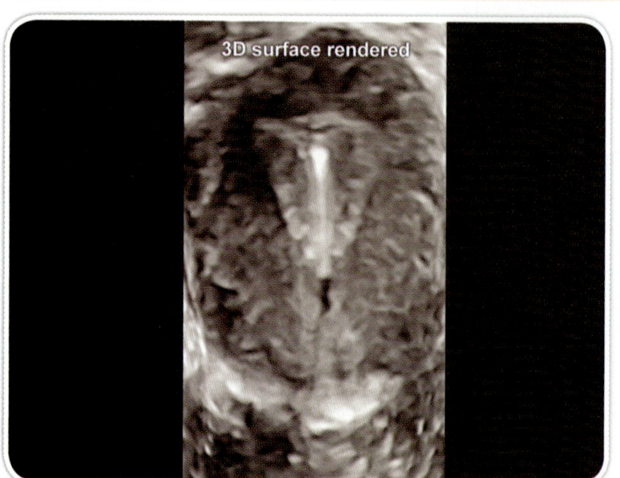

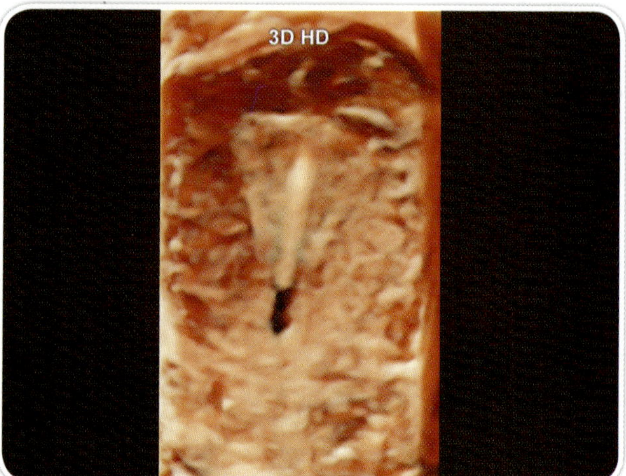

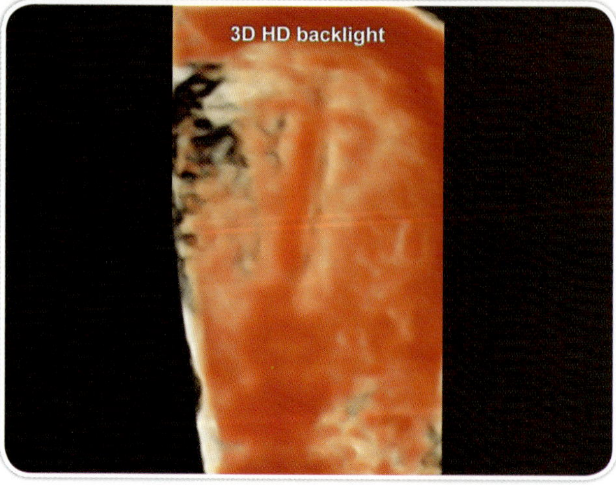

Location of the IUD

- Transvaginal US can help assuring the appropriate location of the IUD in endometrial cavity
- X-ray may be helpful when extrauterine migration is suspected.

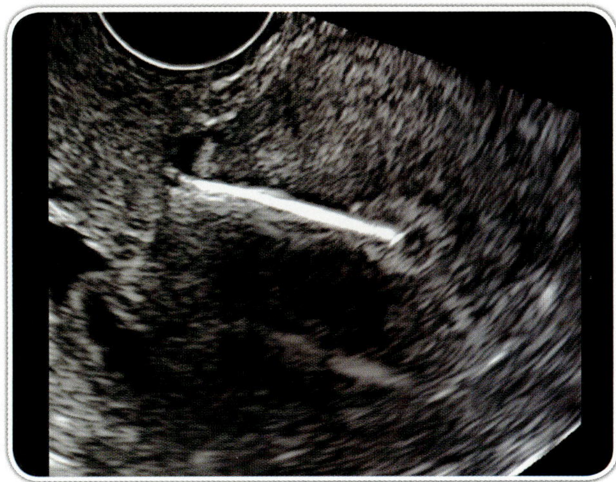

(Peri et al. 2007)

Dislodged Multiload IUD

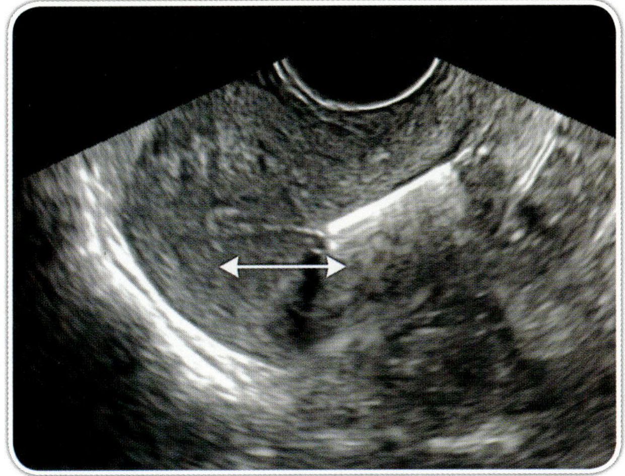

- The IUD has moved down to the lower uterine segment and cervical canal
- It should be removed and replaced, if contraception is still needed

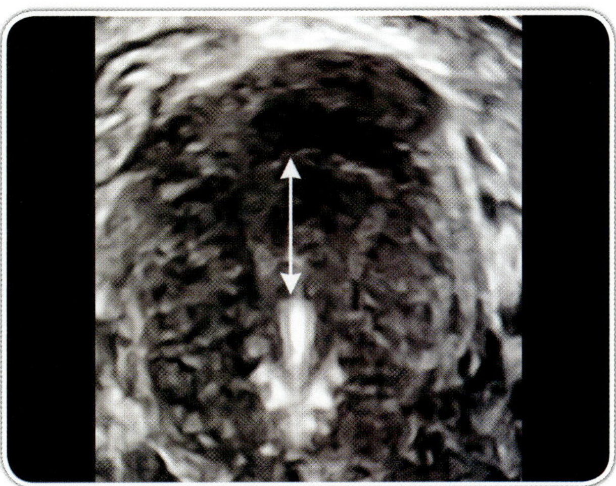

- The IUD has moved down to the lower uterine segment and cervical canal
- Note that the plastic wings are collapsed.

Identification of IUD Type from Single Sagittal Image is Inaccurate

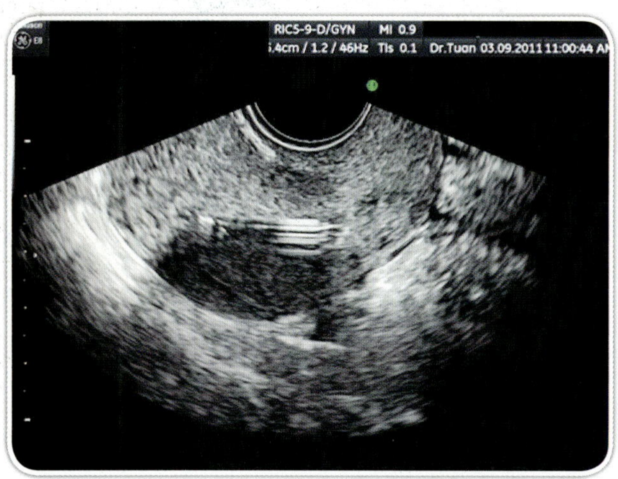

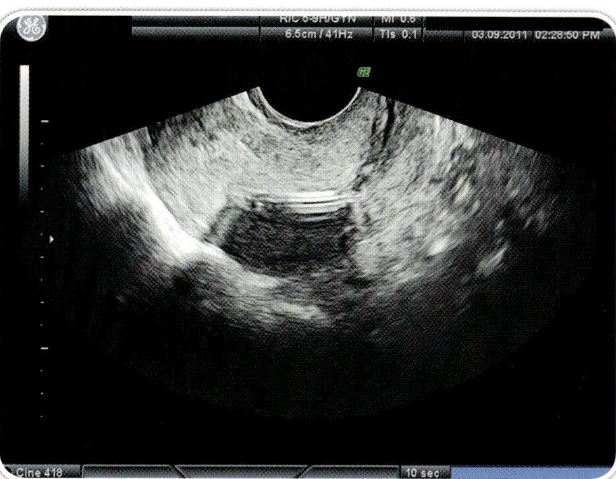

Ring down artifact suggests for metallic content at the rod

Multiplanar Approach Copper-T IUD

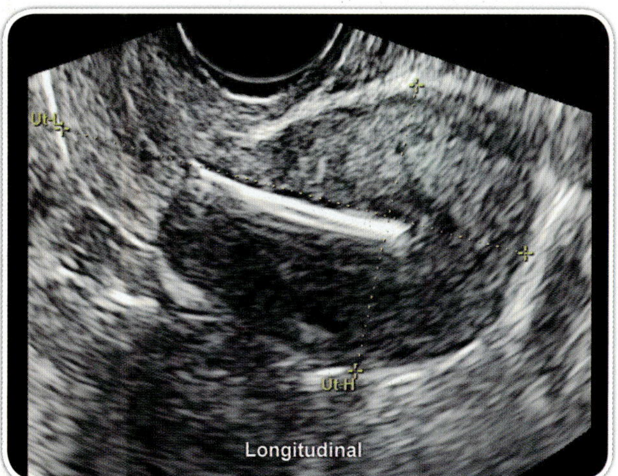

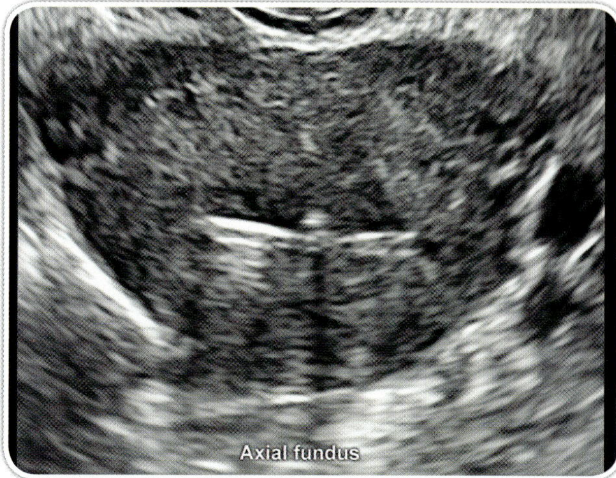

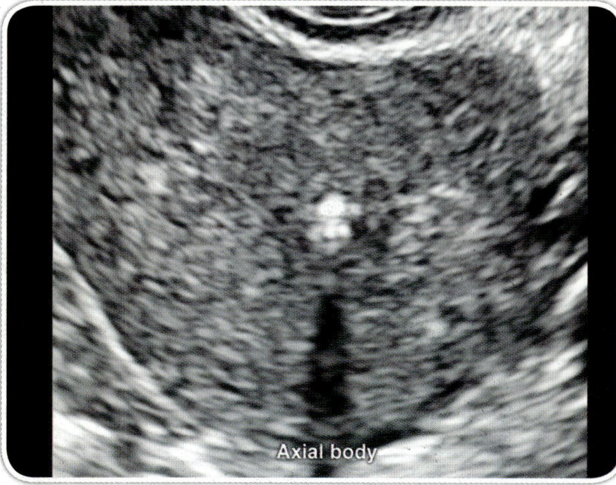

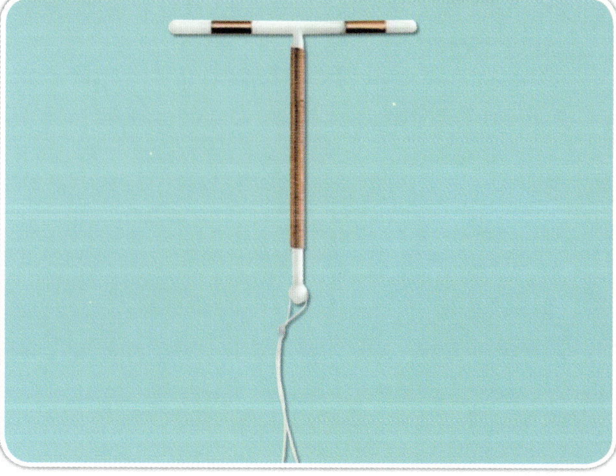

3D TVS can Identify the Type, Location, and Endometrial Cavity at the Same Time

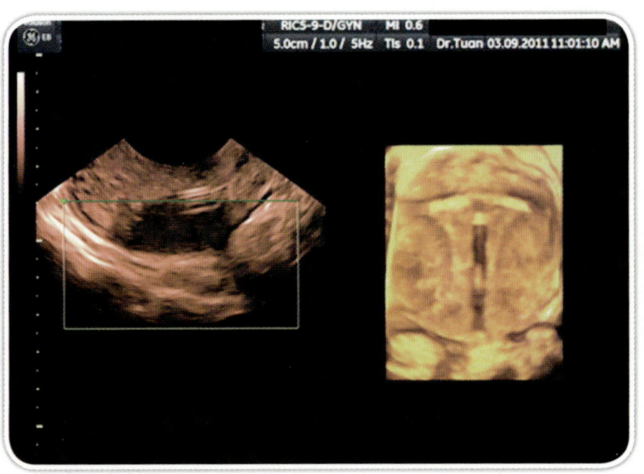

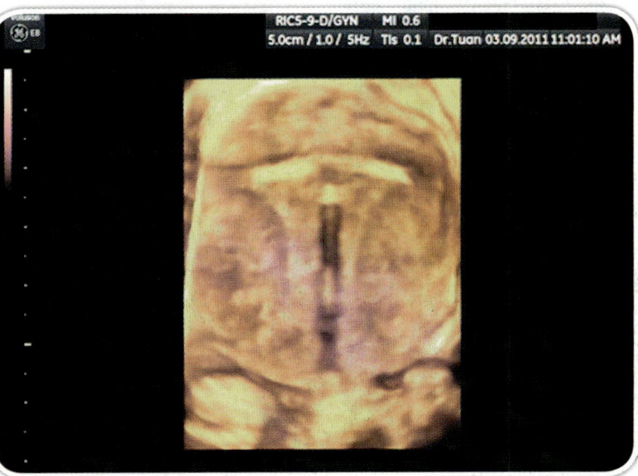

Copper T IUD

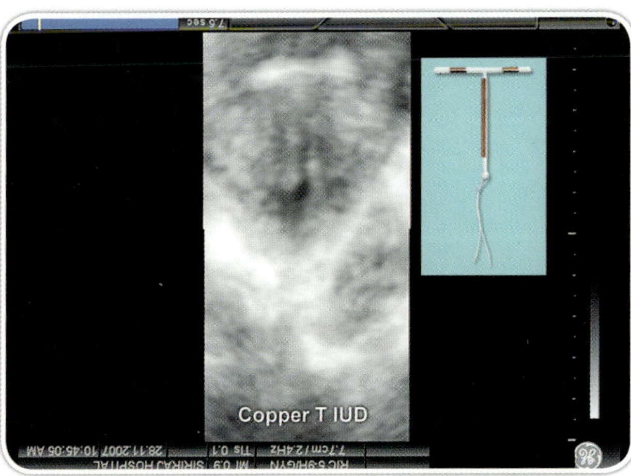

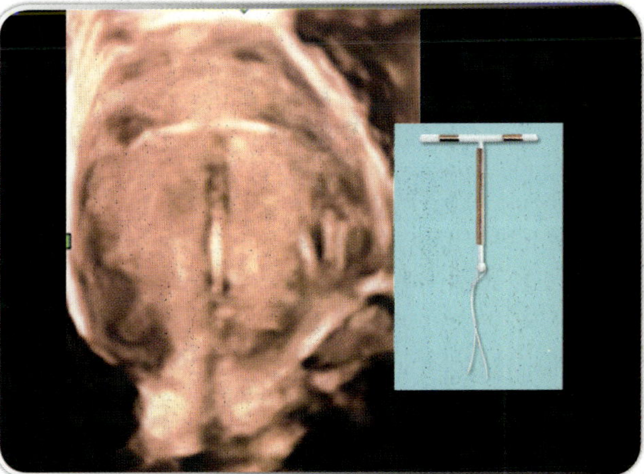

Copper-enhancement is seen on both wings

Transvaginal US; Copper-T IUD

- Location in the uterus
- Uterine cavity
- Wing expansion.

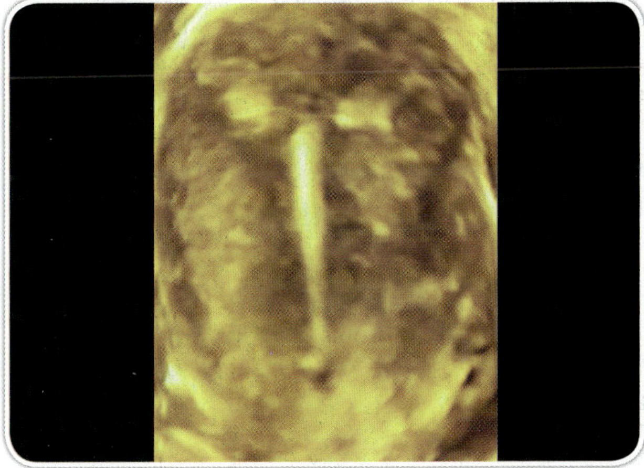

Identification of IUD Type from Single Sagittal Image

Identification of IUD type from single sagittal image is inaccurate, but large-caliber rod without ring down artifact (no metallic components) suggests for **Mirena intrauterine system (IUS).**

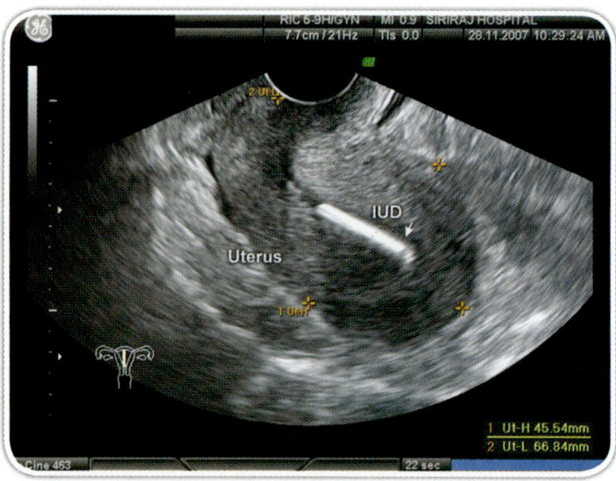

Mirena IUS

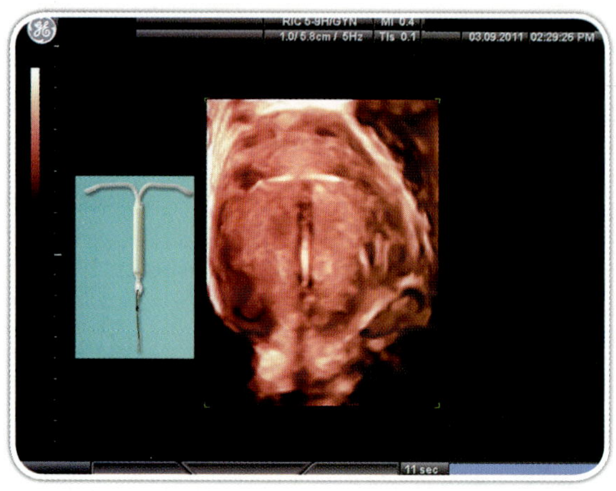

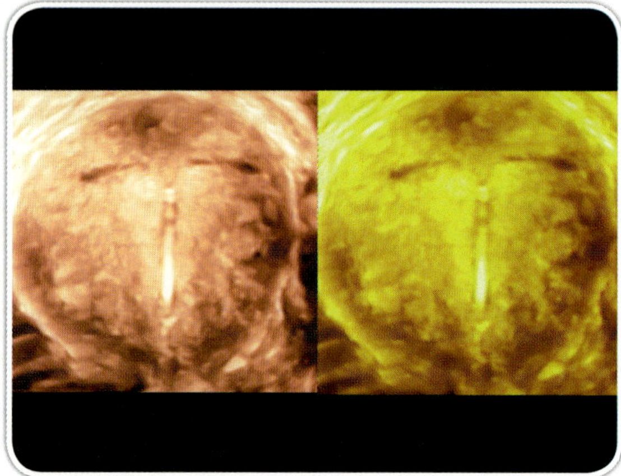

Identification of IUD type from Single Sagittal Image is Inaccurate

- However, note the heavy ring down artifact behind this device.
- Heavy ring down artifact suggests for the heavy metallic content.

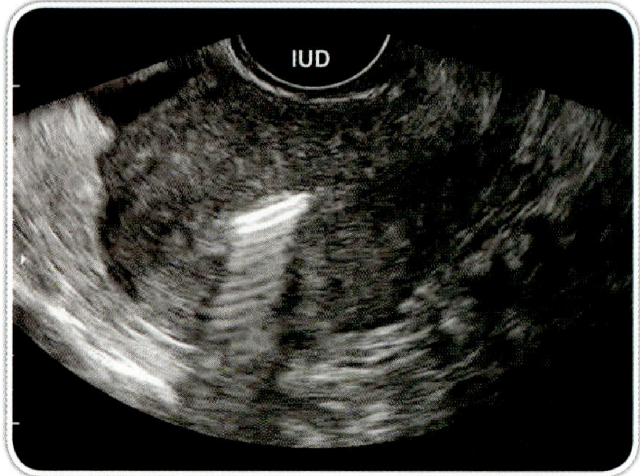

Chinese Ring IUD

- An obsolete permanent contraception in China, no longer available
- Put in right after delivery
- May cause chronic pelvic pain.

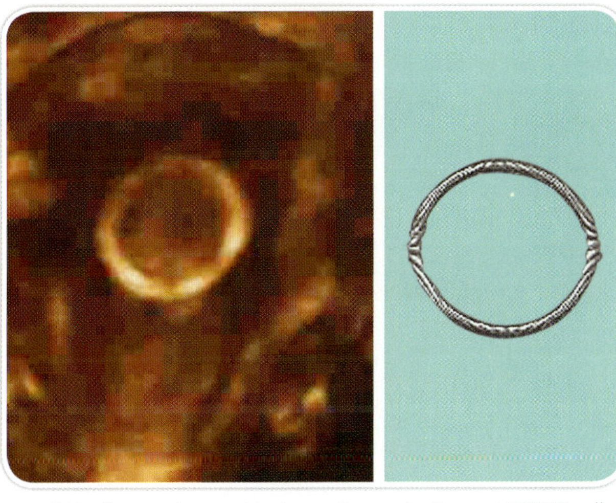

(http://www.obgyn.net/us/us.asp?page=/us/present/9808/Bradley

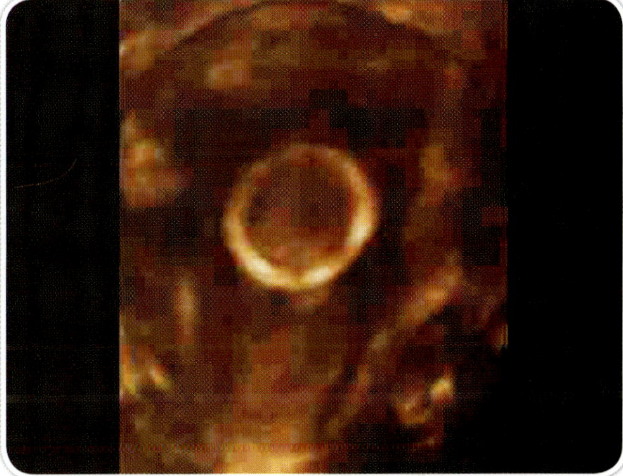

(Wataganara et al. 2008)

Conclusion

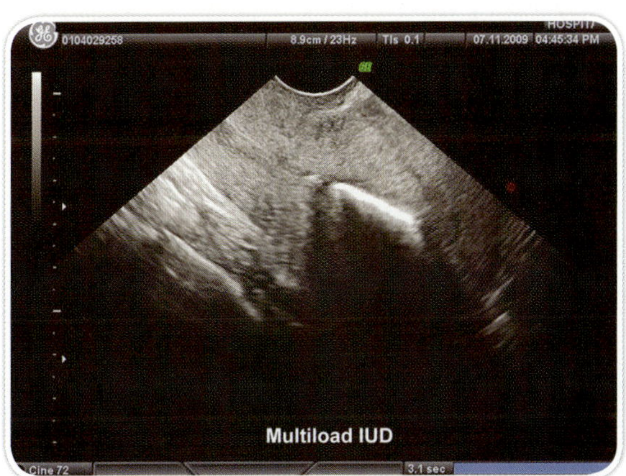

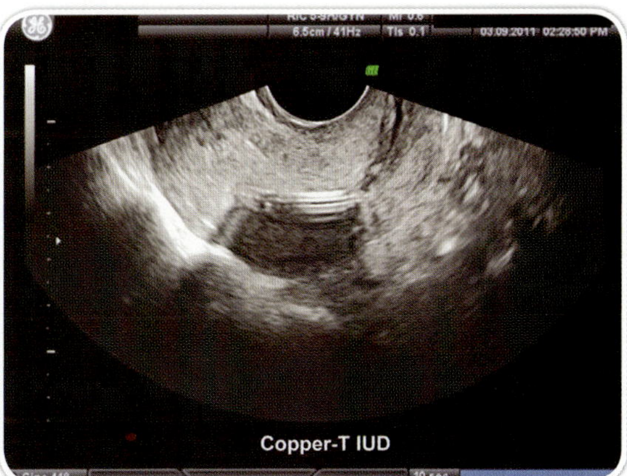

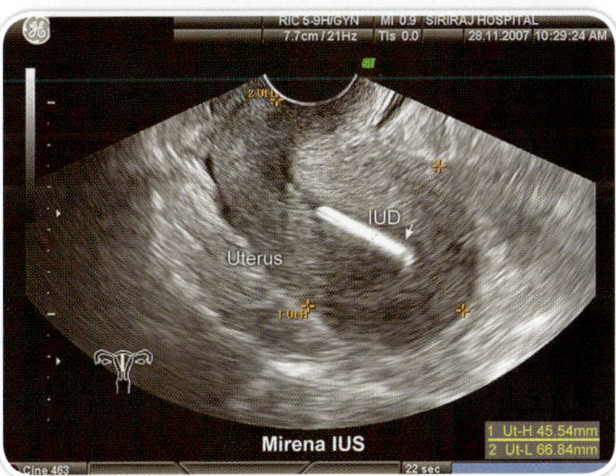

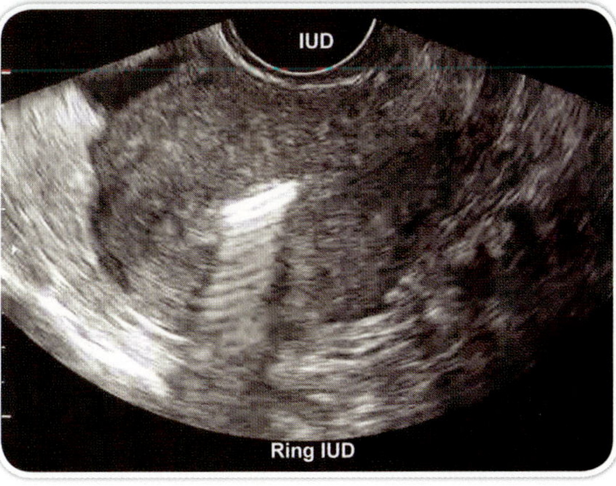

OVARY

Normal Ovary on Conventional 2D Scan

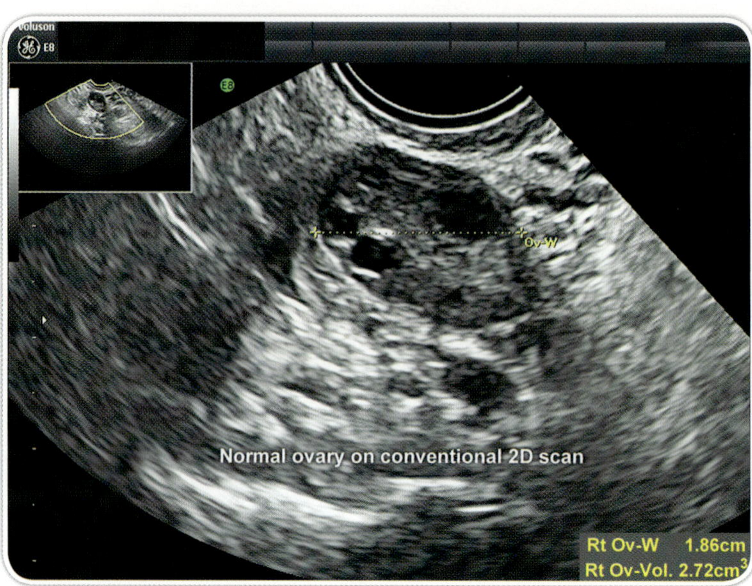

Ovarian Fossa is on Iliac Artery and Vein

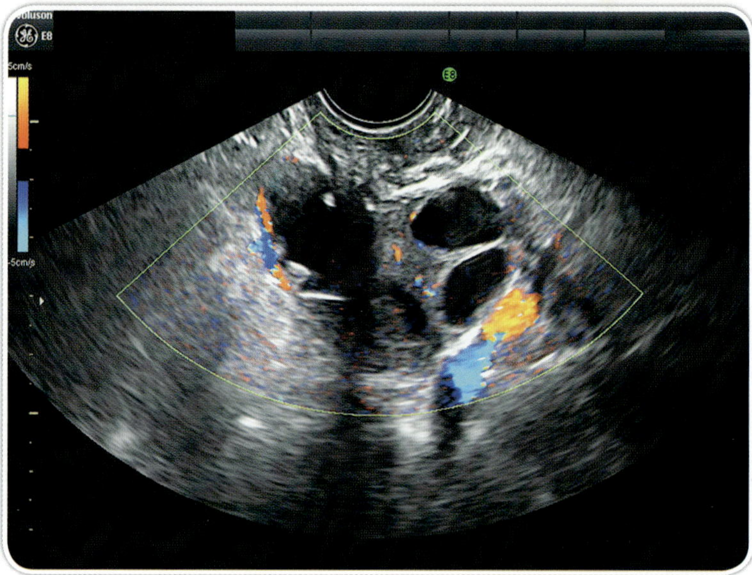

3D US Appearance of the Ovary

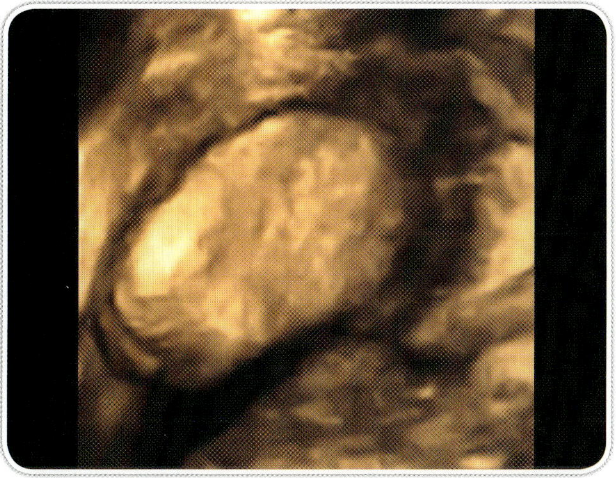
Smooth-surface ovary: Pre-menarche

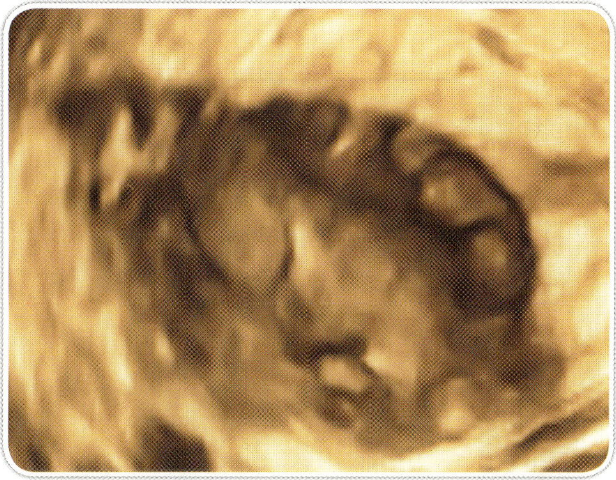
Ovary with growing follicles: Reproductive age

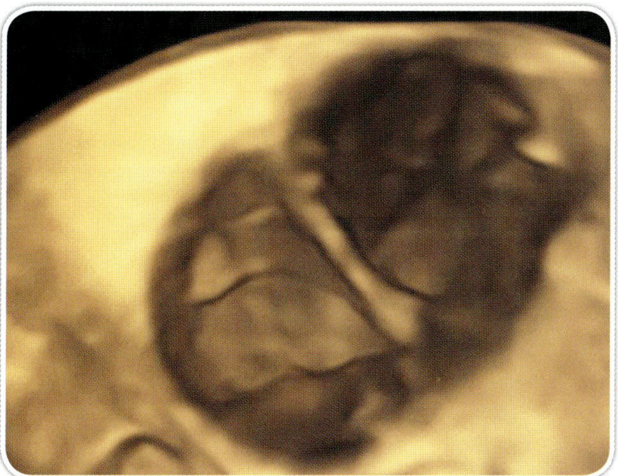
Corpus luteum

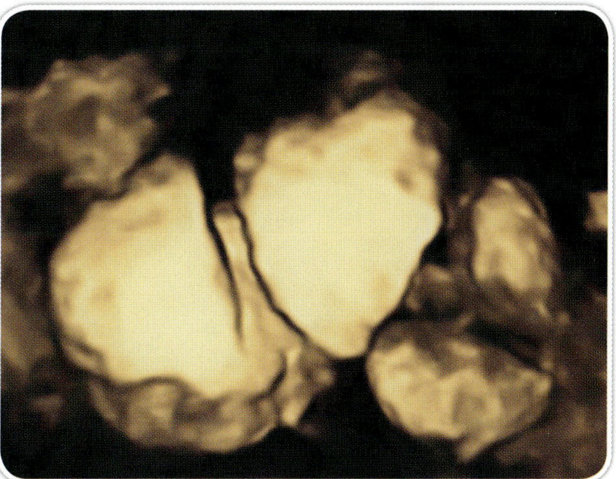
Corpus luteum, Inversion mode

INTERNAL SURFACE OF AN OVARIAN CYST

Simple Cyst of the Ovary

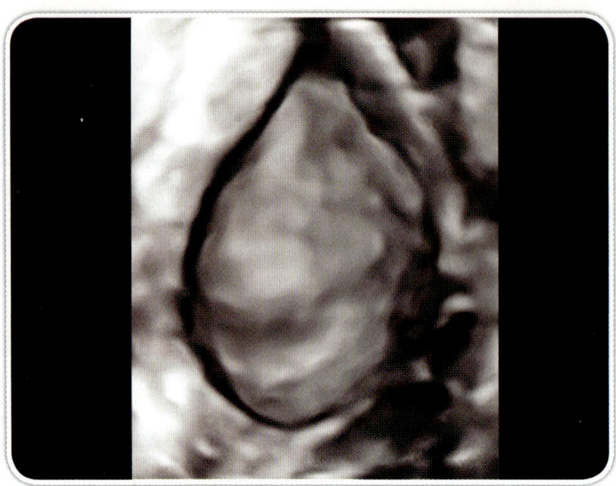

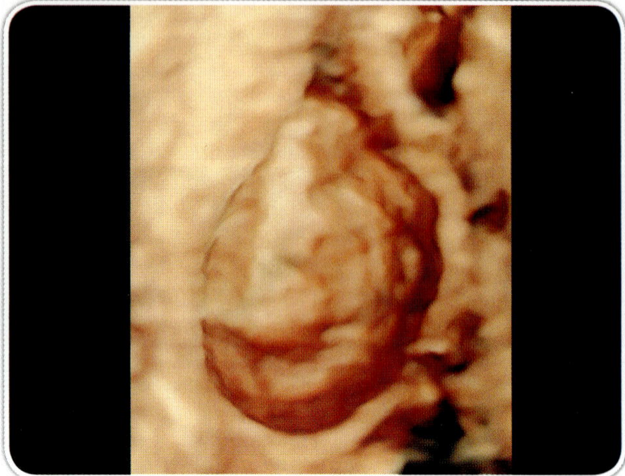

Internal surface on conventional 3D and 3DHD surface rendered

Simple Cyst: Smooth Internal Surface

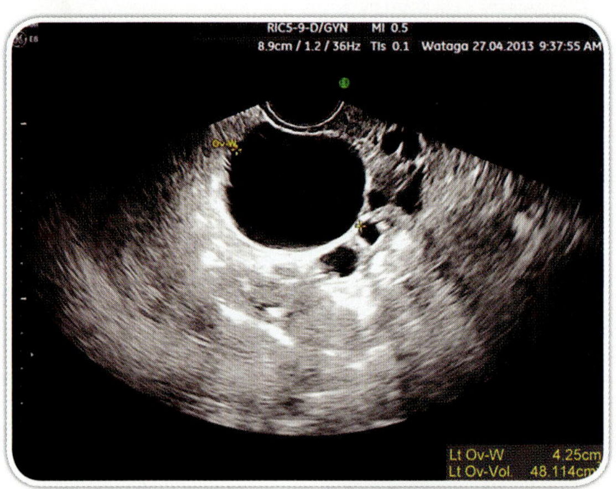

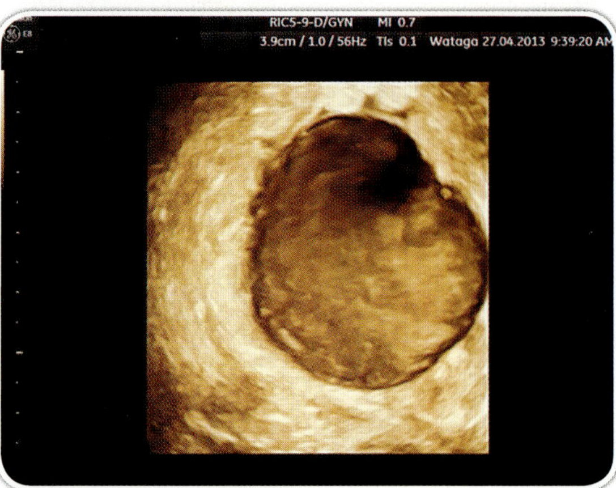

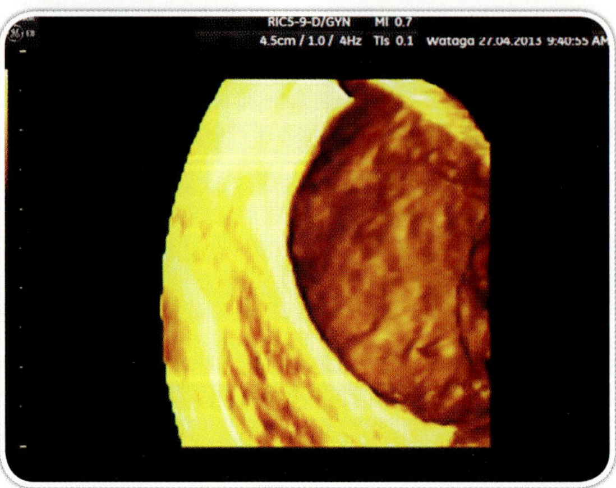

Hemorrhagic Cyst

- Corpus luteum cyst
- Follicular cyst
- Other benign cysts, i.e. endometrioma.

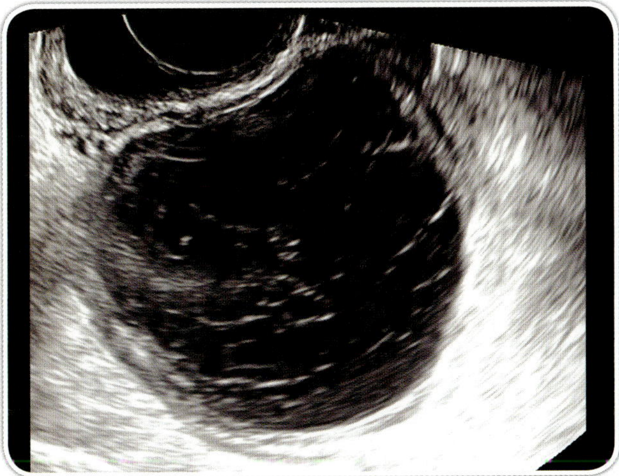

'Lace-like' internal echo

Hemorrhagic Cyst: 3DHD

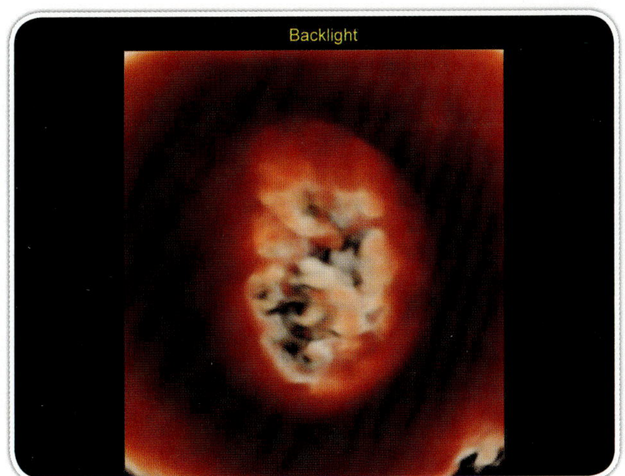

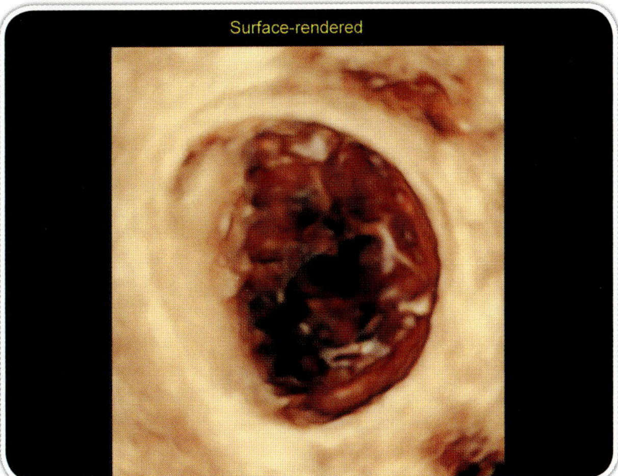

3D 'Lace-like' internal echo

POLYCYSTIC OVARY

Polycystic Ovarian Syndrome (PCOS)

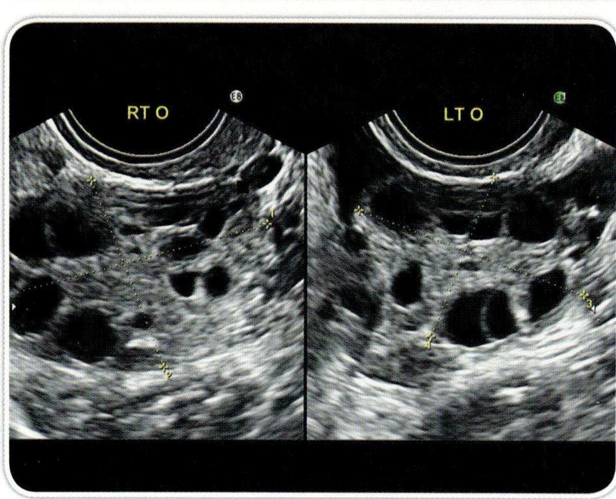

- The Rotterdam consensus
  - $\geq$ 12 or more follicles AND
  - Measuring between 2 and 9 mm AND/OR
  - An ovarian volume >10 cm^3

3D US Surface Rendered to Demonstrate Peripheral Distribution of the Follicles

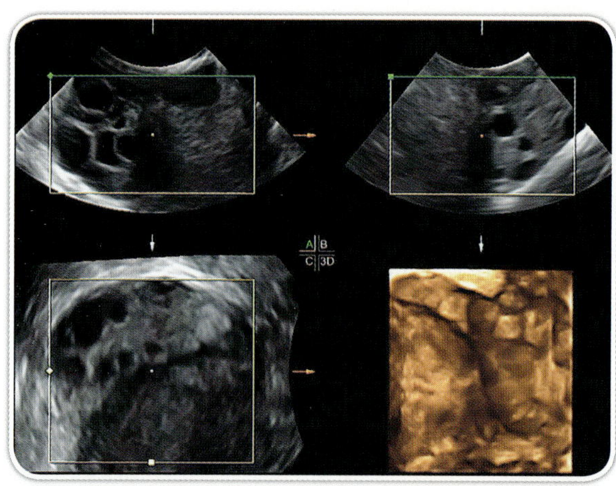

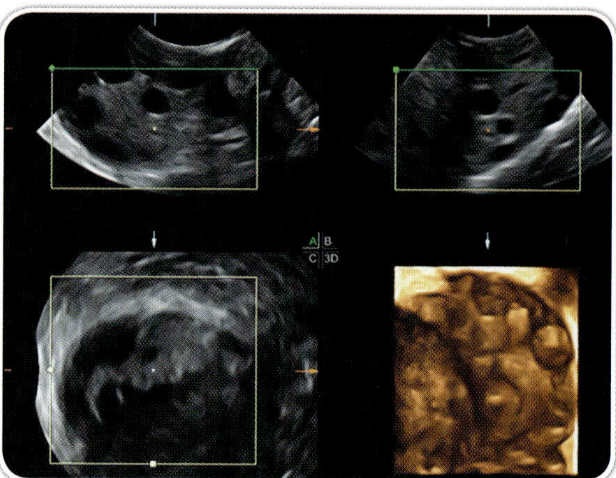

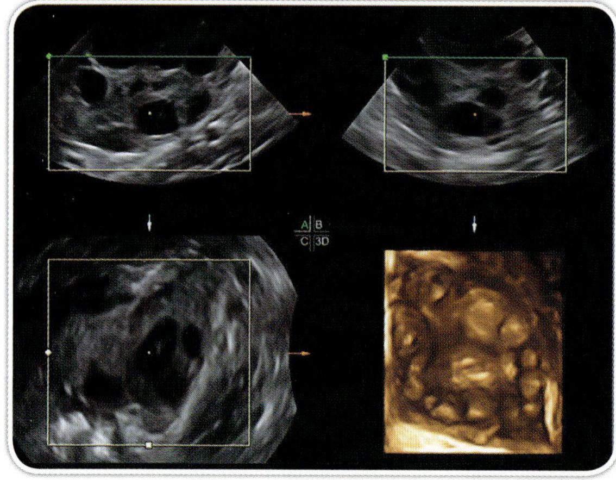

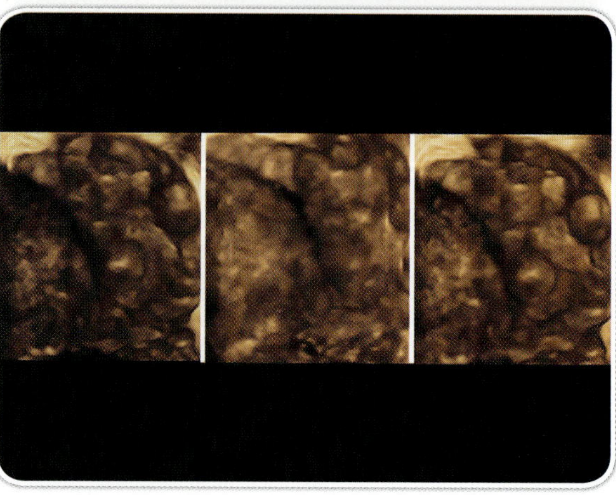

3D US Inversion Mode to Demonstrate Peripheral Distribution of the Follicles

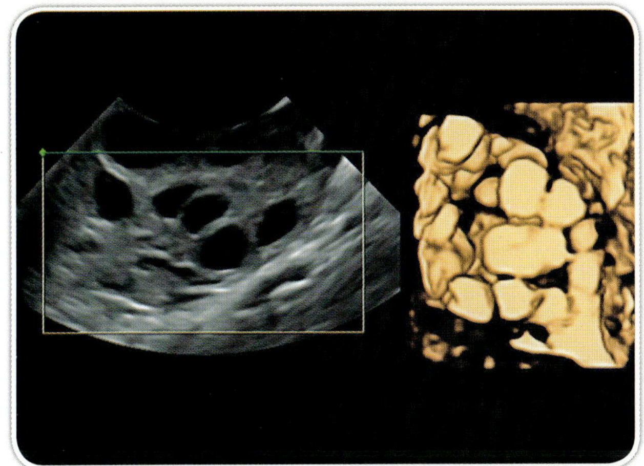

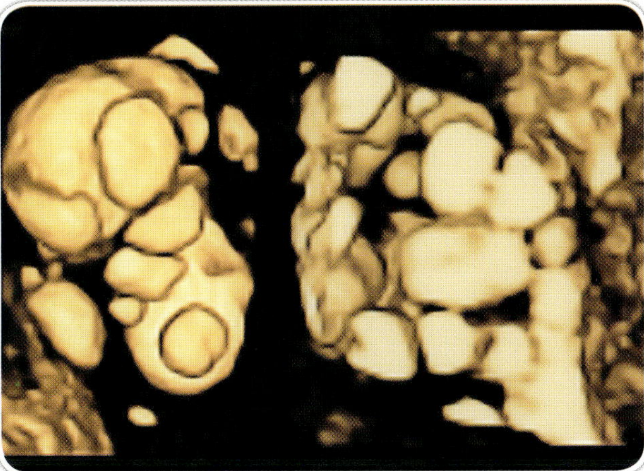

Ovarian vessel

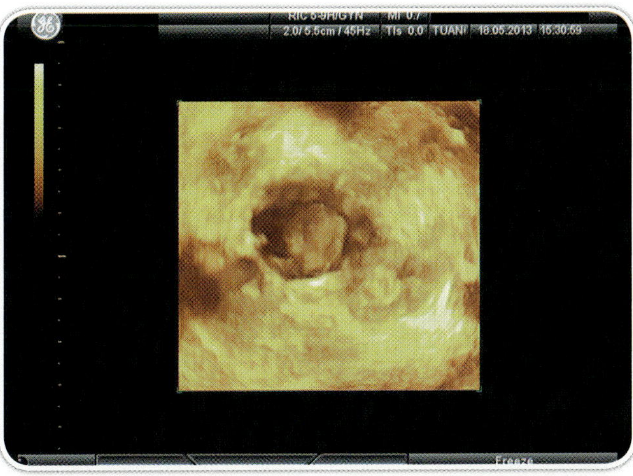

OVARIAN TUMOR

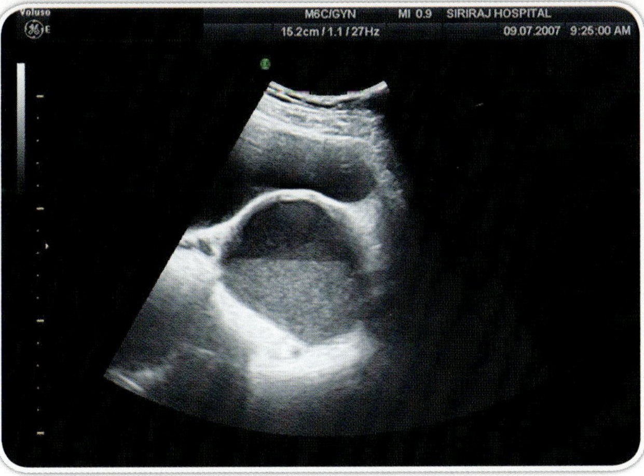

Fat-fluid level

Ovarian Dermoid
2D US Remains the Primary Diagnostic Tool

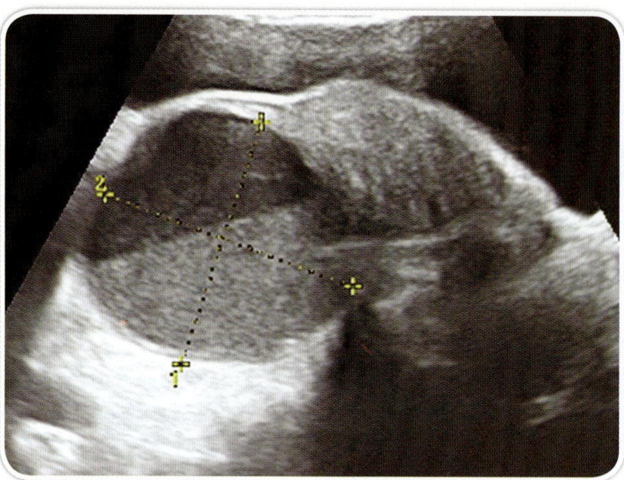

Endometrioma with Internal Solid Fibrous Nodule

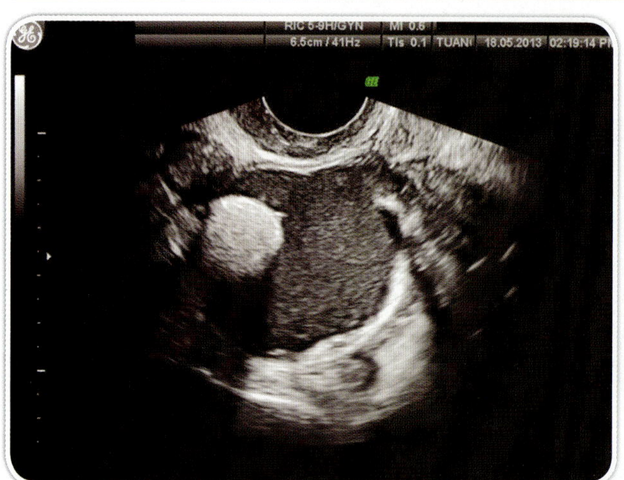

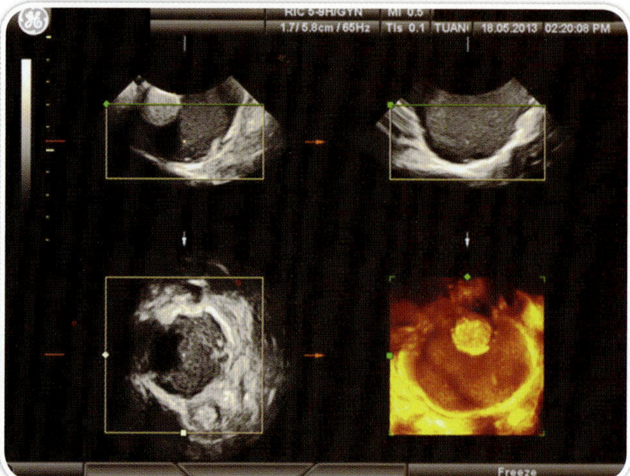

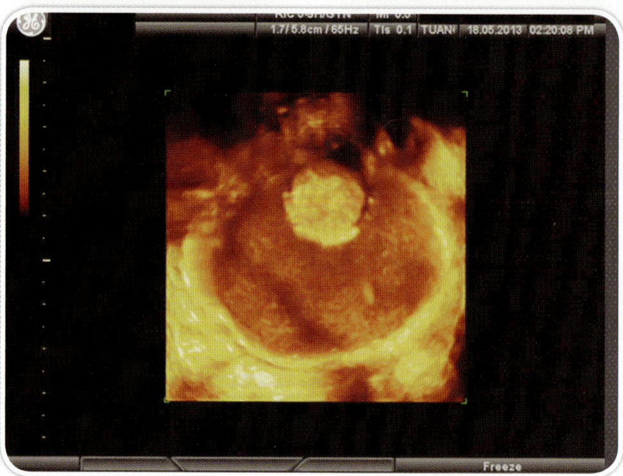

Borderline Serous Cystadenoma

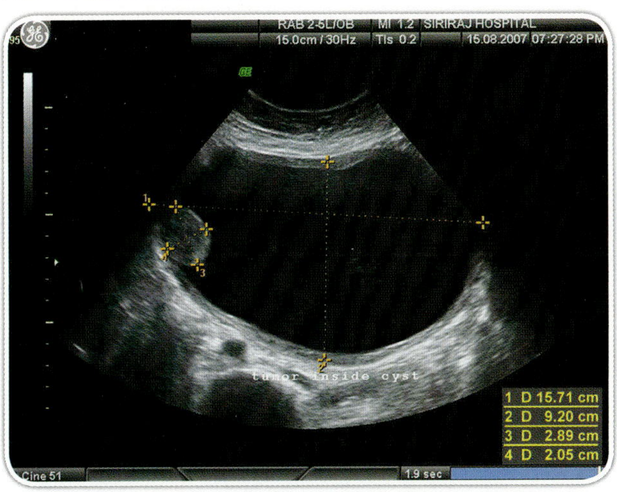

'Pedunculated' solid nodule on the internal surface

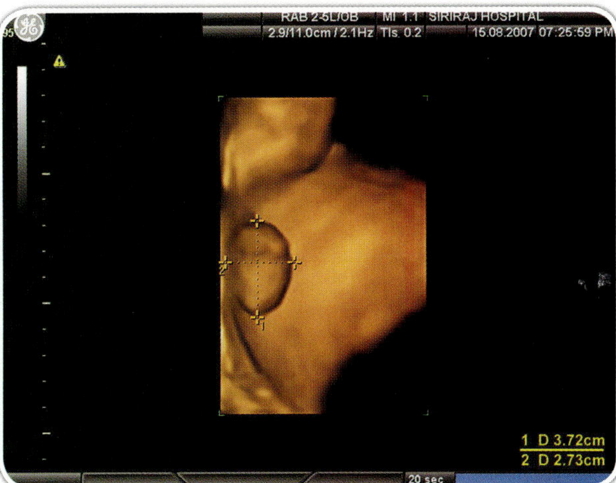

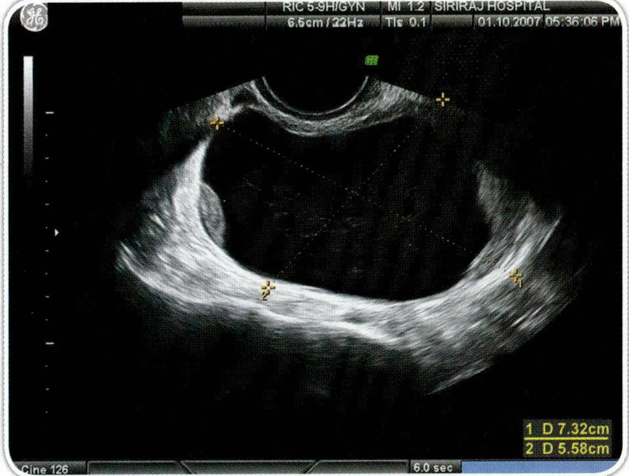

'Sessile' solid nodule on the internal surface

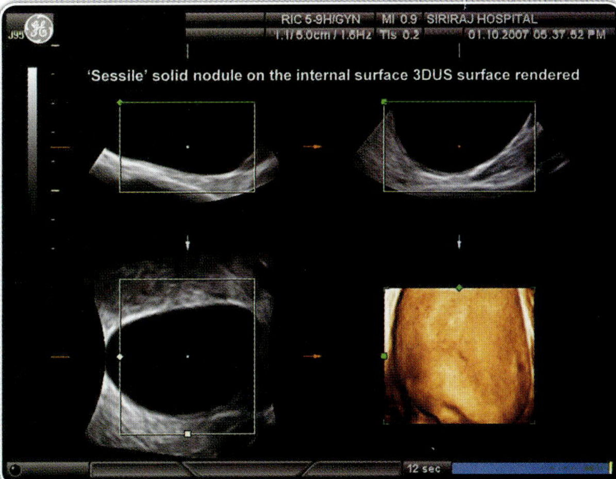

'Sessile' solid nodule on the internal surface
3DUS surface rendered

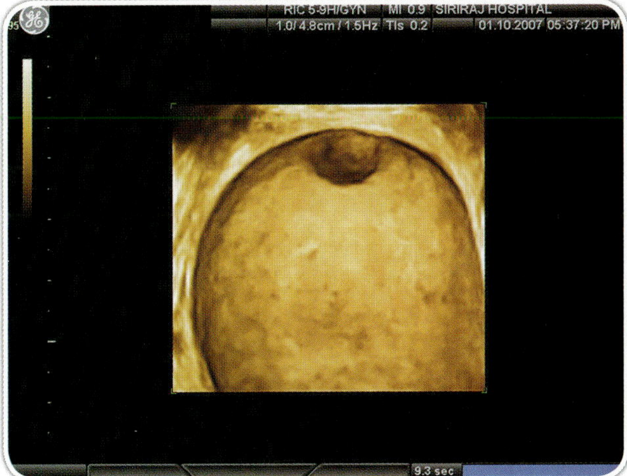

Borderline serous cystadenoma

Borderline Mucinous Cystadenocarcinoma

- Borderline tumor = uni- or multiloculated cyst with some area of cytologic atypia and epithelial stratification
  But NO STROMAL INVASION.

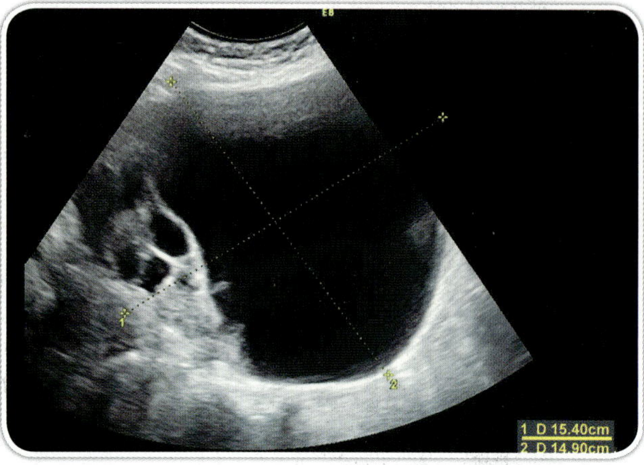

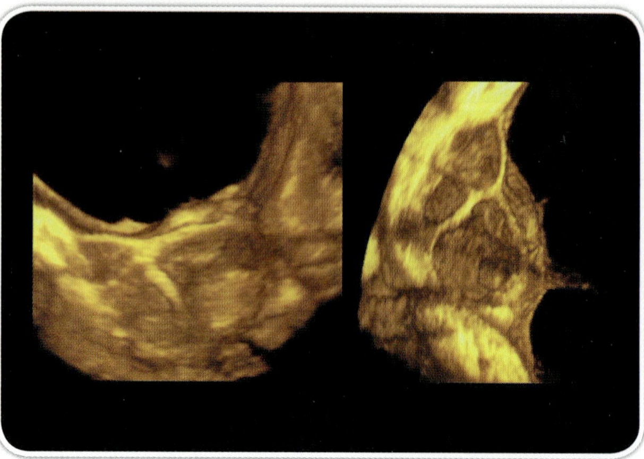

Note the thick internal septation

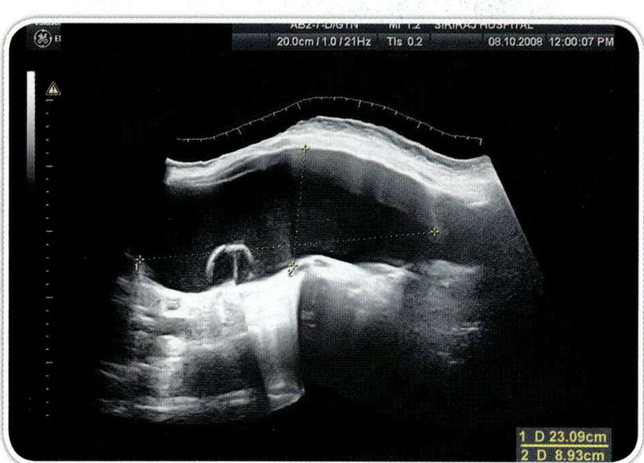

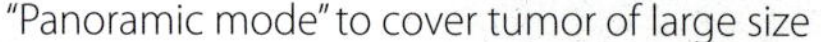

"Panoramic mode" to cover tumor of large size

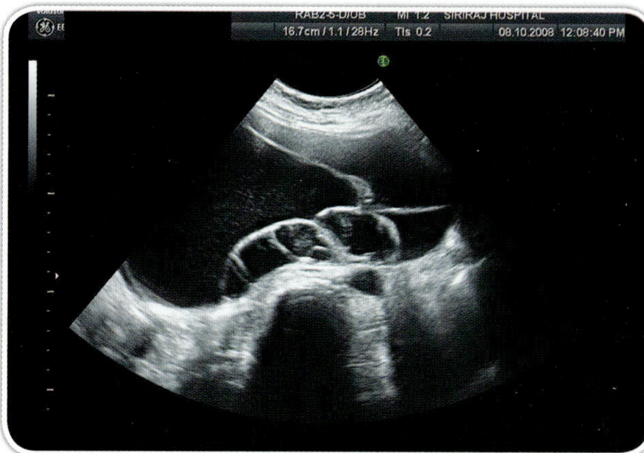

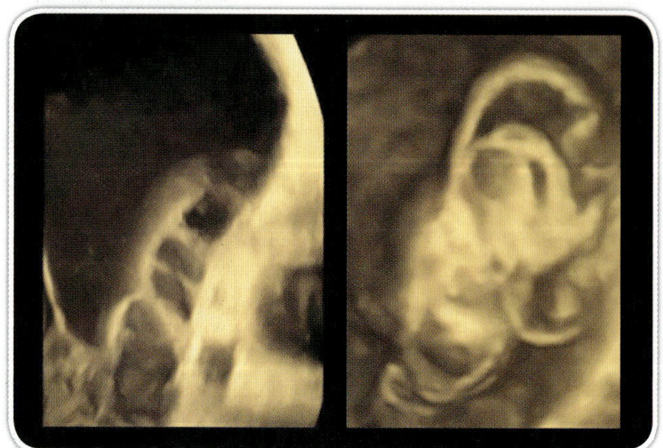

OVARIAN CANCER

Serous Cystadenocarcinoma

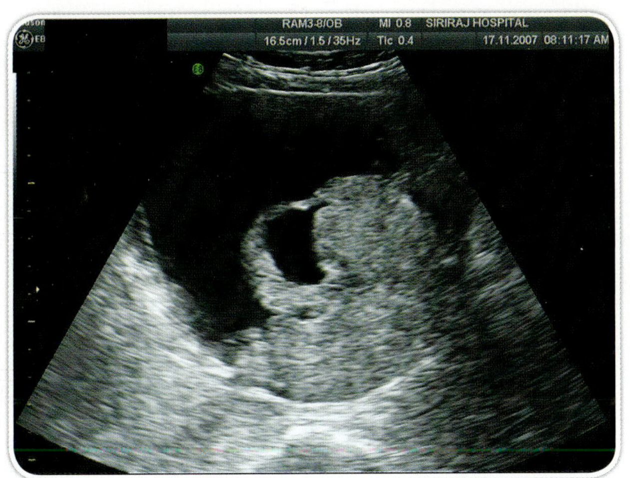

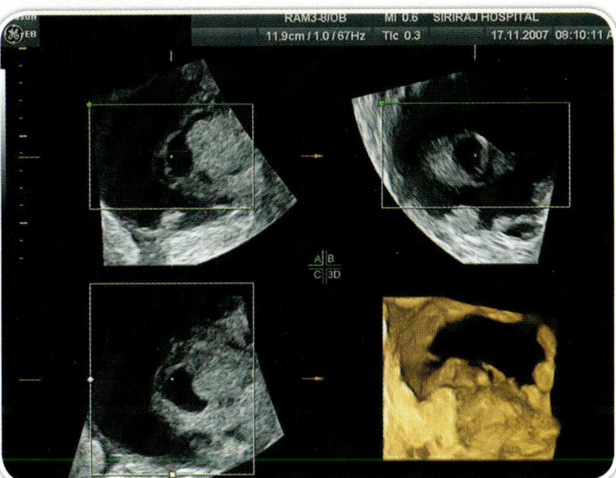

Internal papillary projections

- Most common (50-80%) ovarian cancers
- US findings
  - Papillary projections
  - Thick septations, and/or solid components
  - Ascites
  - ± Doppler indices suggestive for neovascularization.

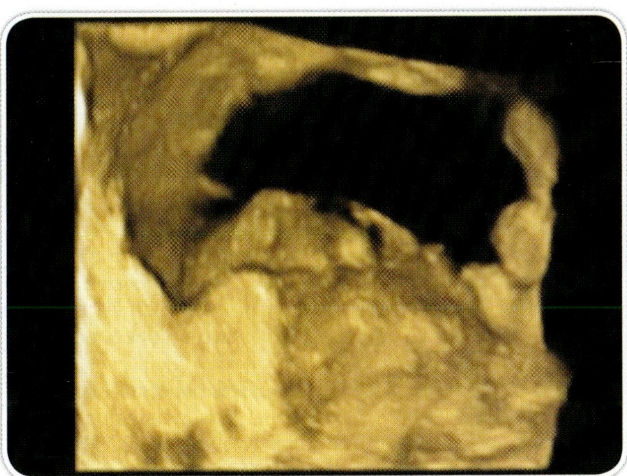

(Jeong et al. 2000)

RECURRENT OVARIAN CANCER

Large Solid Pelvic Tumor

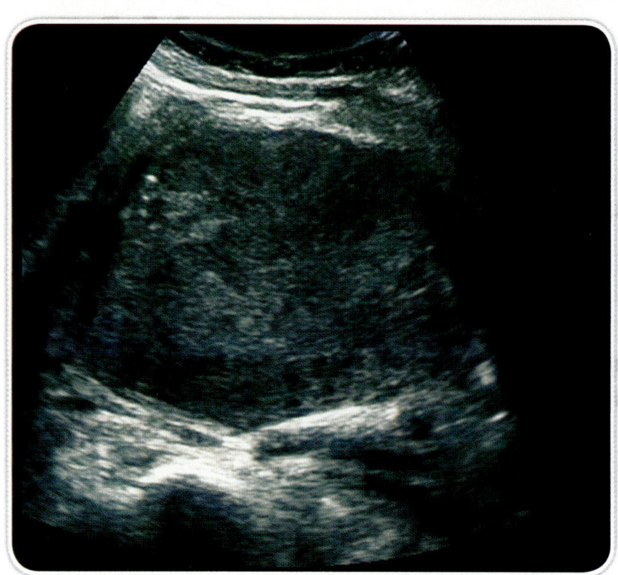

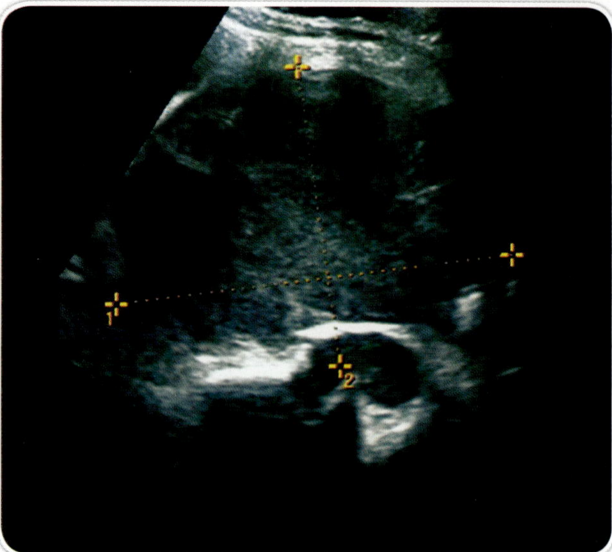

Neovascularization with Low-impedance Flow

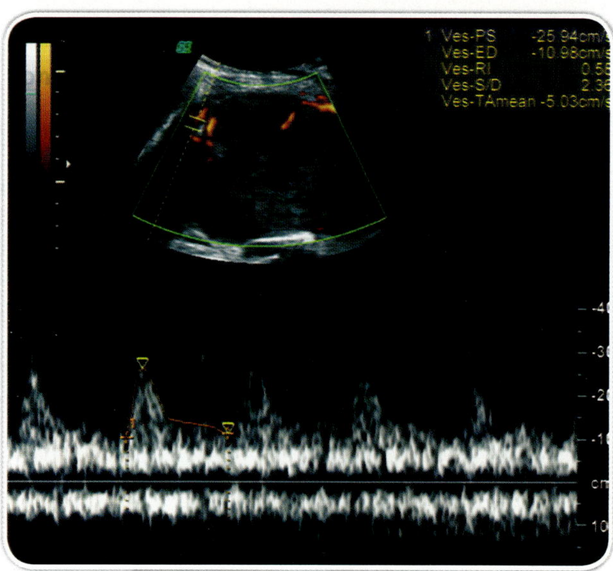

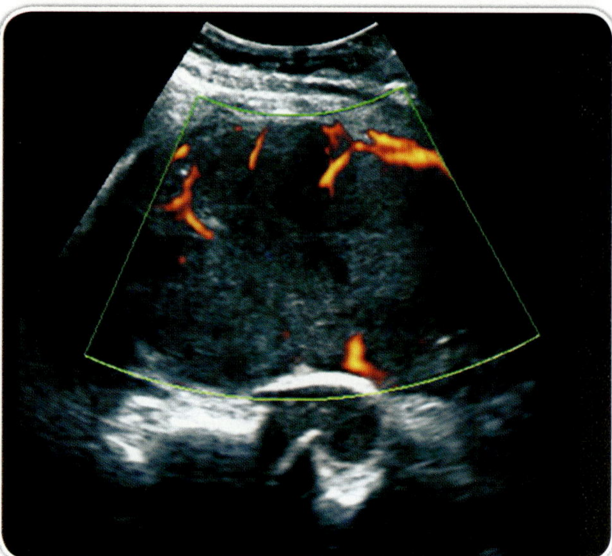

3D Sonoangiogram Shows Rich Vascular Flow

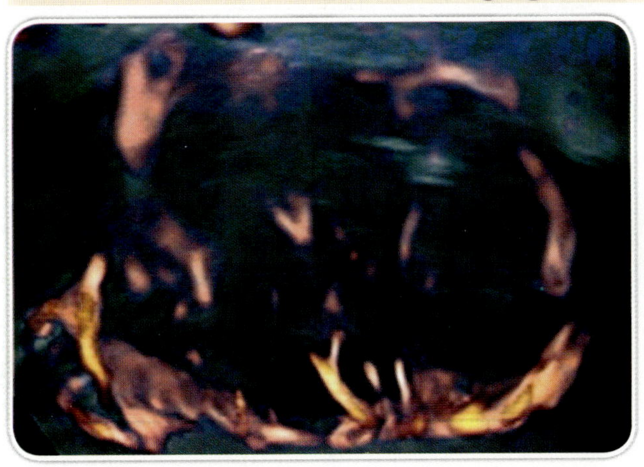

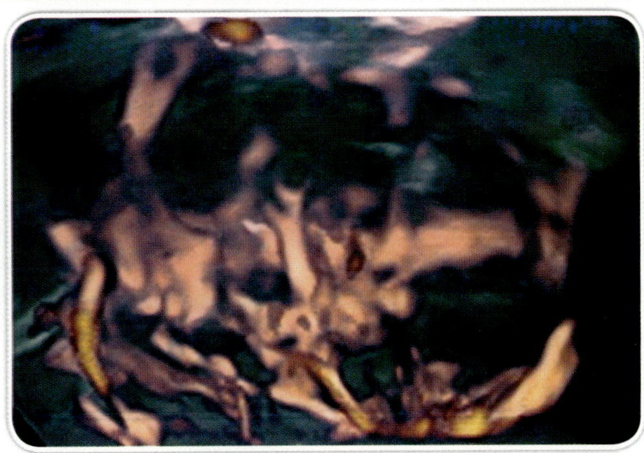

INDICES FOR 3D SONOANGIOGRAM

- Vascularization index (VI)
- Flow index (FI)
- Vascularization flow index (VFI)

Examples from placental 'sonobiopsy'

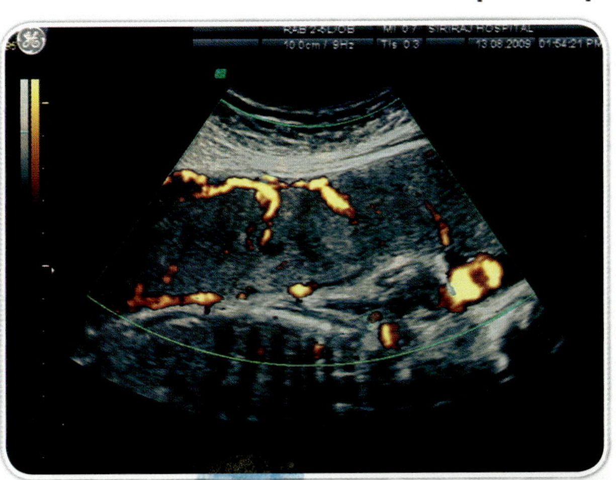

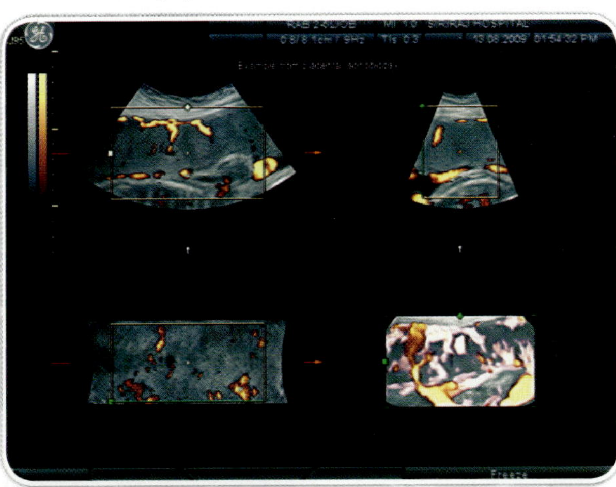

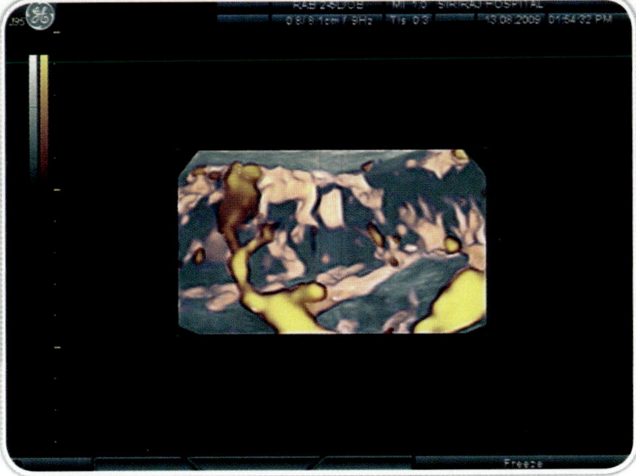

PLACENTAL SONOBIOPSY VASCULARIZATION INDEX (VI)

- Color voxel/total voxel ratio
- Color percentage within the volume of interest (placenta)
- Indicates how many vessels can be detected within the placenta (vascularity).

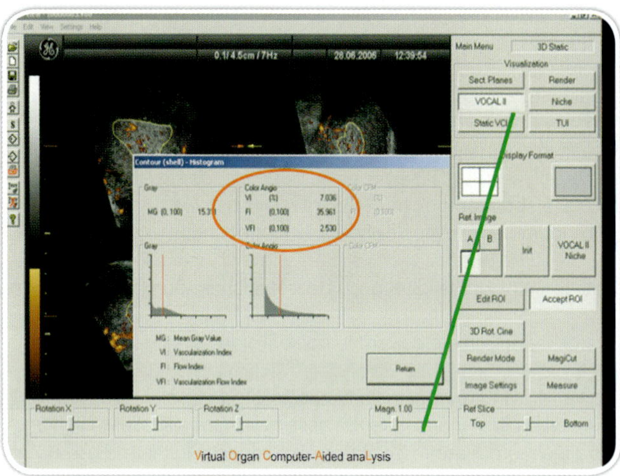

Flow Index (FI)

- Flow index (FI): Weighted color voxel (0-100) / total color voxel ratio
- Amplitude of color signal
- Indicates how many blood cells are being transported at the time of 3D sweep.

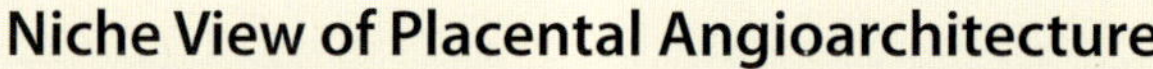

Niche View of Placental Angioarchitecture

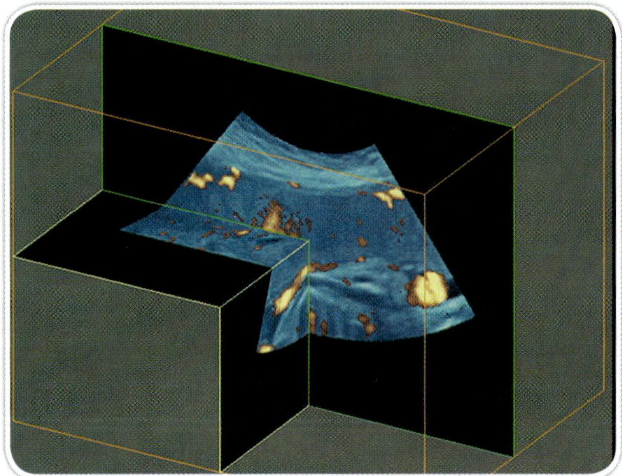

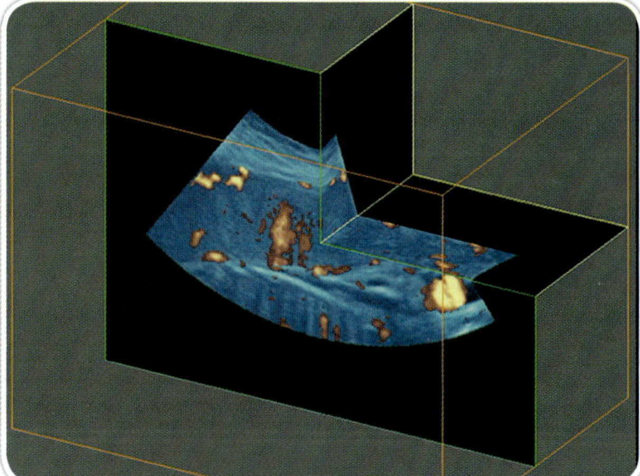

Applications of Placental Sonobiopsy

- Low vascular index has been related with
  - Fetal growth restriction
  - Pre-eclampsia.

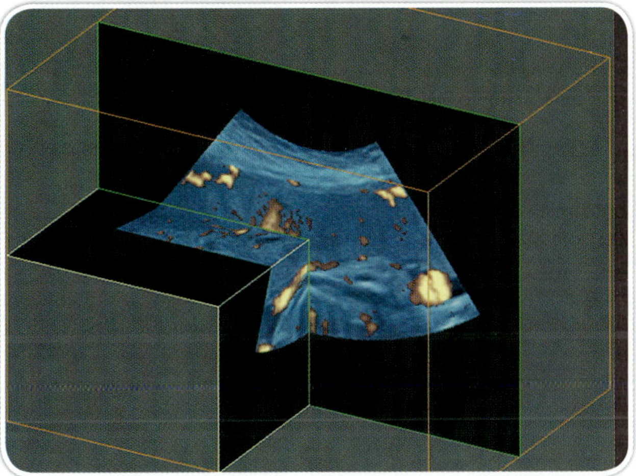

(Noguchi et al. 2014)

PLACENTAL SONOBIOPSY: VASCULARIZATION FLOW INDEX (VFI)

- The weighted color voxel / total voxel ratio
- Combining the information of vessel presence (vascularity) and amount of transported blood cells (blood flow)

Sonobiopsy

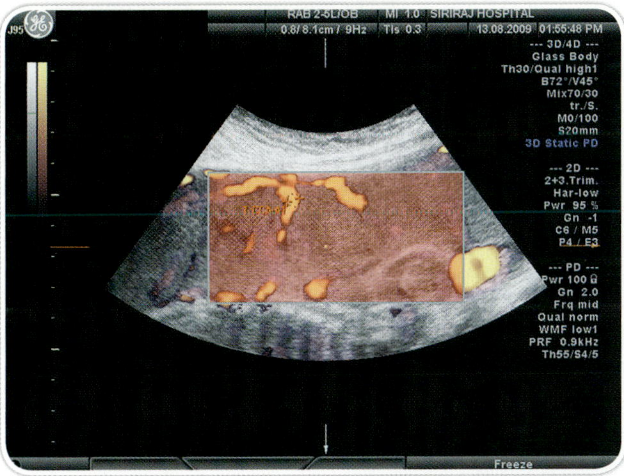

3D volume was sampled for the vascular flow indices

Demonstration of Placental Angioarchitectures

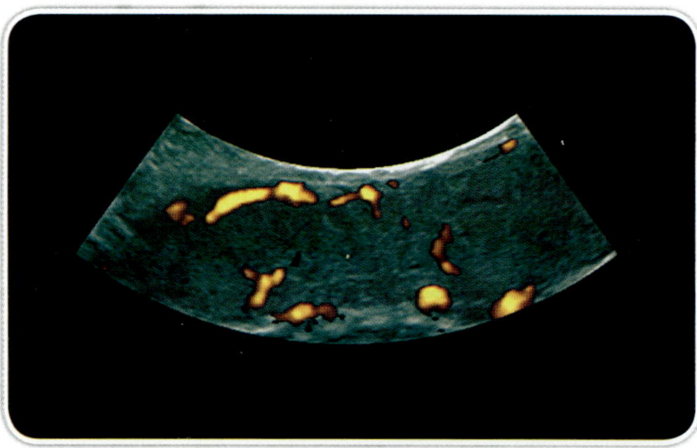

Power Doppler

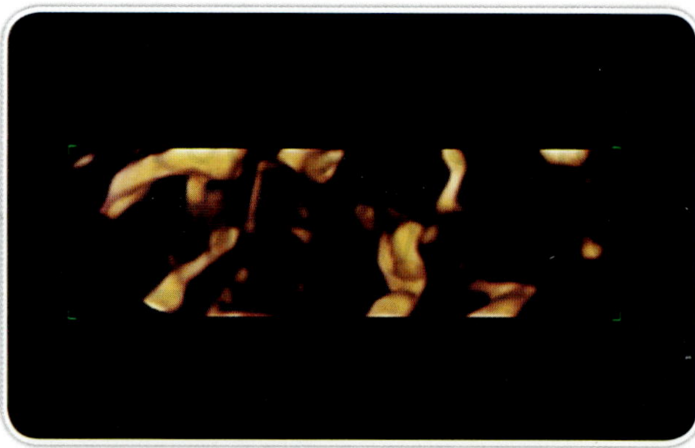

3D Sonoangiogram + Power Doppler

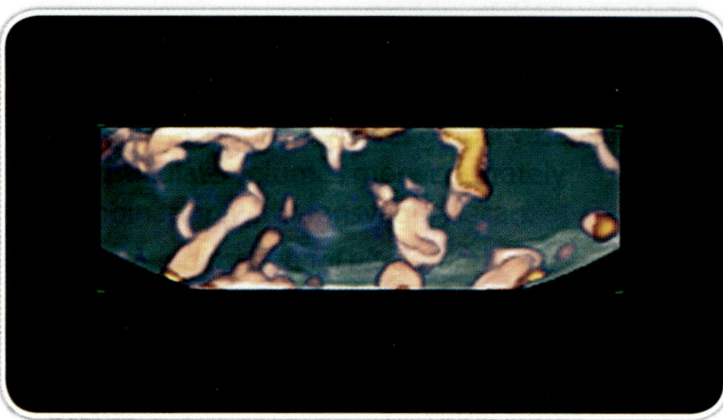

3D Glass Body + Power Doppler

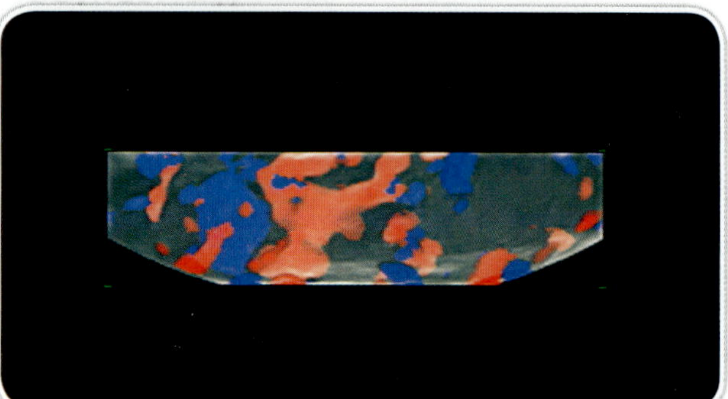

3D Glass Body + Color Doppler

ABDOMINAL PREGNANCY

- **Placental sonobiopsy may be particularly useful in follow up of Abdominal pregnancy**

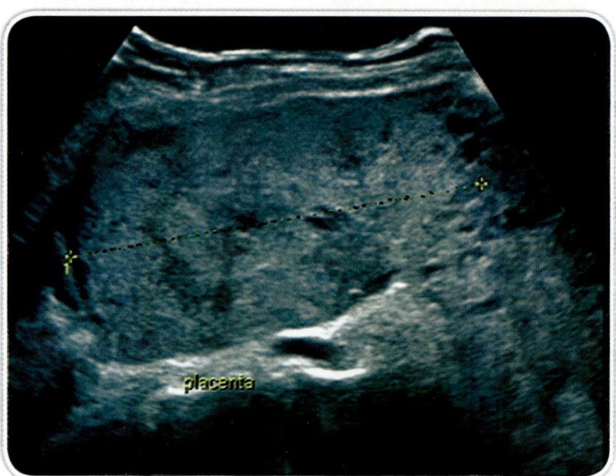

(Poole et al. 2012)

- Life-threatening condition from catastrophic bleeding and infection
- Live born births are possible
- The placenta can be either primarily removed or delayed removal after methotrexate administration.

FOLLOW UP OF PLACENTAL REGRESSION

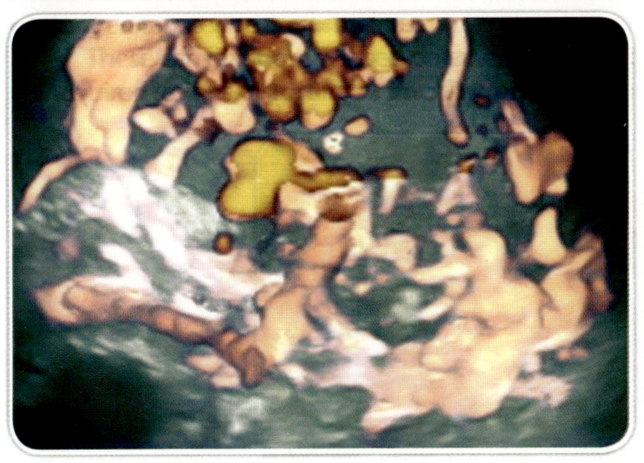

3D Glass Body + Power Doppler

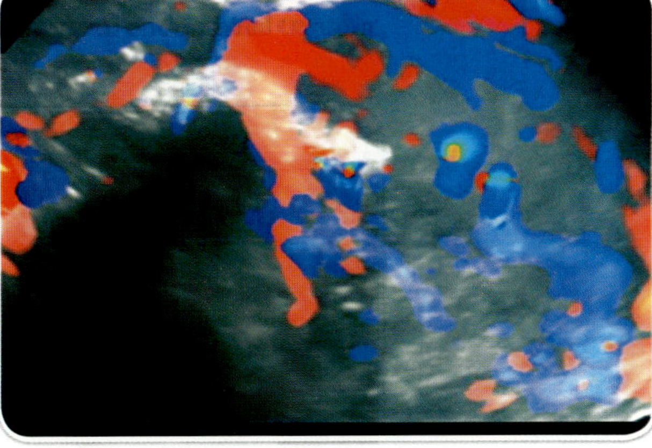

3D Glass Body + Color Doppler

Placental Volume: VOCAL

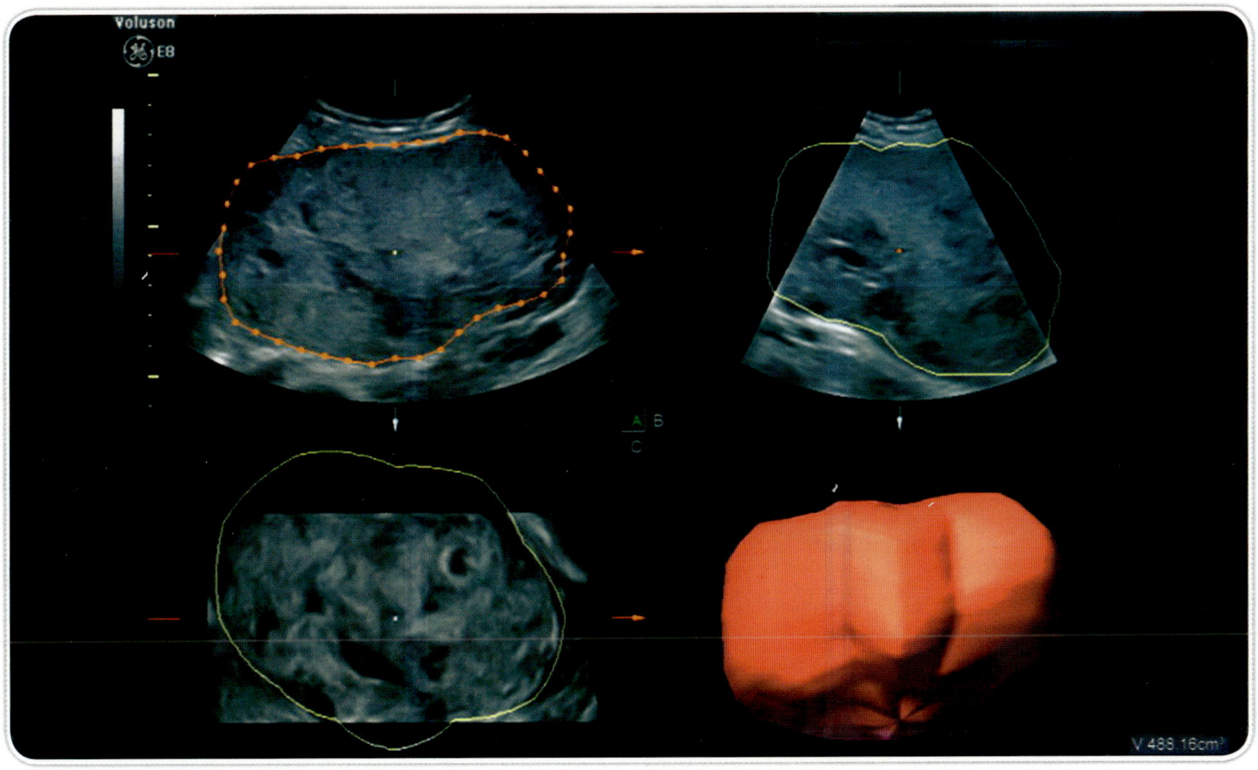

Significantly Decreased Flow After Weeks of Follow Up

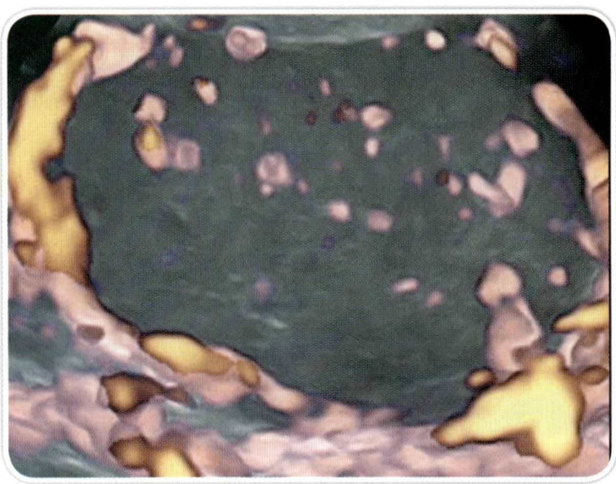

3D Glass Body + Power Doppler

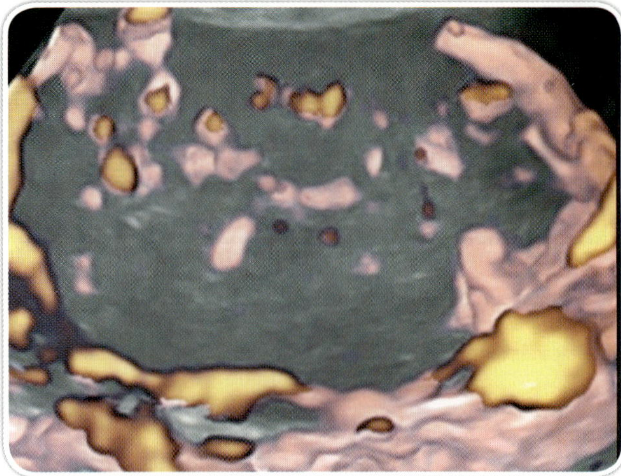

3D Glass Body + Power Doppler

ENDOMETRIAL CANCER

Prediction of Endometrial Cancer

- Postmenopausal uterine bleeding with an endometrial thickness of > 5 mm
- Endometrial volume, VI and VFI are significantly higher in malignant, compared to benign conditions (i.e. hyperplasia or polyp).

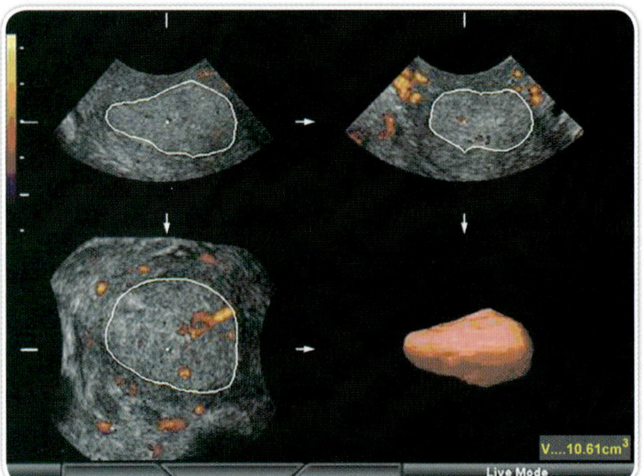

(Odeh et al. 2007)

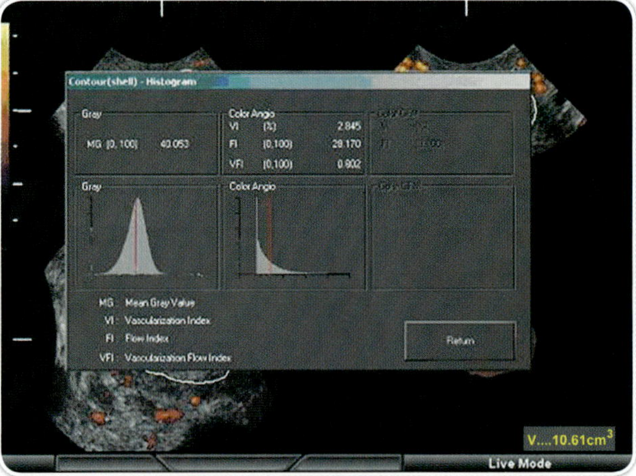

(Odeh et al. 2007)

URINARY BLADDER

Mucosal Invasion of the Urinary Bladder by Cervical Cancer

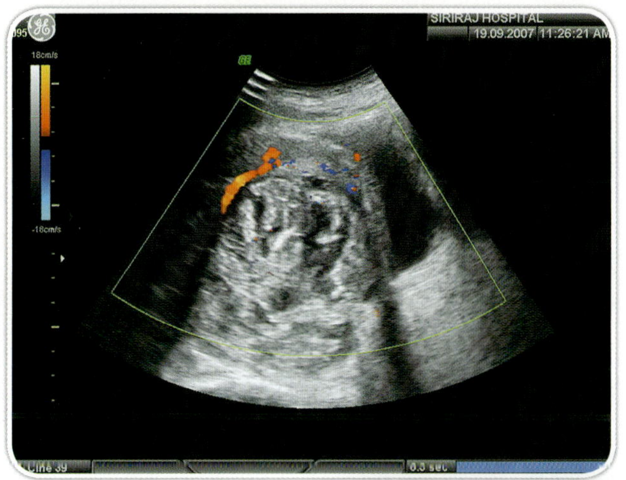

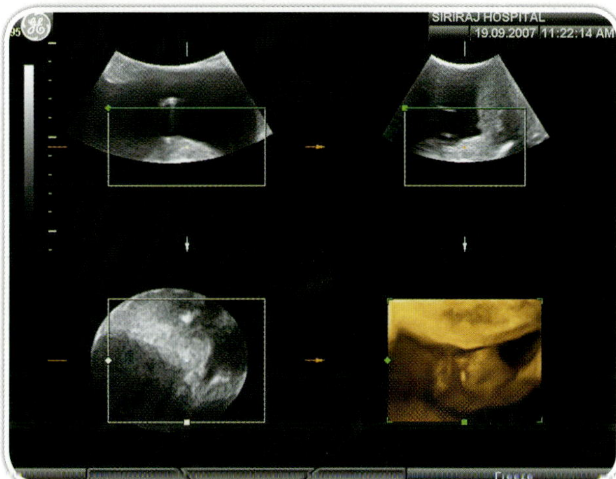

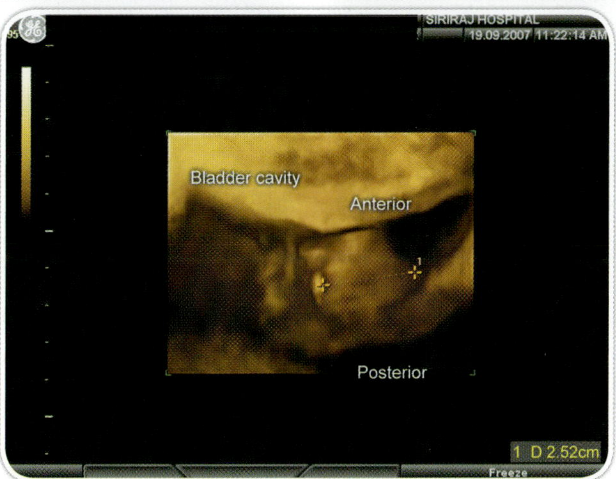

Double-J Stent that was Left for Years

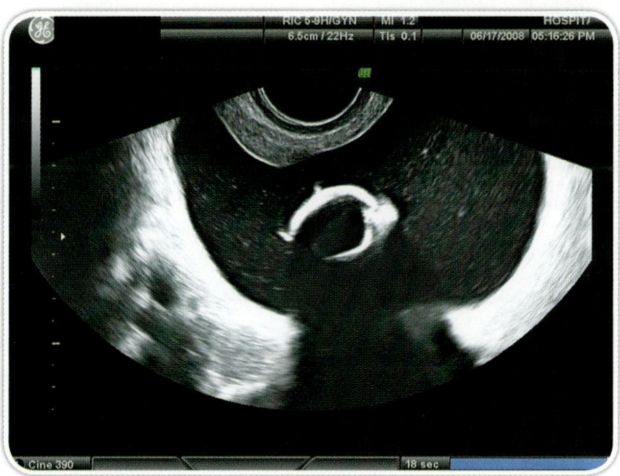

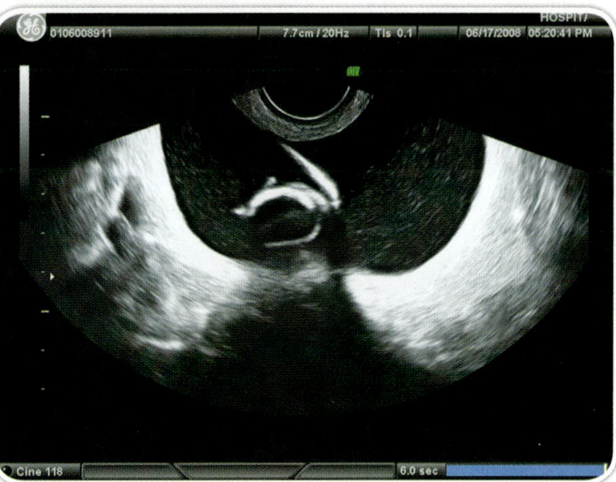

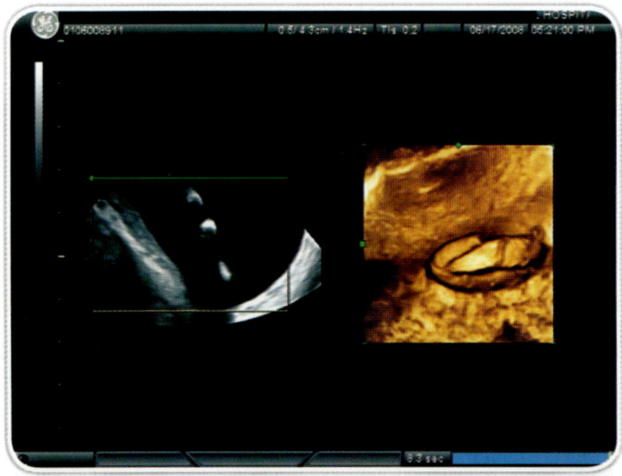

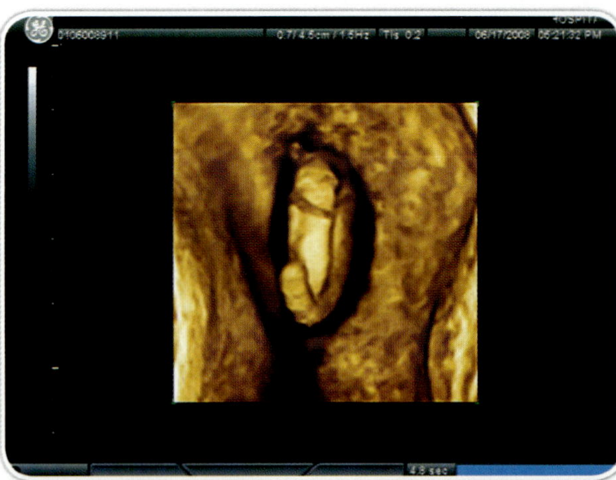

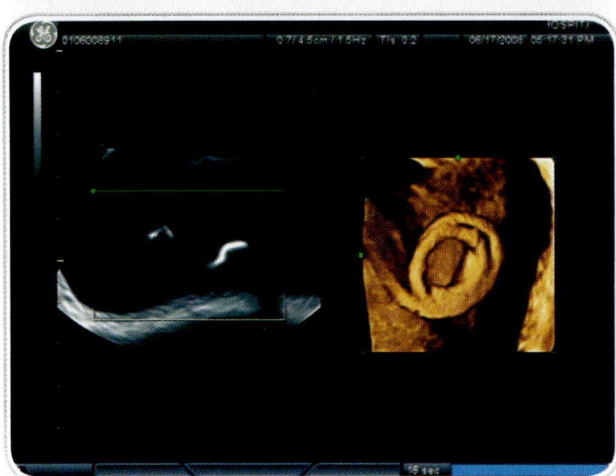

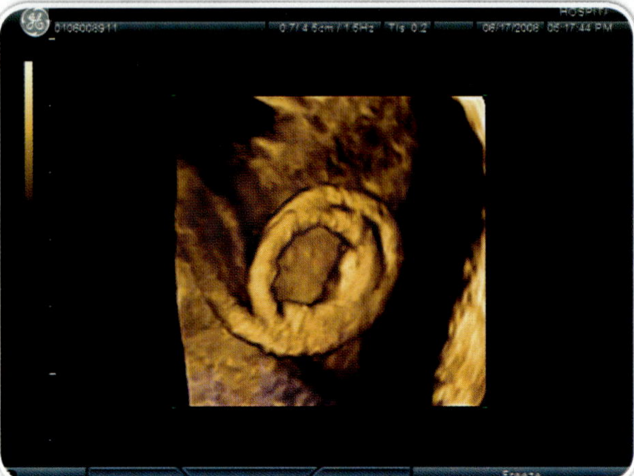

Arcuate Artery

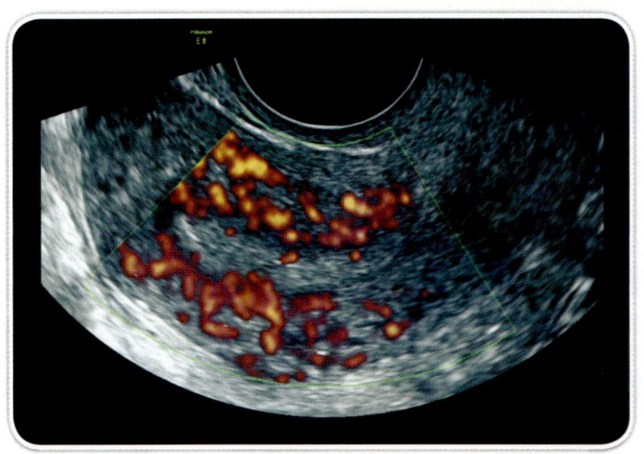

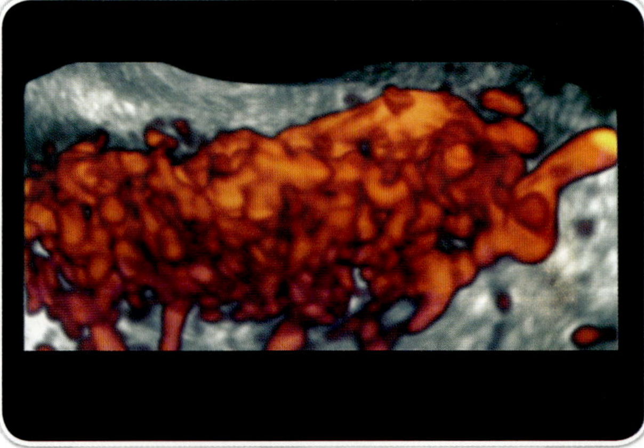

Doppler studies of arcuate artery may help predicting the involution of postpartum uterus.

(Wataganara et al. 2014)

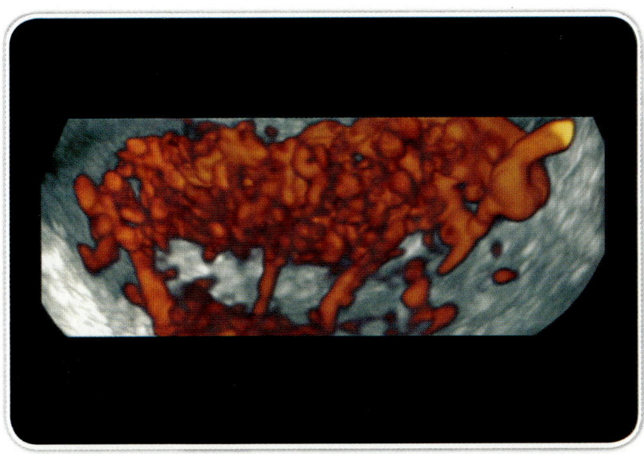

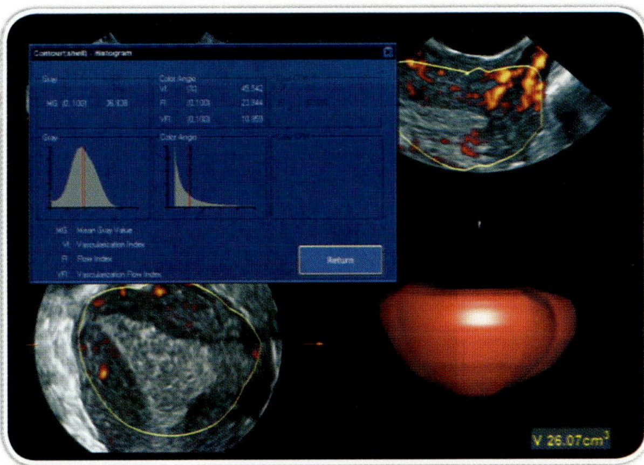

ASCITES

"Virtual Laparoscopy"

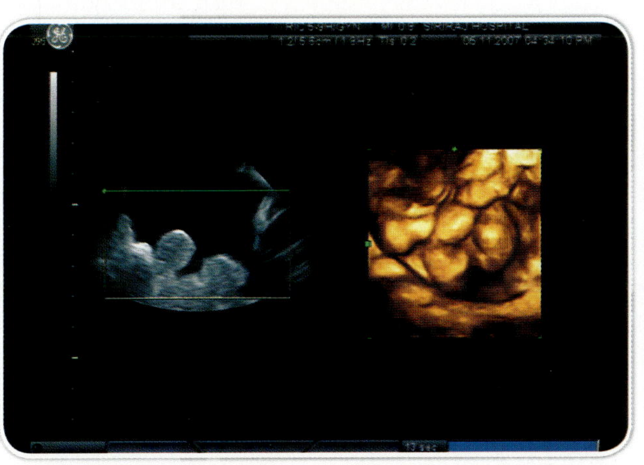

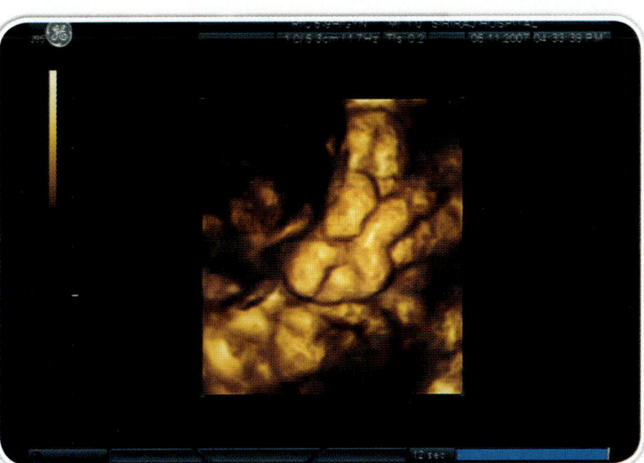

Ascites provides an opportunity to explore intra-abdominal organ

Added Benefits of 3D US in Pelvic Pathology

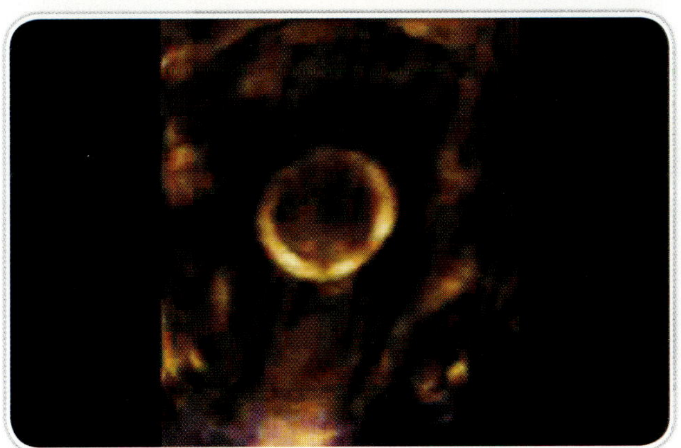

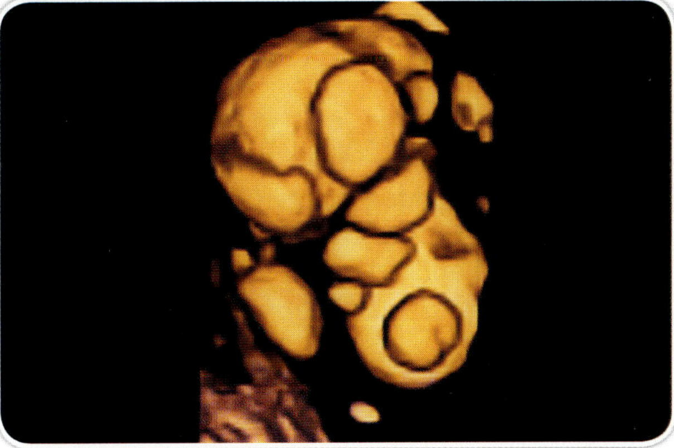

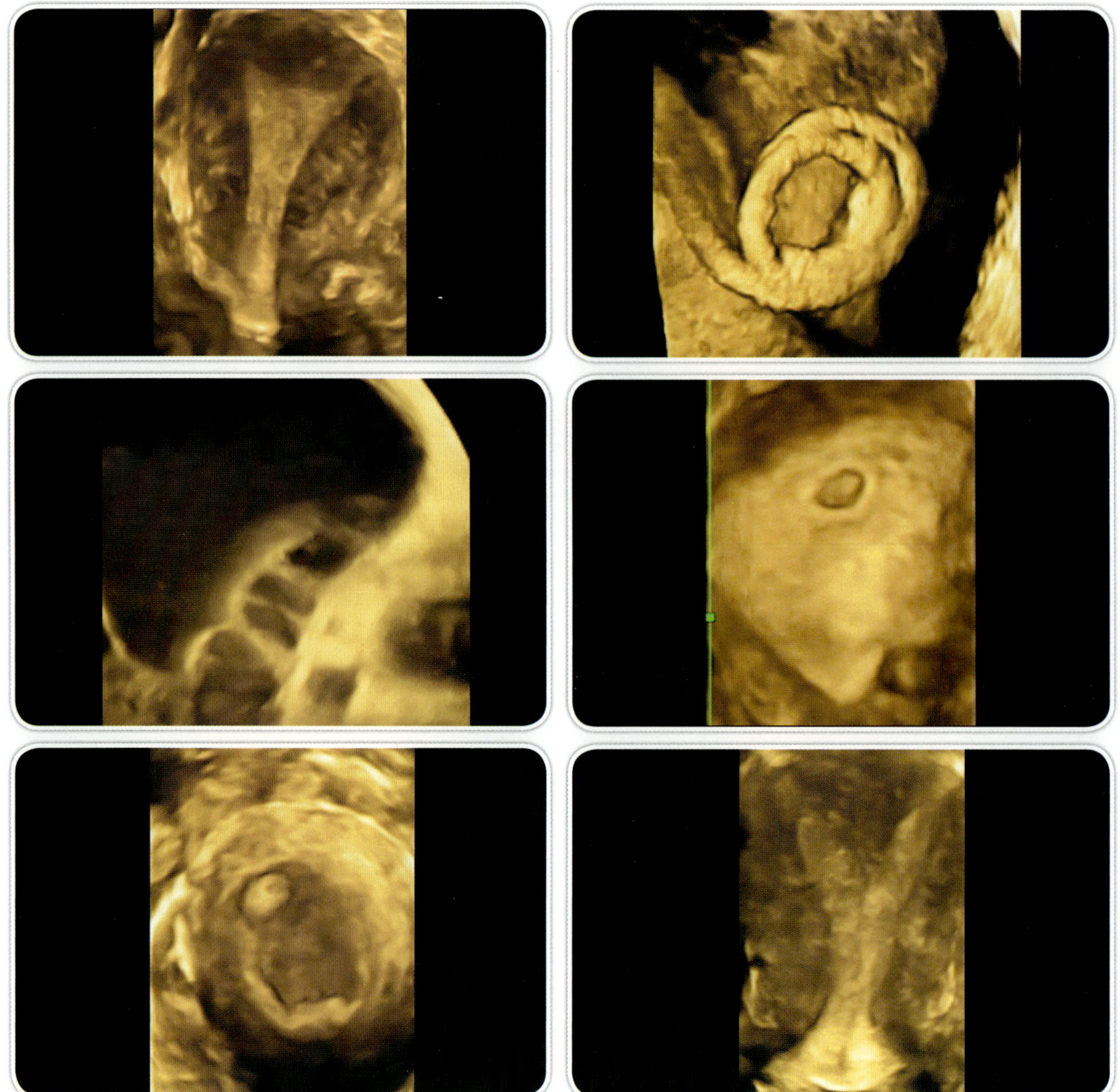

CONCLUSION

- Assessment of endometrial lesions and IUD identification are the unique qualities of 3D US evaluation
- Multimodality approaches of pelvic organs with novel 3D functions may improve an understanding, that can lead to more optimal treatment.

SUGGESTED READING

1. Jayakrishnan K, Menon V, Nambiar D. Submucous fibroids and infertility: Effect of hysteroscopic myomectomy and factors influencing outcome. Journal Hum Reprod Sci. 2013;6:35-9.
2. Jeong YY, Outwater EK, Kang HK. Imaging evaluation of ovarian masses. Radiographics : a review publication of the Radiological Society of North America Inc. 2000;20:1445-70.
3. Lujan ME, Jarrett BY, Brooks ED, et al. Updated ultrasound criteria for polycystic ovary syndrome: reliable thresholds for elevated follicle population and ovarian volume. Hum Reprod. 2013;28:1361-8.
4. Noguchi J, Tanaka H, Koyanagi A, Miyake K, Hata T. Three-dimensional power Doppler indices at 18-22 weeks' gestation for prediction of fetal growth restriction or pregnancy-induced hypertension. Archives of Gynecology and Obstetrics, 2014.
5. Odeh M, Vainerovsky I, Grinin V, Kais M, Ophir E, Bornstein J. Three-dimensional endometrial volume and 3-dimensional power Doppler analysis in predicting endometrial carcinoma and hyperplasia. Gynecologic Oncology. 2007;106:348-53.
6. Peri N, Graham D, Levine D. Imaging of intrauterine contraceptive devices. Journal of Ultrasound in Medicine: official journal of the American Institute of Ultrasound in Medicine. 2007;26:1389-401.
7. Poole A, Haas D, Magann EF. Early abdominal ectopic pregnancies: a systematic review of the literature. Gynecologic and Obstetric Investigation. 2012;74:249-60.
8. Wataganara T, Phithakwatchara N, Komoltri C, Tantisirin P, Pooliam J, Titapant V. Functional three-dimensional sonographic study of the postpartum uterus. The journal of maternal-fetal & neonatal medicine : the official journal of the European Association of Perinatal Medicine, the Federation of Asia and Oceania Perinatal Societies, the International Society of Perinatal Obstet. 2014:1-7.
9. Wataganara T, Talungjit P, Phithakwatchara N, Swasdimonkol S. Three-dimensional sonographic appearances of Chinese ring intrauterine device: a case report and literature review. Siriraj Med J. 2008;60:360-3.

Chapter

39

Ultrasonography in the Evaluation of Pediatric Gynecologic Disorders

Corazon Yabes-Almirante

ADVANTAGES OF US IN PEDIATRIC GYNECOLOGY

- US of children is completely different from that of adults
- Applicable US transducer
  - 3–5 MHz convex transabdominal probe
  - 7.5–8.5 MHz transvaginal probe
  - 8–10 MHz transabdominal linear probe
  - 4–7 MHz 3D transabdominal convex probe.

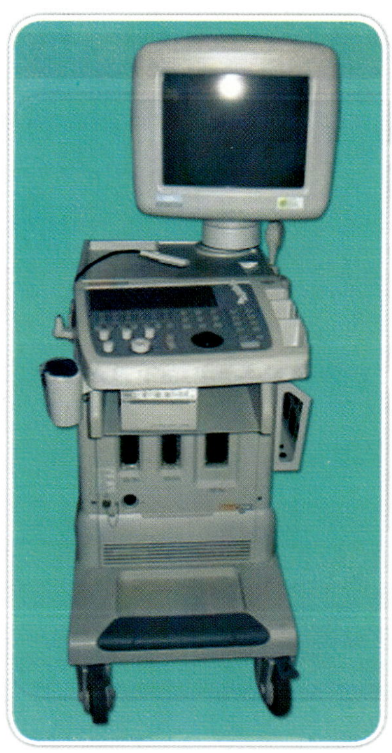

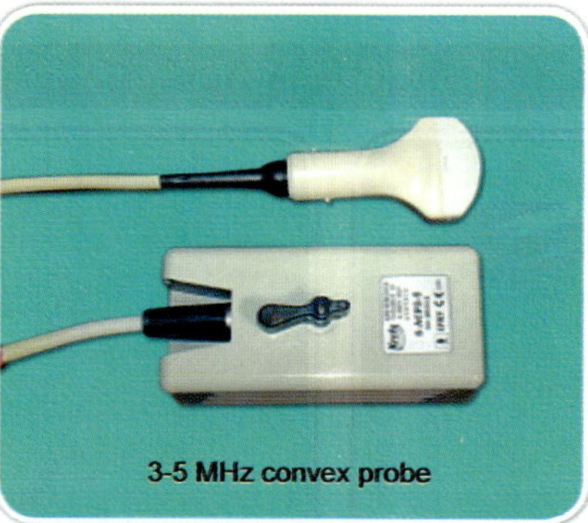

3-5 MHz convex probe

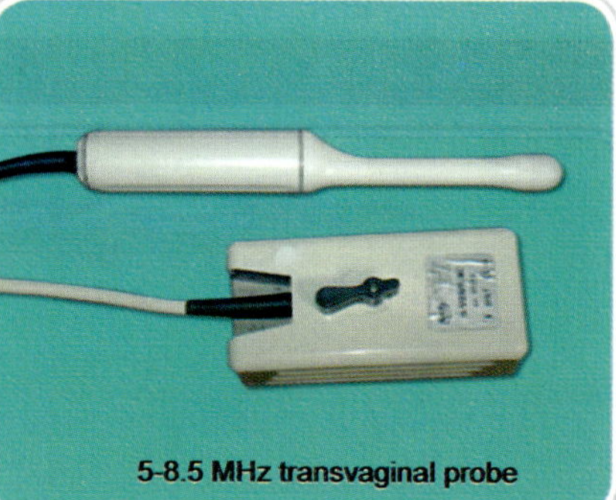

5-8.5 MHz transvaginal probe

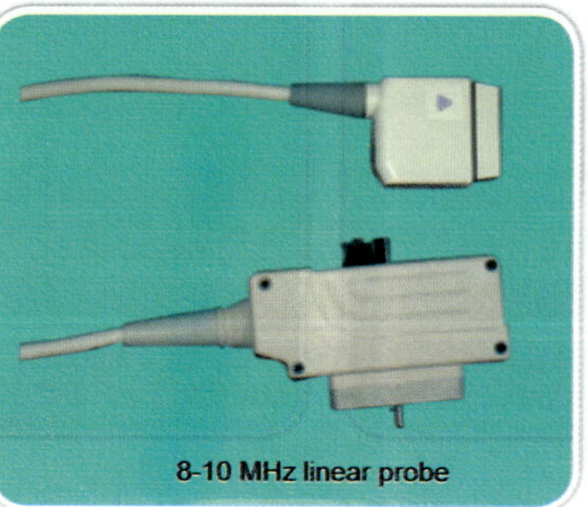

8-10 MHz linear probe

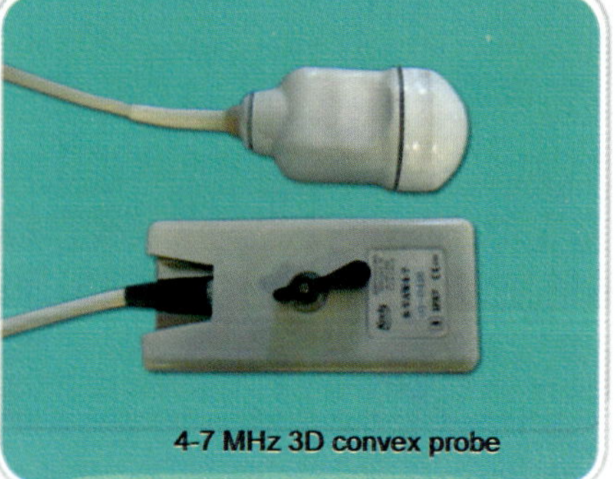

4-7 MHz 3D convex probe

Advantages of US in Pediatric Gynecology

- Fast (especially in emergencies)
- Accurate
- Painless
- Non-invasive
- Widely available
- Few limitations.
- Easy to use
- Less intimidating
- Cheaper than MRI or CT scan
- No ionizing radiation
- No need for sedation

LIMITATIONS OF PEDIATRIC GYNECOLOGIC ULTRASOUND

- Need for full bladder
- Patient movement
- Absence of identifiable reference landmarks
- Vaginal probe cannot be used.
- Abdominal ultrasound may not have best resolution
- Operator/machine dependence

Limitations Overcome By

- Full bladder
  - Replaced by water in vagina (vaginography), rectum, cloaca or utricle or urinary bladder instilled through a catheter
- Movable child
  - Divert attention, show her picture on the TV monitor, give a toy
  - Calm down 30 minutes before examination (full stomach - breast sucking)
  - Mother or guardian should be with the child
  - Cuddling or breast feeding
- Some organs are hard to visualize
  - Use Doppler to identify the blood vessel close to the organ
  - 3DUS help the organ identification (cheaper than a CT Scan or an MRI)
- Transvaginal approach
  - A vaginal probe can be placed transrectally to ensonate the uterus and adnexa
  - Transperineal approach to ensonate the lower genital tract.

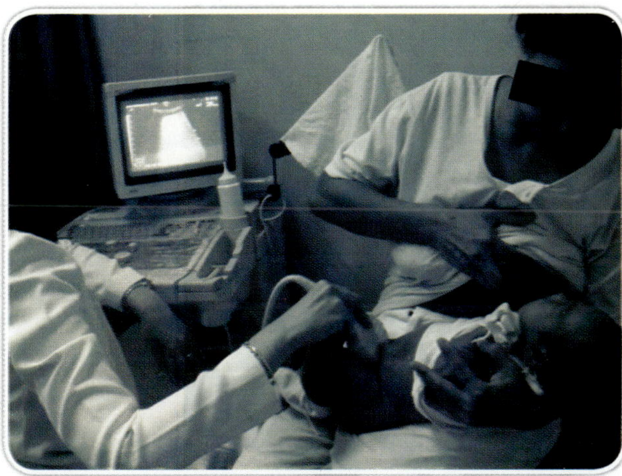

- The baby was being breastfed while US exam is ongoing
- Mother is sitting on the table facing the sonologist
- She cuddles the infant while breastfeeding
- The sonologist places the ultrasound probe on the baby's abdomen.

For complete presentation, please refer the accompanying CD-ROM...

REFERENCES

1. Azurah AG, Zainuddin AA, Jayasinghe Y. Diagnostic pitfalls in the evaluation and management of amenorrhea in adolescents. J Reprod Med. 2013;58:324-36.
2. Granada C, Omar H, Loveless MB. Update on adolescent gynecology. Adolesc Med State Art Rev. 2013;24(1):133-54.
3. Powell J. The approach to chronic pelvic pain in the adolescent. Obstet Gynecol Clin North Am. 2014; 41(3):343-55.
4. Siwe K, Wijma B. The first pelvic examination for an adolescent: is this right passage used to its full potential? Curr Opin Obstet Gynecol. 2013;25(5):357-63.
5. Wang S, Lang JH, Zhu L, Zhou HM. Duplicated uterus and hemivaginal or hemicervical atresia with ipsilateral renal agenesis: an institutional clinical series of 52 cases. Eur J Obstet Gynecol Reprod Biol. 2013;170(2):507-11.

Chapter 40

Ultrasound and the Pelvic Floor

Ashok Khurana

Imaging of the Pelvic Floor

Overview

- Clinical Perspective
- Imaging Techniques
- Pattern recognition and quantitative analysis.

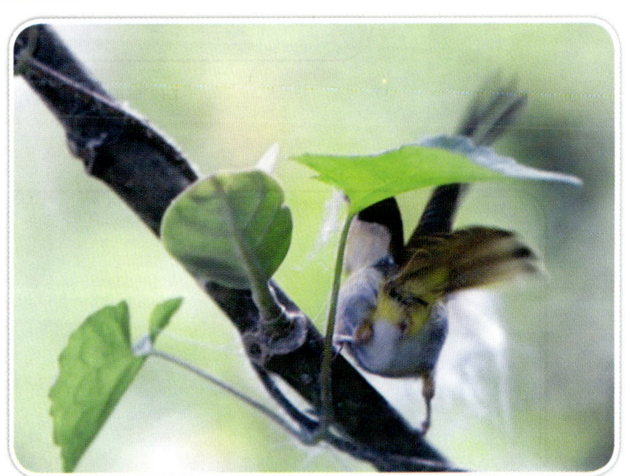

Pelvic Floor Dysfunction

Perspective

- Wide clinical spectrum
- High morbidity and quality of life issues
- Established and evolving treatment options

Clinical Spectrum

- Urinary incontinence
- Recurrent urinary tract infections
- Persistent dysuria/urgency/frequency
- Fecal incontinence and flatus incontinence
- Pelvic organ prolapse (POP)
- Sexual/Orgasmic dysfunction.

Stress Urinary Incontinence (SUI)

Extent of the Problem

- 10% of women 52-65 years
  35% of women >65 years
- Anxiety, depression
  Low self esteem
  Social isolation
  Compromised quality of life.

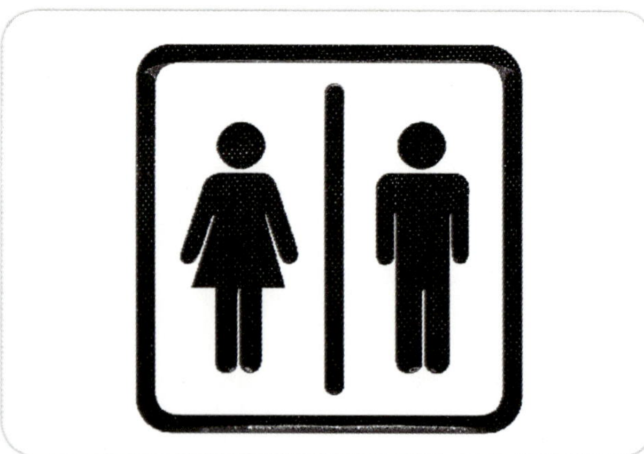

Imaging in Urogynecology

Why Ultrasound (US)?

- Not just because it can be done !
- Because it is now proven to be reliable and possibly superior to other methods (such as clinical and magnetic resonance imaging (MRI)
- Because it answers serious questions.

What Questions?

One Example

- Urethral hypermobility is better handled with a transobturator midurethral sling
- Intrinsic sphincter deficiency is better handled with injectable bioagents.

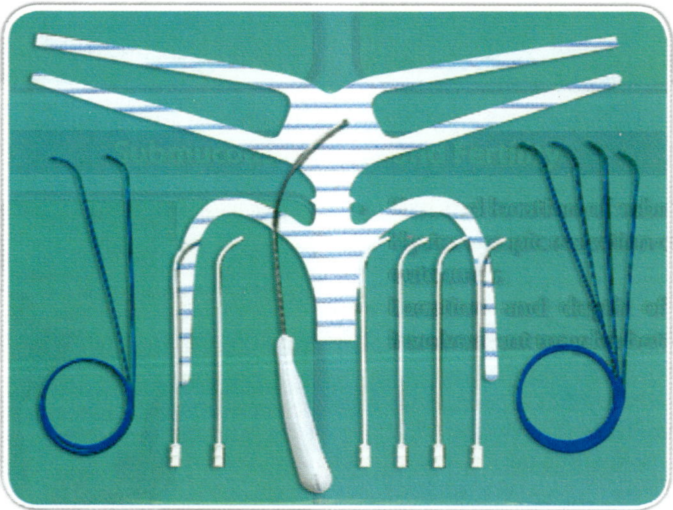

For complete presentation, please refer the accompanying CD-ROM...

SUGGESTED READING

1. Abdool Z, Shek KL, Dietz HP. The effect of levator avulsion on hiatal dimension and function. Am J Obstet Gynecol. 2009;201(1):89.e1-e5.
2. Bader W, Degenhardt F, Kauffels W, Nehls K, Schneider J. Ultrasound morphologic parameters of female stress incontinence. Ultraschall Med. 1995;16(4):180-5.
3. Deindl FM, Vodusek DB, Hesse U, Schüssler B. Activity patterns of pubococcygeal muscles in nulliparous continent women. Br J Urol. 1993;72(1):46-51.
4. DeLancy JOL. Stress urinary incontinence: Where are we now, where should we go? Am J Obstet Gynecol. 1996;175:311-9.
5. DeLancy JOL. Structural support of the urethra as it relates to stress urinary incontinence: the hammock hypothesis. Am J Obstet Gynecol. 1994;170:1713-20.
6. Dietz HP, Clarke B. The urethral pressure profile and ultrasound imaging of the lower urinary tract. Int Urogynecol J Pelvic Floor Dysfunct. 2001;12(1):38-41.
7. Dietz HP, Shek C, Clarke B. Biometry of the pubovisceral muscle and levator hiatus by three-dimensional pelvic floor ultrasound. Ultrasound Obstet Gynecol. 2005;25(6):580-5.
8. Dietz HP, Wilson PD, Clarke B. The use of perineal ultrasound to quantify levator activity and teach pelvic floor muscle exercises. Int Urogynecol J Pelvic Floor Dysfunct. 2001;12(3):166-8.
9. Dietz HP, Wilson PD. The influence of bladder volume on the position and mobility of the urethrovesical junction. Int Urogynecol J Pelvic Floor Dysfunct. 1999;10(1):3-6.
10. Dietz HP, Wilson PD. The 'iris effect': how two-dimensional and three-dimensional ultrasound can help us understand anti-incontinence procedures. Ultrasound Obstet Gynecol. 2004;23(3):267-71.
11. Gordon D, Pearce M, Norton P, Stanton SL. Comparison of ultrasound and lateral chain urethrocystography in the determination of bladder neck descent. Am J Obstet Gynecol. 1989;160(1):182-5.
12. Gosling JA. The structure of the bladder neck, urethra and pelvic floor in relation to female urinary continence. Int Urogynecol J. 1996;7(4):177-8.
13. Howard D, Delancey JO, Tunn R, Ashton-Miller JA. Racial differences in the structure and function of the stress urinary continence mechanism. Obstet Gynecol. 2000;95(5):713-7.
14. Jung SA, Pretorius DH, Padda BS, Weinstein MM, Nager CW, den Boer DJ, et al. Vaginal high-pressure zone assessed by dynamic 3-dimensional ultrasound images of the pelvic floor. Am J Obstet Gynecol. 2007;197(1):52.e1-e7.
15. Khullar V, Cardozo LD, Salvatore S, Hill S. Ultrasound: a noninvasive screening test for detrusor instability. Br J Obstet Gynaecol. 1996;103(9):904-8.
16. Khullar V, Salvatore S, Cardozo L, Bourne TH, Abbott D, Kelleher C. A novel technique for measuring bladder wall thickness in women using transvaginal ultrasound. Ultrasound Obstet Gynecol. 1994;4(3):220-3.
17. King JK, Freeman RM. Is antenatal bladder neck mobility a risk factor for postpartum stress incontinence? Br J Obstet Gynaecol. 1998;105(12):1300-7.
18. Koelbl H, Bernaschek G, Wolf G. A comparative study of perineal ultrasound scanning and urethrocystography in patients with genuine stress incontinence. Arch Obstet Gynecol. 1988;244:39-45.
19. Kohorn EI, Scioscia AL, Jeanty P, Hobbins JC. Ultrasound cystourethrography by perineal scanning for the assessment of female stress urinary incontinence. Obstet Gynecol. 1986;68(2):269-72.
20. Kruger JA, Heap SW, Murphy BA, Dietz HP. Pelvic floor function in nulliparous women using three-dimensional ultrasound and magnetic resonance imaging. Obstet Gynecol. 2008;111(3):631-8.
21. Martan A, Masata M, Halaska M, Voigt R. Ultrasound imaging of the urethral sphincter. Ceska Gynekol. 1997;62(6):330-2.
22. Martan A, Massata J, Halaska M, Otcenasek M. Svabik K. Ultrasound imaging of paravaginal defects in women with stress incontinence before and after paravaginal defect repair. Ultrasound Obstet Gynecol. 2002;19:496-500.
23. Miller JM, Perucchini D, Carchidi LT, DeLancey JO, Ashton-Miller J. Pelvic floor muscle contraction during a cough and decreased vesical neck mobility. Obstet Gynecol. 2001;97(2):255-60.
24. Monga A. Fascia—defects and repair. Curr Opin Obstet Gynecol. 1996;8(5):366-71.
25. Mouritsen L, Strandberg C. Vaginal ultrasonography versus colpo-cysto-urethrography in the evaluation of female urinary incontinence. Acta Obstet Gynecol Scand. 1994;73(4):338-42.
26. Pantazis K, Freeman RM. Investigation and treatment of urinary incontinence. Current Obstetrics and Gynecology. 2006;16(6):344-52.
27. Peschers U, Schaer G, Anthuber C, Delancey JO, Schuessler B. Changes in vesical neck mobility following vaginal delivery. Obstet Gynecol. 1996;88(6):1001-6.
28. Peschers UM, Vodusek DB, Fanger G, Schaer GN, DeLancey JO, Schuessler B. Pelvic muscle activity in nulliparous volunteers. Neurourol Urodyn. 2001;20(3):269-75.
29. Peschers UM, Vodušek DB, Fanger G, Schaer GN, DeLancey JO, Schuessler B. Pelvic muscle activity in nulliparous volunteers. Neurourol Urodyn. 2001;20(3):269-75.
30. Petri E, Koelbl H, Schaer G. What is the place of ultrasound in urogynecology? A written panel. Int Urogynecol J Pelvic Floor Dysfunct. 1999;10(4):262-73.

31. Poon CI, Zimmern PE. Role of three-dimensional ultrasound in assessment of women undergoing urethral bulking agent therapy. Curr Opin Obstet Gynecol. 2004;16(5):411-7.
32. Reddy AP, DeLancey JO, Zwica OM, Ashton-Miller JA. On-screen vector-based ultrasound assessment of vesical neck movement. Am J Obstet Gynecol. 2001;185(1):65-70.
33. Sapsford RR, Hodges PW, Richardson CA, Cooper DH, Markwell SJ, Jull GA. Co-activation of the abdominal and pelvic floor muscles during voluntary exercises. Neurourol Urodyn. 2001;20(1):31-42.
34. Schaer G, Koelbl H, Voigt R, Merz E, Anthuber C, Niemeyer R, et al. Recommendations of the German Association of Urogynecology on functional sonography of the lower female urinary tract. Int Urogynecol J Pelvic Floor Dysfunct. 1996;7(2):105-8.
35. Schaer GN, Koechli OR, Schuessler B, Haller U. Improvement of perineal sonographic bladder neck imaging with ultrasound contrast medium. Obstet Gynecol. 1995;86(6):950-4.
36. Schaer GN, Koechli OR, Schuessler B, Haller U. Perineal ultrasound: determination of reliable examination procedures. Ultrasound Obstet Gynecol. 1996;7(5):347-52.
37. Schaer GN, Koechli OR, Schuessler B, Haller U. Perineal ultrasound for evaluating the bladder neck in urinary stress incontinence. Obstet Gynecol. 1995;85(2):220-4.
38. Schaer GN, Perucchini D, Munz E, Peschers U, Koechli OR, Delancey JO. Sonographic evaluation of the bladder neck in continent and stress-incontinent women. Obstet Gynecol. 1999;93(3):412-6.
39. Tunn R, Perucchini D. Morphologic assessment for diagnosing urogynaecologic disorders. Zentralbl Gynakol. 2001;123(12):672-9.
40. Tunn R, Petri E. Introital and transvaginal ultrasound as the main tool in the assessment of urogenital and pelvic floor dysfunction: an imaging panel and practical approach. Ultrasound Obstet Gynecol. 2003;22(2):205-13.
41. Umek WH, Laml T, Stutterecker D, Obermair A, Leodolter S, Hanzal E. The urethra during pelvic floor contraction: observations on three-dimensional ultrasound. Obstet Gynecol. 2002;100(4):796-800.
42. Unger CA, Weinstein MM, Pretorius DH. Pelvic Floor Imaging. Ultrasound Clinics. 2010;5(2):313-30.
43. Viereck V, Bader W, Skala C, Gauruder-Burmester A, Emons G, Hilgers R, et al. Determination of bladder neck position by intraoperative introital ultrasound in colposuspension: outcome at 6-month follow-up. Ultrasound Obstet Gynecol. 2004;24(2):186-91.
44. Weber AM, Abrams P, Brubaker L, Cundiff G, Davis G, Dmochowski RR, et al. The standardization of terminology for researchers in female pelvic floor disorders. Int Urogynecol J Pelvic Floor Dysfunct. 2001;12(3):178-86.
45. Weinstein MM, Jung SA, Pretorius DH, Nager CW, den Boer DJ, Mittal RK. The reliability of puborectalis muscle measurements with 3-dimensional ultrasound imaging. Am J Obstet Gynecol. 2007;197(1):68.e1-e6.
46. White RD, McQuown D, McCarthy TA, Ostergard DR. Real-time ultrasonography in the evaluation of urinary stress incontinence. Am J Obstet Gynecol. 1980;138(2):235-7.
47. Wijma J, Weis Potters AE, de Wolf BT, Tinga DJ, Aarnoudse JG. Anatomical and functional changes in the lower urinary tract during pregnancy. BJOG. 2001;108(7):726-32.
48. Yang JM, Huang WC. Discrimination of bladder disorders in female lower urinary tract symptoms on ultrasonographic cystourethrography. J Ultrasound Med. 2002;21(11):1249-55.
49. Yang JM, Yang SH, Huang WC. Biometry of the pubovisceral muscle and levator hiatus in nulliparous Chinese women. Ultrasound Obstet Gynecol. 2006;28(5):710-6.
50. Yang JM, Yang SH, Huang WC. Dynamic morphological changes in the anterior vaginal wall before and after laparoscopic Burch colposuspension in primary urodynamic stress incontinence. Ultrasound Obstet Gynecol. 2005;25(3):289-95.

Chapter 41

Ultrasound in Infertility

Sonal Panchal, Jaideep Malhotra, Narendra Malhotra

WHY ULTRASOUND IS USED TO ASSESS INFERTILE COUPLE

- Mainstay of evaluating male and female infertility
- Anatomical diagnosis
- Physiological information by color
- 3D US gives multiplanar information
- Power Doppler gives vascular information
- Intraoperative ultrasound
- Interventional procedures
- As we are discussing the role of ultrasound for assessment of infertility, we shall not include the intraoperative and interventional ultrasound in this presentation
- The discussion otherwise will be divided into two parts:
  - Evaluation of male
  - Evaluation of female.

EVALUATION OF INFERTILITY IN MALES

- Scrotal ultrasound for testis and varicocele
- Penile ultrasound for ejaculatory pathologies
- Transrectal ultrasound for prostate, vas deferens, seminal vesicles and ejaculatory ducts.

Ultrasound of Scrotum

When ??
- Oligoasthenospermia
- Teratospermia

What to look for??
- Varicocele
- Acute/chronic orchiditis
- Testicular tumors
- Testicular torsion
- Epididymal pathologies

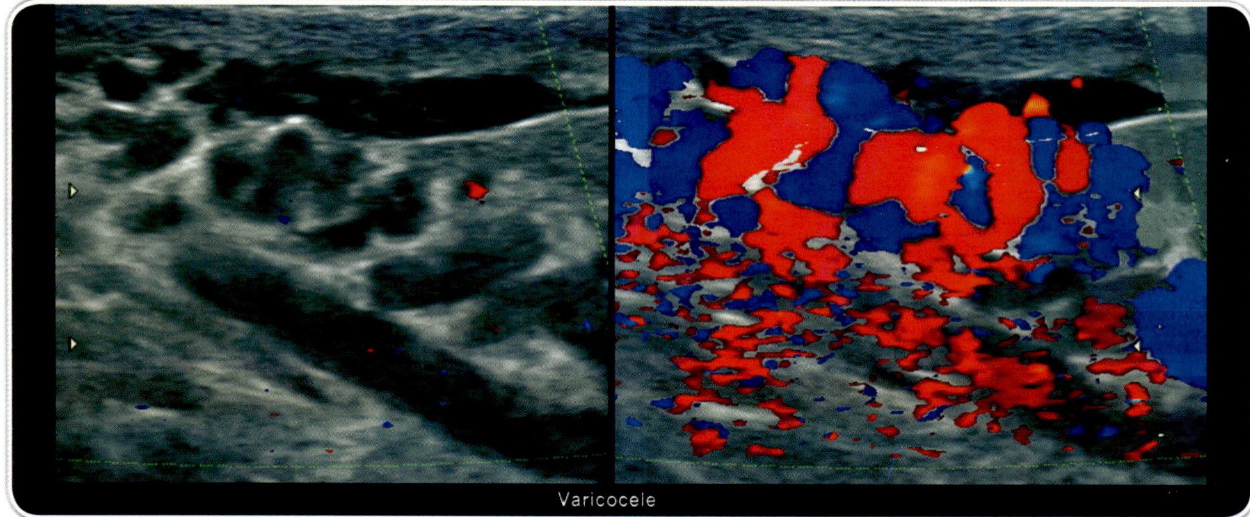
Varicocele

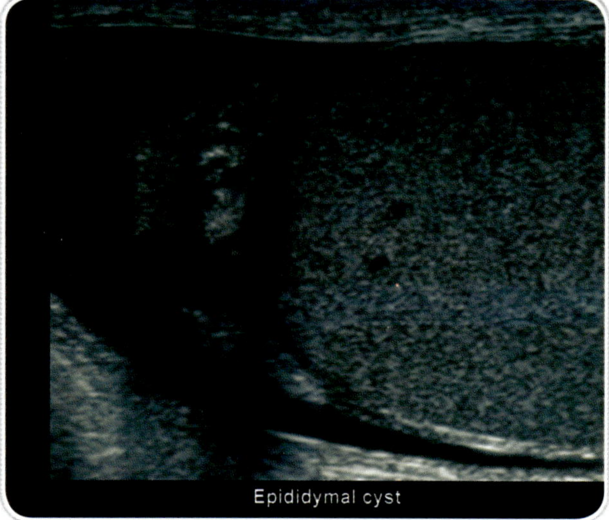
Epididymal cyst

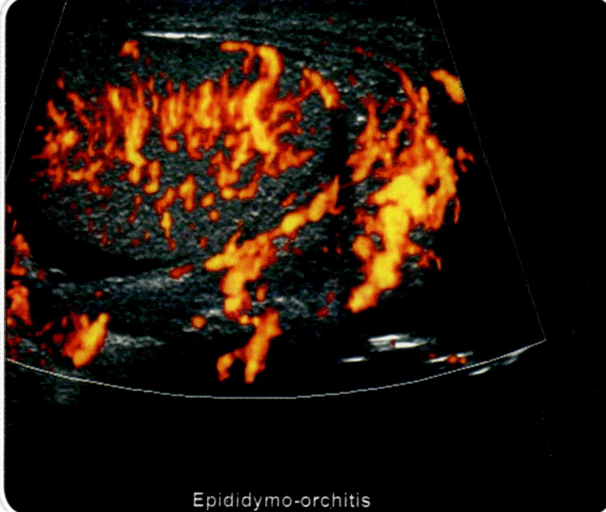
Epididymo-orchitis

For complete presentation, please refer the accompanying CD-ROM...

SUGGESTED READING

1. Cil AP, Tulunay G, Kose MF, Haberal A. Power Doppler properties of endometrial polyps and submucosal fibroids: a preliminary observational study in women with known intracavitary lesions. Ultrasound Obstet Gynecol. 2010;35:233-7.
2. Glock JL, Brumsted JR. Colour flow pulsed Doppler ultrasound in diagnosing luteal phase defect . Fertil Steril. 1995;64:500-4.
3. Jonard S, Robert Y, Cortet-Rudelli C, Pigny P, Decanter C, Dewailly D. Ultrasound examination of polycystic ovaries: is it worth counting the follicles? Hum Reprod. 2003;18:598-603.
4. Kore S, Hegde A, Nair S, et al. Sonography for assessment of tubal patency: our experience. J Obstet Gynecol India. 2000;50:63-6.
5. Kupesic S, Kurjak A. Predictors of IVF outcome by three-dimensional ultrasound. Hum Reprod. 2002;17(4):950-55.
6. Kupesic S, Kurjak A. The assessment of normal and abnormal luteal function by transvaginal colour Doppler sonography. Eur J Obstet Gynecol. 1997;72:83-7.
7. Kupesic S, Kurjak A. Uterine and ovarian perfusion during the periovulatory period assessed by transvaginal colour Doppler. Fertil Steril. 1993;3:439-43.
8. Kurjak A, Kupesic-Urek S. Infertility. In: Kurjak A (Ed). Transvaginal color Doppler. Carnforth, UK: Parthenon Publishing; 1991 pp.33-8.
9. Lamazou AM, Mabille M, Levaillant JM, Deffieux X, Frydman R, Musset O. Real-time transvaginal elastosonography of uterine fibroids. Ultrasound Obstet Gynecol; 2009
10. Lam PM, Jhonson IR, Rainne-Fenning NJ. Three-dimensional ultrasound features of the polycystic ovary and the effect of different phenotypic expressions on these parameters. J Hum Reprod. 2007;22:3116-23.
11. Raine-Fenning N, Deb S, Jayaprakasan K, Clewes J, Hopkisson J, Campbell B. Timing of oocyte maturation and egg collection during controlled ovarian stimulation: a randomized controlled trial evaluating manual and automated measurements of follicle diameter. Fertil Steril. 2009;94(1):184-8.
12. Raine-Fenning N, Jayaprakasan K, Deb S. Three-dimensional ultrasonographic characteristics of endometriomata. Ultrasound Obstet Gynecol. 2008;31:718-24.
13. Raine-Fenning NJ, Lam EP. Assessment of ovarian reserve using the inversion mode. Ultrasound Obstet Gynecol. 2006;27(1):104-6.
14. Salle B et al. Preliminary report of an ultrasonography and colour Doppler uterine score to predict uterine receptivity in an IVF programme. Hum Reprod. 1998;13:1669-73.
15. Sylvester C, Child TJ, Tulandi T, et al. A prospective study to evaluate the efficacy of two and three-dimensional sonohysterography in women with intrauterine lesions. Fertil Steril. 2003;79(5):1222-5.

Chapter

42

3D Ultrasound in Infertility

Radu Vladareanu, Simona Vladareanu, Vlad Zamfirescu

INTRODUCTION

- Transvaginal ultrasound (TV US) and Doppler gives more access to female pelvis
- Three-dimensional (3D) rendering allows for coronal plane reconstruction
- 3D US was first implemented in Obstetrics, now the indications are broadened.

Donal B et al. 2000

3D US in Obstetrics

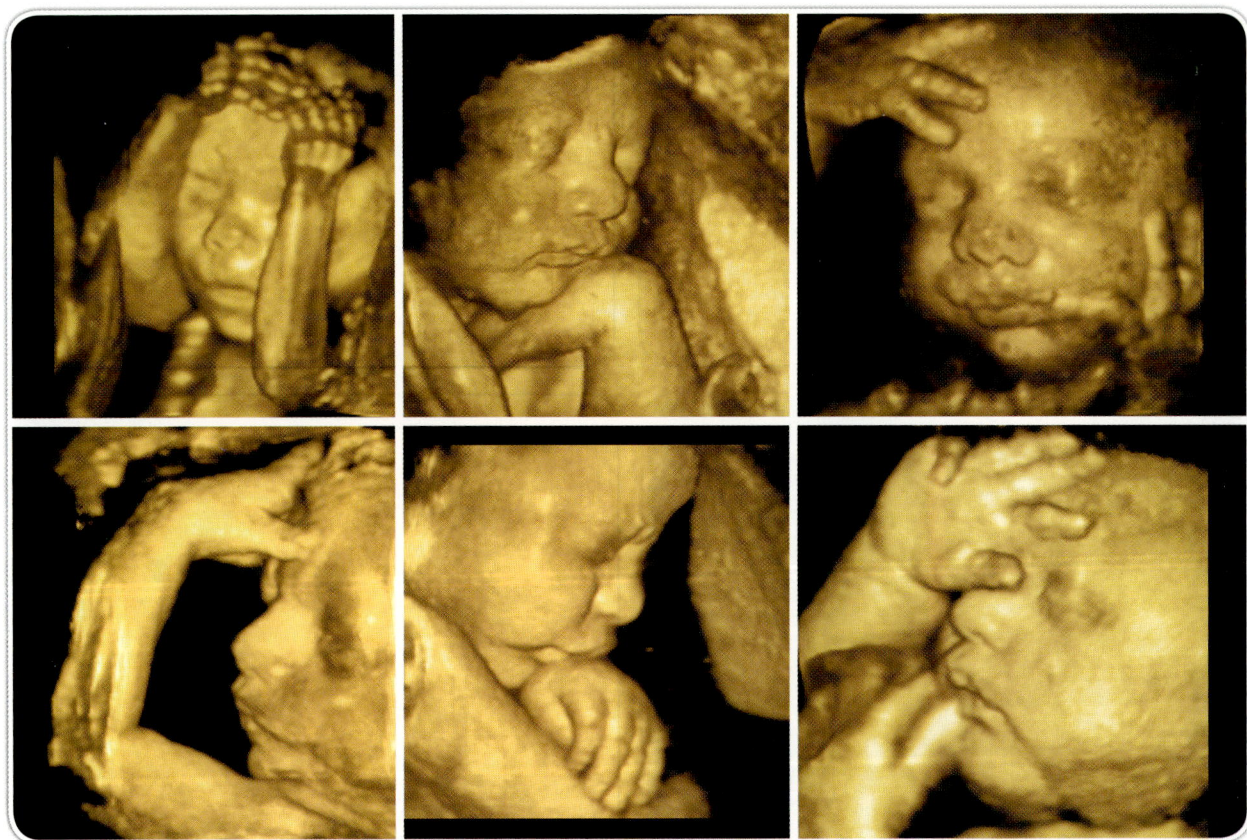

3D US in Gynecology

- Uterine cavity
- Endometrium: volume and vascular pattern
- Adnexal pathology
- Sonohysterogram.

Donal B et al. 2000

Why 3D?

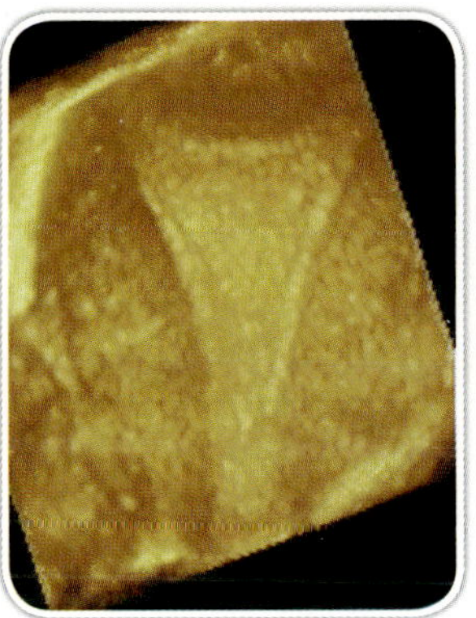
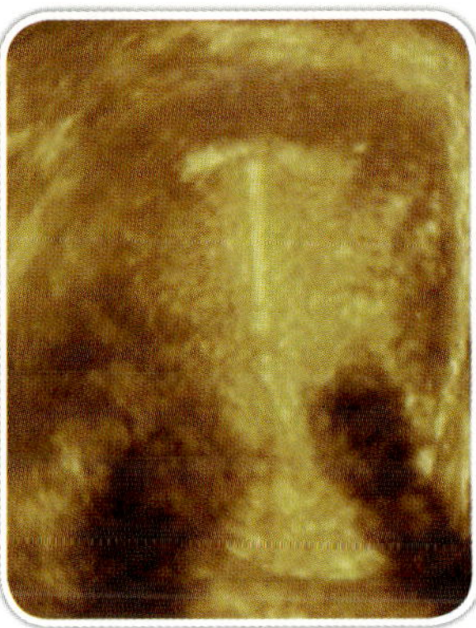
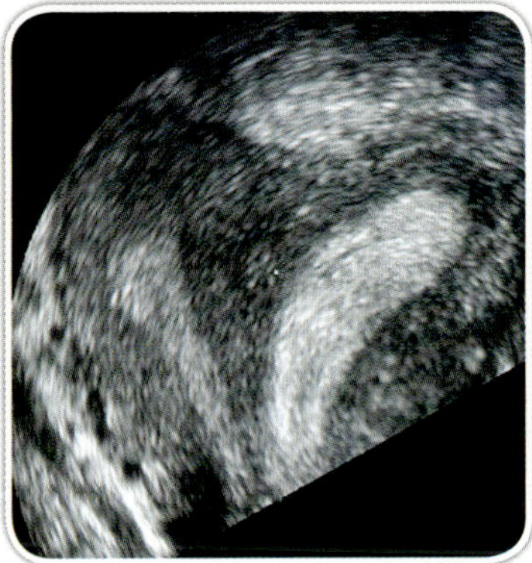
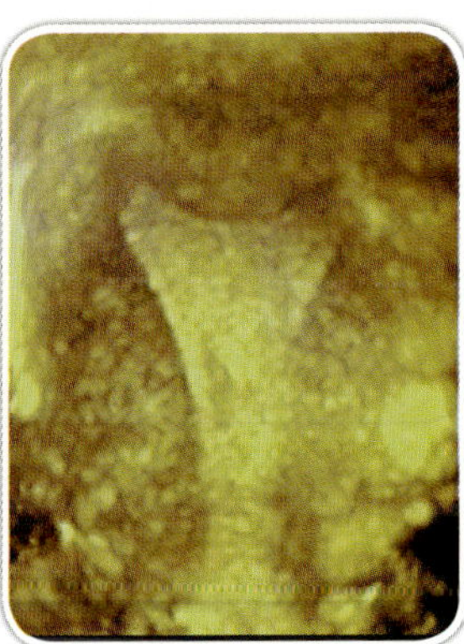

The coronal plane of the image

Normal Uterine Cavity

- Homogeneous texture
- Anterior and posterior wall of equal thickness
- Arcuate +/- spiral vessels.
- Best visualized in secretory phase
- A good 3D image = a very good 2D acquisition

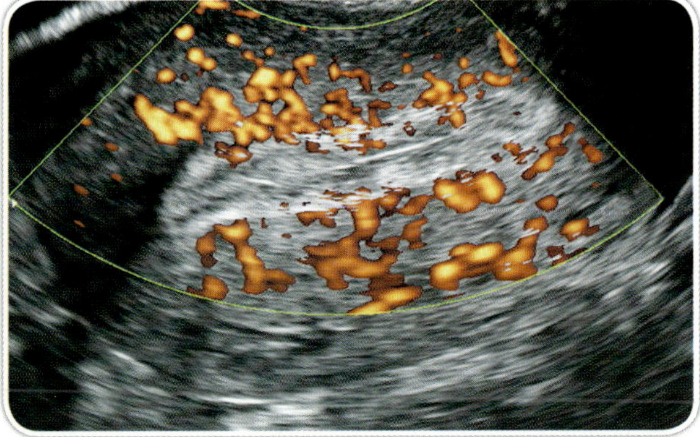

De Kroon CD et al. 2003

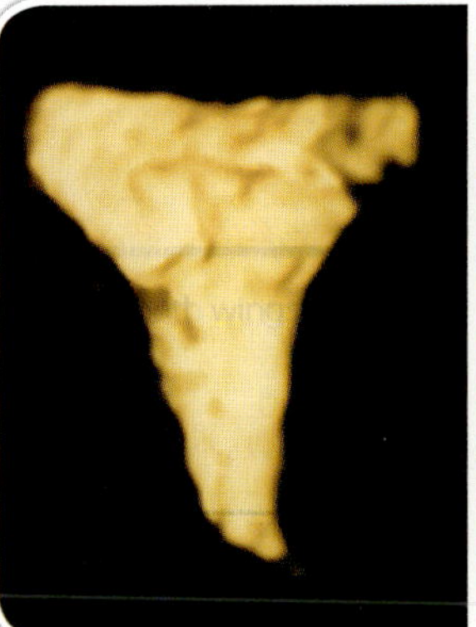
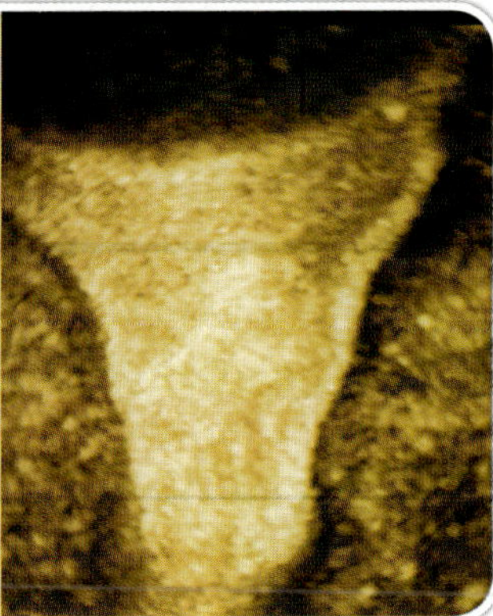

De Kroon CD et al. 2003

For complete presentation, please refer the accompanying CD-ROM...

SUGGESTED READING

1. Acien P; 1997.
2. Baba K. et al. 2000.
3. Benacerraf BR, et al. 2005.
4. Bourne TH, et al. 1996.
5. De Kroon CD, et al. 2003.
6. Desser TS, et al. 2001.
7. Donal B, et al. 2000.
8. Grimbizis GF, et al. 2001.
9. Heinonen PK, 2006.
10. Hill ML, 1992.
11. Ilan Timo -Trisch educational ppt
12. Kupesic S, et al. 2003.
13. Kurjak A, et al. 1991.
14. Kurjak A, et al. 1992.
15. Mercé LT, et al. 2006.
16. Oliveira FG, et al. 2004.
17. Salim Daya, 1994.
18. Salle B, et al. 1999.
19. Soares SR, et al. 2000.
20. Stassart JP, et al. 1992.
21. Troiano RN, et al. 2004.

Index

A

B

C

D

E

F

■ O

■ P

■ Q

■ R

■ S

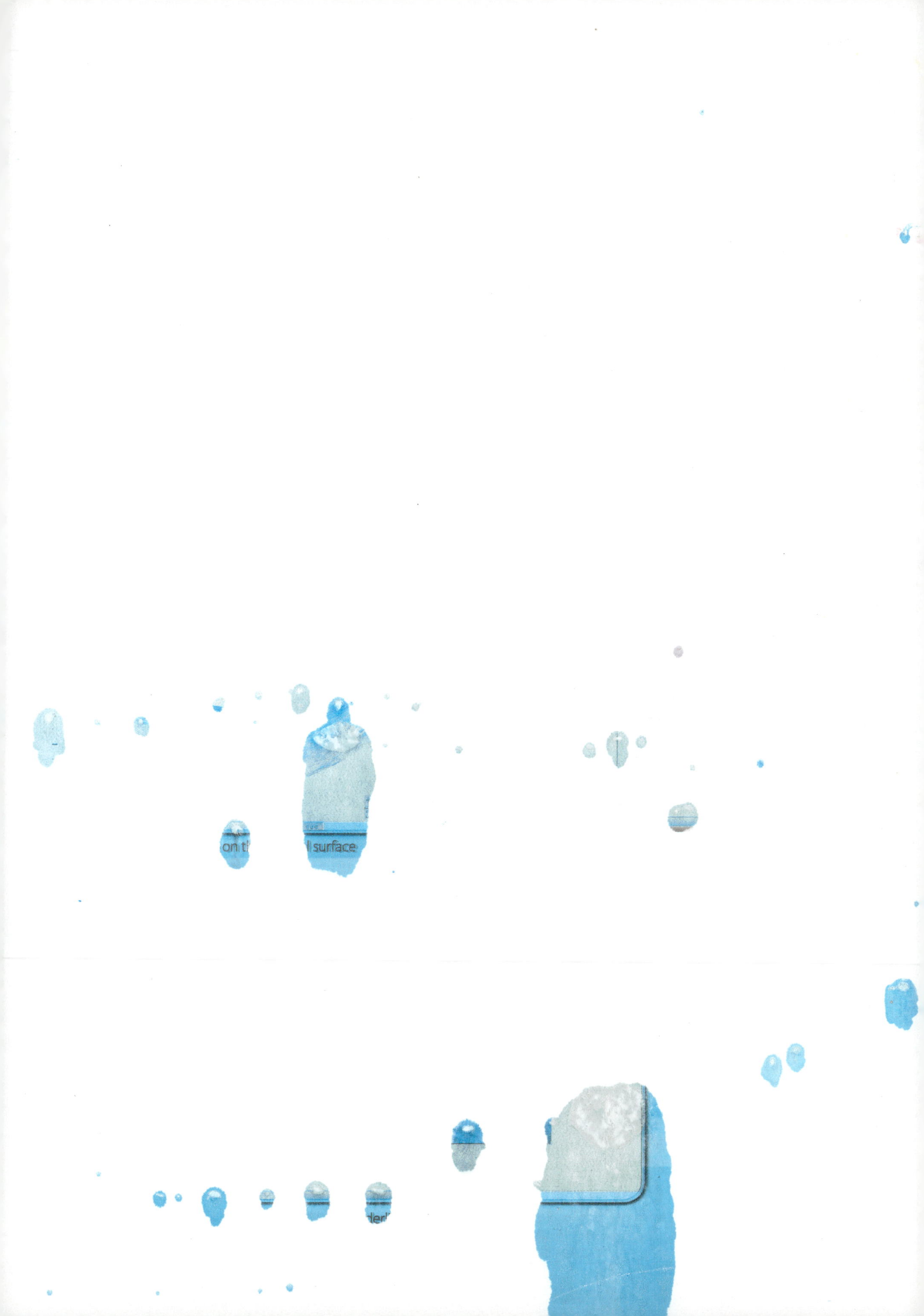